PRAISE FOR

Bhakti Yoga

"Much appreciated for his erudite and comprehensive edition of *The Yoga Sūtras* of *Patañjali*, Edwin F. Bryant has once again done a great service to a wide community of readers, this time by putting into a single volume so much of the history and theology of *bhakti*, judiciously ordered and clearly explained. His discerning selection of texts from the *Bhāgavata Purāṇa* is a welcome addition to the scholarship, making that great text ever more accessible today. Particularly welcome, too, is the inclusion of the *Nārada Bhakti Sūtras* and especially *Śrī* Caitanya's *Śikṣāṣṭakam*, a rare treasure that has long merited closer attention. Teachers and students, scholars and practitioners of religion alike, will be sure to keep this volume on hand in their research and for the sake of practice."

—Francis X. Clooney, S.J., director of the Center for the Study of World Religions, Harvard University

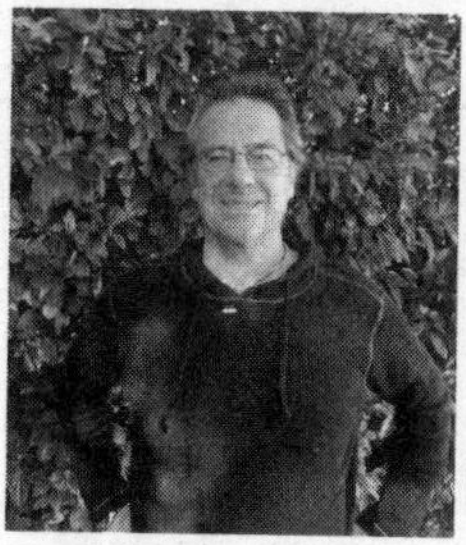

MOHINI BRYANT-EKSTRAND

EDWIN F. BRYANT

Bhakti Yoga

Edwin F. Bryant received his Ph.D. in Indology from Columbia University. He has taught at Columbia University and Harvard University and since 2001 has been a professor of Hindu religion and philosophy at Rutgers University. Bryant has written numerous scholarly articles and published seven previous books, including *The Yoga Sūtras of Patañjali: A New Edition, Translation, and Commentary* and *Krishna: The Beautiful Legend of God*, a translation of the four thousand verses of the tenth book of the *Bhāgavata Purāṇa*. In addition to his work in the academy, Bryant teaches workshops on the *Yoga Sūtras* and other Hindu texts in *yoga* communities around the world. His website is www.edwinbryant.org.

ALSO BY EDWIN F. BRYANT

Free Will, Agency, and Selfhood in Indian Philosophy
(coeditor with Matthew Dasti, 2013)

The Yoga Sūtras of Patañjali:
A New Edition, Translation, and Commentary (2009)

Krishna: A Source Book (editor, 2007)

The Indo-Aryan Controversy:
Evidence and Inference in Indian History
(coeditor with Laurie L. Patton, 2005)

The Hare Krishna Movement:
The Post-Charismatic Fate of a Religious Transplant
(coeditor with Maria Ekstrand, 2004)

Krishna: The Beautiful Legend of God
(translator, with an introduction and notes, 2003)

The Quest for the Origins of Vedic Culture:
The Indo-Aryan Migration Debate (2001)

Bhakti Yoga

Bhakti Yoga

Tales and Teachings from the *Bhāgavata Purāṇa*

EDWIN F. BRYANT

NORTH POINT PRESS
A DIVISION OF FARRAR, STRAUS AND GIROUX
NEW YORK

North Point Press
A division of Farrar, Straus and Giroux
18 West 18th Street, New York 10011

Printed in the United States of America
First edition, 2017

Part 3 was originally published, in slightly different form, in *Krishna: The Beautiful Legend of God*, translated by Edwin F. Bryant (Penguin Books, 2003).

Library of Congress Cataloging-in-Publication Data
Names: Bryant, Edwin F. (Edwin Francis), 1957– author.
Title: Bhakti yoga : tales and teachings from the
Bhagavata Purana / Edwin F. Bryant.
Description: New York : North Point Press, 2017. |
Includes bibliographical references.
Identifiers: LCCN 2016032533 | ISBN 9780865477759 (paperback) |
ISBN 9780374714390 (e-book)
Subjects: LCSH: Yoga, Bhakti. | Krishna (Hindu deity)—Cult. |
Puranas. Bhåagavatapuråaòna—Criticism, interpretation, etc. |
BISAC: RELIGION / Spirituality. | HEALTH & FITNESS / Yoga.
Classification: LCC BL1238.56.B53 B78 2017 | DDC 294.5/436—dc23
LC record available at https://lccn.loc.gov/2016032533

Designed by Jonathan D. Lippincott

1 3 5 7 9 10 8 6 4 2

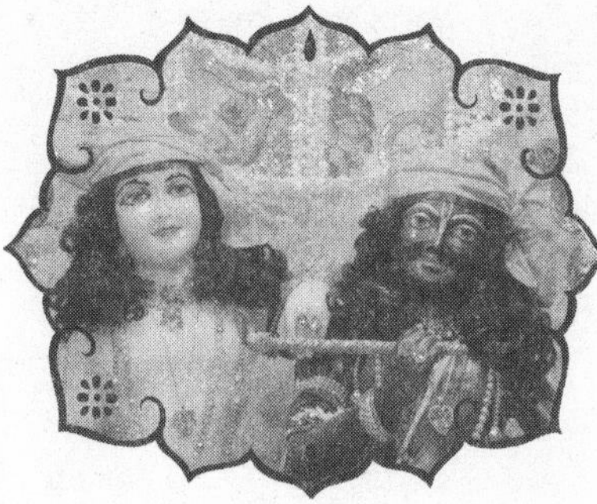

Śrī Śrī Kṛṣṇa-Balarāmābhyāṃ namaḥ

In honor and dear remembrance of my father, George Bryant, MBE, for exemplifying *dharma* long before I encountered the concept in Sanskrit texts. I spent much time in his company as I worked on this text. May he partake of any merit accruing from this work.

To my daughter, Mohinī, in case one day she ever wonders what this piece of her upbringing was really all about.

To my sister, Pia, for all her love and support, that she may gain a clearer understanding of *bhakti yoga*. To Hannah Jackson, in case she ever becomes interested. And to all seekers interested in knowing more about the spirituality associated with the mischievous, lotus-eyed blue boy.

To my teachers and to all the *bhāgavatas* who have recorded, preserved, transmitted, and taught the wonderful *līlās* of *Bhagavān* across the ages. May they accept this little attempt to follow in their footsteps and smile with kindness and good humor at all its imperfections.

And, finally, to Jeff Seroy and the folks at Farrar, Straus and Giroux, for having faith in this project and being a great team to work with.

Contents

Introduction to the Volume

Statement of Purpose: Sources and Scope of the Volume

There are as many variegated expressions of *bhakti yoga* in India as there are sects, languages, communities, lineages, castes, regions, villages, and, indeed, human hearts wherein it ultimately resides. This book is focused on one expression of *bhakti*: *Vaiṣṇava bhakti* centered on *Śrī* Kṛṣṇa as emerges in a sixteenth-century tradition. In this section, we discuss our vision and method for the volume and provide some rationale and contextual background for the texts on *bhakti* that we have chosen to feature. Our discussion in this introductory section may be mildly academic, but we have made every effort in the remainder of the volume to avoid scholarly language and specialized jargon in preference for straightforward prose and concepts accessible for the educated but nonspecialized reader. In this work, we attempt to navigate that unattainable line between producing something that is academically respectable, accessible to the interested nonspecialist, and useful to the intellectually responsible *yoga* practitioner. Since this is an impossible feat, I can only beg the indulgence both of scholars, who may find some of the discussion overly simplistic, and of lay readers, whether personally involved with *yoga* practices or not, who may find it too academic in places. In any event, anyone not interested in this section's technicalities might prefer to proceed to the next section, "Definition of *Bhakti*," where we begin our actual discussion on *bhakti* proper.

Specifically, the tales and teachings in part 2 of this volume are translations from the *Śrīmad Bhāgavata Purāṇa*, the *Beautiful Legend of* Bhagavān [God] (henceforth *Bhāgavata*), as are the stories of Kṛṣṇa in part 3. After much deliberation, we have chosen the translation "legend" here for the Sanskrit term *purāṇa*,[1] with the intention of denoting traditional lore, which presents itself as factual history, is purported to be true by its followers, and has been handed down and believed as such by its adherents across the centuries.[2] The *Bhāgavata* is, as we will suggest later, arguably one of the most important texts on *bhakti yoga*, along with the *Rāmāyaṇa*, in that cluster of traditions that has come to be known as "Hinduism."[3] In addition to the text itself, the systematic analysis of *bhakti yoga*, which will occupy the bulk of part 1, will to a great extent be from the perspective of the commentaries and elaborations on the *Bhāgavata Purāṇa* written by the sixteenth-century theologians Jīva Gosvāmī and his uncle Rūpa Gosvāmī, two of the founding fathers of the Gauḍīya school of Vaiṣṇavism (also known as Caitanya Vaiṣṇavism).[4] We will introduce these sources below. While we will engage a wide variety of other intellectual and theological expressions in India both prior and contemporary to the sixteenth century, our motive will be to compare and contrast these with our chosen case study.

Our aim in this volume is to provide the reader with a modest window into how *bhakti* is understood through the frame of reference of one community of practitioners in the premodern period. Our interest in this book is in the theology of Kṛṣṇa *bhakti*—the beliefs, metaphysics, devotional attitudes, and, most especially, *yogic* practices of this tradition—considered through the tradition's own categories and terminologies as presented by its adherents.[5] We will be directing considerable attention to the soteriological goals of the *Bhāgavata* tradition ("soteriology" is a term used to refer to the nature of religious beliefs pertaining to some sort of perfected afterlife—in the Indic[6] context, *mokṣa*, the liberated state). This is a book intended for anyone with intellectual inclinations interested in exploring an expression of *bhakti* as a lived reality—as a map of how to navigate one's existence in this world, frame its ultimate meaning, and conceive of that which lies beyond.

For my academic colleagues, I feel obliged to point out that this is not an analysis of the social, political, or ideological contexts of

Kṛṣṇa *bhakti*, nor of the material influences that fed into its historical development—concerns that have come to dominate and, in fact, more or less define the study of religion as an academic discipline.[7] These are all essential aspects of the study of any religion, as no tradition, howsoever spiritual, exists in a cultural vacuum, immune from being affected by its sociopolitical environment and devoid of any ideology of its own. But such contexts and agendas will not concern us here. Thus, while our critics may accuse us of naive ahistoricism (that is, extracting a tradition from its historical setting in the real world), we wish to be clear from the outset: our focus is on the theology and practices of a tradition as conceptualized and articulated in the terms and categories of the tradition itself.[8] (I have placed further comments pertaining to how I am framing this work in notes so as not to burden this introduction.)[9]

We thus prioritize premodern traditional sources in this volume (but we have included references to select academic studies in notes). Our hope is that this focus affords an opportunity to glimpse one facet of the traditional Hindu universe of *bhakti* in India as expressed in a very important classical text[10] and a major commentarial tradition prior to its encounter with modernity in the colonial period. Our aim is for scholars and students of religion to gain some understanding of the worldview and principal beliefs of the Kṛṣṇa *bhakta* practitioner of this tradition, and for intellectually responsible *yoga* practitioners to get a better sense of the premodern rationale of a form of *bhakti* as a very specific type of *yoga* practice. As a result of our chosen focus, in addition to engaging an important *bhakti* text, by an exposure to a traditional mode of understanding, interpreting, and reworking sacred scripture (hermeneutics), via Jīva and Rūpa's commentarial writings and interpretations of the *Bhāgavata*, we will explore how an elaborate and sophisticated *bhakti* tradition sets about gaining authenticity for its teachings. Foundational texts such as the *Bhāgavata* in ancient India are almost always studied through the lineage-based commentaries that are written to clarify them, as well as to establish a sect's theological credentials.

Our contention is that there is much that is shared, in both form and experience, in the overlapping but distinct traditions of *bhakti*, and that revealing the worldview and ingredients of one tradition in some depth provides a basic template that can readily be refitted and applied to other expressions, despite important differences. If we analogize "Hinduism" as a universe containing numerous distinct but also significantly overlapping and interacting galaxies, with specific devotional traditions analogous to constellations, then awareness of the constitution and orbits of one constellation provides invaluable information relevant to other constellations, despite important differences. There is thus merit in exploring one *bhakti* universe with some profundity, rather than superficially attempting to cover the entire panoramic multifarious breadth of the vast spectrum of Hindu devotional traditions. Exposure to the metaphysical infrastructure, theological vision, set of practices, mental cultivations, and devotional depths of one tradition provides a useful blueprint that can be readily compared with others.

A further comment here on method: As is obvious from the cover designs, this work was conceived as a follow-up to the author's commentary on the *Yoga Sūtras* of Patañjali. The rationale for that work, given the massive transplantation to the West of practices that have been assigned the name *yoga*, was to attempt to provide some grounding of the actual metaphysics, goals, and practices of classical *yoga* in their most prominent, premodern textual sources. This present project is motivated by similar intentions with regard to grounding *bhakti*. The difference in this work is that owing to the variegation in the *bhakti* traditions, we have focused principally on one lineage-specific expression of *bhakti*. The premodern Patañjali-derived Yoga tradition does not present the same heterogeneity as *bhakti*: there are no distinct lineages that derive from Patañjali's *Yoga Sūtras*,[11] but rather an essentially fairly homogeneous commentarial Yoga tradition, all predicated on the first commentary on the text by Vyāsa, usually dated to around the third century.[12] Because of the canonical nature of Vyāsa, the later primary commentators—such as Vācaspati Miśra, Śaṅkara, Bhoja Rāja, Vijñānabhikṣu, and others—build on and expand on their predecessors, they do not disagree on essential points. Any differences are relatively minor.[13] So we can speak of a fairly consistent "Yoga tradition" without overly generalizing or essentializing (that is, sharing the same Sāṅkhya metaphysics, understanding of mind and of consciousness, set of practices, and the like).

This is not the case with *bhakti*. Just to give a preview of a couple of topics that lie ahead to make this point, *bhakti* is both central to the Vedānta philosophical traditions and to the Purāṇa literary ones. Ontology is the term used in philosophy to refer to the ultimate basic categories of reality (for example, in a typical monotheistic ontology: God, the world of matter, and souls), and there are fundamental differences among Vedānta lineages on essential ontological categories. To name just one we will engage later, is *Īśvara*, God, who is the recipient of *bhakti yoga*, the Ultimate Absolute Truth or a secondary one derived from some higher and even more Ultimate Truth? And there are differences just as significant in the Purāṇas, such as, for our purposes, whether Kṛṣṇa, Viṣṇu, or Śiva is the ultimate source *Īśvara*, with the other divinities secondary or derivative manifestations from this source *Īśvara*. We will, of course, expound on all this in great detail within, but we touch on this now simply to note that it is because of such significant heterogeneity on basic issues pertaining to *bhakti* that we have chosen to enter deeply into one *bhakti* tradition, rather than go broad and superficially attempt to cover multiple traditions. However, we will exemplify our featured tradition through comparisons with others, and hence there will be frequent references to predecessor and contemporary traditions of *bhakti*, especially those of *advaita Vedānta*, Śiva, and other Viṣṇu expressions.

This work is divided into five parts. Part 1 sets out to provide an analytic map of what constitutes the various principal ingredients of *bhakti*. Here, we primarily follow Jīva Gosvāmī's systematic exposition on the *bhakti* of the *Bhāgavata Purāṇa* as expressed in his *Bhakti Sandarbha* (*Analysis of* Bhakti). We also significantly engage Rūpa Gosvāmī's works on *bhakti yoga*, specifically the first part of his *Bhaktirasāmṛtasindhu* (*Ocean of the Nectar of the Experience of* Bhakti) and *Upadeśāmṛta* (*Nectar of Instruction*). We additionally draw from other *bhakti*-relevant texts, especially the *Bhagavad Gītā* (here, too, following in Jīva's footsteps). Our major departure from the textual corpus Jīva invokes is our own profuse referencing to Patañjali's *Yoga Sūtras*. This attention partly reflects this author's own work on the *Yoga Sūtras* (Bryant 2009), but it also allows us to compare and contrast aspects of generic meditative *yoga* (*dhyāna*)—the practice systematized for the first time by Patañjali—with the path of *bhakti*. This is a contrast that surfaces repeatedly as a very important theme in the *Bhāgavata* as will be discovered, and hence we feel justified in frequently referring to the *Yoga Sūtras* of Patañjali (which would be useful but not essential preparatory reading for the present work). This is especially so since, with modern *yogīs* in mind, the selections I have made from the *Bhāgavata* focus on Patañjali-like *yoga*, and I frequently draw attention to common concepts and phraseologies between the two sources.

Part 1 is divided into six sections. After these comments on the methodology of the volume, this section, "Introduction to the Volume," introduces the *Bhāgavata Purāṇa* itself, as well as the commentators who will be our guides. The next section, "Definition of *Bhakti*," provides a definition of our subject matter. This is followed, in "The Practices of *Bhakti*," with an extensive discussion on *bhakti yoga* itself in its various forms of practices and devotional attitudes between devotee and God. "The Practitioner of *Bhakti*, the *Bhakta*" features the devotee, agent, performer, and experiencer of *bhakti* (we note that *bhakti* is the practice and the *bhakta* is the practitioner, in distinction to *yoga*, which is the practice, and *yogī*, the practitioner). "The Object of *Bhakti*: *Īśvara*, *Bhagavān*, *Brahman*, and Divine Hierarchies" discusses the various modes of understanding *Īśvara*, also referred to as *Bhagavān*, God, who is the object or recipient of *bhakti*. Finally, "Concluding Reflections" offers a few of this author's thoughts pertaining to the *Bhāgavata*'s uneasy placement in the modern, post-Enlightenment, intellectual world of our times. Here, we also summarize the Kṛṣṇa tradition's overall soteriology (the nature of the ultimate liberated state) and locate this within the larger framework of some of the Hindu *mokṣa* (liberation) traditions.

The remaining four parts of the volume consist of translations. Part 2 focuses on translations from the first nine books of the *Bhāgavata*, featuring the great exemplars and *yogī* virtuosi of the text—the *bhaktas*, the practitioners of *bhakti*, who have gained pan-Indian status and whose lives and devotional practices serve as inspirational role models for the tradition.[14] The teachings of great *bhakta* sages or of various incarnations of *Īśvara* too are presented here; thus, some of the sections in part 2 are entitled "The Tale of . . ." and others "The Teachings of . . ." The *Bhāgavata*, as we will note below, contains a wide variety of subjects, but we will focus on the *yoga*-related components. Each section is introduced by a brief "*yoga* blueprint," identifying the main *yogic* or theological message and other such distinguishing features being imparted by the narrative. In fact, the first nine books of the text are designed to prepare the reader with the requisite metaphysical, psychological, and other such devotional requirements to encounter with the appropriate attitude and understanding the summum bonum of the work in the tenth book, *Śrī* Kṛṣṇa.

It is in part 3 that we feature the most popular narratives from the tenth book of the *Bhāgavata*, pertaining to the object or recipient of *bhakti yoga* and ultimate goal of all its ingredients: Kṛṣṇa Himself.[15] We will see here that the foundation of this form of *bhakti yoga* is based on the *Bhāgavata*'s narratives of Kṛṣṇa's divine descent into this world as *avatāra*, breaking into human space and time and performing superwondrous deeds (as is the case with other manifestations of *Īśvara* in other *bhakti* traditions). Most especially, we will encounter here the notion of *līlā*, the blissful pastimes Kṛṣṇa inaugurates with His beloved *bhaktas* for their pleasure, which lies at the very heart of Kṛṣṇa *bhakti*: love of God. Here, too, from the many *līlās* featured in book 10, we have extracted those that best highlight Kṛṣṇa's various types of relationships with His *bhaktas* and the corresponding *bhāvas* and *rasas*, emotional states of intense *bhakti*, as it is these that represent the ultimate goals of Kṛṣṇa *bhakti* in the *Bhāgavata*.

In part 4, we present a translation of the *śiksāṣṭaka*, "The Eight Verses of Instruction," composed by Caitanya, teacher of Rūpa and Jīva Gosvāmīs, and the fountainhead of the Gauḍīya tradition, which considers him to be an incarnation of Kṛṣṇa. While Caitanya's teachings were preserved and systematized by the *Gosvāmīs* and his life documented by later hagiographers in a number of works (from which we have extracted here a few illustrations from the *Caitanya Caritāmṛta* and *Caitanya Bhāgavata*), Caitanya himself penned only these eight verses. Finally, part 5 offers a translation of the eighty-four *sūtras* of the *Nārada Bhakti Sūtras*. This is a late text modeled on the *Yoga Sūtras* with the intention of providing a succinct exposition of *bhakti* utilizing the *sūtra* genre of expression. It seems aware of the theology that found its most elaborate expressions in the sixteenth-century writings of our *Gosvāmīs* (and their contemporary,

Vallabha) and so fits harmoniously with the focus of our volume. It is a useful manual for beginners.

With these preliminary comments pertaining to content and method in place, then, we will devote only a few cursory words to introducing the *Bhāgavata Purāṇa*, since we are limited in space here,[16] and a few more introducing Rūpa and Jīva and their tradition.

The *Bhāgavata* as Text[17]

The *Bhāgavata Purāṇa* forms part of a corpus of texts emerging from the late Vedic period known as the Purāṇas. The early Vedic backdrop that spawned not just the *bhakti* of the *Bhāgavata*, but all Hindu forms of *yoga* and philosophies of *mokṣa* (liberation) cannot detain us here in detail (but see appendix 1 to get some sense of the Vedic literary and cultural context from which, and against which, the *Bhāgavata* is establishing its authority).[18] The word *purāṇa,* in Sanskrit, signifies "that which took place in the past"—namely, ancient lore or legend. The Purāṇas are listed as eighteen in number,[19] and it is in this genre of texts that, among many other topics, the stories of the various incarnations and activities of *Īśvara*, God, and of His feminine counterpart, *Īśvarī*, the Goddess, when manifest on earth, are recorded. The Purāṇas also feature the incredible acts of devotion, *bhakti*, toward these manifestations of *Īśvara* by superexemplary *bhaktas*. Thus, since *bhakti* is nothing other than devotion to a form of *Īśvara* or *Īśvarī*, the Purāṇa texts are the mainstay of *bhakti yoga*. The most immediately encountered aspects of Hinduism—the forms, personalities, qualities, deeds, and so on of Kṛṣṇa, Viṣṇu, Śiva, the Goddess, and other divine *Īśvara* manifestations, depicted ubiquitously in the literature and the numerous classical art forms of ancient India—are almost entirely extracted from the Purāṇas (and two epics) and their derivative literatures, as we will see from our case study of the *Bhāgavata*. The Purāṇas as a genre, then, lie as the principal source of almost all forms of *bhakti yoga.*[20]

In addition to these descriptions of the various *Īśvara* forms and their devotees, as well as the sectarian theologies and practices associated with them, these Purāṇas as we have them today are a vast repository of stories about kings and royal dynasties; creation accounts; traditional cosmologies; reworkings of ancient epic and Vedic narratives; *yogic* practices; popular religious beliefs concerning pilgrimages, holy places, and religious rites; information of social and cultural relevance such as caste duties; and even prophetic statements about the future. Almost everything that has come to be associated with "Hinduism" has its roots in the Purāṇas. The eighteen *mahā* (great) Purāṇas[21] are said to contain four hundred thousand verses,[22] and are the largest body of writing in Sanskrit.

There are two main transcendent deities in the Purāṇas, Śiva, and Viṣṇu—three, if we include Brahmā, the secondary creator,[23] but as we will see, as a mortal-created being,[24] he is more of a placeholder and never a serious contender. While we will need to nuance this later, Śiva in the overall Purāṇic narrative is usually associated with the destruction of the universe at the end of each of its periodic cycles, and Viṣṇu, with its maintenance. A number of stories speak of a playful rivalry between these two. A later Purāṇa, the *Devī Bhāgavata Purāṇa*, marks the ascendancy into the Purāṇic genre of Devī, the Goddess, as the supreme matrix. As will be discussed in some detail within, the term "monotheism," when extracted from its historical Abrahamic associations, can, if we wish to adopt it (given our earlier comments about prioritizing Sanskritic terminologies), be applied to certain expressions of the Purāṇic traditions, especially the various orthodox Vaiṣṇava traditions, but also certain Śaiva sects.[25] But this monotheism needs to be understood in the context of a Supreme Being, whether understood as Viṣṇu or Śiva, who can manifest as unlimited other transcendent *Īśvara* and *Īśvarī* Beings, who are thereby derivative from and thus secondary to the original Godhead. This is not polytheism: perhaps we can think of this as a "multiplicity in oneness" parallel of the Christian trinity.

The *Bhāgavata Purāṇa*, consisting of twelve *skandhas* (cantos, subdivisions, or books), occupies itself primarily with Viṣṇu and His incarnations, featuring, most particularly, Kṛṣṇa. This focus is structurally reflected in the fact that Kṛṣṇa is the exclusive subject matter of the tenth book, which disproportionately constitutes about one-quarter of the entire text. It is this tenth book that has caused this Purāṇa to be recognized as the most famous work of Purāṇa literature by far. This tenth book, in my view, along with the *Rāmāyaṇa*, is one of the two most influential texts in Hinduism. This claim can be supported by the enormous amount of artistic and cultural traditions that its narratives have inspired over the last millennium in the form of derivate literature, poetry, drama, iconography, art, and temple sculpture, in addition to a vast array of intellectual and theological treatises from which the work of our *Gosvāmīs* is only one expression.[26] The text's influence can also be gauged by the overwhelming preponderance of traditional commentaries it inspired compared with all the other Purāṇas put together: the *Bhāgavata* has generated eighty-one commentaries currently available in Sanskrit alone, as well as others no longer extant (as a point of contrast, most of the Purāṇas have produced no traditional commentaries at all and others only one or, at most, with the *Viṣṇu Purāṇa*, two). It has been translated into almost all the languages of India, with forty or so translations on record in Bengal alone.[27] Tellingly, it has been neglected by Western scholarship until very recently. This is partly because the Victorian sensibilities of certain nineteenth-century Western Orientalists—and, just as important, early Hindu spokespersons and apologists influenced by Western moral discourses—were outraged by the amorous liaisons of Kṛṣṇa in the *Bhāgavata*, ignorant of their theological significances.[28] Consequently, the Kṛṣṇa of the *Bhāgavata* was jettisoned in favor of the more righteous Kṛṣṇa of the *Bhagavad Gītā* (henceforth *Gītā*)—a text that continues to produce hundreds of non-Indian translations—and still remains relatively unknown in the West.

As an unambiguously Vaiṣṇavite text—that is, adhering to Viṣṇu as the Supreme and Ultimate expression of Godhead (although the *Bhāgavata* will renegotiate Kṛṣṇa's status here), the first nine books of the *Bhāgavata* discuss in greater or lesser detail some of the major incarnations prior to Kṛṣṇa. These pave the way for the tenth book, which comprises about four thousand out of a claimed eighteen thousand total verses of the entire Purāṇa[29] and is dedicated exclusively to Kṛṣṇa. Indeed, it is Kṛṣṇa, under His title of *Bhagavān* (defined later), who gives His name to the whole *Bhāgavata Purāṇa* (literally, *Legend of* Bhagavān), as He does to the *Bhagavad Gītā* (literally, "that which was recited by *Bhagavān*"). Within Vaiṣṇavism, then, the *Bhāgavata Purāṇa* is the Kṛṣṇa-centered text par excellence, to the point that the Kṛṣṇaite theologies that emerged in the sixteenth century[30] use the *Bhāgavata Purāṇa* as scriptural authority to claim that it is not Kṛṣṇa who is an incarnation of Viṣṇu, as He is depicted in the *Mahābhārata* epic and in the other Purāṇas, but rather Viṣṇu who is a partial incarnation of Kṛṣṇa. In the theology of Jīva, Rūpa, and their associates, it is Kṛṣṇa who is the supreme Absolute Truth from whom all other deities, including Viṣṇu, evolve. Thus, Kṛṣṇaism positions itself within the larger matrix of Vaiṣṇavism as a familiar but also distinct expression.

It is an inconclusive task to try to assign specific dates to the Purāṇas, as shown by the considerable variation in the dates proposed by scholars for the *Bhāgavata* itself. Composed for public oral recitation, the Purāṇas are a maleable body of literature that continued to be transformed across the centuries by the fluid processes of transmission and adaptation to time and place as well as sectarian partialities. Any datable piece of information that may be gleaned from the texts may only reflect the historical period of that portion of the text and not necessarily other sections. Moreover, it is impossible to determine how long narratives had been in existence in oral form prior to being committed to writing. Hence Purāṇa scholars such as Rocher (1986) decline to attempt to date them. Accordingly, I will simply note here that the majority of scholars hold that the bulk of the material in most of the eighteen Purāṇas as we find them today reached its full completion and final form by the Gupta period, from about the fourth to the sixth century C.E.,[31] even as many of these narratives had been evolving and handed down for many centuries prior to this.

There is no consensus regarding the date of the *Bhāgavata Purāṇa* itself in its finished form. While most specialists of the Purāṇas from India have opted for a completion around the fourth century C.E. during the Gupta period, some Western scholars have argued that it is the latest of the eighteen Purāṇas, written (depending on the scholar) sometime between the ninth and the thirteenth century C.E. in the south of the subcontinent. There are a number of significant reasons to question such a place of origin as well as time frame, which cause me to wonder whether the *Bhāgavata* too might not have reached its final form by the Gupta period along with the other major Purāṇas.[32] No matter: for our present purposes here, we will only reiterate that whatever date one assigns to the *Bhāgavata* applies only to the final date of the entirety of the text as we now have it, not to the material contained within it or even to portions of the text itself. As with the Purāṇic genre in general, the upper-limit date of the text is one issue, the date of the subject matter recorded in it is another.[33] Be this as it may, there is no question that the story of Kṛṣṇa is far older than the flowering of Purāṇic literature in the Gupta period. The earliest references to the Kṛṣṇa story, including sources outside the texts themselves, such as archaeological ones, take us back to at least the fourth to the fifth century B.C.E.[34]

Needless to say, all such historical considerations of date and provenance are concerns for post-Enlightenment-derived, academic (text-critical) scholarship. Tradition holds the Purāṇa texts to be divine revelations, the *Smṛti*, "that which is remembered," sacred Truths originating from an incarnation of *Īśvara* or empowered sage.[35] Thus the *Bhāgavata* records various different branches of its own earlier stages of transmission[36] prior to its final delivery by sage Śuka to King Parīkṣit that we will find in part 2, including its primordial origins as imparted by Kṛṣṇa to Brahmā at the beginning of creation (II.9.43). Brahmā is deemed to have then imparted it to sage Nārada, from whom it was transmitted to Vyāsa and then on to Śuka.

Moving into this frame of reference expressed in the text itself, in keeping with our own interests, the *Bhāgavata* introduces itself with the claim of being primarily a historical record of the events that transpired when "*Bhagavān*, Kṛṣṇa, performed superhuman activities . . . concealed in the guise of a human" (I.1.20). In other words, it claims to be a record of events that transpired when God descended on earth.

Although the *Bhāgavata* ostensibly presents itself as containing ten topics or subject matters,[37] Jīva points out that actually the real purpose of the text is in fact to provide the reader with the opportunity to encounter Kṛṣṇa, *Bhagavān*, the tenth and ultimate topic. This tenth subject matter is Kṛṣṇa, the *āśraya* (support) of the entire text. As far as the *Bhāgavata* is concerned, "the great souls (*mahātmās*) describe the characteristics of the first nine topics, in order to clarify the tenth" (II.10.2). It is Kṛṣṇa who is the grand finale of all other subject matters.[38] The other nine topics—including the narratives of great kings—are simply to highlight some of *Īśvara*'s potencies and qualities and provide some prerequisite context and preparatory devotional groundwork to enhance the appreciation of the ultimate topic revealed in the tenth book, God Himself:

> These stories of great kings, who spread their fame throughout the worlds and then met their death, have been narrated with the intention of expressing detachment from and insight into [the temporal nature of material grandeur]. They are just a display of rhetoric, they are not the Ultimate Truth. But, on the other hand, the descriptions and qualities of Kṛṣṇa[39] which destroy all inauspiciousness, should always be recited. One desiring to attain pure *bhakti* for Kṛṣṇa should always hear them without interruption. (XII.3.14–15)

Therefore the sages in the forest of Naimiṣa we will encounter in part 2 were interested in hearing about even the saintly king Parīkṣit, Kṛṣṇa's grandnephew, only "if doing so is a basis for stories about Kṛṣṇa" (I.16.5–6).

The other nine topics—including the stories of the great *bhakta* exemplars and their teachings, which will be featured in part 2, as well as accounts of the deeds of Viṣṇu's previous incarnations, along with various related teachings—are covered in the *Bhāgavata*'s books 1–9 and 11–12.[40] The activities of Kṛṣṇa take up book 10, a quarter of the entire Purāṇa's bulk, and are represented in part 3 of this volume. So these previous books are preparatory, providing the necessary theological and metaphysical infrastructure to understand the narrations of Kṛṣṇa, the apex of the entire text. Kṛṣṇa is the summum bonum, the other subject matters providing progressive layers of context for his activities on earth, the *līlās*, Kṛṣṇa's playful pastimes with His beloved devotees.

These *līlā* narratives of this delightful appearance of God have captured the hearts, minds, and intellects of countless Hindus across the centuries and underpin not only much of the aesthetics of Hinduism, but also a good deal of its theologizing. Our concern here is the intellectual textual traditions inspired by the *Bhāgavata*, but the cultural influence of the text has been massive. Anyone who has seen a performance of classical Indian dance, for example, has very likely been treated to an enactment of some *līlā* episode from Kṛṣṇa's childhood, and there is every chance that if one happens upon a Hindu devotional poem or participates in an evening of *kīrtana* (devotional singing), narratives from the text will be featured. Likewise, anyone encountering a collection of traditional Indian paintings will be struck by how many depict scenes from the *Bhāgavata*, such as Kṛṣṇa with His beloved cowherd-women, the *gopīs*, and so forth with other art forms.[41] And, of course, anyone chancing upon a Hindu temple anywhere in India will stand a good chance of encountering a deity of Kṛṣṇa, most typically (at least in the north) with His beloved consort, Rādhā.

The Commentaries

In any event, turning to the scholastic literary tradition, among the eighty-four or so Sanskrit commentaries written on the text's eighteen hundred verses, one was by Jīva Gosvāmī. Jīva was one of six *Gosvāmī* (renounced ascetic) theologians entrusted with intellectually systematizing the popular revival of Kṛṣṇa *bhakti* emerging in the wake of the sixteenth-century charismatic Caitanya. This phenomenon—sometimes considered a renaissance of *bhakti*—took place primarily in East India as well as the Vṛndāvana area in northwest India. Bengal, in East India, was where Caitanya was born, and Vṛndāvana is where the *Bhāgavata* situates Kṛṣṇa's childhood millennia earlier.

Caitanya triggered a wave of Kṛṣṇa devotion across East India featuring meditations on Kṛṣṇa's early-life *līlā* pastimes in the *Bhāgavata*'s tenth book and its derived literature. His movement especially expressed itself through the ecstatic public chanting of Kṛṣṇa's names (we will provide a few glimpses of Caitanya's hagiography in part 1). Caitanya also contributed to the revival of the holy places associated with the *līlās* of the tenth book in Vṛndāvana (also referred to as Vraj herein),[42] which, as a result, developed into the bustling sacred town of today. Here Jīva resided as one of the celebrated six *Gosvāmīs* who settled in this holy place. These *Gosvāmīs* were essentially the intellectual founding figures of the tradition bestowed by Caitanya, producing an entire (and very extensive) canon of literary, philosophical, and aesthetic works dedicated to Kṛṣṇa. They were also responsible for the construction of most of the main temples in the town built on sites sacred to Kṛṣṇa, making Vṛndāvana one of the most thriving pilgrimage places in India today.[43] Thus a school was formed around Caitanya's life and teachings that came to be called the Caitanya Vaiṣṇava tradition, or the Gauḍīya (Eastern) Vaiṣṇava tradition.

Although Caitanya personally recorded only eight verses in writing (see part 4, "The Eight Versus of Instruction"), he inculcated an elaborate theology of Kṛṣṇa *bhakti* to some of His followers, especially Jīva's uncles Rūpa Gosvāmī and Sanātana Gosvāmī.[44] The distinguishing feature of these teachings from the perspective of the greater landscape of the multifarious *bhakti* traditions of the time is their focus on the various types of ecstatic mental states and intimate relationships with Kṛṣṇa that can be cultivated and attained through devotional practices, *bhakti yoga*. These teachings are, to all intents and purposes, a new body of divine revelation purporting to disclose details of some of the most intimate and personal eternal activities of God. Nonetheless, great energy is invested by the *Gosvāmīs* in locating their roots within the larger body of Vedic and Vedic-derived sacred texts accepted by all Hindu schools, the *Śruti* and *Smṛti* (hence the tradition sees itself as a Vedānta tradition, all of which is discussed within and in appendix 1).

Among other things, Rūpa wrote the *Bhaktirasāmṛtasindhu* (*Ocean of the Nectar of the Experience of* Bhakti) on these mental states (*bhāvas*) and relationships (*rasas*). In keeping with this imagery of the ocean, Rūpa divides his *Bhaktirasāmṛtasindhu* into four "quadrants": the Eastern (EQ), Western (WQ), Southern (SQ), and Northern (NQ). These are further subdivided into a sequential numbering of "waves" (for which we have just substituted the numbers). We will be drawing mostly from the Eastern Quadrant here. Rūpa also wrote a small handbook on *bhakti* practice, the *Upadeśāmṛta* (*Nectar of Instruction*), to which we will be referring. But he primarily left it up to Jīva to systematize and articulate the epistemology, metaphysics, and other philosophical ingredients of the tradition and situate it in accordance with the expected criteria of the intellectual milieu of the day. In addition to a considerable body of other writings, including his commentary on the *Bhāgavata* itself, Jīva compiled six treatises, the *Ṣat-Sandarbhas*, which subsequently took their place and remain at the core of the philosophy and *bhakti* systematics of this school.[45] These are essentially thematic analyses of the *Bhāgavata Purāṇa* from the perspective of the Gauḍīya tradition (that is, based on the "revelations" of Caitanya), which was developing in Jīva's time. A Sandarbha is defined as a type of text "which illuminates an esoteric subject matter, expresses its essence as well as its excellence, gives its various meanings, and is worthy of learning."[46] In part 1 of this work, we will be drawing from the fifth treatise, the *Bhakti Sandarbha*.[47]

These six treatises encapsulate the entire philosophical basis—metaphysical, epistemological, ontological, ethical, and soteriological—of Gauḍīya Vaiṣṇavism, which considers itself a Vedānta tradition.[48] The Sandarbhas are designed sequentially, prior volumes providing the epistemological and metaphysical infrastructure precursory to the practice of *bhakti* outlined in the fifth Sandarbha, which itself is precursory to the sixth, the *Prīti Sandarbha*, which deals with the goal of *bhakti*, love of God. So, in the *Bhakti Sandarbha*, Jīva is assuming the reader's familiarity with the previous four Sandarbhas and thus aware of the Gauḍīya position on certain essential issues central to the Vedānta as well as Purāṇa traditions. So by joining Jīva in his fifth Sandarbha, we are leap-frogging over Jīva's own sequential logic. By this point in his Sandarbhas, Jīva has already established why the *Bhāgavata* is to be deemed the paramount scripture on *bhakti* (discussed in appendix 1), and he assumes knowledge of the tradition's ontology (the nature of manifest reality, the individual self within it, and the Absolute Cause from which it emerges), outlined in the first four Sandarbhas. These are extensive domains in their own right, so we can touch only briefly upon such topics when we need to identify the main prerequisite metaphysical presuppositions fundamental to the present study on *bhakti* (especially in the chapter "The Object of *Bhakti*: *Īśvara*, *Bhagavān*, *Brahman*, and Divine Hierarchies"). But we must note that Jīva has argued and defended the tradition's theological fundamentals extensively through scriptural exegesis (interpretation) as well as through reason and argument. He has not simply assumed them.

In terms of the subject matter of these six Sandarbhas, briefly, the first, the *Tattva*, makes some preliminary comments on ontology and then focuses on epistemology (what constitutes a valid source of knowledge).[49] Since the exclusive focus on Kṛṣṇa as Godhead and *bhakti* as the summum bonum of human existence is based on the authority of the *Bhāgavata* tradition, Jīva must begin this first Sandarbha with the epistemological issue of what makes the *Bhāgavata* itself so authoritative. We have represented his arguments from the *Tattva Sandarbha* in appendix 1 so as not to overburden this introduction. The second Sandarbha, the *Bhagavat Sandarbha*, focuses on three transcendent aspects of the one Absolute Reality, with special attention directed toward the ultimate aspect of the personal *Bhagavān*, the Godhead (including monistic and monotheistic expressions). We will elaborate on this in some detail in "The Object of *Bhakti*." The third, the *Paramātma Sandarbha*, features another of these three transcendent aspects: the various manifestations of God derived from Kṛṣṇa in the form of the unlimited Viṣṇus immanent in or associated with the multiplicity of universes in *prakṛti*, the material realm. The fourth, the *Kṛṣṇa Sandarbha*, focuses on the primacy of the form of Kṛṣṇa over other manifestations of *Bhagavān*, such as the multiple expressions of Viṣṇu, a topic also touched on in "The Object of *Bhakti*." Thus, the first four Sandarbhas deal with the relationship between God and His energies, powers, and derivative manifestations. And the sixth, the *Prīti Sandarbha*, occupies itself with the goal, love of God, free from all personal motives. (See Dāsa 2007 for a brief introduction with sample translations from these Sandarbhas.) While we will be drawing on occasion from these other Sandarbhas as noted, in part 1 we are joining Jīva for the fifth, the *Bhakti Sandarbha*, which will outline the manifold ingredients and expressions of *bhakti yoga*. All the Sandarbhas are subdivided into *anucchedas*, thematic or topical sections (henceforth *anu*).

Our aim in this volume has been to open a modest window into the theological underpinnings and devotional practices of one important *bhakti* tradition. We wish to stress once more that the same treatment can be directed to other *bhakti* traditions, Vaiṣṇava, Śaiva, and Devī (Goddess) centered, to which we make frequent references. These all have their own powerful and coherent theological appeal and unique devotional depths. The rich variegation of these traditions reveals the multifarious theistic possibilities and richness of practice stemming from variants of *bhakti yoga* dedicated to the unlimited manifestations of *Īśvara/Bhagavān*. We will consider our meager effort in this regard successful if it inspires the reader to study the primary texts of these traditions directly in order to develop a deeper understanding of their tenets.

Despite our stated focus on attempting to present the tradition in its own terms and frame of references, or perhaps because of it, we would like to hope that this work will be of use to both academics and scholars interested in Kṛṣṇa *bhakti*, as well as practitioners of some of the forms of *yoga*. From an academic perspective, in addition to gaining exposure to an entire devotional worldview and mode of living in the world, by following the logic of the organization and systematization of the textual material by our *Gosvāmīs*, we encounter a good example of sectarian hermeneutics (the methods of scriptural interpretation) committed to promoting a comprehensive view of ultimate reality through a specific *bhakti* lens. This hermeneutics includes the rationale through which certain texts are prioritized and others minimized or ignored, and how, within commonly shared texts, sections or even individual statements conducive to a lineage's sectarian ontologies and hierarchies are prioritized and those less amenable in this regard ignored or assigned secondary meanings.

From the *yoga* practitioners' perspective, we are afforded a window into how a community of *bhaktas* with scholarly gifts and inclinations undertake what they deem to be their service both to their beloved Kṛṣṇa and to humanity at large. For them, this entails promoting, through the established intellectual criteria of their day and age, the metaphysics, practices, goals, and experiences of not just *yoga*, but *bhakti yoga* (an important distinction that we will discuss in detail). Specifically, in this tradition, the summum bonum of human existence is to attain *bhakti rasa*, ecstatic love of a higher *ātman*, *Īśvara*, God. There is no other ultimate meaning or purpose to embodied life: "The rising and setting of the sun simply steals away the life of people other than those whose time is spent in devotion to Kṛṣṇa" (*Bhāgavata* II.3.17). Jīva and Rūpa, along with their contemporary *Gosvāmī* (ascetic) associates, dedicated their lives to revealing to others in a remarkably erudite and intellectually rigorous manner the expressions such devotion takes in its Kṛṣṇa modalities. We encourage those who wish to gain a closer sense of the appeal of *bhakti* as a profound and meaningful worldview and soteriological goal to associate with those dedicated to their practices both in the past, through the literatures they have left behind, and in the present, through their teachings and observing their lifestyles and behaviors. Readers interested in pursuing this subject matter may care to study all the *Sandarbhas* and other *Gosvāmī* works systematically.[50] But first of all, of course, the reader is encouraged to read the entire *Bhāgavata Purāṇa* in its own right.[51]

Oṁ tat sat

PART I

Introduction to *Bhakti Yoga*

Elaborate on that which is called the *Bhāgavata*, such that *bhakti* for *Bhagavān*, Hari, will manifest among people. **—Brahmā to Sage Nārada, II.8.51–52**

Definition of *Bhakti*

We begin with a definition of *bhakti yoga*. But let us first briefly note that the impulse for taking up *bhakti* in the first place is the same as that for any aspiring *yogī* undertaking any path of *yoga*: harassed by the suffering and unfulfillment inherent in embodied existence in *saṁsāra*, the world of birth and death, one seeks to avoid future suffering. Thus, the opening verse of the fourth-century *Sāṅkhya Kārikā* makes awareness of suffering a prerequisite for seeking higher Truth: "It is because of the torment of the threefold sufferings—from one's own body and mind, from other living entities, and from the environment—that the desire to know the means to counteract them arises" (I.1). Adopting a form of *yoga* with serious intent as this entails coming to the realization not just that one is suffering, but that all attempts at finding happiness through the body/mind mechanism, when disconnected from knowledge of the *ātman* (innermost self) or of *Īśvara*—the Supreme Being, God—produces only temporal relief, and even this does not fulfill in any ultimate sense. Hence *Sarvaṁ duḥkham* ("All is frustration") is a central maxim not only of Buddhism, where it is the first foundational Truth of the entire tradition, but of almost all the *yoga* traditions.[1] If one accepts (as did the ancient materialist voices related to Cārvāka[2]) that no doubt there is suffering, but there is also happiness to be sought and found in the pleasures of the world, then one will naturally channel one's energies into pursuing whatever it is that one perceives as being a source of that happiness. In this case, one will not take to a *yoga* path with full dedication or, at least, will not do so in accordance with the presuppositions and commitments of all the classical *yoga*, or *mokṣa* (liberation-seeking), traditions, Hindu, Buddhist, and Jain.

Thus the first dawning of insight, *viveka*, in Yoga (*Yoga Sūtras* II.15)[3] is precisely that *all* is frustration, or at least unfulfilling, when one is under the influence of *avidyā*, ignorance (of the true *ātman* self). Try as one may through the stimulation of the body, mind, and intellect, one cannot shake off a deep-rooted sense of existential malaise and lack of deep-level fulfillment. When that Truth dawns irrevocably, one is ready to sincerely seek alternatives. In *bhakti*, this entails taking refuge of *Īśvara*, God, and it is this devotional surrender to a Supreme Being that lies at the heart of *bhakti yoga*.[4] Rather than pursuing other options such as those of the generic *yoga* or *jñāna* (knowledge of *ātman*) traditions, then, the *yogī* turns to *Īśvara*, but the motive is the same: one has failed to counteract suffering by other known material means.[5]

However, while the practices of *bhakti* are initially performed out of a desire to avoid suffering, *vaidhī bhakti*, they eventually develop into unmotivated, spontaneous, and ecstatic love for God, *rāgānugā bhakti*, as we will see. And it is because of this ultimate result that the *Bhāgavata Purāṇa* follows the *Gītā* in unambiguously asserting that *bhakti* is superior to other *yogas* (for instance, see *Gītā* VI.46–47, XII.2, and throughout). This is both because it is an easier path and more joyfully performed (*Gītā* IX.2) and because it reveals a higher Truth than that revealed by other *yoga* paths. Through other forms of *yoga* one can attain awareness of the *ātman*, the innermost self (the pure consciousness that is the goal of Patañjali in the chapter "The Practitioner of *Bhakti*, the *Bhakta*"), but through *bhakti*, in addition to the *ātman*, one can attain awareness culminating in ecstatic love of *Parama-ātman, Īśvara*, the Supreme *Ātman* beyond the individual *ātman*. In the Vaiṣṇava reading of the *Gītā* and *Bhāgavata Purāṇa*, *Īśvara*, also known as *Bhagavān*, is a Truth beyond that of the *ātman*.[6] And the Ultimate *Īśvara* is Kṛṣṇa. We will return to all this in considerable detail later in "The Object of Bhakti," but for now we can consider *bhakti yoga* as the specific means and practices through which one takes shelter of *Īśvara*, initially—at least for most practitioners—out of material desperation, but eventually out of unrestrainable, intoxicating love.

With regard to a formal definition of *bhakti*, there were, naturally, a variety of overlapping definitions in circulation in textual sources, highlighting its various ingredients and different emphasis given by different sages. The *Bhakti Sūtras* of Nārada (16–19) expresses a few: "*Bhakti* includes attachment to *pūjā* (ritual worship of *Īśvara*), according to sage Vyāsa; love of *kathā* (stories about *Īśvara*'s incarnations) and such things, according to sage Garga; and the offering of all acts to *Īśvara* and the experiencing of extreme distress upon forgetting Him, according to sage Nārada." (We use the gendered pronouns "He" and "Him" and the like, as *Īśvara* is a masculine entity; *Īśvarī* is the feminine form, and were this analysis focused on Durgā, Lakṣmī, Rādhā, or Kālī, as opposed to Kṛṣṇa, we would use feminine pronoun forms.)[7] The *Saunḍilya Sūtra* states that "*bhakti* is supreme devotion (*anurakti*) for *Īśvara*" (I.2).

As discussed in the introduction, Rūpa Gosvāmī and his nephew Jīva Gosvāmī will be our primary guides in our analysis of *bhakti* throughout this part, so we will focus on the definitions they select. In his *Bhaktirasāmṛtasindhu*, Rūpa offers the following definition: "*Bhakti* is said to be service to Kṛṣṇa,[8] by means of the senses. This service is free of all limitations, dedicated to Him and pure [of self-motive]."[9] Jīva opts for a similar definition: "The root *bhaj* means to offer service.[10] Therefore the wise have described *bhakti*, which is the preeminent path of attaining perfection, as service."[11] Thus, putting all these together, *bhakti* is theistic and encompasses such activities as worship; the offering of one's acts to *Īśvara*; reading the stories of His divine incarnations; constant remembrance of Him; and, for Rūpa and Jīva most especially, using oneself in the service of Kṛṣṇa, the ultimate expression of *Īśvara*. We might briefly note here that service is synonymous with love. True love, one can suggest, is nothing other than the experience of complete satisfaction attained from fully dedicating oneself to pleasing one's beloved through acts of devotion and service. And, of course, for love to be true, this devotion and service must be fully reciprocal. We will see in part 3 the unbounded degree to which Kṛṣṇa, despite being supremely independent as the Ultimate Absolute Being, returns the love of His devotees by submitting to them according to their desire.

Bhakti, then, is love of God free of all self-interest. Indeed, Rūpa nuances loving service by defining the "highest type" of devotion (*uttama bhakti*), as "continued service to Kṛṣṇa, which is [performed] pleasingly,[12] is unobstructed by the desire for liberation or enjoying the fruits of one's work in the world, and is free of any other desire."[13] In the words of the *Bhāgavata*:

> The characteristics of *bhakti yoga*, which is free of the *guṇas*, has been described as that *bhakti* to the Supreme Person which is free of motive, and uninterrupted. Such persons [who engage in this] do not accept the five types of liberation[14] . . . even if these are offered, if they are devoid of service to God. (III.29.12–14)

These five types of Vaiṣṇava postmortem liberation will occupy us later, but it is important to note that the very notion of liberation itself, the generic goal of all *yoga* systems, is rejected in the higher stages of *bhakti*, a theme that we will return to frequently. In fact, disinterest in liberation is one of six qualities accompanying *bhakti* identified by Rūpa in another of his works[15] partly because it is still in the realms of self-interest, but also because the bliss *bhakti* bestows far surpasses the bliss of the *ātman*'s immersion in its own nature of pure consciousness, the culmination of the generic path of *yoga*.

The common denominator underpinning all of these definitions of *bhakti yoga* is that they feature the *bhakta*—a type of *yogī* who practices *bhakti*—and *Īśvara*, God, a Supreme Being who is the object of *bhakti*. Thus *bhakti* as a *yoga* process requires at least two entities: the *bhakta* and *Īśvara*. In the next section of part 1 we will turn to the practices of *bhakti yoga* itself, following very closely in the footsteps of our guides, Jīva and Rūpa; in "The Practitioner of *Bhakti*, the *Bhakta*," we will consider some of the characteristics of the *bhakta* as a *yogī*; and in "The Object of *Bhakti*," we will engage some of the ways *Īśvara*, or the term's near synonym *Bhagavān*, has been construed in important *bhakti* traditions of India. We will use the terms *Īśvara* and *Bhagavān* synonymously for now (but will provide some nuance between them in "The Object of *Bhakti*") and note that in the *Bhāgavata*, Kṛṣṇa is presented as the most complete and perfect expression of these terms, the source of all the other unlimited manifestations of *Īśvara/Bhagavān*.

Then, in parts 2 and 3, we exemplify these three aspects of *bhakti yoga* through translations from the *Bhāgavata* itself as source text. We have noted that it is the stories of Kṛṣṇa as *Īśvara/Bhagavān* when He incarnated into the world that have most especially delighted and enchanted *bhaktas* from all Hindu devotional traditions across the ages and that have made the *Bhāgavata* the most devotionally influential text in Hinduism along with the *Rāmāyaṇa*. The innermost core of *bhakti yoga* in the Kṛṣṇa tradition is nothing other than the expression of this enchantment.

The Practices of *Bhakti*

Vaidhī (Prescriptive) *Bhakti* and *Rāgānugā* (Spontaneous) *Bhakti*

In the *Bhakti Sandarbha*, Jīva structures his analysis of *bhakti yoga* around a twofold categorization: *vaidhī bhakti* and *rāgānugā bhakti*. *Vaidhī bhakti* is devotion prompted by rules and prescriptions (*vidhi*)—the injunctions of scripture. In other words, it consists of regulated practices established by tradition—which typically means texts associated with *Īśvara* (for instance, see *Gītā* IV.7–8) or with accomplished predecessor *bhaktas* who attained success in the past and are therefore devotional exemplars and authorities such as our *Gosvāmīs*. *Rāgānugā bhakti* manifests in the case of very rare souls in the form of devotion that has no need for following prescribed or formalized methods but rather results spontaneously from natural innate attraction (*rāga*) for *Īśvara*. In Rūpa's words, *vaidhī* "is born from the prescriptions of the sacred texts, rather than emerging from the development of desire for God," as is the case with *rāgānugā* (*Bhaktirasāmṛtasindhu* Eastern Quadrant[1] 2.6). *Vaidhī* is the method adopted by the vast majority of practitioners who strive to cultivate *bhakti*, while *rāgānugā* stems from inherent attraction unmediated by regulations—at least in this life (in fact, *rāgānugā* usually stems from perfected past-life *vaidhī* practice but can in rare cases be attained by grace).

However, we should immediately note for those familiar with *yoga* concepts that the type of *rāga* in *rāgānugā* (literally, "following" *anugā*, *rāga*) reflects the highest type of *yogic* attainment in this system, since it is focused exclusively on *Īśvara*, as will be discussed in detail later, and is not to be confused with mundane desire—the *rāga* of Patañjali, for example, which, stemming from ignorance, is focused on the body and mind and is an obstacle to *yoga* (a *kleśa* per *Yoga Sūtras* II.4–7). We will first consider *vaidhī bhakti*, which will introduce us to the nine standard practices typically associated with the term *bhakti yoga* and thus with the central theme of this book, and then *rāgānugā*.

The Nine Practices of *Vaidhī Bhakti*

The *Bhāgavata* distills the actual practices of *bhakti* into nine basic activities that constitute the standard classical Vaiṣṇava list of primary *bhakti yoga* processes:

> The nine characteristics of *bhakti* that people can offer to Viṣṇu[2] are: hearing about Him, singing about Him, remembering Him, serving His feet, worshipping Him, glorifying Him, considering oneself His servant, considering oneself His friend, and surrendering completely to Him. (VII.5.23)

Thus, just as the practices for generic or classical *yoga* as articulated in the *Yoga Sūtras* are schematized by Patañjali as consisting of eight limbs, the *aṣṭāṅga* (II.29ff.), even as there were multiple variants and alternative models;[3] and just as some of the Vedānta traditions divide *jñāna yoga*, the path of knowledge, into three (or four) primary activities;[4] so the classical practices of *bhakti yoga* are formalized as comprising these nine, even as this list is certainly not exhaustive or exclusive as we will see. We will discuss these processes one by one.

Śravaṇa (Hearing)

The first actual activity or process of *bhakti*, *śravaṇa*, hearing about *Īśvara*, God, is the starting point from which the other eight processes of *bhakti* develop.[5] Obviously any sort of spiritual practice can begin only when one initially hears or learns something about it. In Jīva's definition: "When the organs of hearing contact the words describing the name, form, qualities, and pastimes [of *Bhagavān*], the term *śravaṇa* is assigned" (*anu* 248). In the time of the *Bhāgavata*, and still in Jīva's time, most people would have received the text orally, since primarily only some members of the *brāhmaṇa* caste were literate, and so the text would typically have been recited by one of them from memory or from a hand-copied manuscript. With the widespread nature of literacy and print media in our day and age, we of course have the facility to read the accounts. Either way, both hearing and reading relate to absorbing the mind in God manifest as sacred Word, and this is the essence of *śravaṇa*.

In fact, the entire *Bhāgavata* sees its own raison d'être as sacred text as being nothing other than the recording and preserving of narratives about *Īśvara* such that they can be formally heard (XII.13.18). These stories, called *līlās*, are deemed so delightful and enchanting that they naturally capture the mind. Just as in conventional love affairs, a person becomes enamored with the form, qualities, and activities of a beloved and, when love is in full bloom, can think of nothing else, so, in *bhakti*, the mind is captivated by *Īśvara* as encountered in the amazing stories contained in texts such as the *Bhāgavata*. When this initial attraction is channeled through the nine practices, devotion and love of God can develop. The *Bhāgavata* is nothing other than concentrated *śravaṇa*, composed so that the seeds of *bhakti yoga* can be planted in the minds of those seeking a relationship with *Īśvara*.

Once the mind becomes attracted to the stories of Kṛṣṇa through *śravaṇa* and, in time, captivated by love for Him, it loses its attachments to this world, which pale in comparison. This too happens naturally. The mind consequently shakes off the grip of mundane desire, which is the fuel perpetuating the cycle of birth and death in all *yoga* traditions. One thereby becomes eligible for liberation from this cycle, *saṁsāra*. *Bhakti*, from the perspective of being a *yoga* process, is nothing other than this. Of course, as we will find out, liberation is not in fact sought by true *bhaktas*, who wish to be immersed in thoughts of Kṛṣṇa rather than in the *ātman*, a state of consciousness devoid of all objects, as per the goal of generic *yoga*. We are repeatedly reminded that, from *śravaṇa*, hearing about Kṛṣṇa, one's mind becomes so enchanted that, to say nothing of interest in material (*prakṛtic*) things, it loses all interest it might have had in conventional *ātman* liberation.[6] This is because conventional liberation deprives the *bhakta* from hearing about the beloved *Īśvara*: "I will never desire even liberation, O Lord, because in that state there is no nectar about your lotus feet, which flows out of the depths of the hearts and through the mouths of the great souls. Please grant me this boon: let me have 10,000 ears [to hear about You]" (IV.20.24). The *Bhāgavata* cannot comprehend anyone not becoming enchanted by Kṛṣṇa: "Who, absorbed in hearing the narrations of Hari, could possibly not develop attraction for them?" (II.3.12).

We will illustrate aspects of the nine processes of *bhakti* with anecdotes from the hagiography of Rūpa's teacher, Caitanya Mahāprabhu, beginning here with a passage pertaining to the effects that can be wrought on the listener by the practice of *śravaṇa* about Kṛṣṇa:

> Then [Caitanya] visited another gentleman's house. . . . Ratnagarbha Ācārya was a great devotee of the Lord, and was very fond of the *Śrīmad Bhāgavatam*. He was at that time reading from the *Bhāgavatam* with great respect and affection. . . . [He read a passage from book X, where the wives of the *brāhmaṇas* meet Lord Kṛṣṇa]. . . . Spoken with great devotion, these words of the *Śrīmad Bhāgavatam* entered the ears of Lord Viśvambhara [Caitanya]. As soon as he heard these words . . . [Caitanya] . . . fell down unconscious overcome with spiritual ecstasy. All the students were amazed at the sight. After remaining in trance for a while, the Lord regained his external consciousness. When he was able to speak, the Lord said to Ratnagarbha Ācārya: "Go on, Go on." He rolled on the ground in ecstasy. The Lord continued to urge him on, saying, "Go on! Go on!" The *brāhmaṇa* continued to read, and everyone floated on the nectarine ocean of love of Kṛṣṇa. Unrestrained tears from the Lord's eyes flooded the entire world. All the ecstatic symptoms like shivering, horripilation, and crying manifested in the Lord's person." (*Caitanya Bhāgavata*, *Madhya-khaṇḍa*, I.300–10)[7]

Since Kṛṣṇa is the source of all bliss, when His presence contained in the *līlās*, stories, enters through the ears by means of *śravaṇa*, the body experiences bliss, and its normal functioning can be disrupted. Indeed, the body can erupt into physiologically aberrant symptoms, such as emiting tears or displaying hair standing on end, owing to contact with this transcendent presence. We will encounter such effects ensuing from the other *bhakti* practices as well. This is the ecstasy of devotion.

Thus, the entire *Bhāgavata* is composed to provide an opportunity for *śravaṇa* and, through that, a vivid and transformational encounter with *Īśvara*, which culminates in falling in love with God:

> For the righteous, who are free of envy, the highest *dharma* is to be found in the *Śrīmad Bhāgavata*, in which all dishonesty (worldly *dharmas*) has been rejected.[8] Composed by the great sage Vyāsa, only the Ultimate Truth is revealed here, which bestows auspiciousness, and uproots the threefold miseries of life.[9] Can *Īśvara* be immediately captured in the heart by anything else? In this text, He is captured in an instant by the virtuous who desire to hear. It is the succulent ripened fruit of the desire tree[10] of the Vedic scriptures. . . .[11] *Aho!*[12] O connoisseurs of divine ecstasy,[13] while in this world drink continuously the spiritual flavors (*rasa*) of the *Bhāgavata*—love of God—to your full satisfaction. (I.1.2–3)

Indeed, as we will see in his tale, prior to his composition of the *Bhāgavata*, the despondency of the great sage Vyāsa—whom tradition ascribes to be the divider of the one Veda into four, the compiler of the one Purāṇa into eighteen Purāṇas totaling four hundred thousand verses, the recorder of the immense one-hundred-thousand-verse *Mahābhārata* epic (and even the primary commentator on the *Yoga Sūtras*)—was precisely because, despite this prolificacy, he had not adequately described the *līlā* narrations of *Bhagavān* Kṛṣṇa in all this massive output of knowledge. His heart was thus dry from lack of *rasa*, devotional ecstasy. From the perspective of *bhakti*, all these other texts deal with mundane subject matters or, at best, in the case of the *mokṣa* (liberation) traditions of generic *yoga*, spiritually incomplete topics:

> Sir, for the most part, you have not described the spotless fame of *Bhagavān*.[14] I consider any knowledge, which does not satisfy the Lord, to be barren. You have not described the

> greatness of Vāsudeva (Kṛṣṇa), to the same extent that you have glorified the four mundane goals of life—*dharma*, civic duty; *artha*, material prosperity; *kāma*, fulfillment of desires; and *mokṣa*, liberation of the *ātman*.[15] Those who dwell in the lovely abode of Kṛṣṇa *bhakti* do not find attractive those words, even if replete with literary embellishments, that do not describe the glory of Hari [Kṛṣṇa], which purify the world—just as the swans from the celestial Mānasa lake do not dwell in the ponds frequented by crows. (I.5.8–11)[16]

Thus, the entire *Bhāgavata*, and especially its tenth book, is nothing other than *śravaṇa* about Kṛṣṇa, the summum bonum of existence. And *bhakti yoga* is nothing other than the mind becoming attracted to the *līlās*, pastimes, through *śravaṇa*, and then subsequently engaging itself in the remaining eight processes of *bhakti* such that this blissful encounter with Kṛṣṇa can be cultivated into an active relationship and ceaselessly deepened.

Before proceeding to the remaining practices of *bhakti*, Jīva presents a sequence of focus pertaining to *śravaṇa*, hearing about Kṛṣṇa, which also applies to the next two processes of *bhakti*. He notes that the ideal progression in the order of aural topics is, optimally, first to hear about Kṛṣṇa's names, then to hear about His forms, then His qualities, and finally His *līlās*, pastimes, in that order (*anu* 256). While hearing about any of these and in any order can lead to perfection, he states that generally the process starts with hearing the names of Kṛṣṇa. This cleanses the mind, allowing it sufficient purity to begin to comprehend the second item of focus, Kṛṣṇa's form: "Entering through the ears, that form becomes imprinted on the minds of the saints and never escapes" (XI.30.3). Once the form manifests in the mind, then, in turn, one can better hear about the qualities associated with Kṛṣṇa's form. Each step of this process purifies the mind further, until finally Kṛṣṇa's *līlās*, pastimes, which of course feature and highlight His form and qualities, can be experienced, as we will discover in part 3.

Kīrtana (Chanting)

Kīrtana refers to singing, chanting, or reciting the names and deeds of *Īśvara*. As with all the nine processes, "*bhakti* for *Bhagavān* will arise in one who sings, hears about, and rejoices in Him" (X.69.45).

Although *śravaṇa* is the primary and foundational practice of *bhakti*, it is, in a sense, a passive activity. *Kīrtana* is the preeminent active spiritual practice promoted by the *Bhāgavata*,[17] and is the most accessible process for attaining immediate personal contact with *Īśvara* for most practitioners.

This is so because sacred names are considered identical to *Iśvara*: "the Lord . . . takes the form of mantras" (I.5.38). *Mantras* are divine presence, not symbols or names representing something beyond themselves as with normal language. They embody actual immediate Divinity. Conventional names and words, such as "book" or "pot," are representational sounds, established by social consensus for the purpose of communication. And they differ from one language group to another: the English word "book" is *pustaka* in Sanskrit, *libro* in Italian, *kitab* in Hindi/Urdu, and so on (and one could just as well invent a new word for book, such as "umma-gumma," if one could convince other people in one's social sphere to start adopting it). So conventional words are different from the actual objects to which they refer;[18] one's thirst cannot be quenched by saying "water," since the word "water" is different from the substance water, nor will the contents of this book be internalized simply by repeating its title. The name of Kṛṣṇa, in contrast, *is* Kṛṣṇa personally and immediately present in sonic form. Therefore, God can be directly experienced by reciting His name:

> The Name [of Kṛṣṇa] is absolute and it is pure, because there is no difference between the Name, and that which it denotes. The Name *is* Kṛṣṇa Himself in His form of pure consciousness.[19] It is eternally liberated. It is a wish-granting gem.[20] The Name, etc.,[21] of *Śrī* Kṛṣṇa cannot be grasped by the material senses: Kṛṣṇa Himself manifests [by His own accord] on the tip of the tongue, which has been applied to service [in the form of chanting]. (*Bhaktirasāmṛtasindhu* Eastern Quadrant II.233–34)

That Kṛṣṇa can actually personally appear in the form of the Name (sometimes written with a capital "N" to stress its nondifference from the person God) is just a sonic parallel of the claims, discussed later, that He can also appear before the eyes in a perceivable form.[22] As a vision of Kṛṣṇa is visual divine presence, the sound "Kṛṣṇa" is sonal divine presence. In both cases, this presence is perceived or not perceived in proportion to the purity and devotion of the *bhakta* or not. Hence, since Kṛṣṇa fully manifests His personal presence for advanced practitioners, such *bhaktas* can exhibit extreme ecstatic states in *kīrtana*. This is because whenever the psychophysical mechanism contacts Kṛṣṇa manifest in any form such as sound, the ecstasy the mind and body experience from this direct encounter causes them to erupt into abnormal physical symptoms. Kṛṣṇa is the embodiment of ultimate bliss, and extreme bliss can wreak havoc on the conventional functioning of the body/mind mechanisms. These bodily reactions can sometimes be quite startling to conventional perception. Consider the dramatic ecstatic symptoms produced by *kīrtana* that were exhibited frequently by *Śri* Caitanya Mahāprabhu (Prabhu, below):

> Mahāprabhu danced . . . deeply absorbed and the people all around him were wet with the tears of *prema* [divine love] of Prabhu. Prabhu raised his arms and said, *"Bol! Bol!"* ["Chant! Chant!"] and the people floating in *ānanda* [bliss] raised the sound of Hari. Now he fell in a faint, and he had no more breath; and suddenly he stood up again and shouted. He was like a *śimūlī* tree, thick with gooseflesh: sometimes his body blossomed [with it], and sometimes it abated. Blood sweat came out of every pore of his body, and he stuttered. . . . It seemed that each of his teeth were separately trembling; his teeth chattered so, it seemed that they would fall out on the ground. As time went on Prabhu became increasingly absorbed in *ānanda*. The third watch came, and still the dancing was not ended. A sea of *ānanda* welled up in all the people, and everyone forgot their bodies, their selves, and their homes. (*Caitanya Caritāmṛta Antya-līlā* 10.66–73)[23]

I sometimes analogize such states as comparable to an electric appliance designed for one voltage system, blowing its mechanisms when contacting a much higher voltage system.

Mantra, then, sometimes called *nāma-avatāra*, sonic incarnation, is "infused with specific power, either by the Lord or great sages, and establishes a unique relationship with the Lord," says Jīva (*anu* 284). In the words of the *Bhāgavata*, "The Lord of worship is without material form, but He takes the form of *mantras*. By worshipping Him by means of the forms of these names, a person becomes a sage and his or her perception becomes perfect" (I.5.37–38). As fire permeates an iron bar, which becomes "fire-ized" and nondifferent from fire because of such permeation, so *Īśvara* manifests within *prakṛti* in various forms, one of which is sound, such that it becomes *Īśvara*-ized, so to speak. And, as wherever there is fire there are the qualities of heat and light, so wherever *Īśvara* is present, there is, in addition to ecstasy, purity as well. Hence, in addition to its bliss-bestowing potential, *kīrtana* is especially effective in removing impure influences from the mind (the *kleśas*):[24]

> A sinful person is not purified by the acts of atonement and vows prescribed by the experts in Vedic knowledge as much as by the reciting of the syllables of the name of Hari. . . . For even when atonement is performed, it is not really accomplished if thereafter the mind once again runs along the path of unrighteousness. For one who desires to eliminate all *karma*, the repetition of the names and qualities of Hari truly makes the mind pure (*sāttvika*) [and hence one loses the desire to perform further unrighteous acts]. (VI.2.11–12)

Other purificatory processes may eliminate the negative *karmic* consequences of unrighteous action, but they do not eradicate the initial impulses or desires, called *saṁskāras* in Yoga psychology, that prompted such behavior in the first place. Hence, those *saṁskāras* (not to be confused with *saṁsāra*[25]) can activate again. This is sometimes compared with an elephant taking a bath in the river only to emerge from the water and then roll in the sand again. *Kīrtana* eradicates the *saṁskāras* themselves, not just their *karmic* consequences, and hence is considered the supreme purifier.

The reason for this is that since *Īśvara* is nondifferent from the name, it is *Īśvara* who actually manifests personally within the mind of the sincere chanter, and where *Īśvara* is present, there can be no impurity: "*Bhagavān* quickly enters the heart of one who faithfully hears and constantly recites His activities. Entering through the portals of the ears, Kṛṣṇa purifies all impurities from the lotuslike heart of His devotees, like Autumn does to the waters" (II.8.4–5). Consequently: "A thief; a drunkard; a murderer of friends; a killer of *brāhmaṇas*; one who defiles his *guru*'s bed; a murderer of a woman, king, parent, or cow; all these and other types of sinners—indeed for every kind of evil person—the chanting of the name is the best atonement; the mind of Viṣṇu [is attracted] by that sound" (VI.2.10–11).

Of course, since *kīrtana* is initially a *vaidhī* practice, and thus typically initiated by self-centeredness (albeit of the right sort) rather than pure love of God, it may take some time for these impurities to clear such that the consequent natural sweetness of the name can manifest, and ecstasy be experienced, as Rūpa notes: "Even though the name, activities and so forth of Kṛṣṇa may be sweet, they may not be relishable to a tongue which is afflicted by the bile of ignorance. Nonetheless, if chanted every day diligently, it destroys the poison at its roots, and its nectar slowly becomes pleasurable" (*Upadeśāmṛta*, 7). But once the heart (the seat of the mind) has been cleansed through *kīrtana*, and *Bhagavān* has begun to reveal His presence, the ecstatic effects of *kīrtana* can be quickly felt: "When one's love is awakened and one's heart has melted while chanting loudly the names of one's beloved Lord, one laughs, one weeps, one cries out, one sings and one dances like a madman, completely indifferent to social norms" (XI.2.40). Thus *kīrtana* embodies both *yoga* as method—clearing all impurities (*kleśas*)—and *yoga* as goal—ecstatic love of God.

In fact, the *Bhāgavata*, along with other Purāṇas,[26] considers *kīrtana* to be the *yuga dharma*, the recommended spiritual practice for *Kali yuga*, the present and most degraded of the four ages (*yugas*):[27]

> Although the age of *Kali* is a breeding ground of faults, O king, it does have one great quality: merely by performing Kṛṣṇa *kīrtana,* one is freed from attachments and attains the supreme. The goal that was obtained in the *yuga* of *Satya* by meditation (*dhyāna*), in the *yuga* of *Tretā* by worshipping through ritualistic sacrifices (*yajña*), in the *yuga* of *Dvāpara* by deity worship (*paricaryā*), is attained in the *yuga* of *Kali* by *kīrtana*. (XII.3.52)[28]

Consequently: "The noble Āryans,[29] who are connoisseurs of quality and extract the essence of things, extol the age of *Kali*, because in that age, all desired objects are obtained merely by *saṅkīrtana*"[30] (XI.5.36).

The practice of *japa* is also situated under the rubric of *kīrtana*. Where *kīrtana* is a public congregational practice, *japa* is the personal, private, and meditative recitation of *mantra*. The verb *jap* means to repeat something softly. The term has its origins in the Vedic period[31] and, by the Upaniṣads, the earliest mystico-philosophical texts in the Vedic corpus, becomes associated with the repetition of *oṁ*. *Oṁ* in these texts is identified with *Brahman*[32]—*Brahman* is the name given to the Absolute Truth in the Upaniṣads—and both *oṁ* and *Brahman* in turn become identified with *Īśvara*, the personal feature of *Brahman*.[33] (The various ways *Brahman* is construed in the main schools derived from the Upaniṣads, and exactly how it correlates with the term *Īśvara* is a topic that will occupy our attention in "The Object of *Bhakti*.") As *bhakti* practices superseded the old Vedic rituals, the term *japa* increasingly referred to the soft (or silent) repetition of *Īśvara*'s name—that is, the absorption of the mind in the Deity's sonic *mantra* form, or sound presence. Thus, Kṛṣṇa states in the *Gītā* that He is *oṁ*,[34] and of all ritual offerings, He is *japa* (X.25). Likewise, in the *Yoga Sūtras*, *Īśvara* is presented as the most important object upon which to fix the mind in order to still it, and one does this through performing *japa* on *oṁ*, His signifier, "keeping its meaning in mind" (I.28; we will consider a *bhakti* reading of this phrase below). In the more developed theisms of Śaivism and Vaiṣṇavism, *oṁ* is retained but expands into the more personal *mantras* associated with *Īśvara* as Śiva and Viṣṇu. The two *mantras* explicitly expressed in the *Bhāgavata* are *oṁ namo Nārāyaṇāya*, the *mantra* for Viṣṇu (VIII.3.32), and *oṁ namo Bhagavate Vāsudevāya*, that for Kṛṣṇa (I.5.37, IV.8.54, VIII.16.39). The corresponding *mantra* in Śaivism is *oṁ namo Śivāya*. In Jīva's Gauḍīya tradition, *japa* becomes the primary practice of personal meditation, and Caitanya popularized the chanting of the by now well-known Kṛṣṇa *mahāmantra* (great *mantra*): *Hare Kṛṣṇa, Hare Kṛṣṇa, Kṛṣṇa Kṛṣṇa, Hare Hare*; *Hare Rāma, Hare Rāma, Rāma Rāma, Hare Hare.*

Mantra japa is optimally performed first thing in the morning—ideally an hour or so before the sun rises. This is called the *brāhma-*

muhūrta (*Brahman* time).[35] At this time, the mind is rested and no longer in a state of lethargy (*tamas*), and the activity of the day has yet to commence with the awakening of living creatures and life's duties along with the rising sun (*rajas*). This *brāhma-muhūrta* is the optimal time for *yogīs* serious about meditation, as it is the period most favorable for concentration, detachment, and calmness.

In *japa* meditation, all the generic rules of classical Patañjali-type meditation apply: the mind is to be fixed without deviation on the *mantra* (*Yoga Sūtras* I.28 and 32), and this practice requires prolonged regular effort (I.12–13). However, this is ideally performed in a mind imbued with love for *Īśvara*, *bhāva*, discussed below, rather than just mechanically.[36] Additionally, the *japa* is uttered in a mood of total dependency on *Īśvara*'s grace as opposed to one's own willpower and *yogic* virtuosity. In advanced stages, the *bhakta*'s mind is naturally permeated with love and surrender to the beloved *Īśvara*. However, these attitudes of love and surrender while performing *japa* are flavors of the meditating mind, they must not agitate it into active thought. The rules of meditation remain the same—the mind must strive to remain fixed without deviation on the repetition of the *japa*: "From wherever the mind wanders, due to its fickle and unsteady nature, one must control it and bring it back under the control of the higher self" (*Gītā* VI.26). So *japa* is not prayer. Of course prayer is most definitely a *bhakti* activity—in fact, Jīva places under this category of *kīrtana* reciting prayers to *Īśvara*, along with expressing feelings of humility and revealing one's desires to Him (*anu* 276). But prayer is conventionally a practice that involves an active mind; *japa* is a practice of *citta-vṛtti-nirodhaḥ*, the complete stilling of all the thoughts of the mind upon the *mantra* (*Yoga Sūtras* I.2, applied to I.27–28).

In Jīva's tradition, the *nāma-ācārya*, or exemplar of *japa*, is Haridāsa Ṭhākura. Perhaps the most famous Gauḍīya story featuring *japa* involves a young prostitute sent by a malicious king, Rāmacandra Khān, to allure and entice the ascetic Haridāsa away from his *japa* practices. Seeking to secure her spiritual well-being without humiliating her by spurning her advances, the compassionate Haridāsa promises to fulfill her seductive proposals, just as soon as he has finished his daily chanting practice. This, however, consisted of three hundred thousand repetitions of the Hare Kṛṣṇa *mantra* noted above, which took all day and night to complete, leaving no time for any liaison with the prostitute. So the promise was renewed the next day. The young lady waited patiently and respectfully, while this went on for three days. On the third day:

> Bowing to the Ṭhākura and to the *tulasī* (plant sacred to Kṛṣṇa),[37] she sat in the doorway and listened to the names, saying, "Hari Hari." "The names will certainly be finished today," said Haridāsa, "and today I shall fulfill your desire." And while he was still at *kīrtana*, the end of the night came. And in the company of the Ṭhākura, the prostitute's mind was turned. Bowing deeply she fell at the feet of the Ṭhākura, and humbly told him the story of Rāmacandra Khān. "As a prostitute I have committed infinite sins; be merciful and save me, wretched as I am." Ṭhākura said: "I know all about the Khān. He is ignorant and stupid, so I do not take offense from him. That day [when you came] I was going to go from this place, but I remained for three more days to save you." The prostitute said, "Be gracious and instruct me; what should I do, that the agonies of *saṁsāra* pass from me?" Ṭhākura said, "Give the goods of your house to a *brāhmaṇa*, then come to this house and remain here. Take the name incessantly and serve *tulasī*, and quickly you will gain the feet of Kṛṣṇa." So the prostitute took the orders of her guru. . . . She shaved her head and remained with one cloth in the house, and night and day she took the name three lakhs [three hundred thousand] times. She served the *tulasī*, fasted, [only] chewing; and as she controlled her senses, *prema* [love of God] manifested itself. She became a famous Vaiṣṇava, a very great person, and many great Vaiṣṇavas went to have *darśana* [a visit] of her. (*Antya-līlā* 3.120–34)

Here we see the portrayal of the purifying effects of *mantra* even on those who happen to be merely in the vicinity of the chanter.

Thus although these terms have porous boundaries (as we see with the usage of *kīrtana* in the Haridāsa narrative above, for what is more typically considered *japa*), *kīrtana* usually represents the communal and congregational chanting of *mantras*, the names of *Iśvara*, or brief repeated devotional phrases about *Īśvara*'s activities. *Saṅkīrtana* features this even more so—indeed, in the hagiography of Caitanya, the *saṅkīrtana* points to public chanting in the streets accompanied by music and dancing (popularized in the West by a modern branch of the Gauḍīya tradition, ISKCON, better known as the Hare Krishna Movement[38]). In contrast, *japa*, which focuses on very short *mantras*, is personal, quiet, meditative, and performed in a more secluded and private manner. We can also mention here another term, *bhajana*, which overlaps in significance and content with the term *kīrtana* and is also often a public practice but tends to refer to devotional hymns—that is, entire phrases, sentences, or even long narrative sequences that flow from verse to verse—about the stories of *Īśvara* inspired by the epics and Purāṇas (such as, in the case of Kṛṣṇa, from the *Bhāgavata*'s tenth book). These are often set to more intricate devotional *rāgas* (melodies) and may be accompanied by more sophisticated instrumentation than is the case with *kīrtana*. *Kīrtana*, in partial contrast, tends to feature the basic names and *mantras* associated with the various *Īśvara* forms or very short, simple, and succinct phrases connected with their activities. These are encapsulated in less elaborate melodies repeated over and over again to simple musical accompaniment that involves the participation of larger numbers of people than typically is the case with *bhajana*. But all these terms overlap considerably.

Finally, since, as with all processes of *bhakti*, the goal is to develop love of *Īśvara*, one should chant the specific names that one holds dear, says Jīva, so that this love (*rāga*) can develop (*anu* 263). In other words, the *mantra* one selects should correspond to the manifestation of *Īśvara* toward whom one is attracted. We will discuss some of the ways such attraction may develop later. Also, as with the first *bhakti yoga* process of *śravaṇa*, the focus of chanting optimally also revolves around the progression of names, forms, qualities, and pastimes.

Smaraṇa (Remembering)

Jīva quotes the following *Bhāgavata* verse as best defining *smaraṇa*, the third practice of *bhakti yoga*: "*Yoga* has been taught . . . as being that by which the mind is withdrawn from everything else, and fixed on Me [Kṛṣṇa]" (XI.13.14). In other words, in *smaraṇa* one thinks of (remembers) Kṛṣṇa at all times. Absorbing all of one's thoughts in God[39] is actually the ultimate goal of *vaidhī bhakti* and repeatedly stressed as the ultimate goal of all *yoga* in the *Gītā*: "Of all *yogīs*, the one who performs *bhakti* to Me with his innermost self absorbed in Me is the best of all those engaged in *yoga* (VI.47); "Listen once more again to my highest, most intimate of all teachings. . . . Fix your mind on Me and become My *bhakta*" (XVIII.64–65).[40] Jīva notes that remembrance is possible only if the heart is pure—that is, freed from mundane desires—hence *kīrtana* as a purifying practice is an essential prerequisite to being able to keep *Īśvara* in one's thoughts at all times. But when the mind is withdrawn from mundane engagements and fixed on God in this way, "Kṛṣṇa . . . gives His own self to one who remembers Him" (X.80.11). Thus, where *śravaṇa* is the initiator of *bhakti*, and *kīrtana* the primary active purificatory practice, constant *smaraṇa* is the actual goal.

A comment about the psychological mechanisms of *smaraṇa*: *bhakti* meditation, as with any other type of activity performed by the mind, is a mental construct—that is to say, it consists of creative imaging made of *saṁskāras*. *Saṁskāras* are nothing other than impressions of previous sense experiences. Since the senses cannot perceive the divine forms of *Īśvara* (for example, see *Gītā* 11.8), the practitioner can only imagine a form made from the imprints of conventional experience. This, incidentally, is why we will find the *Bhāgavata* so frequently provides vivid and colorful personal descriptions of Kṛṣṇa's forms and ornaments, which become standardized by dint of constant repetition. Such repetition aids in the process of mental imaging during *smaraṇa*. The actual divine form is, of course, made of *Brahman* "stuff" (called *suddha sattva*) transcendent to the senses, but the *yogī* can still construe a form made out of *prakṛtic saṁskāras* (*cintāmaya*) that best corresponds to these descriptions. As with any form or deity, as we will see later in the practice of *arcana*, worship, *Īśvara* can manifest personal presence in that mentally constructed form (which is in fact a deity made of mind stuff) if the endeavor—the *smaraṇa*—is permeated with *bhakti*. Nonetheless, in terms of the psychological mechanics involved, if the text informs us Kṛṣṇa is blue like a monsoon cloud (which is closer to black than blue),[41] we can meditate on Kṛṣṇa's color only by utilizing a blue of our *prakṛtic* experience. Likewise with His flute, the ingredients in His *līlās*, or anything else—one can draw only from our repertoire of mundane experiences to attempt to conceive of these or to construct a visual narrative when engaging in *smaraṇa* type practices, until one attains an actual vision of God.

However, such practices are no different from that of *jñāna yoga*, where one has to keep the *saṁskāra* of one's ultimate *ātman* nature always in mind, until the *ātman* is perceived in its own right (*Yoga Sūtras* I.3). This too can only involve fixing the mind on the "idea" of an *ātman*. Even Patañjali's *citta-vṛtti-nirodhaḥ*, "stilling of all states of mind"—namely, the proposal to transcend mental imaging altogether—is (until experienced) a mental construct, idea, or ideation. Any thought occurring in the mind can be made only of *saṁskāras*, which are in turn made of *sattva guṇa*—one of the three base metaphysical components of *prakṛti*. The thoughts themselves are not *Brahman* stuff. Likewise with *Īśvara smaraṇa* in *bhakti*. We will discuss this further in "Hierarchies of Bliss" and also the notion of divine presence permeating some form made of a *prakṛtic* substance—be it a mental form, as in *smaraṇa*, or a form made of some other substance including metal or stone—in the process of *arcana*, deity worship, the fifth of the nine practices.

Also, readers familiar with the *Yoga Sūtras* may be reminded here of Patañjali's *Īśvara-praṇidhāna*, "dedication to *Īśvara*" (I.23–27). *Īśvara* is highly recommended in the *Yoga Sūtras* as the best object upon which to fix the mind after it has been withdrawn from everything else[42] (although the *bhakti* element in the *Yoga Sūtras* is what I sometimes refer to as *Bhakti* Lite in comparison with the *bhakti* XXX Extra-Strength of the *Bhāgavata*!). In fact, Jīva expands *smaraṇa* into a five-step sequence that closely mirrors the three highest limbs of the progressive eight-limb (*aṣṭāṅga*) schema in the *Yoga Sūtras*, except with bolstered devotional flavorings (*anu* 278). *Smaraṇa* itself, to think of *Īśvara* according to one's inclination, initiates Jīva's fivefold sequence. This is followed by the second step, *dhāraṇā* (Patañjali's sixth limb), withdrawal of the mind from external objects and focus of it on *Īśvara* in a general way; then the third step, *dhyāna* (Patañjali's seventh limb), contemplation on *Īśvara*'s name, form, qualities, and pastimes; the fourth step, *dhruvānusmṛti*, fixed remembrance of *Īśvara* flowing without interruption like a continuous flow of nectar (interjected between Patañjali's sixth and seventh limbs);[43] and eventually the fifth and final step, *samādhi* (Patañjali's eighth limb), when only the object of awareness is manifest, without any subjective or self-awareness. However, and very important, unlike the general understanding of *samādhi* as reflected in the *Yoga Sūtras*,[44] where the ultimate goal is for awareness to be immersed in its own nature (*svarūpa*, *Yoga Sūtras* I.3, the *ātman/Brahman* of Vedānta), the ultimate object of awareness in *bhakti samādhi*, as in all its preliminary stages, is exclusively *Īśvara*. In other words, in the state of *samādhi*, says Jīva, a person may have a direct vision of *Īśvara*. This is not a mental image made of *saṁskāras*, but a direct perception or experience of *Īśvara* as a personal distinct Being with full transcendent form and qualities made of pure *Brahman*[45] appearing present as an object of consciousness (internally and/or externally, as we will see in the Tale of Prince Dhruva) before the awareness of the meditating *bhakta*. The *bhāgavatas* claim that the bliss ensuing from such a vision far eclipses the bliss experienced when awareness becomes reimmersed in its own nature, which is the goal of generic yoga.

Thus, raising a theme we will later discuss at length, Vyāsa preferred to immerse his consciousness in Kṛṣṇa's pastimes than in the bliss of the *ātman*: "Although he was fixed in the bliss of the self and was devoid of any other thought, his heart was attracted to the enchanting *līlās* of the infallible Kṛṣṇa" (XII.12.68). When Nārada urges Vyāsa to "recall, by means of *samādhi*, the activities of Kṛṣṇa" (I.5.13)—in other words, to engage in *smaraṇa*—Vyāsa does so, and "in his mind, which, completely purified by the practice of *bhakti yoga*, was fully concentrated, he saw that perfect Person" (I.7.4).[46] This direct vision of God is the fifth and final stage of *smaraṇa* and, hence, of *bhakti yoga*, in Jīva's five-stage sequence.

Perhaps the most visually replete and startlingly extreme example of such visions in Kṛṣṇa literature is, again, exhibited by Caitanya Mahāprabhu (Prabhu, below). We should note that while some of the ecstatic bodily symptoms that he exhibits appear almost grotesque to conventional perception, they are physical manifestations of the highest states of internal ecstasy—as we noted previously, the material body is poorly equipped to handle unfamiliar dosages of ecstatic experience:

> The whole night long, Prabhu sang *kīrtana* loudly. Suddenly Prabhu heard the sound of Kṛṣṇa's flute, and absorbed in his *bhāva* [devotional meditation], he left that place. Though the doors were barred, absorbed in that *bhāva* Prabhu went outside. . . . Then Svarūpa Gosvāmī, taking the *bhaktas* with him, lit a lamp and searched for Prabhu. Searching here and there, they went eventually to the lion-gate, where they found Prabhu among the cows. His hands and feet were pulled into his stomach; he had the shape of a tortoise. There was froth on his lips, his whole body trembled, and there were tears in his eyes. Fallen unconscious, he was like a *kuṣmāṇḍa* fruit; externally he was stiff and rigid; inwardly he was overwhelmed with *ānanda* [bliss]. . . . Many tried hard, but he remained unconscious. The *bhaktas* raised Prabhu up and brought him home. Loudly in his ear they sang Kṛṣṇa *saṇkīrtana*, and after a long time Mahāprabhu regained consciousness. When he came back to consciousness, his hands and feet came out again, and his body was as it had been before. Getting up, Prabhu sat down and looked this way and that, and said to Svarūpa, "Where have you brought me? I heard the sound of the flute and went to Vṛndāvana, and I saw in the pasture Vrajendranandana [Kṛṣṇa] playing his flute. By the sound of the flute, he secretly brought Rādhā to the *kuñja*-bower, and Kṛṣṇa went to the *kuñja* to play there. I followed after him, and my ears were conquered by the sound of his ornaments. There he sported with the *gopīs*, laughing and joking, and hearing the sound of his voice, my ears were thrilled. Then you all came, making a great uproar, and took me away by force." (*Antya-līlā* 17.8–26)[47]

We will see that Kṛṣṇa's eternal divine *Brahman* realm called Goloka, where Caitanya's consciousness was transported in this account, both is coextensive with this realm of *prakṛti* and transcends it. It is *Brahman* (pure consciousness), but an expression of *Brahman* with divine forms and qualities (*saguṇa Brahman*). We will discuss this later in detail, but for now we will just note that such accessing of the *saguṇa Brahman* dimension and direct perception of God is the highest stage of *samādhi* in the Kṛṣṇa tradition. This is a very far cry from the contentless self-awareness of the *ātman* that is the goal of generic Patañjali-type *samādhi* and most *jñāna* traditions.

Pāda-sevana (Service to *Īśvara*'s Feet)

Pāda-sevana, the fourth practice, has various synonyms, Jīva points out, such as *sevā* and *paricaryā*, all of which denote service to *Īśvara*. He does not have much to say about what this fourth category of *bhakti yoga* comprises in terms of specifics, but we can recall from "Definition of *Bhakti*" that most of the definitions of *bhakti* scattered in various texts featured the ideal of service, which we noted is synonymous with love. While the word "service" sometimes carries a negative connotation associated with servitude, we can understand from our own human relationships that the more we deeply love another person, the more we try to please him or her with service.

Since in traditional Sanskrit theological exposition all practices must be supported by reference to the sacred texts, Jīva, as always, strives to illustrate the practice of *pāda-sevana* by quoting the *Bhāgavata*: "For one who is faithful and desires to hear, attraction to the stories of Vāsudeva (Kṛṣṇa) develops by means of service to the sages and assisting great saints, and dwelling in holy places" (I.2.16). The *Gītā* also uses the term *sevā* specifically in reference to service rendered to the accomplished practitioners in gratitude for receiving guidance and instruction: "Through humble submission, inquiry and service, the wise, those who have perceived the Truth, will instruct you in knowledge" (IV.34). Service to such *guru* figures who impart knowledge is all-important in almost all *bhakti* traditions, but service to the *bhaktas* in general is also greatly stressed, as will be discussed in a later section. Jīva adds to this various other activities that constitute service: seeing, touching, and circumambulating the Deity; following the Deity in temple processions; and visiting *Īśvara*'s temples, the *Gaṅgā* river, and holy places associated with *Īśvara*'s incarnations and deeds. These types of *pāda-sevana* activities are some of the most visible expressions of *bhakti* in India, as is the case with other devotional traditions of the world.

A much-loved example of service in the hagiography of Caitanya Mahāprabhu was demonstrated by King Pratāparudra of Orissa (East India) during the famous annual cart festival in the town of Purī. Here, Kṛṣṇa in the form of the massive Jagannātha Deity leaves His temple and is transported on gigantic chariots (from which derives the English-borrowing "juggernaut") to the Guṇḍicā temple, in reenactment of Kṛṣṇa's meeting with the *gopīs* in Kurukṣetra:[48]

> Pratāparudra himself, with his ministers, was among the followers of Mahāprabhu to see the *vijaya* [triumphal procession]. There were powerful personal attendants [of Jagannātha], strong as mad elephants, who with their hands brought Jagannātha out for the *vijaya*. . . . Who has the strength to cause . . . Jagannātha to move? By his own desire he went on his pleasure-trip [to the Guṇḍicā temple]. . . . Then Prataparudra performed his personal service: with a golden broom he swept the path. He moistened the path with water and sandal-wood; he performed these menial tasks [even though] he sat on the royal lion-throne. Though he is elevated, the king performs menial services, and thus is a receptacle for the grace of Jagannātha. Seeing these services, Mahāprabhu was delighted, and because of these services, [the king] gained the grace of Mahāprabhu. (*Madhya Līlā*, 13.3–17)

The descendants of the king still reenact this service of sweeping the road before the procession every year.

As with the previous three processes of *bhakti*, service is purifying: "The attraction to serve His lotus feet, growing day by day, immediately washes away from the ascetics the dirt accumulated over unlimited lifetimes, just like the *Gaṅgā* river does" (IV.21.31). And service, too, like all forms of *bhakti*, is fully satisfying, hence *bhaktas* "do not desire any favor other than the service of Kṛṣṇa's feet" (X.51.55).[49] We wish to repeat here that the notion of service, which may carry with it negative connotations in other contexts, is almost synonymous with love and devotion in the *Bhāgavata*. To love is to render acts of devotion that please the beloved. *Pāda-sevana* is essentially this. And true love must be reciprocal between lover and beloved. Consider, in this light, the following verses spoken by Viṣṇu, which we will encounter in the Tale of King Ambarīṣa:

> O *brāhmaṇa*! I am under the control of my *bhaktas*—it is as if I have no independence. My heart has been captured by the saints (*sādhus*) and *bhaktas*, and I, in turn, am dear to the *bhakta* community. Without My *bhaktas* and the *sādhus*, I do not desire even My own self, O *brāhmaṇa*, nor Śrī, the Goddess of Fortune, who is very intimate to Me. I am the supreme goal for My *bhaktas*. They have renounced spouse, home, sons, great wealth, and their very life and approached Me for shelter. How am I capable of rejecting them? The *sādhus*, who see all beings with equal vision, have their hearts bound to Me. They control Me with their devotion, just as a chaste wife controls a true husband. Satisfied by My service, they do not even desire the four types of liberation,[50] which are available through service, to say nothing of any other temporal thing. The *sādhus* are My heart, and I am the heart of the *sādhus*. They do not know anything other than Me, and I can barely think of anything other than them. (IX.4.63–68)

Arcana (Worship)

Arcana here refers specifically to deity worship, certainly the most visible aspect of *bhakti* and of Hinduism in general. Jīva spends some time on it:

> [Worship is] the faithful effort in installing, either alone or in coordination with others, My Deity (*arcā*); the work of [providing them with] gardens, groves, pleasure grounds, and the construction of temples and towns; rendering service to My temples sincerely like a servant by cleaning, plastering with cow-dung, and creating ornamental designs; and in being free from ego and pride, and not advertising one's acts. . . . Whatever is considered desirable in the world, and whatever is held most dear to the self, that should be offered to Me [manifest as the Deity]. By this, one attains the eternal. (XI.11.38–41)

The primary traditional Sanskrit textual sources that deal with the prescriptive details of deity worship extensively are genres called the *Āgamas* and *Pañcarātras*. The various procedures described in these texts begin with invoking (*āvāhana*) the presence of *Īśvara* into the Deity and thereafter caring for Him with love and devotion. Here, again, an important metaphysical consideration that needs to be established before considering the specifics of *arcana* is that the Deity—as with the *mantra*—is considered nondifferent from *Īśvara*'s own form. It is not a symbol, substitute, or some sort of mental prop: *Īśvara*'s actual presence is invoked in *āvāhana*. This is somewhat similar to the notion of "transubstantiation" in Catholicism, where the bread and wine are considered to be transformed into the body and blood of Christ actually, not figuratively. Similarly, *Īśvara* is considered to be personally present within the Deity, by permeating or "merging" (*līna*) into it. Jīva quotes the *Hayaśīrṣa Pañcarātra*, here: "Whatever may be Your transcendent nature, and whatever may be Your form made of pure consciousness (*jñāna-māyā*), may all that together, merged into this [Deity] body, awaken"[51] (*anu* 286). The Deity, he continues, is a special seat within which *Īśvara* manifests (*anu* 289).[52] We should thus avoid using terms such as "statue," with its implication of a lifeless representational object made of inert matter such as marble that copies or represents something beyond itself—or worse, "idol," with its Abrahamic implication of a false god.

The typical objection to all this raised by, for example, certain missionaries in colonial India was that the Supreme all-pervading Godhead cannot surely be reduced to a meager lifeless stone or material representation; God is unlimited and infinite. How can one presume to imagine that the all-pervading infinite transcendent Being has been confined within a limited, inert, base material substance?

> What is idolatry but a practical treason against Reason, the royal crown of our manhood, the setting up of the sensuous Imagination in its stead? If, then, any vision of God, as the Being who transcends all sense, be possible in any degree to man, it must be attained through the inner and not through the outer eye. . . . Thought, not sense, must eventually be recognized as the true organ of religion. . . . The Infinite

and the Eternal, however they are to be apprehended, cannot possibly be represented in finite form by even the most perfect efforts of human art. . . . If ever man could construct a material image of God, it would only be possible if He showed the pattern of Himself on the highest mount of inspiration, but the Hindoo idolmaker has had no such vision . . . and can only draw the forms of his imagery out of himself, and his images can only at the best represent his own subjective moods of feeling or aspiration, and not the known, transcendent, divine reality. (Hastie 1882, 15–17)

The Hindu response to this, predictably, is that it is Hastie's assumptions that limit God: it is precisely because God is unlimited that, in addition to manifesting in thought as Hastie would require, He can not only become manifest to the sensual eyes, should He so choose, but also become manifest in stone, and disallowing this possibility is itself curtailing the omnipotency of the Supreme Being. As Jīva puts it, although *Īśvara* is all-pervading, he particularizes Himself in the form of the *śālagrāma* stones,[53] and other such forms (*anu* 294). And, again, it is *Īśvara*'s very unlimitedness that allows Him to manifest in unlimited deities simultaneously, while still maintaining a full presence and personal form in His unlimited divine *Brahman* realms of Vaikuṇṭha and Goloka (or, more precisely, unlimited divine presences in unlimited divine realms, as we will discover). And at the same time, *Īśvara* is both omnipresent and omniconstitutional in all things of *prakṛti* (*Gītā* X.41). Of course, even the stone is a product of *prakṛti*, Kṛṣṇa's impersonal *śakti* ("power"), and in this sense also Kṛṣṇa, but the Deity is more than this. This is not some Hindu variant of pantheism. While the stone substance of the Deity is made of Kṛṣṇa's *śakti*, Kṛṣṇa as *Śaktimān* ("possessor of *śakti*")—the distinct personal Godhead who is the source of all powers, as will be discussed in "The Object of *Bhakti*"—enters into and transforms the metaphysics of the stone, converting it into a vehicle of divine presence. Yet *Īśvara* is not confined by this act of grace, simultaneously remaining a distinct independent Being.

We might add here one other consideration raised by a Hindu more or less contemporary with Hastie against the latter's assumption that "thought, not sense, must eventually be recognized as the true organ of religion." Bhaktivinoda Thakur's argument here is subtle:

> The Supreme Lord does not have a material form, but is endowed with a transcendent spiritual form called *sat-cit-ānanda-vigraha*.[54] The fullest manifestation of this transcendent form cannot be perceived by the conditioned *jīvas* [*ātmans*]. For this reason, in whatever fashion man conceives of God in this world, his conception must assume a degree of idolatry . . . Śri Kṛṣṇa can be perceived in the heart, to some extent, through the help of divine love. When this form is perceived in the mind . . . it assumes a greater degree of phenomenality, while being served through the body and senses in physical form, *Śrī Mūrti* [the Deity] assumes the greatest level of phenomenality (quoted in Das, 192).

To understand the full import of this statement, we must bear in mind that throughout much of Indic thought, the mind is considered to be a nonconscious material element extraneous to the real self. In the Sāṅkhya metaphysics of the *Bhāgavata* (which, with some sect-specific taxonomic variants here and there, became the dominant metaphysical and physical descriptive model of reality of the Vedānta and Purāṇa traditions), mind and intelligence are material substances that do not differ in ultimate essence from the other material substances—the gross elements of earth, water, fire, air, and ether—except that they are more subtle in nature (which simply means they contain more of the *sattva guṇa* and less of the *tamas*, discussed in the next section). They are all *prakṛti*, matter, and external coverings of the *ātman*.

So Bhaktivinoda's argument, then, is that *any* statement or notion emanating from human thought pertaining to God—such as that God is "love," or "good," or "all-powerful," or "almighty," or "just," or "beyond human comprehension," or anything whatsoever including "God is," all and any such declarations—is idolatry, if one is to adopt the logic of those theistic traditions critical of Hindu deity worship. This is because all such attributes are constructions formed by the mind or intellect, and the mind and intellect are *prakṛtic* matter in *Bhāgavata* metaphysics; they merely contain more of the *sattva guṇa* than the *tamas guṇa*.[55] Indeed, conceiving of God *in any way whatsoever* means, by definition, constructing a conceptual (that is, a mental or intellectual) material image of Him, but this is still subtle matter distinct from the Deity. Thus, for Bhaktivinoda, whether the image is made of the material elements of stone or whether it is a conceptual image made of thought, "there is no difference between the two because even mind and thought are material" (Das, 193). Therefore, taking this to its logical conclusion, *there is no other way to conceive of, or discuss, God except through image worship*: "Image worship is therefore the foundation of human religion" (ibid.). Hindus construct a variety of images of stone and other denser material substances in addition to constructing the variety of intellectual images of God evidenced in the elaborate theologies of the subcontinent; other theistic traditions have restricted themselves to worshipping intellectual images: both are worshipping images.

In any event, returning to the logic of *arcana* from the point of view of its adherents, just as our own *ātman* permeates our physical body made of the material elements and animates it with consciousness, so *Īśvara* the Supreme *Ātman* permeates the physical form of the Deity, which is also made of the elements, and animates it with divine presence. The difference, of course, is we are forced into a body not by any immediate choice of our own, but according to our *karma*,[56] whereas *Īśvara* enters the Deity as an act of grace bound only by *bhakti*. This act of grace is so that the *bhakta*, enveloped in matter and thus unable to perceive his or her own *ātman*, to say nothing of perceiving the Supreme *Ātman*, can worship *Īśvara* directly in a very immediate personal manner when *Īśvara* manifests in a material form. It is to facilitate *arcana*, worship, that *Īśvara* does so, and indeed, in the twelfth-century South Indian Vaiṣṇava tradition stemming from the theologican Rāmānuja, *Iśvara* in the Deity (*arcā-vigraha*) is one of the five types of *avatāra* (divine descent). In his *Laghu-Bhāgavatāmṛta*, Rūpa defines *avatāra* as a form of the Lord "manifesting in the universe to accomplish a new purpose either personally or through some other agency" (II.1.2).[57] And as is the case with *mantra*—which is a sonic *avatāra* (*nāma-avatāra*), and indeed all forms of *bhakti yoga*—*Īśvara* reveals His presence in the Deity in proportion to the sincerity of the *bhakti* rendered. And the same, of course, holds true for the Goddess *Īśvarī* forms.

In fact, it is very common in India, almost ubiquitous, in fact, to find stories associated with local temples, where the Deity interacts with His or Her devotees in various active and very personable ways. One of the best-known stories in Jīva's tradition, for example, is that of Sākṣī-Gopāla (Kṛṣṇa the "Witness"). The context of the story is of a promise that was made before the Gopāla (Kṛṣṇa) Deity in Vṛndāvana between two *brāhmaṇas* from the south of India, while on pilgrimage in the north. Upon their return home down south, this promise was unwillingly broken because of family pressure by the elder *brāhmaṇa*. The younger *brāhmaṇa* therefore returns north to request that the Deity come back south to his village in order to bear witness to the promise made such that the elder *brāhmaṇa* would not incur the sin of breaking a promise. Note the very personal and almost banterlike tone between the devotee and Deity in the following passage—the *brāhmaṇa* even admonishing the Deity not to commit a sin! This is typical of the relationship between devotee and Deity and so reflective of the intimate "real life" relationship with *Īśvara* that lies at the heart of *bhakti yoga*:

> Then the younger *brāhmaṇa* went to Vṛndāvana and bowing to the ground he related the whole tale [to the Deity of Kṛṣṇa] . . . "that the promise of a *brāhmaṇa* be broken—this is very bad. Knowing these things, bear witness . . . he who knows and does not bear witness commits a sin." . . . Kṛṣṇa said: "No one has heard of an image moving." The *brāhmaṇa* said, "[In that case], as an image, how do you speak words? You are not an image, you are the manifest Vrajendranāndana[58] [Kṛṣṇa]. Will you do this thing, which is not done, for the *brāhmaṇa*?" Laughing, Gopāla [Kṛṣṇa] said, "Listen, O *brāhmaṇa*, I shall follow after you. Do not turn around to look at me; if you look at me I shall remain in the place [where you looked]. You will only hear the sound of my ankle bells, and from that sound you will know that I am moving." The next day, having begged leave, the *brāhmaṇa* departed, and Gopāla followed after him. . . . Moving in this way, the *brāhmaṇa* came to his own country, and nearing

> his village, he reflected in his mind . . . "I shall go and say to the people that the witness has come." . . . Reflecting thus, the *brāhmaṇa* turned around and looked; and smiling Gopāla . . . was there . . . when they heard of it, all the people were astonished. They all came to see the witness, and when they saw Gopāla, they bowed to the ground. . . . And the king of that country came, hearing of the wonderful thing, and he gained the highest pleasure when he saw Gopāla. The king built a temple there, and caused the service to be instituted. It was called Sākṣīgopāla [Gopāla the witness], and it became famous. (*Madhya Līlā* V.86–117)

Countless temples on the subcontinent, both majestic and pan-Indian, as well as humble and local, have such narratives associated with them.

Deity worship lies at the very core of all forms of *bhakti* practices of real-life Hinduism, in terms both of the private practices of dedicated individuals and, more visibly, of practices in temple settings. Its description thus merits quoting at length:

> One who wishes to speedily cut away the knot in the heart [desire] of the transcendent *ātman* should worship Lord Keśava (Kṛṣṇa) according to the prescriptions expressed in the Tantra texts.[59] Upon receiving the permission of the *ācārya* (*guru*), and after having received instruction from him, one should worship the Supreme Being in a Deity form that reflects one's personal preference. In a clean state, seated facing [the Deity], after purifying this lump of a body by *prāṇāyāma* (breath control) and other practices, as well as protecting it by invoking various names of *Īśvara* into different body parts (*nyāsa*), one should worship Hari. One should prepare the paraphernalia, surface, oneself, and the Deity; consecrate the seat; perform *nyāsa* to one's heart and other parts of the body;[60] and prepare the ingredients for worship such as water for washing the feet, etc. Then, with concentration, one should invoke the presence of the Divinity either in the Deity or in the heart, and perform worship with the *mūla-mantra*.[61] One should worship the various limbs of

> the Deity, as well as His associates,[62] with: the *mantra* corresponding to that Deity's specific form;[63] foot washing water, welcome beverage, and mouthwash, etc.; then bathing, clothing, and ornaments; then scents, flowers, unbroken grains, and garlands, as well as incense and ghee lamps. Having completed the *pūjā* (ritual worship) according to the prescriptions, one should offer obeisance to Hari. Meditating on oneself as made of Him,[64] one should worship the Deity form (*mūrti*). One should place the remnants on one's head, and respectfully replace the Deity back in its place.[65] In this way, one who worships *Īśvara*, the soul of everything, in fire, the sun, water, and other such natural phenomenon, and in the guest, or in one's own heart, is quickly liberated. (XI.3.47–55)

This may all sound rather complex and ritualistic, but the whole idea is to develop *prema*, divine love (XI.27.32). Ultimately, it is not rituals and offerings that count (since *Īśvara* owns everything anyway), but *bhakti*. As Kṛṣṇa states in the *Gītā* (twice repeating the word *bhakti* in the same verse for emphasis): "If one offers Me a flower, leaf, fruit, or water with *bhakti*, I accept that offering of *bhakti* from one sincerely devoted to Me" (IX.26). Or, in the words of the *Bhāgavata*: "Even just water offered to Me faithfully with *bhakti* is dear to Me . . . but even great abundance offered by one who is not a *bhakta* does not cause satisfaction" (XI.27.18–19). It is the internal meditation of love that is the goal, not the external forms of *pūjā*.[66]

In fact, despite the ritualistically elaborate, caste- and gender-exclusivistic, "high" forms *arcana* can take in elite Hindu orthopraxy, its expressions are, in fact, highly flexible, allowing anyone, anywhere, to engage in some form of this practice in modest, intimate modes. So, for example, the Deity can be made from any among eight substances most readily available, with a mental option ensuring that there is no one who cannot partake of this process even if deprived of all material facilities: "There are eight kinds of deities (*pratimā*); they may be made of: stone, wood, metal, sandalwood or mud, paint [a picture], sand, mind, or precious gem." If one has material facilities, then one should offer one's beloved the very best one can afford, but if one is utterly impoverished, a mere offering of heartfelt *bhakti* is perfection: "My worship in the Deity should be performed with the choicest articles, but it can be performed by my sincere *bhakta* with whatever is available, or even just in the mind" (XI.27.15).[67] The important thing is to engage worship as a practice to assist in the cultivation of *bhakti*, not for ostentatious display.

Arcana is especially recommended for householders, says Jīva: "This path, by which the Supreme Person is worshipped faithfully with one's wealth obtained by pure means, brings good fortune to the householders" (X.84.37). This is so because householders are usually more challenged in keeping the mind always fixed on *Īśvara* than those who have renounced all worldly possessions, for obvious reasons. And channeling their wealth into deity worship helps them curb the tendency to become miserly, says Jīva. Moreover, if undertaken according to the prescriptions, deity worship assists them in cultivating the mental *yogic* discipline of strict regulation (*anu* 283).

As with *bhakti* in general, worship can either be performed purely, with no motive other than to cultivate devotion for *Īśvara*, or be mixed with *karma*, desire for some personal material gain. We will discuss this type of "mixed *bhakti*" later, but Jīva notes at this point that those whose worship of the Deity is mixed tend to be people who are merely blindly following social norms picked up from here or there, or following family traditions and so forth (*anu* 284). However, the ideal, as Kṛṣṇa Himself states, is to become free of personal desire and seek only *Īśvara*: "It is through the practice of *bhakti yoga* without motive, that one attains Me" (XI.27.53). Either way, whatever be the motive: "Worshipping Me in the above ways through the path of *kriyā yoga* by means of either Vedic or Tantric[68] rites, a person attains from Me the desired success, both in this life and the next" (XI.27.49).

There are many other practices subsumed under the category of *arcana*, says Jīva, such as celebrating festive days like Kṛṣṇa's birthday, observing vows during the months of *Kārtika*,[69] fasting from grains on the bimonthly *ekādaśī* days,[70] wearing *tilak* sacred clay,[71] and others (*anu* 298–99). We can briefly mention residence in sacred places or the very commonly undertaken activity of pilgrimage to them. We have discussed how *Īśvara* can manifest in sound and in the Deity, so, similarly, in many Hindu *bhakti* traditions, places associated with *Īśvara* represent yet another type of divine manifestation: "Lord Hari is eternally present in Mathurā [where He took birth]" (X.1.28); "Even today, out of affection, Lord Hari appears to His devotees who reside in that holy place, in whatever form that they desire" (V.7.2). Indeed, so beneficial is living in holy places to the development of *bhakti* that Rūpa, who personally resided in Kṛṣṇa's childhood abode of Vṛndāvana (Vraj), along with Jīva and the other *Gosvāmīs*, wrote the following in his *Upadeśāmṛta*: "Living in Vraj, and following those who are attached to Kṛṣṇa, one should spend all one's time gradually engaging one's mind and tongue in remembering and chanting the name, form, and deeds of Kṛṣṇa. This is the essence of spiritual instruction" (8).

One further element that Jīva discusses under the rubric of *arcana*, which is very much stressed in this tradition, is not offending the *bhaktas*: "Hari . . . does not accept worship from those who commit offense to the righteous [devotees] who want nothing [but Him]. The intelligence of such people is perverted due to intoxication from learning, wealth, family, or accomplishments" (IV.31.21). Such offenses "destroy everything," says Jīva (*anu* 301). The Tale of King Ambarīṣa in part 2 will illustrate this point. The *bhakta* is as dear to *Īśvara*—and *Īśvarī*—as they are to the *bhakta*. Of course, Kṛṣṇa favors no one, as He states in the *Gītā*, but this indicates that no one is excluded from the opportunity of becoming a *bhakta*. If one avails oneself of this opportunity by choosing to turn to Him in a devotional manner, one is favored, hence the frequent statements that *bhaktas* are especially dear to Kṛṣṇa (*Gītā* IX.29–32).

But, in fact, while the *bhaktas* are as dear to *Īśvara* as He is to them, all living entities are nothing other than manifestations of *Īśvara*. Hence, Jīva adds to all this that the highest form of *arcana* is the worship of all living entities.[72] He points out that worshipping the Deity while offending other living entities is useless:

> Therefore, some perform worship to Hari (Kṛṣṇa) faithfully and reverentially in the form of the Deity, but, despite being performed, worship does not provide any benefit for one who hates his fellow beings. The bodies of men, animals, sages, and celestials have been created by Hari, and it is He who then

dwells in these bodies (*pureṣu*) in the form of the *jīva*; hence He is called *puruṣa*. (VII.14.37–40)[73]

The idea here is that the *ātman* within all beings is a part of *Īśvara*, as is the body within which the *ātman* is embodied. To recognize *Īśvara* in the Deity but not in all beings because of ignorance is offensive to *Īśvara*. Kṛṣṇa ends the *Uddhava Gītā* in book 11 on a similar note, stressing that seeing all beings as nothing other than *Īśvara* is in fact the highest form of worship:

> One should perceive Me as manifest in all beings and in oneself. . . . A *paṇḍita* is considered to be one who sees everything equally, whether it be a *brāhmaṇa*,[74] a member of the *Pukkaśa* tribe, a thief, one devoted to *brāhmaṇas*, the sun, a spark of fire, the gentle or the cruel. Rivalry, envy, abuse, and ego quickly disappear from a person who constantly reflects upon the essence of all people as being Me. . . . Until [the ability] to see Me as the essence of all living beings develops, one should worship Me with the activities of the body, mind, and speech. . . . I definitely consider this [attitude]—that the essence of all living entities is in Me—to be the most efficacious of all practices involving the activities of one's body, speech, and mind." (XI.29.12–19)

Vandana (Offering Respect)

Jīva has little to say about this limb, noting that *vandana* overlaps with the previous practice of worship. *Vandana* is the attitudinal and functional equivalent of genuflection in Catholicism and usually refers to bowing or offering prostrations to *Īśvara* (as manifest, for instance, in the Deity, sacred text, or holy place) or to the *guru* or the *bhaktas*. He comments that there are some *bhaktas* who simply feel unworthy of directly serving the Deity, and these prefer to meditate on Him and engage in the practices of *vandana*.[75] The humble *bhakta* perceives *Īśvara*'s compassion in all situations and thus becomes blissful, says Jīva.

As an aside, one can still find ascetics today who circumambulate the holy town of Vṛndāvana, where Kṛṣṇa spent His childhood, by performing *vandana* along the entire circumference. The distance is approximately ten kilometers, and there are those who perform obeisance to this form of Kṛṣṇa manifest as sacred space by means of a full *daṇḍavat*: an elongated prostration on the ground with arms extended. They place a stone where their fingers reach and then begin the next prostration from that spot, this time placing the stone at the new spot reached by the fingers at the next *daṇḍavat* (approximately six or seven feet farther). They thus circumambulate the entire circumference of the holy place, performing an ongoing sequence of fully prostrated *vandanas* in this way, and may spend weeks before finishing (one can see extreme versions of this where a person performs a *vandana* of 108[76] *daṇḍavats* in one spot before moving to the next). While this is a form of *tapas* (austerity) and may also, perhaps more often than not, reflect the "mixed" *bhakti* of which Jīva will speak later (that is, performed in the hope of some boon), it nonetheless is still a form of *vandana* to *Īśvara* present as holy place.

Dāsya (Servitorship)

Here too Jīva has little to say, as this practice overlaps with the others—in fact, we may have noticed by now that these nine practices of *bhakti* have porous boundaries between them. He defines *dāsya* as considering oneself to be a servant of Viṣṇu. As an example of the attitude of servitorship, Jīva selects Uddhava's statement: "We are your servants, and, since we partake of your remnants—the garlands, ointments, clothes, decorations, and food enjoyed by you—we will surpass *māyā*" (XI.7.46). The remnants of the Deity, such as the garlands and other items mentioned here, are highly valued tokens of divine grace in *bhakti* practice. Typically, any person visiting a temple and having *darśana* (seeing the Deity) will receive some consumable item from the officiating *brāhmaṇa* (priest), if only a few drops of sacred water. For more fortunate visitors, a garland or more lavish array of foodstuffs that had been previously offered to the Deity might be forthcoming, or some other item such as mentioned in the verse. In sum, *dāsya* is an attitude of service and, as practice, perhaps best understood as the mental vigilance invested in cultivating this attitude. Where the fourth practice of *bhakti*, *pāda-sevana*, refers to actual physical acts of service, *dāsya*—and the next practice, friendship—refers more to states of mind. Perhaps we can consider these two to be internal practices that are expressed externally through the other practices. We will again touch upon *dāsya* in the discussion on *bhāva* (loving mood) below and will find illustrations of it in the stories from the tenth book in part 3.

Sakhya (Friendship)

As with *dāsya*, servitorship, the practice of *sakhya*, friendship, involves a state of mind (*bhāva*), which in general terms, says Jīva, entails wishing someone's well-being. In *bhakti* it is reciprocal, as Hari is the well-wisher of all by supplying material facilities for the needs of the internal and external senses, as well as by bestowing pure love for God. It is thus not very difficult to perform, continues Jīva, because *Īśvara*'s feelings of well-being for His *bhaktas* are eternal (*anu* 306). We will discuss the theology of *bhāva*, which will include the *bhāvas* of both *sakhya* and *dāsya*, in more detail under *rāgānugā bhakti* below, drawing from Rūpa's *Bhakti-rasāmṛtasindhu*. We will also encounter the delightful exemplars of *sakhya* in some of the stories we have included in this volume from the tenth book. At this point, Jīva simply draws our attention to a couple of quotes mentioning *sakhya*, as per his method in exemplifying all the elements of *bhakti* he selects for analysis with verses from the *Bhāgavata*: "See the good fortune, O just see the good fortune of Nanda the cowherder and the residents of Vraj! Their friend is the supreme bliss, the eternal absolute *Brahman*!" (X.14.32); "The friends of the infallible Kṛṣṇa, who are peaceful, equanimous, pure, and affectionate to all beings, easily attain Kṛṣṇa's abode" (IV.12.37).

Ātma-nivedana (Self-Surrender)

The last on the list of nine practices, self-surrender, says Jīva, entails "offering everything to the Lord, from one's body to one's pure *ātman*" (*anu* 309). This means the cessation of any self-striving, and dedicating all one's activities to, and focusing one's efforts on *Īśvara*. It can be compared with the selling of a cow, he continues: once sold and given away, the seller invests no more effort in its maintenance, as this has become the responsibility of the purchaser (*anu* 309). Likewise, the devotee considers himself or herself the property of *Īśvara* and has full faith and dependence on *Īśvara* for all material necessities. In such a state of surrender to *Īśvara*, says Jīva, bodily functions, dressing, and so on are undertaken simply for service, not for any personal interest or motive (see *Gītā* V.9–10 for an expression of this state).

Rukmiṇī, one of Kṛṣṇa's queens, is selected by Jīva as exemplifying the mood of this ninth practice of *bhakti*: "I have clearly chosen You as a husband, dear Kṛṣṇa, and I have hereby surrendered myself to You as wife" (X.52.39). But perhaps the more classic passage viewed as most representative of the extensiveness of *ātma-nivedana*, this state of total self-surrender, is one we will find in the Tale of King Ambarīṣa:

> He engaged his mind in [meditating on] the lotus feet of Kṛṣṇa; his words in describing the qualities of Vaikuṇṭha, Viṣṇu's divine *Brahman* adode; his hands in cleaning the temple of Hari and other such acts; and his ears in hearing the beautiful accounts of Acyuta [Kṛṣṇa]. He engaged his eyes in seeing the temples and deities of Mukunda [Kṛṣṇa], the limbs of his body in touching the bodies of the servants of God, his sense of smell in the fragrance of the beautiful *tulāsi* plant [offered to] the Lord's lotus feet, and his sense of taste in [the food] offered to God. He used his feet in frequenting the places touched by the feet of Hari, his head in offering obeisance to the feet of Hṛṣīkeśa [Kṛṣṇa], and his desire in service rather than in the fulfillment of sensual desires. He did this to develop affection for those who have taken shelter of Viṣṇu, whose glories are supreme. (IX.4.18–20)

After outlining similar examples of those who have attained *bhakti* for Him through this ninth practice of *ātma-nivedana*, Kṛṣṇa Himself concludes: "What other goal is there left for such a person to attain?!" (XI.19.24).

We remind the reader that Jīva has divided *bhakti yoga* into *vaidhī*, rule regulated—the nine processes in this preceding section—and *rāgānugā*, spontaneous, which will occupy us later. There is, of course, much more that can be said about *vaidhī bhakti*. Just as there were variant taxonomies of *yoga* practices in addition to the eight limbs promoted in the *Yoga Sūtras* (there are references in other texts to five limbs as well as six limbs of *yoga* even as the eight limbs became the "classical" model in later times),[77] so there were various taxonomies of *bhakti* practices in addition to the nine formally presented in texts such as the *Bhāgavata*, which were to become standardized and normalized. Jīva acknowledges that he has not covered everything connected with *vaidhī*, and, in fact, his uncle Rūpa lists sixty-four *bhakti* practices in his *Bhaktirasāmṛtasindhu*. Indeed, Rūpa deemed even this much more expansive list incomplete, referring his readership to the *Hari-Bhakti-Vilāsa*[78] for even more extensive coverage of other ingredients of *bhakti*.

Worthy of mention from these sixty-four (in addition to the first three pertaining to the *guru*, which will be discussed later) are the last five, since Rūpa specifies them as all-important (some, but not all, of which correspond to the practices in the classical list of nine):

> Love for service to the lotus feet of the Deity; . . . relishing the meanings of the *Bhāgavata*; . . . association with *bhaktas* who have the same inclination as oneself; . . . singing the holy names; . . . and residing in the environment of [Kṛṣṇa's birthplace] Mathura . . . these five are so difficult to comprehend and possess incredible power, that faith in them is hard to find; but even a little connection with them produces love, *bhāva*, in the pure mind. (*Bhaktirasāmṛtasindhu* Eastern Quadrant II.225–38)

Indeed, only passing comments have been made by Jīva about residing in a holy place, for example, or about pilgrimage. In this regard, in his *Upadeśāmṛta*, Rūpa states: "Here is the essence of all instruction (*upadeśa*): one should pass all one's time in this manner: residing in Vraj following those who are devoted to Hari,[79] while increasingly engaging one's mind and tongue in remembering and reciting the name, forms, and activities of Kṛṣṇa" (8). Both the *Gosvāmīs* and Caitanya spent the rest of their days in holy places, the former in Vṛndāvana, the latter in Jagannāth Pūri.

This might be the place to quote Rūpa's list of the primary qualities favorable to devotion: "*Bhakti* is made successful by these six things: enthusiasm, confidence, patience, engaging in various activities, rejection of mundane association, and following the saints" (3). Additionally, while *vaidhī*, of course, nurtures *bhakti*, it seems relevant to note Rūpa's identification in the *Upadeśāmṛta* of six activities that endanger it: "*Bhakti* is destroyed by these six things: excessive eating, over-endeavoring, idle chatter, not following *niyama* regulations,[80] association with worldly people, and avariciousness" (2).

By way of a conclusion to all this, the main point is that

> although among these practices more importance is given to one over others in one place, while a different practice is emphasized somewhere else, there is no contradiction, as these reflect different dispositions and jurisdictions. They are to be understood in the same way as the prescription of medicine [different remedies being pertinent to different ailments]. (*anu* 310)

Indeed, any one single practice, performed with pure devotion and unmixed intention, can bestow the goal of *bhakti*: Kṛṣṇa *prema*, love of God. The purpose of all or any one of these practices is this and nothing else.

Bhakti Mixed with Attachment to *Dharma* and *Jñāna*

As a contrast to the higher stages of *bhakti* discussed next in *rāgānugā*, and to better highlight it, Jīva spends some time offering observations about Kṛṣṇa *bhakti* that are mixed with motivations other than just pure devotion. He makes a distinction between devotionality free of any self-interest that is performed without any ulterior motive other than to attain pure devotion (*akaitavā bhakti*)—in other words solely to please *Kṛṣṇa*—and *bhakti* that is performed in order to gain some other type of personal benefit (*sakaitavā bhakti*, *anu* 217).[81] Needless to say: "Hari is pleased by pure *bhakti*. Anything else is just show" (VII.7.52). The *Bhāgavata* sees even *karma yoga* and *jñāna yoga* practices as compromised—while not denying their ability to bestow the respective fruits claimed by them, the realization of the *ātman*—since they are motivated by personal desire, albeit in the form of liberation.[82] Nonetheless, since almost all *bhakti* in any theistic tradition of the world is performed with some sort of personal self-interest at heart, it is important to understand the mindset associated with *sakaitavā bhakti*, motivated devotion, so as to better contrast it with pure devotion, the *rāgānugā bhakti* of the next section, which is the ultimate goal of Kṛṣṇa *bhakti*.

With a view to getting a better sense of the relationship between action in the world and the specific types of desires or self-interests underpinning the performance of motivated *bhakti*, we will first discuss the relationship between *bhakti* and *dharma*, then that between *bhakti* and *karma*. We remind the reader of our commitment, outlined in the "Introduction to the Volume," that our interest in this work is with the theology of *bhakti* and thus with *dharma* as related to the transcendental goal of that theology (Kṛṣṇa *prema*). Therefore, the attitude of the *Bhāgavata* to nondevotional *dharma* in the material world, a very important topic in its own right, lies beyond the scope of our focus. In this, we follow the *Gosvāmīs*, who show very little interest in their voluminous writings to issues pertaining to mundane *dharma*. So we will simply mention in passing that where it does touch on such things (for instance, in the eleventh canto), the *Bhāgavata* is an orthodox, socially conservative text upholding the conventions of the *varṇāśrama* (caste and stage-of-life) social order and gender dynamics in accordance with the standard *dharma śāstras* of its time (such as those of Manu).[83]

Bhakti and *Dharma*

The term *dharma* in social contexts refers to duty—the everyday obligations incumbent on any form of familial and civic life.[84] There are, surely, duties inherited simply by dint of living in this world: in fact, people have multiple *dharmas*—professional, family related, gendered, cultural, stage of life, and so forth—so the term is context-specific. In the idealized Vedic social system, there are four *varṇas*, professional occupations: *brāhmaṇa*, priestly/intellectual and religious specialist; *kṣatrīya*, warrior/administrator; *vaiśya*, merchant/landowner; and *śūdra*, employee of the other *varṇas*. There are also four *aśramas*, progressive stages of life: *brahmacārya*, celibate student; *gṛhaṣṭha*, householder; *vanaprastha*, married renunciant retiree; and *saṅnyāsa*, solitary renunciant. In terms of profession, ideally—as is explicit in the *Bhāgavata* and (arguably) implicit in the *Gītā*—occupational *dharma* reflects not the accident of birth, but the natural disposition of a person's psychophysical nature that lends itself most effectively to a particular type of activity—teaching, statesmanship, business, craftsmanship, and so forth.[85] Since any expression of *dharma* reflects nothing other than this temporal *guṇa/karma* configuration of a particular body/mind mechanism in any one embodiment, a person's *dharma* completely changes from one birth to another.[86] *Dharmas* are thus temporal, as they pertain only to one particular birth; they are not ultimate or connected to the *ātman* per se.

In accordance with the *Gītā* (II.41–46), the *Bhāgavata* opposes the mind-set typically underpinning conventional *dharma* (although not necessarily the performance of the *dharma* itself)—namely, it criticizes the performance of *dharma* to fulfill selfish and personal desires, such as those aimed at satisfying the body and mind. In fact, conventional *dharma* undertaken in the pursuit of material happiness is not the goal of human life for *yoga* in general, as it has nothing to do with the *ātman*, unless performed as *karma yoga* as in the *Gītā*,[87] where it entails the selfless performance of *dharma*, with no attachment to the results of the actions, or, in *bhakti yoga*, as an offering to *Iśvara*.[88] Indeed, like the *Gītā*, while the *Bhāgavata* certainly promotes the performance of mundane *dharma* in conventional contexts,[89] it is clear that this should be coupled with the pursuit of Truth for it to be meaningful from an ultimate point of view. In fact, a good number (but by no means all) of its exemplars represented in this volume completely renounce *dharma* at some point or, at least, again in accordance with the *Gītā*,[90] are prepared to renounce it for their beloved Lord. This is exemplified most dramatically in the story of the simple cowherding *gopī* women, as we will see, who are heralded as the greatest *yogīs* of all.

Irrespective of whether one remains active in the world or chooses to renounce it, the ultimate *dharma* in the *Bhāgavata* is *bhakti* for *Īśvara*, which is eternal (that is, continues in the liberated state); everything else is no better than toil and tribulation:

> The highest *dharma* is that through which *bhakti* for Kṛṣṇa [is born]. It is through this—performed without motive and uninterrupted—that the mind becomes completely satisfied. . . . If *dharma*, howsoever perfectly performed, does

> not produce attraction for the stories of Kṛṣṇa, then it is simply brute labor. (I.2.6–8)

Here and elsewhere, the *Bhāgavata* completely reconfigures the meaning of the term *dharma*: "Whatever activity is dedicated to Me, the Supreme, without self-interest, even if it be useless and performed out of fear or other such things, is *dharma*" (XI.21.29); and again: "It is this alone which has been handed down as the ultimate *dharma* for humankind in this world: *bhakti yoga* for *Bhagavān* by taking His name and other such devotional activities" (VI.3.22). The ultimate *dharma*, then, is to connect with *Īśvara* in devotion.

We need to touch briefly on Vedic ritualism. The regularized performance of sacrifice, *yajña*, was also considered a *dharma* in ancient Vedic orthopraxy, as it was considered essential for upholding the natural order of things. Vedic *yajña* was the mainstream form of religion on the sociocultural landscape at the time of the *Bhāgavata* (as also the *Gītā*), and, as we will suggest, it provided the same function as most forms of religiosity today. Vedic *yajña* was also a kind of *bhakti* to celestial beings, *devas*. But it was, in essence, ritualized business—rites performed with extraordinary meticulousness and attention to protocol, but always in the expectation of soliciting boons.[91] Items were offered into the sacred fire, *yajña*, to be transported to the *devas*, the demigods, whom we have been referring to as celestials (so as not to confuse them with the manifestations of *Īśvara*),[92] in return for material well-being—typically, for the Vedic Āryans, cows, offspring, and victory in battle. It is this mercantile mentality associated with the ritualized Vedic devotionalism of the day that is targeted by the *Bhāgavata*, as by the entire Yoga tradition in general,[93] as an inferior form of religiosity.

To understand the *Bhāgavata*'s critique of the lusty mind-set underpinning this ritualistic *dharma* from the perspective of our modern religious attitudes, we can equate Vedic ritualism with materialistic religiosity in general in terms of the desires and expectations that motivate it. By materialistic religiosity, I intend the performance of any religious activity that, rather than seeking ultimate transcendent Truth (whether knowledge of the self or devotion to God), is performed for obtaining temporary benefits for the material body and mind by soliciting higher powers. Thus whether these rituals involve lighting candles, offering prayers, ringing bells, performing prostrations or circumambulations, and other such forms of worship—or, in the Vedic case, offering oblations into the sacred fire—and whether that higher power is conceived of in the form of the celestial recipients of Vedic ritualism (*devas*), or in some notion of God, or angels, saints, *Boddhisattvas*, spirits, or any superhuman entity, the mind-set motivating those activities is essentially the same: the soliciting of some boon. Keeping this in mind, the following quote has perennial relevance:

> The goal of the *dharma* which leads to liberation is not compatible with [that *dharma* performed for] the goal of material gain:[94] the goal of the *dharma* which is devoted to the One Supreme Being is not taught in the sacred texts as the desire for material attainment. In fact, the purpose of desire is not to fulfill the gratification of the senses, but to fulfill as much as is necessary to sustain life. And the purpose of life in this world is inquiry into Truth, not to engage in actions dedicated to *karma*, material gain. . . . Thus, . . . the ultimate perfection of *dharma*, performed diligently by people according to the divisions of the *varṇas* and *āśramas* (professions and life stages), is the satisfaction of Hari [Kṛṣṇa]. Therefore, *Bhagavān*, the Lord of the *Sātvatas* [Kṛṣṇa], should constantly be heard about, glorified, meditated upon, and worshipped with a concentrated mind. (I.2.9–14)

Thus, as is typical of the *bhakti* traditions in general, while the *Bhāgavata* certainly does not undermine *dharma* related to the *varṇāśrama* caste system in terms of its social stratifications and work-related expectations in the real world of *prakṛti*,[95] it subverts it in the context of *bhakti*. Indeed: "A dog-eater whose life resources, endeavors, words, and thoughts are devoted to *Bhagavān* is better than a *brāhmaṇa* endowed with the twelve characteristics of the *brāhmaṇa* caste,[96] who is averse to the lotus feet of Hari. . . . The former purifies his lineage; not so one who thinks himself to be important" (VII.9.10[97]). In the tenth book, the *brāhmaṇas* themselves lament their caste-induced spiritual myopia: "Curses on that birth which is threefold,[98] curses on vows, curses on extensive learning, curses on our family lineage, and curses on skill in rituals, because we still remain averse to Kṛṣṇa" (X.23.40). And as a very important aside, of relevance to the modern Indian context, it merits repeating that the *Bhāgavata* explicitly states that caste (as in profession) should be determined by one's innate nature, not by birthright (VII.2.31, 35).[99]

Gender hierarchies, too, are subverted (but, importantly, only in the context of *bhakti*),[100] with the illiterate, forest-dwelling, simple-hearted *gopī* cowherd women extolled as the greatest of all *yogīs*, simply by dint of their devotion:

> These *gopī* women are the highest embodied beings on the earth: their love for Govinda [Kṛṣṇa], the soul of everything, is perfected. Those who are fearful of the material world aspire to this, and so do the sages, and so do we ourselves. . . . *Aho!* May I become any of the shrubs, creepers, or plants in Vṛndāvana that enjoy the dust of the feet of these women. They have renounced their own relatives, who are so hard to give up, as well as the *Ārya* code of conduct, and worshipped the feet of Mukunda [Kṛṣṇa], the sought-for goal of the sacred texts of revelation. . . . I pay eternal homage to the dust from the feet of the women of Nanda's Vraj. (X.47.58–63)

And further, in marked contrast to the pure/impure concerns so central to Vedic orthopraxy, even foreigners and those entirely outside the Vedic construct of *dharma* are eligible to practice *bhakti*: "By taking shelter of those devoted to Him, the tribes of the *kirātas*, *hūṇas*, *andhras*, *pulindas*, *pukkaśas*, *ābhīras*, *kaṅkas*, *yavanas*, *khasas*, etc.,[101] as well as others who are sinful, become purified" (II.4.18), as do even animals (II.7.46).[102] Indeed, one of the very earliest archaeological evidences for Kṛṣṇa *bhakti* is a metal column, constructed circa 100 B.C.E. by a Greek, Heliodorus, who refers to himself as a *bhāgavata*. (Western devotees of Kṛṣṇa may thus have a long antiquated predecessor!)

Bhakti, then, is the ultimate *dharma* and hence the summum bonum and very goal of life, as the five-year-old Prahlāda convinces his fellow students:

A wise person should practice the *dharma* of *Bhagavān* from childhood. A human birth is rare, and even though it is temporary, it can bestow the goal of life. Therefore, a person in this world should approach the feet of Viṣṇu: He is one's *Īśvara*, the dearest friend, and beloved of all beings. (VII.6.1–2)

The *Bhāgavata* urges us to appreciate this rarity and hence urgency of the human opportunity and its potential: it is only in the human form, attained after countless previous births, that one can attain liberation. This is not possible in the higher or lower realms, says Jīva, "because there is complete immersion in sense enjoyment among those born as celestials[103] and an absence of discrimination (*viveka*) among animals" (*anu* 55). And what is to be lost from at least trying? "If a neophyte, after renouncing conventional *dharma* falls down [from the standards] while worshipping the lotus feet of Hari, what harm is there in that for him? On the other hand, what [ultimate] benefit is attained for one following one's conventional *dharma* but without worship?" (I.5.17). As Kṛṣṇa assures the hesitant Arjuna in the *Gītā* with regard to *yoga* in general, the fallen *yogī* takes a celestial birth in the next life, then returns to this realm and picks up the practices where he or she left off, "as if spontaneously" (VI.37–47). This simply means that the previous birth's *saṁskāras*, latent memories, subconsciously reactivate in the mind, and one is automatically reattracted to the path, seemingly without (or despite) conscious deliberation.

Bhakti Mixed with *Karma* and *Jñāna*

Continuing the theme of *bhakti* performed out of some personal motivation, let us further fine-tune our understanding of conventional action in the world, but here with a focus on *karma*, action performed for the fulfillment of desire (where the focus of *dharma* is more on the moral and dutiful dimension of action). *Karma* is a theme to which Jīva frequently returns in his *Bhakti Sandarbha*, as, naturally, how to act in the world is of paramount concern to most, given that the vast majority of people do have desires that they pursue and are not inclined to renounce the world to become ascetics. This discussion overlaps considerably with the previous one on *dharma* and, indeed, the terms *karma* and *dharma* are sometimes used synonymously. But they have been separated since, whereas the focus in the previous section was on *dharma* as action—the nature of the acts themselves—we now consider action in the world from the perspective of its motive: the desire for outcome.

The definition of *karma* presented by Kṛṣṇa in the *Gītā* is "the creative force which gives rise to the desires of living beings" (III.8). It is action in pursuit of fulfilling desires. When the pursuit of these desires is undertaken by means of actions performed in accordance with the Vedic legal codes and injunctions, it is *dharma* and begets good fruits (VI.1.40). In classical times, the specifics of what kinds of actions constituted right *dharma* were outlined in a genre of texts, the *Dharma sūtras* or *Dharma śāstras* such as those of Manu.[104] Thus action, *karma*, is to all intents and purposes more or less synonymous with *dharma* (social, professional, or familial duties), when these activities dedicated to the fulfillment of desires are performed within the contours of Vedic norms and regulations.

When desires are pursued disregarding these codes, *karma* becomes *adharma*, non-*dharma* (unrighteousness), and begets bad fruit. In both cases, *karma* is action prompted by desire and, as the *Yoga Sūtras* inform us, determines the *jāti*, future birth; *āyur*, future life span; and *bhoga*, future quality of life, good or bad, of the agent (II.13–14). These fruits or effects are pleasurable or distressful—good or bad birth, long or compromised life span, and good or bad quality of life and access to resources (and all their intervening shades)—depending on whether their initial causal actions fell into the category of *dharma* or *adharma*.[105] The important point is that it is action prompted by desire that generates seeds of *karmic* reaction, irrespective of whether *dharmic* or *adharmic*, and it is thus action that perpetuates reincarnation (as one must take future births, good or bad, to receive the fruits of such actions). These basic principles of the mechanisms underpinning reincarnation are shared by all the *mokṣa* schools, including Buddhism and Jainism. But this leaves open the possibility of action performed free from desire, which does not plant seeds of reaction. As readers familiar with the *karma yoga* and *bhakti yoga* teachings of the *Gītā* will recognize, it is the mind-set underpinning the performance of action that is in question here—the yearning for material profit, fame, or other such benefit: in other words, desire—not necessarily the actions themselves. It is action performed with desire that perpetuates *saṁsāra*. Action performed without desire does not breed reaction.

This seed of reaction, good as well as bad, can also be eradicated when *karma* is offered to Kṛṣṇa: "Whatever action you perform, whatever you eat, whatever sacrifices you perform, whatever you give in charity, whatever austerities you undertake, do that as an offering to Me, O Arjuna. In this way, you will be freed from the bondage of the fruits, whether auspicious or inauspicious" (*Gītā*, IX.27–28). In other words, acts of *karma/dharma* may contain varying degrees of self-interest, but they are accepted as *bhakti* when offered to *Īśvara*, and, importantly, this act of offering them erases the very desires that spawned them, along with their reactions.

So in *bhakti yoga* routine duties need not be abandoned but can become *bhakti* when offered to *Īśvara*: "Whatever one does naturally with one's body, words, mind, senses, intellect, or heart should all be offered to the supreme Nārāyaṇa" (XI.2.36; another theme strongly emphasized in the *Gītā*, such as in IX.27). In fact, according to one verse, one can not only perform one's *dharma* in the world, but cultivate economic well-being and even satisfy desires while offering these to *Īśvara* and cultivating the various practices associated with *bhakti*, at least until pure *bhakti* devoid of all personal desire is eventually attained: "A faithful person listening to, reciting and remembering the narrations about Me, which are auspicious and purify the worlds, and enacting My birth and deeds [for example, in dance, poetry, art, drama, and the like], while pursuing [the conventional goals of life] *dharma*, *artha* (prosperity), and *kāma* (desire) for My sake after taking shelter of Me, attains unwavering *bhakti* for Me, the Eternal" (XI.11.23–24).

The idea here is that by dint of focusing the mind on *Īśvara*, any unwholesome desires underpinning one's actions are eventually eradicated: "For those who worship Him, even though they do not aspire for it, He bestows His own lotus feet, and these extinguish all desire" (V.19.26). In this way, says Jīva, "even through offering one's worldly activities one can somehow or other still attain perfection" (*anu* 217). Put differently, *karma* is removed by *karma*: "That which causes disease for living beings, cannot [under normal circumstances] be the remedy for that very disease. But it can cure when used as medicine: the performance of all actions (*karma*), which are the causes of bondage for people, when performed for the Supreme become capable of destroying themselves" (I.5.33–34). In Kṛṣṇa's words, "The desire of those whose minds are absorbed in Me, does not produce desire" (X.22.26).

In point of fact, as we will see much more prominently in the case of Śiva, Kṛṣṇa, too (although much less stressed), is not averse to fulfilling the desires of His devotees on occasion, albeit with a higher goal in mind: "It is true that, when solicited, the Lord fulfills that which has been requested by men; but He is not really bestowing true benefit by this, as more requests are then again made" (V.19.26). Paraphrasing the *Gītā* (X.11), it is *Īśvara*, situated in the heart, who removes ignorance and desire: "All the desires in the heart of a wise person who continuously worships Me through the *bhakti yoga* I have imparted, are destroyed by Me situated in the heart" (XI.21.29); Patañjali's *Īśvara-praṇidhāṇa* aspect of *kriyā yoga*, designated as that which removes the impurities, *kleśas*, such as desire, and brings about *samādhi*, can also be read in this light (II.1–2; II.45).[106] Therefore, the bottom line is: "Irrespective of whether one is free of desire, full of all desires, or desirous of liberation (*mokṣa*), if one is intelligent, one should intensely worship the Supreme Person through the practice of *bhakti yoga*" (II.3.10).

And more, even if one is addicted to unwholesome behavior, *adharma*, one is still not excluded from performing *bhakti*. Jīva advises such people to offer even these unwholesome deeds to *Īśvara* accompanied by the following prayer: "May the Lord who is full of compassion bestow compassion upon seeing my suffering due to my bad inclinations which are the cause of this suffering" (*anu* 217). Thus, no one is denied access to *bhakti*: "If even the performer of the most evil deeds worships Me with undivided devotion, he will quickly become righteous and is to be considered saintly, for his determination is perfect" (*Gītā* IX.30–31).

Nonetheless, Jīva notes, there is obviously a difference between genuinely offering one's *karma* for *Īśvara*'s satisfaction and offering it incidentally as an afterthought. He notes that there might be three motives in the offering of one's *karma*: the fulfillment of one's own material desire, to become free from the bondage of *karma*, or pure devotion to *Īśvara* (*anu* 224). In the first two, says Jīva, the underlying motive is actually an aspiration to be free from suffering, and this is self-interest—any devotion to *Īśvara* is merely "a semblance." The offerings are still efficacious, as has been noted, insofar as they eventually eradicate self-interest and desire, but only the third type of motive, wherein only the satisfaction of *Īśvara* exists, is pure *bhakti*. An example of *bhakti* performed with personal desires is perhaps Dhruva, who will be encountered in his tale in part 3.[107] The child prince performed astonishing *tapas*, austerity, while fixing his mind on Viṣṇu, but his intention was gaining a kingdom greater than that of his father, who had offended him. Once Viṣṇu appears to him, he realizes the foolishness of this aspiration: "Alas! Like a foolish person who, because of little merit,[108] requests chaffed rice from a sovereign, I, because of illusion, requested for my pride [to be upheld] from the Lord who was offering me His own personal abode." (IV.9.35)

In addition to such "devotion mixed with personal sensual desires" (*sa-kāmā bhakti*), Jīva discusses "devotion mixed with a desire for liberation"[109] (*kaivalya-kāmā bhakti*). This is a theme to which we will return frequently in the next section, as it expresses an important subtext of the *Bhāgavata*. This type of *bhakti* refers to those who devote themselves to *Īśvara*, but with the intention of gaining *mokṣa*, liberation (also known as *kaivalya*)—that is, realization of the *ātman*, the goal associated with the path of *jñāna*. The liberation-seeking type of *bhakta* uses a *bhakti* method for the purpose of realizing the *ātman* rather than engaging in *bhakti* out of love for *Īśvara*.[110] In other words, the *yogī* here is worshipping *Īśvara* so as to be purified and in the hope that experience of the *ātman* will be bestowed by *Īśvara*. This type of practice resonates with the role of meditation on *Īśvara* in Patañjali's system, *Īśvara-praṇidhāna*, which results in *samādhi-siddhi* (II.45)—namely, "the immersion of the seer in its own pure essence" (I.3). The important point is that seeking the *ātman* through *bhakti* methods is not the goal of pure *bhakti*, as *Īśvara* is a higher Truth beyond the *ātman*, as we will discuss from a metaphysical perspective in "The Object of *Bhakti*." Thus the practitioners of these two types of *bhakti* mixed with *karma* or *jñāna* seek goals other than pure devotion for *Bhagavān*. While neither of these is the pure unmotivated *bhakti* that we will encounter in *rāgānugā*, they are both nonetheless efficacious by dint of being connected with *Īśvara* on some level.

Finally, all of these compromised or "mixed" forms of practicing *bhakti* can also be conceptualized according to the *guṇa* schema—that is, different expressions of *bhakti* are also reflective of the different *guṇas* prominent in the mind of the *bhakta*:

> *Śrī Bhagavān* said:
>
> "One who performs *bhakti* for Me full of anger, for the purpose of inflicting violence, out of pride or envy, with a divisive mentality, is in *tamas*. One who worships My Deity form for the purpose of sense indulgence, fame, or power, with a mentality that sees difference, is in *rajas*. One who [worships Me] for the purpose of becoming free from *karma*, as an offering to the Supreme, or because worship is something that ought to be done, yet still entertaining a mentality that sees difference [from Me], is in *sattva*." (XI.29.7–10)

In sum, concluding all this using more familiar modern frames of references, praying to God in any place through any mode of worship for anything other than pure devotion—for one's daily sustenance, for help in a crisis, for victory in war or sport, for the cure of a loved one—soliciting God for any material, emotional, social, cultural, political, humanitarian, or even soteriological reason, is considered *bhakti* performed under the influence of the *guṇas*. Obviously, appealing to God for humanitarian concerns toward the suffering of others is much higher (*sattva*) in the scheme of "mixed" *bhakti* than praying to God for one's own successes (*rajas*) or to assist one in harming an enemy (*tamas*). But pure *bhakti* has full faith in and surrender to *Īśvara*'s supreme will and omniscience in all things and thus does not presume to request for some petty tinkering of material affairs for temporary *prakṛtic* gain. Indeed, as we noted, true *bhaktas* do not even request liberation, the goal of all other Indic soteriological (*mokṣa*) systems—even liberation of the personal sort, which maintains a postmortem devotional relationship with *Bhagavān* in Vaikuṇṭha or Goloka, and thus is deemed acceptable to Vaiṣṇavas, unless service to their beloved Lord is its central feature:

> The characteristic of *bhakti yoga*, which is free of the *guṇas*, has been described as when the mind flows toward Me, who am seated in the heart, unimpeded, simply from hearing about My qualities, like the waters of the *Gaṅgā* river into the ocean. It is that *bhakti* to the Supreme Person, which is free of motive, and uninterrupted. Such persons do not accept [the five types of liberation]—residing in the same abode as Viṣṇu (*sālokya*); having the same opulence as Him (*sārṣṭi*); being close to Him (*sāmīpya*); having the same form as Him (*sārūpya*); and merging into Him (*ekatvam*)—even if they are offered—without service to Me. That type of *bhakti yoga* has been described as uninterrupted. By following it, one transcends the three *guṇas* and attains to My nature. (III.29.11–14)

By way of a rather succinct yet apropos conclusion to all this, and as a segue into the next section, there are as many varieties of *bhakti* as there are *bhaktas* who practice it: "The path of *bhakti yoga* assumes many forms, my dear lady. It manifests variously, according to the permutations of the *guṇas* manifest in people's nature" (XI.29.7).

Rāgānugā Bhakti

Vaidhī is clearly the *bhakti* performed by the vast majority of practitioners, but exceptionally advanced practitioners—which generally entails those who have cultivated *vaidhī bhakti* for numerous preceding lifetimes[111]—may immediately experience an irrepressible attraction, *rāga*, toward Kṛṣṇa upon first encountering narratives about Him. This is an attraction that appears spontaneous—*rāga-anugā*, "conforming to one's [devotional] innate desire." Before proceeding, we must note that, where the previous discussion on *vaidhī bhakti* contains the basic types of practices recognized and adopted by most schools or expressions of Hindu *bhakti*, even as each tradition tinkers with such practices uniquely and has its own flavorings and details, the following discussion on *rāgānugā* is specific to the Kṛṣṇa theologies of the sixteenth century that emerged with Caitanya and his contemporary Vallabha (in whose tradition these practices are called the *puṣṭi mārga*).[112] Therefore, for reasons that will become clear, in order to understand *rāgānugā bhakti*, we need to establish some theological infrastructure pertaining to the nature of *mokṣa*, liberation, distinctive of Vaiṣṇava/*Bhāgavata* theology in general. This involves Viṣṇu's divine realm, Vaikuṇṭha, as well as, more particularly still, Kṛṣṇa's realm, Goloka.

The Divine *Brahman* Realms of Vaikuṇṭha and Goloka

As we will discuss from a philosophical and theological perspective in the chapter "The Object of *Bhakti*," *Īśvara* is an eternal Supreme Person in the Vaiṣṇava traditions, the *ātmans* are also not only eternal but eternally individual parts of *Īśvara*, and *bhakti* too between these individuals is eternal and not simply a means to some higher end. Where, then, does *bhakti* transpire between *Īśvara* and His *bhaktas* who have attained *mokṣa*, in the postmortem state? And in what manner does this take place, given that liberation entails becoming free from the *prakṛtic* body and mind? The answers to these questions are an essential trademark feature of Vaiṣṇavism, defining and distinguishing its ultimate goals vis-à-vis other *yoga* systems. They are also indispensable to understanding *rāgānugā bhakti*.

In *Bhāgavata* cosmology, or rather beyond it, in the trans-*prakṛtic* dimension of pure *Brahman*, there are innumerable divine realms called Vaikuṇṭha. These realms have nothing to do with the temporary realms in *prakṛti* and so are not to be confounded with the celestial realms within *saṁsāra* (*svārga*), the abodes of the *devas*—celestial beings or demigods—which are the destination of those with requisite amounts of good *karma* (which, sooner or later, expires). They are eternal transcendent realms made not of the three *guṇas* of *prakṛti*, discussed later, but of *Brahman* stuff—namely, pure consciousness (*cit-śakti*). They are real, not *māyā*. These constitute the eternal "Kingdom of God" in Vaiṣṇavism, the abodes of Viṣṇu and His devotees.

The *Bhāgavata* provides a few glimpses at the nature of Vaikuṇṭha. It is adorable to all the worlds (X.12.26); the highest realm where Viṣṇu, also known as Nārāyaṇa, resides (XII.24.14); the highest region (IV.I2.26); beyond the world of darkness and *saṁsāra* (the cycle of birth and death; IV.24.29, X.88.25); the destination of those who have transcended the three *guṇas* (XI.25.22); and beyond which there is no higher place (II.2.18, 11.9.9). The peaceful ascetics who reach that place never return (IV.9.29, X.88.25–26). The residents of Vaikuṇṭha have "pure" forms, not material bodies (VII.1.34). These forms are like that of Viṣṇu (III.5.14ff.).[113] One passage notes that

> Viṣṇu/Nārāyaṇa resides in Vaikuṇṭha with Śrī, the Goddess of Fortune, in palaces with crystal walls. The parks there shine like final liberation itself, and contain wish-fulfilling trees [that can fulfill any request made], which blossom all the year round. There are fragrant winds, and creepers dripping with honey near bodies of water. Cries of exotic birds mingle with the humming of bees, and magnificent flowers bloom everywhere. Devotees of Viṣṇu along with their beautiful wives travel in aerial vehicles made of jewels, emeralds, and gold, but the beautiful smiling residents of this realm cannot distract the minds of the opposite sex, since everyone is absorbed in Kṛṣṇa (III.15.14–25).

Again, all forms in Vaikuṇṭha are made of *Brahman* (*cit-śakti*), not of the ever-changing stuff of *prakṛti*. And the Gauḍīya tradition holds that Śiva has his own transcendent realm as well, where he resides with those who prefer to worship *Īśvara* in that form.[114]

As a theological aside, a typical default response to the notion of a personal Godhead with a divine abode possessing form and quality is that any such imagining is an anthropomorphic construction—the projection of qualities known to humans upon a transcendent Godhead beyond all such qualities and mental constructions. But from a Vaiṣṇava perspective, rather than Vaikuṇṭha being an anthropomorphic projection, the reverse holds true: it is actually this world that is a "theopomorphic" projection. That is to say, there can be forms and personages in our world only because they are temporary and *prakṛtic* reflections and imitations of the eternal *Brahman* protoforms. This world, as an effect, must owe its dynamic personalized qualities and characteristics to its cause; so this cause, too, must have qualities.[115] "Man is made in the image of God" is a coherent inference in personalist theology.[116]

In any event, according to the Kṛṣṇa branches of Vaiṣṇavism,[117] among the Vaikuṇṭha realms of Viṣṇu there is one specific to Kṛṣṇa called Goloka, the most supreme realm of all (the exact relationship between Kṛṣṇa and Viṣṇu is discussed in the chapter "The Object of *Bhakti*"). This transcendent abode of Kṛṣṇa is not described in detail in the tenth book, even though Kṛṣṇa reveals it to the *gopas* (X.28.14), but we are told that it is beyond darkness and is pure, eternal, unlimited, conscious, and effulgent *Brahman* and that the *gopas*, cowherds-men, were overwhelmed with the highest ecstasy upon seeing it (X.28.14–17).[118] In fact, for the Gauḍīya tradition, the description of Kṛṣṇa's own transcendent *Brahman* realm of Goloka corresponds to the descriptions of the landscape of Vraj in the *Bhāgavata*'s tenth book that we will encounter in part 3. Goloka is the divine protoversion of this or, more accurately, the Vraj depicted in the tenth book is a *prakṛtic* version of the true *Brahman* realm. In fact, Jīva outlines in the *Kṛṣṇa Sandarbha* that there are two manifestations of Vraj: the one visible to the senses and the one perceivable only in deep states of *bhakti* meditation. The *prakṛtic* Vraj is thus a portal to the divine realm with which it coexists—hence Rūpa's advice to aspiring *bhaktas* to reside there quoted earlier. Thus, despite such descriptive frugality in its source text, according to the Gauḍīya tradition, expanding, as always, on hints in the *Bhāgavata* itself, when He descends within this world, Kṛṣṇa opens a window into the eternal *Brahman* realm of Goloka. The stories in the tenth book that we will encounter in part 3 about Vraj, where Kṛṣṇa spent His childhood, and indeed, the very landscape with its flora and fauna, are actually, to again borrow some phraseology, something akin to the Kingdom of God on Earth. Not only does Kṛṣṇa descend, He brings His divine abode and even certain associates from Goloka with Him. More than this, and fundamental to understanding *rāgānugā bhakti*, the various relationships we will find between Kṛṣṇa and His beloved associates in Vraj replicate some of the relationships the liberated souls can have with Him for all eternity in the eternal realm within *Brahman*, Goloka.

In fact, the text suggests that Kṛṣṇa's incarnation has, in reality, two motives: one is the "official" motive expressed in the *Mahābhārata* (I.35–60) and the *Gītā* (IV.4ff.), as also the *Bhāgavata* (X.1.15–22)—namely, to protect the righteous and free the earth from the intolerable buildup of demoniac military power. But the one of interest to us in the context of *rāgānugā bhakti* is to attract the souls lost in *saṁsāra* to the possibility of eternal *līlā*, loving relational pastimes, with God in the transcendent eternal Goloka abode of Vraj, as revealed in the tenth book. These various relationships, discussed next, are deemed so attractive that even just hearing about them enchants the listener away from his or her attachments to the self-centered indulgences of this world of *saṁsāra,* which simply perpetuate the cycle of *karma* and thus of repeated birth and death (XI.1.6–7, XII.3.14–15). *Samādhi,* in Kṛṣṇa *bhakti*, is nothing other than initially fixing the mind in contemplating these *līlās* until, ultimately, consciousness is eligible to become absorbed in them directly, even while still embodied. Just as *jñāna yoga*, the path of knowledge, involves fixing the mind on the idea or notion of the *ātman* until consciousness is eligible to become reabsorbed in its own *ātman* nature experientially, *bhaktas* opt to fix their minds on *līlās* until they become eligible to participate in them directly. They are not interested in the static passive state of self-awareness offered by the *jñāna* paths and prescribed by Patañjali in the *Yoga Sūtras* (even as they acknowledge their factual availability), but seek spiritual reembodiment in a form made of pure *Brahman* and an active dynamic state of relationship with God. The mechanics and metaphysics underpinning the differences in both these practices and their respective goals are discussed in "The Object of *Bhakti*" and "Concluding Reflections."

With all this as a necessary preliminary backdrop that will become clearer as we proceed, in order to understand the workings of *rāgānugā bhakti* we also still need to understand two further concepts more clearly: *līlā*, pastime, and the divine power that facilitates it, *yogamāyā*.

Līlā and *Yogamāyā*

In the *Bhāgavata*, the term *līlā* refers to pure play or spontaneous joyful pastime with intimate *bhaktas*.[119] It is an exchange of love between God and devotee. The noun *līlā* is used frequently in the tenth book of the *Bhāgavata* when God is playing as a child with His friends in the beautiful idyllic forests of Vraj, where He spent His childhood, interacting with His beloved *bhaktas*—the *gopī* and *gopa* cowherding community—free of any sense of mission or purpose, other than to engage in *līlā*. The term is never used in the *Bhagavad Gītā*, where Kṛṣṇa is portrayed as God playing the role of a teacher imparting spiritual knowledge to Arjuna. But in the Vraj section of the tenth book, we are granted a vision of God at play, God reciprocating playful, loving exchanges with His most intimate *bhaktas*.

Indeed, a number of the usages of the noun *līlā* in the tenth book suggest that Kṛṣṇa has assumed a body for the sake of *līlā*[120] (in contrast with the *jīvas,* the souls in the world, who are helplessly injected into bodies as a result of their *karma*, propelled along by forces beyond their control). Of course, the *Bhāgavata* resonates with the discussion of the Vedāntins in insisting that God is *aptarāma*, self-satisfied, and requires nothing. So His decision to engage in *līlā*, then, points to a spontaneous expression of His blissful nature, not to some lack.[121] But most of all, it is an expression of His love for His *bhaktas*, for whom He makes himself amenable so that they can love Him through different roles and relationships according to their devotional desires (*rāga*). All this will become clearer as we discuss the specifics of these relationships.

Kṛṣṇa's *līlā* completely enchants the residents of Vraj, who have earned by the purity of their unshakable *bhakti* over numerous lives this privilege of having their unique personal relationship with Him as friend, parent, or lover (X.8.52). *Līlā* is how Kṛṣṇa and His *bhaktas* express their blissful and spontaneous reciprocation of love according to the devotees' *bhāva*, mood (discussed below). Understandably, the great fortune of the residents of Vraj who were able to engage so intimately with Kṛṣṇa in His *līlā* is stressed prominently throughout the text: to be an intimate associate of God is the highest possible perfection of human existence in the *Bhāgavata* (X.47.58). The ecstatic states of love exhibited by Kṛṣṇa's associates in Vraj are not paralleled by other paradigmatic devotees anywhere else in the entire *Bhāgavata*.

A corollary concept essential to understanding *līlā* is *yogamāyā*, the power of "divine illusion." This nominal compound appears, at first glance, to be an oxymoron. We know in Hindu thought in general that the term *yoga* has positive valences denoting that which connects the *yogī* with the innermost *ātman* (and, in the case of *bhakti yoga*, with *Īśvara*, the Supreme *Ātman*). But we also know that the term *māyā* has negative ones, as that which does precisely the opposite by preventing the practitioner from realizing his or her own *ātman* and also from recognizing *Īśvara*, the *Paramātman*. *Yoga* is the set of practices that redirects the awareness of *ātman* back to its original pure *Brahman* source (*Yoga Sūtras* I.3), where *māyā* does precisely the contrary; it is the power that prevents the *ātman* from realizing both its nature as pure eternal consciousness and the presence of *Īśvara*. *Māyā* diverts consciousness instead into identifying with the instrumentation of the external bodily and psychic coverings and then outward into the things of this world as objects of desire.[122] *Māyā* is the illusory power that keeps the *ātman* bewildered by the sense objects of this world and consequently ensnared in *saṁsāra*,[123] while *yoga* is the means to free the *ātman* from these. How then can the oxymoron *yogamāyā* be rendered coherent?

As with her *saṁsāric māyā* counterpart, *Yogamāyā* indeed deludes the pure liberated souls participating in the *līlā* with her power of concealment so that they do not perceive Kṛṣṇa as Supreme Godhead. But, like *bhakti yoga*, she does this so that the souls can connect with *Īśvara* intimately by perceiving Him, rather, as their friend, lover, or child (etc.) instead. Otherwise, if souls realized Kṛṣṇa's true nature as Supreme *Īśvara*, they would consequently be incapable of interacting with Him in *līlā* in these intimate modes because they would be overwhelmed by His majesty and supremacy. Hence the term preserves the valence of illusion, but an illusion that manifests only at the highest stage of *bhakti*. Unlike that of her *saṁsāric* alter ego, *Yogamāyā*'s power of illusion is a highly coveted one experienced only by the most qualified *yogīs*. Although even great *ṛṣis* (sages) are anxious to *avoid* the illusory power of the conventional *māyā*, the greatest sage of all, Nārada, by contrast, is very eager to *experience* the power of the divine *yogamāyā* (X.69.19ff.). While the regular *māyā* can *disappear* only by devotion to Kṛṣṇa, the divine *yogamāyā* can *appear* only by devotion to Kṛṣṇa (X.69.38). Just as entrance to the mundane world of *saṁsāra*, an undesirable state of affairs, depends on the pure knowledge of the *jīva* being enveloped by the influence of the *saṁsāric māyā*, entrance into the transcendent world of *līlā*, a desirable state of affairs, depends on the pure knowledge of the *jīva* being enveloped by the influence of the divine *yogamāyā*.

Kṛṣṇa relishes these personal informal associations far more than the conventional formal worship in awe and reverence that results from the awareness of His position as Lord and Creator of everything.

Kṛṣṇa doesn't want to be exclusively *Īśvara*—God on high, so to speak—He also wants to enjoy *līlā* with His friends as an equal or with His parents as a subordinate: "For those who could understand, *Bhagavān* Kṛṣṇa manifested the condition of [submitting] himself to the control of His dependents in this world" (X.11.9). But how could God truly play spontaneously and unceremoniously with anyone in the role of a son or friend, if everyone knew He was really God? It is *Yogamāyā* who ensures, with her illusory but divine devotional spell, that the *ātmans* in Kṛṣṇa's *līlā* remain unaware of Kṛṣṇa's real nature.[124] Indeed, even Kṛṣṇa himself becomes so involved in His *līlā* that He sometimes also seems to prefer to forget His own supremacy.[125]

The *Bhāgavata* vividly illustrates *yogamāyā*'s essential role in the world of *līlā* when, as we will see in part 3, Kṛṣṇa's foster mother, Yaśodā, looks into her son's mouth to see if He has eaten dirt but sees the entire universe there instead (X.8.36). Becoming enlightened as to the real nature of both herself and Kṛṣṇa, she finds that her ability to interact with Him as His mother is immediately shattered and, instead, she begins to bow down at His feet, spouting lofty Vedāntic rhetoric and eulogizing Him as the Supreme Being (X.8.40ff.). Kṛṣṇa immediately deludes her with His *yogamāyā,* erasing her memory of the event so that she can again place Him on her lap, nurse Him, and continue with her maternal duties in pure love, thinking of Him as her adorable infant dependent on her care.[126] This divine illusion, of course, is appropriate for the perfected souls who have attained God in these ways by their past-life *vaidhī bhakti*, but we, the audience (or, nowadays, reader), are constantly reminded of who Kṛṣṇa is: "Do not consider that Kṛṣṇa is His father's offspring; He is the *Īśvara* or all *ātmans*, the Supreme imperishable Being. But He has concealed His majesty in the form of a human being by His *māyā* power" (XI.5.49).[127]

Being subject to the influence of *yogamāyā*, and hence able to play such intimate roles in God's *līlā*, then, is the highest and most rare boon of human existence. The *Bhāgavata* repeatedly states that not even the celestials, or most elevated personalities, or even Viṣṇu's eternal consort, the Goddess of Fortune herself, enjoy the grace bestowed on the residents of Vraj (X.9.20). Kṛṣṇa's foster mother, Yaśodā, was able to chase Kṛṣṇa in anger, to spank Him whom the greatest *yogīs* of all cannot reach even in their minds (X.9.9). So elevated are the residents of Vraj that Kṛṣṇa Himself becomes subservient to their love, "like a wooden puppet . . . controlled by them" (X.11.7). They are able to engage in these unique modes with Kṛṣṇa, whom *yogīs* cannot reach even after many births of austere disciplines (X.12.12). All this is possible by the power of *Yogamāyā*. Without her, there could be no *līlā* and, hence, no intimate, nonmajestic relationship of love with *Īśvara*. And without such relationships, there could be no *rāgānugā bhakti*.

Rāga, *Bhāva*, and *Rasa*

Connecting all this with our present purposes of understanding *rāgānugā bhakti*, when Kṛṣṇa's associates absorb themselves in their particular *līlās* with their Lord under the spell of *yogamāyā*, these relationships are expressions of their specific *rāga*, devotional desire, and *bhāva*, loving mood. *Rāga* and *bhāva* are two out of three terms that overlap and are central to understanding the spontaneous *bhakti* to which we will now turn our attention in this section, the other term being *rasa*. With regard to *rāga*, we will also need to differentiate *rāgānugā bhakti* from the protomodels upon which it is based: *rāgātmikā bhakti*.

Rāga, desire, is one of the five *kleśas*, obstacles to Yoga, which must be overcome in almost all Hindu, Buddhist, and Jain *mokṣa* traditions in order to realize the *ātman* (see, for instance, *Yoga Sūtras* II.4–7).[128] It stems from *avidyā*, ignorance, defined in the *Yoga Sūtras* as considering oneself to be the temporal, impure, suffering-prone body and mind, rather than the eternal pure blissful *ātman* (II.5). *Rāga* is defined as *sukha-anuśayī*, the pursuit of material pleasure (II.7). The *Nyāya Sūtras* identifies its synonym *icchā* as that which prompts actions (III.2.305), and the *Gītā* gives yet another synonym, *kāma*, as contemplation of and attachment to sense objects (*viṣaya* II.62). All these terms denote the motivational trigger that prompts action aimed at fulfilling some material need or want. Jīva defines *rāga* similarly, as the "innate overwhelming desire to contact a sense object (*viṣaya*) by one who is attracted to that sense object" (*anu* 310), and Rūpa as "being completely and innately absorbed in the object of desire" (II.272). In all such *yogic* contexts, desire is directed toward the satisfaction of the body/mind self due to ignorance of the true self, and hence it generates *karma*, which is the cause of bondage, *saṁsāra*. In other words, desires underpin actions, and all actions, whether good or bad, when performed in ignorance of the true *ātman* self, generate corresponding reactions, and so one has to take rebirth to experience these reactions, good or bad. Desires are insatiable, says the *Mahābhārata*, and "there has never been, nor will there ever be anyone born in this world who has been able to satisfy them" (*Mokṣadharma* 177.22); hence desires are "fetters" to this world (*Mokṣadharma* 251.7). Indeed, the *Gītā* considers mundane desire "the all-consuming enemy in this world, impelling one to impious deeds" (III.36–37).

However, when *Īśvara* is established as the object (*viṣaya*) and desires are channeled toward Him, everything changes, even as such desires are likewise also called *rāga*. The obvious difference is that self-centered desires seeking to gratify the body and mind with the sense objects of *prakṛti* end up perpetuating suffering and *saṁsāra*, the cycle of birth and death, instead.[129] Attraction for Kṛṣṇa, on the other hand, eradicates mundane desires and attachments and ultimately leads to bliss and liberation (*Gītā* IX.34).[130] As Kṛṣṇa Himself puts it: "The desire of those whose minds are absorbed in Me, does not produce desire, just as grain which is cooked or fried is not generally capable of sprouting" (X.22.26). Even in the stoic *Yoga Sūtras*, dedication to *Īśvara* removes obstacles such as mundane *rāga* (II.1–2) and causes liberation (II.45).

Nonetheless, the underlying psychological principles of *rāga*, whether stemming from ignorance (the *kleśa*s) or of the *bhakti* variety, are identical. Let us consider this with more focus: in conventional Yoga psychology, *rāga* is initiated by the senses encountering an object that produces a pleasant experience. This experience becomes recorded as an imprint (*saṁskāra*) on the mind (*citta*), as all experiences do, which can then emerge at a later time as a pleasant memory. This memory can be caused either from reencountering that same (or a similar) object, which triggers the memory, or just from idle daydreaming, when one sieves through one's reservoir of *saṁskāras*, patching *saṁskāras* together in fantasy and reverie. Desire is nothing other than contemplation on this memory with a wish to re-create the experience of which it is an imprint. As outlined in the *Gītā* (II.62–63), if the memory is entertained long enough, it develops into desire, which in turn morphs into an impulse for action—to reexperience or reacquire that sense object. This is the psychological (or, actually, metaphysical[131]) underpinning of desire and its variants, such as greed and lust, in Yoga.

So, for example, let us suppose that one samples chocolate for the first time, and as a result of this experience the tongue registers a pleasant sensation of taste as a *saṁskāra* in the *citta*. Now, when one happens by the chocolate store some other day and the eyes encounter the chocolate display in the window, one's memory of the previous taste of chocolate is activated—in this case, a pleasant recollection.[132] That previously existing *saṁskāra* becomes classified as *rāga* when it causes one to wish or decide to reattain the experience underpinning it—that is, to obtain some chocolate on another occasion. So the longer one gazes through the window, the stronger is the likelihood of desire—the impulse to reattain that experience or taste—developing and growing. And aversion works in exactly the same way: the senses encounter an object that creates an unpleasant experience, and this is also recorded as memory. On reencountering that object in some future time (or simply in one's anxious imaginings), one strives to avoid or eliminate it. Fear, anxiety, hatred, anger, and other such mental states are variants of *dveṣa*.

Kṛṣṇa too is a sense object,[133] whether encountered through the narratives of the *Bhāgavata*, as in our case—that is, by means of the sense of hearing via the ears through *śravaṇa*, the first process of *bhakti* (or, if reading the text, via the eyes)—or whether encountered personally during His incarnation (through the eyes, ears, and all the senses in the case of the residents of Vraj). The *Bhāgavata* holds that howsoever encountered, Kṛṣṇa leaves an impression on the mind, which, like any other sensual imprint, remains as a memory. Unless the mind is consumed by an inordinate degree of *tamas* or *rajas* (see discussion in "Meditation in Hate and Lust"), this memory can be enchanting and keep resurfacing, prompting the devotee to continually reseek the experience of Kṛṣṇa through some of the processes of *bhakti* we have discussed—*śravaṇa*, *kīrtana*, *smaraṇa*, and so on. This is the psychological mechanics of *bhakti yoga*.

In fact, this dual applicability of the term *rāga* is just a *bhakti* variant of the binary distinctions between the *kliṣṭa-akliṣṭa vṛttis* (detrimental and nondetrimental states of mind) in Patañjali (I.5) or of the mind's potential to be either the friend or the enemy of the *yogī* in the *Gītā* (VI.6). Any *yoga* practice takes place in the mind. When the mind is used in ignorance of the true self (*Yoga Sūtras* II.4ff.) and dedicated to the pursuit of bodily and mental desire in the realm of *prakṛti*, rather than the quest for the *ātman* or *Īśvara*, it is detrimental, an obstacle, an enemy, because it is ignorance that perpetuates frustration, unfulfillment, *karma*, and hence *saṁsāra*. But when the functions of the same mind—the *vṛttis* of Patañjali, the object of its thought in the *Gītā*, or, in the present context, its *rāgas*—are directed to the goals of *yoga* of any stripe, the mind is transformed into a *yogic* one: "The wise say that this mind is the cause both of lower experience under the influence of the *guṇas*, as well as of higher existence, liberation, the state beyond the influence of the *guṇas*. If the mind is influenced by the *guṇas*, it leads the living beings to calamity. If it transcends the *guṇas*, it leads to liberation" (V.11.7–8). In other words, love of God, wisdom, discrimination, knowledge, enlightenment, and all or any other such *yogic* attainments refer to nothing other than states of the mind when the mind is manifesting its higher potentials—they are not states of *ātman* in the metaphysics of the *Bhāgavata*.

So, likewise, in the context of *bhakti*; when *rāga* is devotional—that is to say, when the mind is manifesting and channeling feelings of desire and love directed toward Kṛṣṇa, the ensuing state of mind is called *rāgānugā* (*Bhaktirasāmṛtasindhu* Eastern Quadrant II.272).[134] We can note that this is one major difference between classical *yoga* and *bhakti*: in generic *yoga* one essentially strives to suppress all states of mind completely (*citta-vṛtti-nirodhaḥ*, *Yoga Sūtras* I.2) and weaken their underlying impulses such as *rāga* (*kleśa-tanū-karaṇa* II.2). In *bhakti*, devotees have no interest in *nirodhaḥ*, suppressing the mind; *bhaktas* endeavor to fully activate the mind's states and impulses such as *rāga* but to channel them exclusively and entirely toward *Īśvara*.

As touched upon above, these feelings toward *Īśvara* take different forms: "I [Kṛṣṇa] am their intimate soul, the son, friend, teacher, well-wisher, and beloved Deity" (III.25.38).[135] Simply put, when Kṛṣṇa incarnates, He does so in a familial and social context, as we will see later from the tales of the tenth book. He is thus a son or brother to someone, a husband to someone else again, a friend to others, and so on. And *rāga* in the devotional context is a specific *bhakta*'s spontaneous desire to be Kṛṣṇa's servant or, for another, to be His friend or, for someone else again, to be His parent or lover, the intense attraction underpinning that specific relational mood. It is a desire for Kṛṣṇa molded into the specifics of a relationship unique to the *bhakta*.

Where *rāga* is a specific type of desire, *bhāva* is the mind-set that accommodates it—the mood, thoughts, feelings, and associations nurtured by that desire. A *bhāva* is natural, says Jīva, and unique to each individual "as a distinctive *bhāva* that reflects a *bhakta*'s sense of self" in terms of his or her unique personal relationship with Kṛṣṇa (*anu* 310).[136] These relationships will be discussed in the next section, but one's *bhāva* can be to consider oneself Kṛṣṇa's parent or friend or lover—to experience the convictions and emotions associated with this sense of self vis-à-vis Kṛṣṇa. It is an unbreakable conviction that Kṛṣṇa is one's very own intimate child, friend, and the like.

Bhāva is the first state of *prema*, which is a more intense level of love of God, the ultimate stage of *bhakti* itself: "When this *bhāva* takes on a very intense nature and is characterized by a sense of 'my-ness'[137] [a feeling of Kṛṣṇa belonging to onself], this stage is called *prema* by the wise" (*Bhaktirasāmṛtasindhu* Eastern Quadrant IV.1). This sense of "my-ness" reflects the unbreakable bond the *bhakta* has established with Kṛṣṇa. It is free of all the self-centered motives that we have discussed as "mixed" *bhakti* and hence wins over Viṣṇu (*Bhaktirasāmṛtasindhu* Eastern Quadrant IV.13). Just as the last three limbs (*aṅgas*) of Patañjali's *aṣṭāṅga* (eight-limbed) *yoga—dhāraṇā*, *dhyāna*, and *samādhi*—are simply deepening degrees on the same spectrum of concentrative focus (III.1–3), so *prema* is a more intense form of *bhāva*. According to Rūpa, "The progression in the manifestation of *prema*, love of God, for those engaging in *bhakti* is: first faith; then the association of saints; then acts of devotion; then the cessation of all obstacles;[138] then becoming fixed in practice; then *bhāva*;[139] then detachment; and then finally *prema* manifests" (*Bhaktirasāmṛtasindhu* Eastern Quadrant IV.15–16).

Additionally, although *bhāva* and *prema* appear in the mind—permeating it as fire permeates a metal bar—they are divine powers that are distinct from the mind (as fire is distinct from the bar) according to Gauḍīya theology. They are, in fact, bestowed by Kṛṣṇa as a gift from His own personal nature of pure bliss to His devoted *bhaktas*.[140] They are bestowed either as a result of devotional practice, *vaidhī bhakti* (*sādhana*), which is how they are most commonly attained, or, more rarely, for those who are fortunate, simply by the grace of the already perfected *bhaktas* or of Kṛṣṇa.[141] Already at the state of *bhāva,* the preliminary ecstatic symptoms of love in the form of tears and goose bumps begin to manifest,[142] and by the stage of *prema* a person's behavior is unpredictable and hard to comprehend;[143] we have seen in the example of Caitanya the degree of divine madness and the extremeness of the ecstatic bodily symptoms that the highest states of *prema* can wreak on the *bhakta*.

The reader will, at this point, perhaps be gaining some sense of the richness of the Gauḍīya analysis of the various stages and ingredients of love of God, which are excavated in far greater detail in the technical literature of the tradition, but we still do not yet have all the ingredients in hand to understand *rāgānugā bhakti.* We must briefly touch upon *rasa*—anyone interested in pursuing further advanced study in Kṛṣṇa *bhakti* will soon encounter the term (and it is the central term in the title of Rūpa's work *Bhakti-rasa-amṛta-sindhu*, *Ocean of the Nectar of the Experience of Bhakti*).[144] Rūpa describes *rasa* as follows: "When love for Kṛṣṇa has become a fixed state of mind, it becomes *bhakti rasa*. By hearing the stories of Kṛṣṇa, it generates a relishable taste in the heart of the *bhaktas*" (II.1.5). *Rasa* is the "taste" or actual experience of love itself. In other words, while all these terms overlap considerably, and are interdependent and coexistent, *rāga* is the specific desire to relate to Kṛṣṇa in a particular way, *bhāva* is the corresponding mind-set that accommodates and nurtures it, and *rasa* is the specific devotional taste or actual ecstatic experience of love in the heart that ensues from these. There are five primary *rasas* ensuing from what the tradition identifies as the five principal personal relationships a *bhakta* can have with God.[145] From these we have already encountered *dāsya*, servitorship, and *sakhya*, friendship, as the seventh and eighth of the nine processes of *vaidhī bhakti*. Now we will find them incorporated as the second and third of these five major *rasas*, the modes of interaction the *bhakta* can have with Kṛṣṇa.

The first of the five *rasas* discussed by Rūpa is *śānta*, peaceful. Here, the *bhakta* is attracted to "the form of *Īśvara*" but not to active participation in the *līlās* enjoyed in the other *rasas* discussed next (*Bhaktirasāmṛtasindhu* Western Quadrant I.6). There is no *yogamāyā* here, *śānta rasa* stems from awareness that Kṛṣṇa is the Supreme *Ātman* (*Parama-ātman*), so there is no sense of the "my-ness" found in the more intimate *rasas* that are devoid of any awareness of God's majesty, and there is no attitude that one is intimately bound to Kṛṣṇa through an active relationship. In other words, one finds one's complete existential fulfillment beholding the majesty of God, rather than thinking of God as "my son," "my friend," and so forth. Rūpa adds that "it is similar to the happiness found in the *ātman* by the *yogīs*, except that the happiness of the *ātman* is incomplete, and the happiness that is connected with *Iśvara* is complete. . . . Therefore, when the two eyes behold Kṛṣṇa's form, the minds of the great enlightened sages abandon the path of the impersonal *Brahman* [synonymous with *ātman*]" (*Bhaktirasāmṛtasindhu* Western Quadrant 1.5–8). So while this is a passive form of devotion, where the *bhakta* is fully content in the bliss of beholding a vision of the personal Godhead, it is nonetheless an experience that far surpasses the bliss of absorption in one's *ātman*, which is sometimes referred to as an experience of impersonal *Brahman* (as we will discuss in "The Object of *Bhakti*").

Rūpa makes another interesting comment here pertaining to one category of *yogī* cultivating *bhakti* through this *śānta bhāva*: "There are ascetics who are completely immersed in renunciation with an unshakable desire for liberation, and who perform worship to *Īśvara*, thinking: 'Liberation is attained without difficulty through *bhakti*' " (*Bhaktirasāmṛtasindhu* Western Quadrant I.15). In other words, for this category of *yogī*, *bhakti* is performed functionally in the motivated manner Jīva described as "devotion mixed with the desire for liberation"[146]—namely, to attain an experience of *ātman*/*Brahman* rather than to achieve unmotivated love of *Īśvara* or experience a relationship with Him. In other words, *Īśvara* is approached as a benefactor, but for an alternative goal, realization of one's *ātman*, not for the real goal of *rāgānugā bhakti*, which, as we know, is prema—love for *Īśvara* and nothing else, not even liberation itself. We will discuss this further, but here we can recall the role of *Īśvara* in the *Yoga Sūtras*: *samādhi siddhiḥ*, to bestow *samādhi* (experience of the *ātman*, II.45), and perhaps Rūpa, too, has this in mind. Nonetheless, even such *ātman*-seeking *yogīs* may be in for a surprise, as Kṛṣṇa Himself notes: "When I am obtained by a *yogī* who is in the state of *samādhi* (*ātman* absorption)[147] their bodies tremble [in ecstasy] by My *līlā*" (*Bhaktirasāmṛtasindhu* Western Quadrant I.36). Along the same lines, Rūpa notes that "when the great occasion of Hari's *līlā* was sung by Nārada on his *vīṇā* stringed instrument, trembling occurred in the body of sage Sanaka, even though Sanaka had attained absorption in *Brahman*" (*Bhaktirasāmṛtasindhu* Southern Quadrant V.19). This, according to another such *yogī* he quotes, is because "the intensity of that bliss that appeared in *samādhi* after all ignorance had been completely destroyed increased a millionfold when Kṛṣṇa, the Lord of the Yādavas, personally appeared to me"[148] (*Bhaktirasāmṛtasindhu* Western Quadrant 1.37). In comparison with this *Īśvara*-related bliss, "the long time spent in the bliss of the *ātman* seemed useless" (*Bhaktirasāmṛtasindhu* Western Quadrant 1.34). After seeing Kṛṣṇa's form, "the mind does not relish the inner *ātman* as it did before" (*Bhaktirasāmṛtasindhu* Western Quadrant I.40). In fact, "after discarding the experience of liberation . . . [the] mind longs to see the higher aspect of *Brahman* (*para-Brahman*,[149] beyond the *ātman*), which is that adorable Kṛṣṇa, who is as beautiful as a dark rain-cloud" (*Bhaktirasāmṛtasindhu* Southern Quadrant V.20). Ultimately, "for Kṛṣṇa *bhakti*, it is this vision of God that is the true goal of the eight-limbed *yoga*" (*Bhaktirasāmṛtasindhu* Western Quadrant 1.39); in comparison with this, the experience of the *ātman* pales into insignificance (*Bhaktirasāmṛtasindhu* Western Quadrant I.40).

We have dwelled at some length on the *śānta rasa*, as the reader will soon become well aware that one of the main subthemes of the *Bhāgavata* is this diminution of the goal of classical *yoga*, the experience of one's *ātman* (*mokṣa*/*mukti*/*kaivalya*/*nirvāṇa*[150]), namely, consciousness absorbed in its own nature,[151] in comparison with the bliss of any type of personal encounter, relationship, with Kṛṣṇa. The remaining four *rasas* express such personal relationships, each one consecutively increasing the level of bliss experienced by the *bhakta* immersed in that *rasa*.

The second *rasa* is *dāsya*, which we know from its occurrence as the seventh of the nine processes of *bhakti* is experienced by "those who identify themselves as the servants of Kṛṣṇa" (*Bhaktirasāmṛtasindhu* Western Quadrant II.5). What distinguishes this relationship vis-à-vis the three *rasas* that will follow is "knowledge of Kṛṣṇa's supreme majesty" (*Bhaktirasāmṛtasindhu* Western Quadrant II.16). *Yogamāyā* is less present here. But *dāsya*, in turn, differs from the previous first *rasa* in that *dāsya* is an active relationship rather than the passive one of *śānta*. The defining characteristic of *dāsya bhaktas* is that they consider themselves to be incredibly favored by Kṛṣṇa but nonetheless to be His inferiors (*Bhaktirasāmṛtasindhu* Southern Quadrant V.27). Rūpa identifies various categories of servants, from which, again in keeping with this main subtheme, we can mention those who formerly followed the path of *jñāna*, knowledge, seeking the experience of the *ātman*, but "renounced *mokṣa* after hearing about your sweetness from the saints" (*Bhaktirasāmṛtasindhu* Western Quadrant II.22). The servants are encountered in the selections in part 3 from the tenth book of the *Bhāgavata* exhibiting their devotion as Kṛṣṇa's attendants and personal servants, fully content with the ecstasy they experience from this relationship.

The third *rasa* is *sakhya*, friendship (again, these sequential positionings of Kṛṣṇa's *rasas* reflect the increasing intensity of *rasa*, love, experienced by the *bhakta*). Rūpa defines it as "the affection that exists between two people who are more or less equals; its nature is one of trust and an absence of respectful deference" (*Bhaktirasāmṛtasindhu* Western Quadrant III.105). This intimate sense of equality characterizes this *rasa*, contrasting it with the *rasa* of *dāsya*, where inferiority is felt by the *bhaktas* owing to awareness of Kṛṣṇa's majesty. *Sakhya* manifests in such things as laughing and joking (Southern Quadrant V.30). So here, as with the following two *rasas*, Kṛṣṇa conceals His majesty (through *yogamāyā*) and in this *rasa* assumes the role of an equal for those who choose to relate to Him in this way. In all of this, God, out of love, reciprocates with and conforms to the specific nature of the *bhaktas*' love for Him.

As with all the *rasas*, there are various subcategories of friendship—including that of Arjuna from the *Bhagavad Gītā*. From these varieties, the Vraj friends are preeminent: "The friends in Vraj, who always roam about with Kṛṣṇa and are miserable if they do not see Him even for a split second, devote their lives to Him alone. Therefore, they are considered the best among Kṛṣṇa's friends" (*Bhaktirasāmṛtasindhu* Western Quadrant III.16). Arjuna's friendship, while certainly intimate, is comparatively more formal and deferential, as can be gauged from the *Gītā* and *Mahābhārata*. We will encounter the *sakhya bhakti* of these most intimate of friends in Vraj in part 3.

The fourth *rasa* is *vātsalya*, parental. Since in this *rasa* Kṛṣṇa submits to accepting protection and support from His *bhaktas* who are in the roles of His parents or senior guardians and well-wishers, here, too, His majesty is even more concealed (*Bhaktirasāmṛtasindhu* Western Quadrant IV.5). Rūpa defines *vātsalya* as "that love, devoid of all awe and reverence, directed to Kṛṣṇa as one who needs sustenance by someone who provides sustenance" (*Bhaktirasāmṛtasindhu* Western Quadrant IV.52). Those who experience this *bhāva*, in addition to Kṛṣṇa's actual parents and foster parents, are the elderly cowherd-women and -men of Vraj as well as certain sages (*Bhaktirasāmṛta sindhu* Western Quadrant IV.10–11). As we will see in part 3, under the influence of *yogamāyā*, those in this *rasa* are fully convinced that Kṛṣṇa is dependent on their protection and support for His well-being, and it is this phenomenon of guardianship that characterizes *vātsalya*.

Finally, exhibiting the most intense expression of love, the fifth *rasa*, *madhura*, amorous, is also the most easily misunderstood. Rūpa defines it as "the pleasure exchanged between Kṛṣṇa and the fawn-eyed women" (*Bhaktirasāmṛtasindhu* Southern Quadrant V.36). The two major expressions of *madhura* are romantic love in separation from the beloved and love in union (*Bhaktirasāmṛtasindhu* Western Quadrant V.24). The tradition considers the love-stricken behaviors and maddened ramblings of the *gopīs* when their beloved disappears from their midst, examples of love in separation (*virāha bhakti*), to be a more heightened state of ecstatic love than when Kṛṣṇa appears and satisfies their amorous desires. The *gopī* chapters from part 3 portray some sense of the flavor of these modalities of *madhura*. And from all those whose love for Kṛṣṇa is expressed through this *rasa*, "the most excellent of Hari's beloveds is Rādhāraṇi, the daughter of King Vṛṣabhānu" (*Bhaktirasāmṛtasindhu* Western Quadrant V.7).

Although Rūpa acknowledges that the expressions of *madhura* are vast, and in fact dedicates a separate treatise, the *Ujjvalanīlamaṇi*, to this *rasa*, his treatment of it in the *Bhaktirasāmṛtasindhu* is curt. This is "because of its intimate nature, because it is difficult to comprehend, and because it is of no interest to those who are renounced [that is, who seek the *ātman*]" (*Bhaktirasāmṛtasindhu* Western Quadrant V.2). In terms of this last comment, Jīva' elaborates[152] that the *jñānīs* (*ātman*-seeking *yogīs*) who confound this *rasa* with mundane romance are uninterested in it, even though it is connected with *Bhagavān*. The roots of this difference in understanding between the Vaiṣṇavas and certain *ātman*-seeking *jñāna* traditions will become clearer in the chapter "The Object of *Bhakti*," which examines how *Īśvara* is conceived in the various traditions.

The misunderstanding of *madhura* in fact prevailed into the colonial era, but for different reasons, and it was to a great extent this aspect of the Kṛṣṇa tradition that caused the Kṛṣṇa of the *Bhāgavata Purāṇa* to be severely impugned and jettisoned in favor of the seemingly more righteous Kṛṣṇa of the *Bhagavad Gītā* in both colonial and Hindu apologetic neo-Vedantin moral discourses.[153] But of course *madhura* is divine love and has nothing to do with mundane eroticism (indeed, Rūpa, Jīva, and all the *Gosvāmīs* were celibate and highly orthodox renunciants).

Given the extensive nature of the subject and the parameters of our focus, we can do no more than briefly note here that almost all Kṛṣṇa worship in India is Rādhā-Kṛṣṇa worship, at least in the north, even as Rādhā, Kṛṣṇa's eternal consort in Gauḍīya theology, is not explicitly mentioned in the *Bhāgavata*. This worship is an enormously important feature absolutely central to the highest stages of Kṛṣṇa *bhakti*. Rather than attempting an inadequate or cursory treatment of this most intimate form of love of God, we follow Jīva and Rūpa's example in not covering this in a preliminary treatise on *bhakti* and in advising the reader to engage this topic in subsequent reading (for example, see Rūpa's *Ujjvalanīlamaṇi*).[154]

Rāgātmikā Bhakti

Jīva next introduces yet another related and overlapping concept indispensable for our purposes: *rāgātmikā*, the last ingredient we must discuss in order to understand *rāgānugā*, since *rāgānugā* is modeled on *rāgātmikā*. When the *bhāvas* and *rasas* discussed previously are exhibited by Kṛṣṇa's eternal family and associates in the divine Goloka (Kṛṣṇa's eternal *Brahman* abode beyond *prakṛti*), they are called *rāgātmikā bhakti*. *Rāgātmikā* means that the very nature of the spiritual mind[155] (*ātmika*) expresses a particular *rāga* for Kṛṣṇa; this *rāga* does not need to be cultivated through practice, as we will see is the case with *rāgānugā*; it is inherent. In other words, it is the specific *rāga* for Kṛṣṇa eternally present in His liberated associates living in Goloka. As we know, this *rāga* produces and sustains the corresponding natural *bhāva*, mood, such as friendship or parenthood, reflecting every *rāgātmika bhakta*'s unique, constant, and natural relationship with Kṛṣṇa. It is spontaneous and completely independent of rules and prescriptions (*vaidhī*) and thus, being natural, is not considered a practice (*sādhana*).[156] In Rūpa's words, "That form of *bhakti* when *rāga* is utterly absorbed naturally in the beloved is called *rāgātmikā*" (*Bhaktirasāmṛtasindhu* Eastern Quadrant II.272).

Rāgātmikā is also found in those *bhaktas* eligible to take their last birth in *prakṛti* prior to their attaining the eternal *Brahman* Goloka, which they do during Kṛṣṇa's incarnation as part of His entourage.[157] These *rāgātmikas* then participate in Kṛṣṇa's *līlā* when He incarnates. We should always keep in mind, when we read the Vṛndāvana (Vraj) section from the tenth book in part 3 of this volume, that the rustic illiterate cowherd folks among whom Kṛṣṇa appears during His incarnation did not just randomly end up being born by chance at the right time and place. They are all *rāgātmika bhaktas*. His simple-hearted mother, Yaśodā, His hardworking father, Nanda, His boisterous youthful *gopa* (male cowherd) companions and enamored *gopīs* (female cowherds)[158] are all highly accomplished *rāgātmikas* from previous lives: "What did Kṛṣṇa's father, Nanda, do to obtain such great fortune? And what did the greatly fortunate Yaśodā do, that Hari drank from her breast?" (X.8.46). What Nanda and Yaśodā in fact did in their previous lives in order to obtain the fortune of having Kṛṣṇa as their son, according to the *Bhāgavata*, was to devote themselves to intensely austere practices of *vaidhī bhakti*, including enduring extremes of temperature and subsisting only on leaves and air (X.3.2–8). It is as a result of this that "Nanda is the most fortunate person in the world of men; the sages who purify the worlds visit [his] house, because the Supreme *Brāhman* Himself, disguised by the characteristics of a human being, resides there" (VII.10.48). The cowherd boys who had the opportunity to roam about with Kṛṣṇa had "accumulated an abundance of merit" (X.12.11), and the *Bhāgavata* cannot even describe the penance that must have been performed previously by the queens of Dvārakā who were able to massage the feet of Kṛṣṇa as their spouse (X.90.27).

It is through remarkable previous-life *vaidhī yoga* practices that some *bhaktas* become eligible to take birth during Kṛṣṇa's incarnation, and the fruit of this previous practice is that their *rāga* at this point manifests spontaneously; "it is perfected" and arises "like the waves of the *Gaṅgā*" (*anu* 310). They too have attained the stage of *rāgātmikā bhakti*. Like the already eternally liberated souls in the *Brahman* realm of Goloka, those who are born in intimate proximity to Kṛṣṇa during His descent into the world also no longer need to perform practice, *sādhana*, and follow the rules of *vaidhī*, because their devotion has already attained the *sādhya*, the perfected goal of *sādhana*. Hence *rāgātmikā*—as well as *rāgānugā*, which conforms to it—does not come under the heading of *vaidhī bhakti*. But how specifically does *rāgānugā bhakti* differ from *rāgātmikā bhakti*?

The Development of *Rāgānugā Bhakti*

We now have all the pieces in place required to understand *rāgānugā bhakti*. *Rāgānugā* begins after a *bhakta*'s mind has been sufficiently purified of the *kleśas* (mental impurities, such as material desire) by the practice of *vaidhī bhakti*. At this point, he or she begins to develop a preliminary attraction for one of these *rāgas* exhibited by the *rāgātmika bhaktas* encountered in the narratives in part 3 from the tenth book of the *Bhāgavata*. It is the prequel to becoming a *rāgātmika* oneself, but a stage when the *bhakta* has not yet attained the eternally inherent, perfected, and exclusive love of the actual *rāgātmikas* in Goloka. It is an initial spontaneous attraction conforming to a particular *rāga*, but one that has not yet developed into the intense, all-consuming, uncontrollable love of the *rāgātmikas*. Let us quote Jīva directly here before discussing this further, as, unlike the nine processes of *bhakti*, this level of *bhakti* is inferred from, but not explicitly articulated in, the *Bhāgavata* itself:

> Now *rāgānugā* will be discussed. When an attraction for a specific type of *rāga* as discussed previously has arisen, but not the actual specific *rāga* itself, the mind becomes like a crystal, reflecting the rays of the moon of that *rāga*. By hearing from the sacred texts and teachers, an attraction arises for the behavior of that *rāgātmika* who has that same *rāga*. That attraction seeking that same *rāga* that manifests in the practitioner is *rāgānugā*. (*anu* 310)

Rāga-anuga literally means "conforming to" or "following" a *rāga*. As the crystal can "conform" or reflect the moon's rays, and so capture some of its rays, even though not containing the actual moon, so a *bhakta* accomplished in *vaidhī bhakti* begins to reflect the mood of the chosen *rāgātmika* to whom he or she is attracted, even as his or her own *rāga* in that mood is still preliminary and not yet fully developed. In Rūpa's words, "When devotion models itself on the *rāgātmikā bhakti* that radiates visibly through the residents of Vraj, it is known as *rāgānugā*" (*Bhaktirasāmṛtasindhu* II.270).

Rāgānugā thus is a preliminary stage where a particular *rāga*, a particular yearning to relate to Kṛṣṇa in a specific *bhāva*, mood—as a child, friend, lover, and so forth—has begun to stir in the heart of the *bhakta* that has been purified by *vaidhī bhakti*. What Jīva intends by "modeling itself on the *rāgātmika*" is that this fascination or stirring draws the *bhakta* to further and more deeply study and increasingly restudy the specific narratives associated with that particular *rāga*—that is, the relevant narratives in the tenth book of the *Bhāgavata* and its derivative literatures that feature the *rāgātmikas* who exhibit that *rāga*. The aspiring *bhaktas*' thoughts and moods start to conform to those of the favorite *rāgātmikas* in the narrative. These *rāgātmikas* thus become the exemplars that the *rāgānugā bhaktas* seek to emulate.[159]

So, for example, if one is intrigued by and drawn to Kṛṣṇa as a young boy in the mood of the *sakhya bhāva* of friendship, one will especially relish those specific narratives where Kṛṣṇa goes to the forest with His companions of the same age, frolicking and playing games, such as those we will find in the *līlās* of Kṛṣṇa with the cowherd boys in part 3. One never gets tired of reading these sections of the narrative but finds oneself becoming more and more enchanted with each reading and wondering about this or that detail. Now, within such narratives, the friends of Kṛṣṇa, who already have the full-blown eternal love for Kṛṣṇa in that *sakhya rāga,* are the *rāgātmikas*. They are *rāgātmikas* because their *rāga* is their very nature (*ātmika*). It is inherent, not something that needs to be further cultivated, as is the case with the *rāgānugās*. So they serve as the role models for the *rāgānugās*, the readers[160] who are beginning to experience a spontaneous attraction to these particular episodes and to feel an inclination to mold their own *bhāva* on these exemplars.

This principle is fairly standard even in conventional behavior: if one wishes to become, say, a popular singer, one will likely spend much time imitating and copying the songs of others who "have made it" in the particular style of music to which one is drawn and seek every detail about the life and behaviors of one's idols that one can possibly glean, before one develops one's own identity in that genre. So with *rāgānugā*:

> Those are eligible for *rāgānugā* who are eager to attain the *bhāva* of those residents of Vraj who are fixed exclusively in *rāgātmikā*. The sign of the emergence of that desire is that, when hearing the sweetness of that *bhāva*, the intelligence has no regard for the [prescriptions of] sacred texts or logic. However, one [whose devotion has not yet manifested sufficiently and hence who is more appropriately] eligible for *vaidhī bhakti* should follow the prescriptions of the sacred texts and also engage the type of logic that is favorable [to *bhakti*] until the *bhāva* manifests. (*Bhaktirasāmṛtasindhu* Eastern Quadrant II.291–93)

Vaidhī bhakti is weak compared with *rāgānugā*, says Jīva, as it is based on the prescriptions of the sacred texts, where *rāgānugā* is independent of rules and irresistible. Scriptural injunctions, says Jīva, are intended only for those who do not have natural attraction for *bhakti*. Prescriptions and regulations are there so as to at least somehow or other initiate some form of practice by training the mind in a way that gradually leads to it becoming absorbed in devotion; otherwise it is overwhelmed by the material disturbances (*kleśas*) endemic in embodied life. But they are not required for one who actually has *bhāva*, because such a person will naturally and spontaneously be absorbed in thoughts of the Beloved, irrespective of theological scriptural pronouncements and prescriptions: "Sages who are situated in the state beyond the *guṇas*, have desisted from rules and regulations and relish the qualities and stories of Hari" (II.1.7). In fact, we know that such spontaneous and irrepressible love transcends consideration or awareness of even who Kṛṣṇa is in the grand scheme of things: "Whether one knows or does not know who I am, or the nature or extent of My Being, if one worships Me with undivided *bhakti*, I consider that person to be the best of all *bhaktas*" (XI.11.33).

However, Jīva preemptively quickly adds that this type of spontaneous devotion is very rare, and if one imagines oneself out of conceit (or, worse, nefarious motives) to have attained this as an excuse for disregarding scriptural injunctions, then one is simply deluding oneself and others out of foolish pride. Indeed, to minimize the possibility of being exploited by charlatans posing as *rāgānugā bhaktas* so as to transgress moral social norms or befool the public, Jīva recommends real *rāgānugā bhaktas* to nonetheless combine their spontaneous unrestrained devotion with *vaidhī* prescriptions and practices so as to set an example for others, even if they themselves have transcended the need for *vaidhī* (*anu* 132).

We are reminded here of a parallel situation in the *Gītā*, but there in the context of following duty and social prescriptions (*dharma*). Kṛṣṇa tells Arjuna that even though it is true that "for a person who delights in the *ātman*, is satisfied in the *ātman*, and is content in the *ātman*, there is no *dharma*," by the same token, even as "there is no gain to be had from performing work, there is also no gain to be had from not performing work" (IX.17–18). Therefore, he recommends that Arjuna "should perform work to uphold the social order . . . as whatever acts a great person does, people will follow" (IX.20–21). Even He Himself acts, says Kṛṣṇa, despite being the supreme unrestrained Lord, otherwise people would try to imitate His example (IX.22–23). Very relevant here, too, is Patañjali's (unusually) emphatic assertion that there are absolutely no exceptions to the following of the *yama* moral obligations, predicated on neither birth, time, place, nor circumstance of any sort (such as level of spiritual attainment).[161] Thus, any aspiring *yogī* approaching a *guru* figure who claims to have transcended the need for moral codes in the name of some higher esoteric spirituality should know that such claims are not in line with the classical *yoga*, Vedānta, *jñāna*, Vaiṣṇava, Śaivite, or *Bhāgavata* traditions (or, indeed, any Indic tradition, including Buddhism, Jainism, and right-handed Tantra[162]).

To conclude this section, then, the prescriptions of the sacred texts, including those of *vaidhī bhakti*, are designed to train the mind of the aspiring *bhakta* toward an increasing absorption on Kṛṣṇa—specifically, on His names, forms, qualities, and pastimes. When Kṛṣṇa sees the sincerity of the practitioner, He cleanses the mind of all impurities—such as the *kleśas*, ignorance, ego, *rāga* for sensual indulgences, and so on (*Yoga Sūtras* II.3ff.). As the mind becomes pure, it loses its *rāgas* for the sense objects of *prakṛti* and begins to replace these with the beginnings of a particular *rāga* for

Kṛṣṇa. This *rāga* can take various forms—an attraction to Kṛṣṇa as a master, child, friend, or lover, the five *bhāvas*, or *rasas*. As this *rāga* deepens, one becomes drawn to the liberated *rāgātmika bhaktas* who spontaneously embody this particular *rāga* with their entire being in their intimate interactions with Kṛṣṇa during His *līlās*. One encounters such *rāgātmikas* within the texts that record and depict them—with the *Bhāgavata's* tenth book as canonical and paramount in this regard. Through study and instruction on the *Bhāgavata Purāṇa*, one strives to enter deeper and deeper into the *bhāva*, mood, of this role model *rāgātmika*, spontaneously modeling ("conforming," *anuga*) one's own thoughts upon his or hers. This practice is natural rather than prescribed (and therefore, in a sense, if not artificial, somewhat forced), as is the case with *vaidhī*. This is *rāgānugā bhakti*, the goal of Kṛṣṇa *bhakti* as a *yoga* process prior to liberation, but the penultimate goal of *bhakti* itself. The ultimate grand-finale stage is to oneself attain a role as a *rāgātmika* in Kṛṣṇa's divine *Brahman* realm of Goloka (or as a *rāgātmika bhakta* during Kṛṣṇa's next incarnation in *prakṛti*, and then, after that last birth, continuing that *rāgātmikā bhakti* for all eternity in Goloka). For this, as will be discussed further, one is endowed with a divine *Brahman* body and mind bestowed by Kṛṣṇa upon shedding the *prakṛtic* body (for example, see I.6.28 and IV.12.29) that can facilitate that requisite *bhāva*.

Pertinent to all this, in *Bhāgavata* theology, it is the *bhakta* who chooses the *bhāva* toward *Īśvara* corresponding to his or her desire and preferences. There is free will here.[163] In the *Gītā*, Kṛṣṇa states that "in whatever way people resort to Me, I reciprocate in that way" (IV.11). As always, the *Bhāgavata* is a bit more expansive and visual in exemplifying this:

> Kṛṣṇa went to the arena with his elder brother. He was perceived by the wrestlers as a lightning bolt; by men as the best of men; by the women as Kāma (Cupid) personified; by the *gopas* as their relative; by the unrighteous rulers of the earth as the chastiser; by His mother and father as a child; by Kaṁsa, the king of the Bhojas, as death; by the ignorant as the manifest universe; by the *yogīs* as the Supreme Truth; and by the Vṛṣṇi clan as the Supreme Divinity. (X.43.14)

While ultimately *bhāva* is bestowed by Kṛṣṇa (Eastern Quadrant III.4), it reflects the free will of the *bhakta*. For those who have attained the stage of *rāgānugā*, Kṛṣṇa is just as keen to reciprocate and serve His *bhaktas* as they are to offer their loving service to Him. Love involves reciprocal submission and service between individuals: it cannot be unidirectional. As we will see in the *līlā* stories in part 3, even though supremely independent, and even though He is *svarati*, one whose pleasure is self-contained and needs no external stimulus (X.33.23), Kṛṣṇa relishes submitting to His beloved devotees: "The quality of submission to His devotee was demonstrated by Hari, despite the fact that He is only constrained by His own free will" (X.919). "He becomes subservient to His servants such as the Pāṇḍavas, acting as friend, messenger, and guard," says Jīva (*anu* 327).

Meditation in Hate and Lust

Those familiar with the *Yoga Sūtras* will recall that *rāga*, desire, the third of the five *kleśas*, obstacles to *yoga*, has a flip side: *dveṣa*, aversion, the fourth *kleśa* (II.3–8). Indeed, the mechanisms underpinning these two *kleśas* are identical. In the *Bhakti Sandarbha*, Jīva discusses an interesting counterpart to being spontaneously absorbed in adoring thoughts of Kṛṣṇa's attractive qualities: one can obsessively despise Him and still attain liberation. The *Bhāgavata* makes a point of stressing that one does not even need to be favorably devoted to Kṛṣṇa, as long as the mind is intent upon Him. In other words, *dveṣa* can be directed toward Kṛṣṇa, just as *rāga* can. Our discussion on this is followed by point of contrast with some further comments on *rāga* directed toward Kṛṣṇa, but in this case *rāga* that stems from sensual lust for personal sexual gratification. And this, in turn, is compared with the *rāgānugā* of the *gopīs* touched upon above.

Meditating in Enmity: Kṛṣṇa and the Demons

The *Bhāgavata* highlights in numerous narratives that even adversaries and demons (*asuras*) out to kill Kṛṣṇa attain liberation, simply by dint of their minds being absorbed in Him, albeit in psychopathic hatred: "Even [the demoness] Pūtanā, in the guise of a good person, attained You, O God" (X.14.35, X.6.35). Since she was a devourer of infants who attempted to murder Kṛṣṇa, "it is astonishing that the wicked Pūtanā attained the destination of Kṛṣṇa's mothers, even though she offered Kṛṣṇa her breast smeared with poison desiring to kill Him. Who else is more merciful than He?" (III.2.23). We will see in part 3 that when the serpent demon Agha was killed, "an amazing great light rose up from the thick coils of the snake, illuminating the ten directions with its splendor. It waited in the sky for the Lord to emerge, and then entered into Him before the very eyes of the residents of the celestial realms" (X.12.33). This type of liberation[164] is attained by all the demons such as Śiśupāla (X.74.45) and Dantavakra (X.78.9–10), who "could not tolerate Kṛṣṇa from the time they began babbling as babies!" Kṛṣṇa's mortal enemy Pauṇḍraka, like the demon king Kaṁsa, had his bondage destroyed "through his unceasing meditation on *Bhagavān*." He was awarded liberation, because "even Kṛṣṇa's sworn enemies attain the highest destination" (X.66.24, X.87.23).[165]

King Yudhiṣṭhira asks Nārada how all this can possibly be so—how, rather than being cast into hell, can Kṛṣṇa's murderous enemies attain a destination even the saintly *jñāna yogīs* who seek their *ātman* do not achieve? The sage replies that Kṛṣṇa cannot be touched by anger. Anger, as Patañjali tells us, stems from ignorance of the true self (*Yoga Sūtras* II.12)—that is, from misidentifying with the temporal *prakṛtic* coverings of body and mind. Clearly *Īśvara*, the Supreme *Ātman*, is not subject to ignorance.[166] Therefore, everything *Īśvara* does is for the ultimate welfare of His creation and not out of the *kleśas*—ignorance and its by-products, such as anger and revenge (*dveṣa*). Demons (*asuras*) too are nothing other than *ātmans* temporarily covered by inordinately dense *tamas* and *rajas* due to past misdeeds. But beneath those layers they are also *Īśvara*'s *aṁśas* (parts) and eligible to burn up their afflicted *karma* and attain liberation like any other embodied being. And anyone, friend or foe, coming in contact with Kṛṣṇa becomes purified.

But for our purposes of understanding the mechanics of *bhakti* as a *yoga* process, from a *samādhi* point of view, Kṛṣṇa's enemies may have been unconventionally devoted—devoted to killing Kṛṣṇa—but this is still a mental absorption so intense that it was nonetheless a type of undeviating concentration on *Īśvara*. Patañjali defines *samādhi* as "when only the object of meditation shines forth alone, and [the mind] is devoid of its own [reflective nature]"

(III.3). Put differently, when one is not aware of anything other than the object of meditation in conventional *samādhi*, then that object constitutes one's universe.[167] Consider, in this light, Kṛṣṇa's archenemy: "Whether sitting, resting, eating, or moving about the land, Kaṁsa thought of Kṛṣṇa. He saw the whole universe pervaded by Kṛṣṇa" (X.1.24). For the *Bhāgavata*, this qualifies as an expression of *samādhi*—after all, in order to attain *samādhi*, Patañjali allows that one can fix the mind on anything, *yathābhimatā-dhyānād vā* (I.39), as long as it is undeviating. In fact, says sage Nārada, these adversaries' fear and hatred may sometimes translate into an even deeper state of *samādhi* than that of the pious *bhaktas*: "Just as an insect, trapped in a pot by a wasp, and thinking of him in anger and fear, attains the same form as the wasp [in the next life]."[168]

Of course, Jīva (and Rūpa) hasten to note that despite the liberation awarded to Kṛṣṇa's adversaries, their type of meditation is not considered part of the *Bhāgavata dharma*. Obviously *bhakti yoga* promotes a loving intentionality as that underpinning the mind's absorption in *Īśvara*. And needless to say, if those inimical to Kṛṣṇa are involuntarily liberated just by coming into contact with Him, irrespective of their motives, then "what to speak of those who offer something of highest value to Kṛṣṇa, the Supreme Soul, with faith and devotion like His mothers did?!" (X.6.36). Put more elaborately: "[The adversarial] kings, thinking in enmity of Kṛṣṇa's gait, appearance, and eye movements, while sleeping, sitting, and engaging in other acts, had their minds molded by Him, and so attained oneness with Him—what then to speak of[169] those whose minds are full of love for Him?!" (XI.5.48).

The following passage sums up the psychological principles involved here:

> One should fix one's mind on Govinda [Kṛṣṇa] and not think of anything else, whether out of enmity, friendship, goodwill, fear, affection, or lust. . . . [His] enemies had their sins cleansed from thinking of Kṛṣṇa, who is *Īśvara*, *Bhagavān*, and has taken the form of a human through his *māyā* potency. Many have attained His abode after becoming freed from sin and absorbing their mind in *Īśvara* out of desire, enmity, fear, affection, or *bhakti*: the *gopīs* out of desire, Kaṁsa out

of fear, the king of the Cedis out of enmity, the Vṛṣṇi clan out of friendship, you [Pāṇḍavas] through friendship, and we [Nārada and others] through *bhakti*." (VII.1.25–30)

Anything coming into contact with *Īśvara* even mentally becomes purified, just as anyone contacting electricity becomes electrified, irrespective of who that person is or what his or her motive might be: "Kṛṣṇa bestows the devotional path [to one who even] once internalizes a mental image of Kṛṣṇa's body" (X.12.39); "By meditating on, hearing, and reciting Your name, by worshipping and remembering you, even a dog-eater from anywhere is made fit to perform the *soma* ritual pressing;[170] what then to speak of one who has had a direct vision of You, O *Bhagavān*?" (III.33.17). As Kṛṣṇa is supreme purity, nothing in contact with Him can remain impure.

Meditating in Passion: Kṛṣṇa and the *Gopīs*

Jīva then proceeds to engage the very same principles in considering the amorous desire that the *gopīs*, Kṛṣṇa's adoring cowherd maidens, directed toward their beloved (*anu* 320), which we will encounter in their narrative in part 3. Isn't their attitude a *rāga*, the flip side of *dveṣa*, enmity/aversion from Patañjali's five *kleśas*, obstacles to *yoga*? The *gopīs' rāga* is rather different from the *dveṣa* of Kṛṣṇa's adversaries, as, in Jīva's opinion, unlike the latter, they had no self-interest in their undeviating absorption on Kṛṣṇa, even as they are attracted to Kṛṣṇa as a gorgeous male. We will return to the *gopīs* in a moment. Perhaps the ointment maker Kubjā, who unabashedly solicits Kṛṣṇa when the latter enters the capital city, Mathurā, is a better counterexample of the *dveṣa*, aversion, phenomenon of Kṛṣṇa's enemies, as her intentions are clearly lusty and geared toward her own sensual impulse: "Kubjā pulled the end of Kṛṣṇa's outer garment and spoke to Him smiling. Kāma (Cupid) had awakened in her heart: 'Come, hero, I am unable to leave you here—let us go home! You are the best of men; oblige a woman whose mind has been aroused by You!' " (X.42.9–10). Kṛṣṇa obliges because of her simple act of devotion in offering Him her choicest perfumes. Thus, while her intentions were not selfless as Jīva considers those of the *gopīs* to be, nonetheless, because Kubjā's *rāga* was directed toward *Īśvara*, rather than some object of *prakṛti*, she attained the highest goal of life, and in this represents the flip side of the *dveṣa* principles of Kṛṣṇa's adversaries outlined above.

The *rāga* of the *gopīs*, in contrast, is heralded in Kṛṣṇa *bhakti* as the highest, purest expression of simple and unrefined, selfless love. While it was love reflected through an amorous or conjugal *bhāva*, it was centered on abandoning all personal considerations for Kṛṣṇa's satisfaction: "We gently place Your tender lotus feet on our rough breasts with trepidation. You wander in the forest on them and our minds are disturbed: What if they have been hurt by small stones? Your Lordship is our life" (I.31.19). Kṛṣṇa Himself appears stumped by the purity of their love: "You have broken the enduring shackles of the household, and have served Me. You are full of goodness and without fault, and I am unable to reciprocate. . . . Therefore, let your reward be your own excellence" (X.32.22). Love for anything other than *Īśvara* simply "shackles" one to the institutions of *saṁsāra* such as the household, where love for Kṛṣṇa liberates one and entitles one to attain the divine realm of Vaikuṇṭha/Goloka. And of all those who love Kṛṣṇa, the illiterate simple-minded *gopīs* are deemed the topmost *bhaktas* in the *Bhāgavata*.

One passage is worth quoting at length in this regard for the insights it expresses with regard to the unsurpassed *bhāva* of these female *rāgātmikās*:

> When Uddhava saw how moved the *gopīs* were in their preoccupation with Kṛṣṇa, he was extremely pleased. Paying homage to them, he spoke as follows: "These *gopī* women are the highest embodied beings on the earth: their love for Govinda [Kṛṣṇa], the soul of everything, is perfected. Those who are fearful of the material world aspire to this, and so do the sages, as do we ourselves. What is the use of births as Brahmā [the highest celestial being], for one who has a taste for the infinite stories [of Kṛṣṇa]? On the one hand, these women are forest dwellers tainted by deviant behaviors, yet, on the other, they have developed a love for Kṛṣṇa, the soul of everything. Truly, the Lord personally bestows blessings on the person who worships Him even if that person is not learned. . . . He bestowed His favor on the beloved women of Vraj, who were accorded the honor of having their necks

embraced by his long arms. Such favor was not bestowed on the most loving Śrī, the Goddess of Fortune, who [resides] on His chest, nor on the celestial women, who have the beauty and the scent of lotuses—not to mention other women. *Aho!* May I become any of the shrubs, creepers, or plants in Vṛndāvana that enjoy the dust of the feet of these women. They have renounced their own relatives, which are so hard to give up, as well as the Āryan code of conduct,[171] and worshipped the feet of Mukunda [Kṛṇṣa], the sought-for goal of the sacred texts of revelation." (X.47.58–61)

And once again, let us not forget, when we contemplate who it is that takes birth as a female who gets to experience intimate association with Kṛṣṇa, that "how can one describe the penance [they must have performed in previous lives]?" (X.90.27). Jīva quotes the *Kūrma Purāṇa* here: "The sons of Agni [in a previous life], great souls, attained a female form [as *gopīs*] through great austerity (*tapas*), and thereby Kṛṣṇa, the son of Vāsudeva, the unborn, all-pervading source of the universe, as their husband."[172] In fact, the text presents the *gopīs* as the most accomplished beings in the entire universe.[173] It is essential to note that the *rāga* one develops toward Kṛṣṇa has nothing to do with one's temporary gendered embodiment in any particular birth: it transcends the sexual orientations of any temporal body or mind-set, which changes from birth to birth. Males too can be drawn to an amorous physical *rāga* toward Kṛṣṇa. Rūpa quotes a verse in the *Padma Purāṇa* similar to the reference in the *Kūrma Purāṇa* noted above, but here about other sages in the Daṇḍaka forest from a previous age mentioned in the *Rāmāyaṇa*, who became enamored with Rāma, a previous incarnation, and so in a subsequent birth they too took birth in Vṛndāvana as *gopīs*.[174]

This brings us to the topic of our next section. How does one become a *bhakta* of one sort or another to begin with? We have seen some of the various permutations that *bhakti yoga* can take—what are some of the characteristics of the various categories of *bhakta*?

The Practitioner of *Bhakti*, the *Bhakta*

The First Step in *Bhakti*: Association with a *Bhakta*

We now turn our attention to the *bhakta* as the performer of *bhakti*. One of the first questions Jīva raises in this regard in the *Bhakti Sandarbha* is: How does one become a *bhakta*? Put differently, if a *bhakta* is one who performs *bhakti yoga* out of devotion for *Īśvara*, then how is the initial devotional attraction, *rāga*, to *Īśvara* prompting a *yogī* to initially take up the path of *bhakti* developed in the first place? While, as we know, this *rāga* toward *Īśvara* is the cause of liberation and has nothing to do with the mundane attachments to the temporal personages or objects of *prakṛti*, it is still a *rāga*—a *saṁskāra*, or "mental imprint," of something pleasing to the mind. Thus, although we are dealing with a unique sort of *rāga*, the psychological metaphysics and mechanisms are the same: whether mundane or devotional, *saṁskāras* do not self-manifest; they enter into the *citta* from external sense impressions, and *bhakti* is no different. So from where do the very first external impressions originate to then enter the mind to eventually form *saṁskāras* of *rāga* for *Īśvara*?

Jīva notes that some souls are already born with the *saṁskāras* of *bhakti* that were cultivated in a past life (see *Gītā* VI.37–47 for an exposition on this and the Tale of King Bharata in part 2 for a narrative example). These *saṁskāras* are triggered in the subsequent life when coming in contact with a *bhakti* environment, at which time such persons appear to be endowed with a natural or spontaneous attraction to *bhakti*; but this is, in fact, an attraction born of the reactivation of past-life *saṁskāras*. For such rare souls "who are already eager to hear, *Īśvara* is immediately captured" (I.1.2). Such individuals do not necessarily need a *bhakti yoga* path since their devotion appears spontaneous. But even then, the same question remains here, too: From where did the original seed of *bhakti* in some past life first originate?

For most, *bhakti* needs to be cultivated, requiring conscious and determined work owing to the presence of mundane desire and other spiritual defects that occupy and dominate the mind. We can locate the vast majority of *bhaktas* in this category given that even Prahlāda, one of the great *mahājana* (exemplar) devotees of all time,[1] who will be encountered in part 2, laments: "O Viṣṇu, Lord of Vaikuṇṭha, my mind does not take pleasure in narratives about You: it is completely corrupt, impious, agitated, overwhelmed by lust, and tormented by joy, sorrow, fear, and desire. How then, with such a mind, can a wretch like me contemplate your nature?" (VII.9.39). It is for those with minds like this whose attraction is not spontaneous that a process is required; hence the efforts of theologians such as Jīva and Rūpa in composing voluminous literature outlining the path of *bhakti yoga*. But the question still remains: Whether in this or a past life, whether spontaneously or cultivated, how is anyone inspired to take up the process at all in the first instance? Whence the very first *saṁskāra* of attraction?

For the majority of newcomers to the path of *bhakti*, this first impulse is due to the grace of a *bhakta*, also known as a *bhāgavata*, an advanced practitioner of *bhakti*, who plants a deep seed of *bhakti* in the disciple's mind, which overwhelms it. (The term *bhāgavata* refers both to the *Bhāgavata Purāṇa* as text and to the practitioner of its contents, that is, the devotee of *Bhagavān*; the former is differentiated from the latter herein by a capital letter.) At the beginning of the *Bhāgavata* (I.2.16–22), the sage Sūta outlines (what Jīva identifies as) the basic five-step process through which this beginning seed of *bhakti* is first attained and then cultivated—in other words, the method by which one typically becomes a *bhakta*. This sequence perhaps functions as a sort of minipreview of the role that the *Bhāgavata* itself is attempting to accomplish as its own raison d'être, which is precisely this planting of the seeds of *bhakti*.

First: "Attraction to the stories of Vāsudeva (Kṛṣṇa) develops for one who is faithful and desires to hear by means of service to the sages and assisting great saints" (I.2.16). The seed of *bhakti* is attained by associating with those who already have that seed. Here, Jīva points to the importance of holy places in Hinduism, as sages and saints—*bhaktas*—congregate in those sacred environments that are reminiscent of their beloved deity and thereby supportive of their meditative practices (as is still the case today), such as Kṛṣṇa's childhood home, Vṛndāvana. And *bhaktas*, says Jīva, naturally discuss their beloved *Īśvara* among themselves (*anu* 11):

> In that place where there are *bhāgavata* devotees, O king, who are saints with pure hearts and minds eagerly hearing and reciting the narratives and qualities of *Bhagavān*, there, rivers of the nectar of narrations about Viṣṇu recited by the great souls flow everywhere. Those who imbibe these narrations with inundated ears without getting satiated, O king, are never affected by illusion, sorrow, fear, or hunger. (IV.29.39–40)

Holy places thus provide a locus where *bhaktas* can be encountered, and it is by associating with such persons, hearing from them, admiring their character and devotion, and assisting them in their service to *Īśvara* that one's own very first seed of *bhakti* is born: "From association with saints, realization of My power arises. Then, these narratives of My activities become pleasing to the ears and the heart. By enjoying them, faith, love, and devotion quickly manifest consecutively on the path to liberation" (III.25.25). Thus the association of *bhaktas* is, in essence, nothing other than *śravaṇa*, hearing, the first of the nine processes of *bhakti*: "Among such souls, discussions of the qualities of Viṣṇu are relished and mundane topics avoided. By cultivating these discussions daily, the pure mind of the seeker of liberation becomes inclined toward Vāsudeva [Kṛṣṇa]" (V.12.13). One's first step to becoming a *bhakta*, then, is through fellowship with other *bhaktas*.

As a result of this association, in the next step, the *kleśas*, impediments to *yoga*, such as ignorance, ego, desire, and so on, are purified, as they must be cleared from the mind for higher Truths to manifest therein. This is the case with all *yoga* practice—for instance, the *kriyā yoga* practice of the *Yoga Sūtras*, performed "to weaken the *kleśas* so as to bring about *samādhi*" (II.1–2ff.). *Bhakti* is no different (in the chapter "Definition of *Bhakti*," we noted that the removal of the *kleśas* is one of the six accompanying qualities of *bhakti* identified by Rūpa), and Jīva here situates this process as the second step in attaining the seed of *bhakti*. It is the following of the practices of *bhakti* that removes the impediments to the actual manifestation of *bhakti* itself: "Just as gold, when heated by fire, relinquishes its impurities and attains again its original nature, so the mind, through the performance of *bhakti yoga*, is purified of its accumulation of *karma* and attains to Me" (XI.14.25). As throughout the *Gītā*,[2] and hinted at in the *Yoga Sūtras*,[3] such purification is gained by grace: "To those who hear His narratives, Kṛṣṇa, who is the friend of the truthful and is situated within the heart, cleanses inauspicious things. Hearing about Him and performing His *kīrtana* are purifying" (I.2.17).[4] The aspirant is at this stage deepening the process of becoming a *bhakta* in his or her own right.

As a consequence of purification, the third step, the dawning of *bhakti*, can then ensue: "When almost all inauspicious things are destroyed by means of constant service to the *bhāgavatas*, then unshakable *bhakti* for *Bhagavān*, who is praised in the best of verses, manifests" (I.2.18). The word "almost" here indicates that *bhakti* appears even while there are still traces of ignorance and *prakṛti*-related desires, says Jīva (*anu* 13).[5] In the fourth step, after all desires have been completely destroyed, "then the mind, situated in *sattva* and not being agitated by states of *rajas* and *tamas*—lust, greed, and so on—becomes content" (I.2.19). In *bhakti*, when the mind becomes joyful by the practices, it automatically abandons lust, simply by dint of a higher taste (*Gītā* II.59). Experiencing the bliss of *bhakti*, one's status and self-identification as a *bhakta* have now pervaded deep into one's very being. The practitioner's mind in this penultimate step is in a state of pure *sattva* and "becomes qualified for direct experience (*sākṣātkāra*) into the nature of *Bhagavān*" (*anu* 16).

Finally, in the fifth step, this actual direct encounter with *Īśvara* can take place, and any residual imperfection at this point is completely destroyed. As with the *mokṣa* traditions in general,[6] the claim here is experience: "Direct realization of the Truth of *Bhagavān*[7] manifests for one whose mind is content and who is free from attachment through the practice of *bhakti yoga* in this way. When *Īśvara* is seen (*dṛṣṭa*) within oneself, the knot [of ego] in the heart is broken, all doubts are destroyed, and *karma* is weakened for that person" (I.2.20–21). The practitioner's status as a *bhakta* can now never be shaken or compromised. We need to stress again that this "direct experience" of *Īśvara* is visual (although *Īśvara* can also manifest sonically and in other ways, as we discussed). The ultimate cherished goal of the *bhakta* is a "vision" of God—the personal God with form and qualities discussed previously. This vision can manifest within the "heart" of the practitioner, or externally to the senses, as we will see in the Tale of Prince Dhruva:

> Viṣṇu, on account of the intensity of Dhruva's mature *yoga* practice, appeared in the lotus of Dhruva's heart, effulgent as lightning. After this, Dhruva observed that He suddenly disappeared. [Opening his eyes,] Dhruva then saw Him standing outside in the same position. Seeing that vision, Dhruva was thrown into confusion. He prostrated his body on the ground like a stick[8] and offered obeisances. Beholding Lord Viṣṇu, the boy was as if drinking Him with his eyes, kissing Him with his mouth, and embracing Him with his arms. (IV.9.1–2)

The "lotus of Dhruva's heart" refers to the mind: the heart has been identified as the locus of both the *citta* and the *ātman* since the Upaniṣads.[9] Since the mind, *citta,* is external to consciousness, *Īśvara*'s form can manifest in the mind, subtle *prakṛti*, just as it can manifest in gross *prakṛti*. Both layerings of *prakṛti* are in fact external to consciousness itself, even as one appears to be "internal" and one "external" from the perspective of the sensual apparatus of the physical eyes (see *Yoga Sūtras* III.7–8). We have discussed how such visions can deepen into witnessing not just Kṛṣṇa's form and qualities, but His active pastimes (*līlā*) and the possibility of eventually personally participating in them for all eternity in the liberated state. The spiritual (*Brahman*) body and mind required for this will be discussed later.

Returning to the five consecutive stages of *bhakti*, Jīva recognizes that until direct experience transpires, there cannot be complete and utter freedom from doubt (*anu* 16).[10] One risks the danger of fanaticism if one does not entertain some level of doubt about that which one has not experienced. But after direct experience, doubt evaporates and there is nothing left to do but remain immersed in the bliss of continued *bhakti*: "After *Īśvara* is seen within oneself, the poet-sages always engage in great ecstasy in *bhakti* for *Bhagavān* Vāsudeva, which satisfies the mind" (I.2.21–22). In any event, for our present purposes, in answer to the question we initially raised, the first seed of *bhakti*, which eventually culminates in the fruit of this type of direct experience of *Īśvara* and subsequent immersion in the bliss of a *bhakti* relationship with Him—in other words, the process of becoming a *bhakta*—is triggered by an initial encounter with an advanced *bhakta* or *bhaktas*. This is repeatedly stressed throughout the *Bhāgavata*: "Someone wandering [in the cycle of *saṁsāra*] who encounters a holy person, O Kṛṣṇa, attains the end of material existence. Such an encounter allows an inclination to take root toward You" (X.51.54).[11]

Such encounters reflect the compassion of advanced *bhaktas* who, rather than enjoying their ecstasies in seclusion, make themselves available: "Auspicious devotees of Kṛṣṇa wander around out of compassion for those unrighteous and very miserable people who, out of misfortune, have become averse to Kṛṣṇa" (III.5.3). As with the Buddhist *Bodhisattva* tradition, some sages, such as child Prahlāda, even renounce their own liberation so as to help others in their spiritual quest: "Often, O God, sages, desirous of their own liberation, cultivate silence in a solitary place; they are not concerned with the welfare of others. But I have no desire for liberation for myself alone, abandoning these unfortunate souls. Other than You, I see no other refuge for one wandering [in *saṁsāra*]" (VII.9.44).

In sum, the role of the *bhaktas* in the planting of the first seeds of *bhakti* in others is indispensable. Kṛṣṇa informs Uddhava that "neither the practice of *yoga*, nor the study of Sāṅkhya, nor the pursuit of *dharma*, nor study of sacred texts (*svādhyāya*), nor austerities (*tapas*) and renunciation, nor ritualistic performances, nor charity, nor vows, nor sacrificial hymns, nor visiting holy places, nor the moral abstentions and observances (*yama* and *niyama*) attract

Me as much as the association of saints" (XI.12.1–2). As mentioned, the reason for this is that *bhaktas* are constantly immersed in meditating on the activities and qualities of *Īśvara*:

> Narrations about Me are always taking place among those greatly blessed souls, and these narrations purify the vices of those who hear them. Those who attentively hear them, recite them, and delight in them, holding Me as their Lord with faith, attain love for Me. I am *Brahman* of unlimited qualities, and My nature is blissful experience. What else is there to be desired for those saints who have attained *bhakti* for Me? Just as cold, fear, and darkness are dispelled for one taking shelter of fire, so it is with service to the saints. (XI.26.28–31)

The tale of the genesis of his own spiritual journey is recounted by sage Nārada in part 2, and exemplifies how one who became the greatest *bhakta* of all[12] began his devotional journey by dint of the fact that his mother was a maidservant to a community of sages. This afforded the young Nārada the opportunity to hear from and serve these great souls:

> Permitted by the sages to eat the remnants of their food, I partook of it once daily, and from this all my sins were destroyed.[13] Engaged in this manner, with purified mind, a personal interest in their religion developed firmly in me. From this, by their kindness, I went on listening to the captivating narrations of Kṛṣṇa's pastimes that were recited by them. Listening attentively to every word of those narrations with faith, an attraction arose in me for Kṛṣṇa. Hearing about Him is so pleasing to the heart, O great sages! Then, once I had developed this attraction, my mind became firmly fixed in Kṛṣṇa. Narrations about Him are so relishable. As a result, I could perceive that due to my illusion, this gross and subtle reality had been imagined to be in me, whereas I am actually the Supreme *Brahman*. (I.5.25–27)

In fact, the entire *Bhāgavata* text is spoken under this principle of great devotees transmitting the seeds of *bhakti*. The imparting of the teachings of the *Bhāgavata* in the first place is triggered by King Parīkṣit, who has seven days left to live, encountering sage Śuka. As a consequence, Śuka imparts the *Bhāgavata* to him, to the gratitude of the king:

> The king said:
>
> "*Aho!* The human birth is the most excellent of all births. What good is there in other births—even in that other world [the celestial realm]—if there is not the abundant association of great souls, whose minds are purified by the glories of Kṛṣṇa? There is nothing to be amazed at in the fact that sins are destroyed, and pure *bhakti* to Kṛṣṇa occurs from the dust of Your lotus feet. My ignorance, rooted in false reasoning, has been destroyed by a moment of Your association." (V.13.21–22)

Indirectly, then, the *Bhāgavata* as text positions itself as embodying this association with advanced *bhaktas* in the form of recording and preserving their narratives as well as the descriptions of Kṛṣṇa's *līlās*. Thus, just as those fortunate enough to have taken birth when Kṛṣṇa incarnated on earth attained perfection, the text claims that "those born after Kṛṣṇa's departure to His abode who are fortunate enough to encounter the *Bhāgavata Purāṇa*, listen to it, read it, and contemplate it with a devoted heart, will likewise attain liberation" (XII.13.18). Reading the *Bhāgavata* thus constitutes a powerful means of initially beginning (or, if begun, deepening) one's devotional life.

Satsaṅga and the *Guru*

Within this context of receiving the first seeds of *bhakti* from the fellowship of other *bhaktas*, called *satsaṅga* (literally the "coming together of saints"), Jīva then focuses more specifically on the figure of the *guru* as the most important element of this *satsaṅga*. He notes that there are two types of neophytes (or, perhaps more precisely, approaches adopted by newcomers) when encountering the association of *bhaktas* (*anu* 202). The first, which I venture to state is by far the most common, is that a beginner, inspired by a particular *bhakta* or association of *bhaktas*, accepts a person from their ranks as spiritual teacher. Typically, one subsequently becomes interested in hearing about *Īśvara* in the mode *Īśvara* is understood in that tradition. In other words, one is initially attracted by a community or by a charismatic and then simply inherits the form of *Īśvara* and, we can add, sectarian metaphysical and theological specifics through which *Īśvara* is received in that community (such as those that will be touched upon in "The Object of *Bhakti*"). The newcomer eventually worships that form in the specific ritualistic manner, filtered through the philosophical and theological categories, that defines that community. As an aside, we see this phenomenon clearly from the examples of the lineage-embedded Hindu teachers who came to the West in the 1960s. Their disciples were initially attracted by the *guru*'s charisma, and only subsequently, sometimes after many years, did some of these students begin to excavate more fully the specificities and complexities of the teacher's lineage tradition—be it Kaśmir Śaivism, *advaita Vedānta*, Gauḍīya Vaiṣṇavism, or others (and in some cases, such as in some of the Krishnamācārya-derived *yoga* schools, have for the most part still to seriously engage with, in this case, the twelveth-century theologian Rāmānuja's lineage, Śrī Vaiṣṇavism, with its philosophical tradition, *viśiṣṭādvaita Vedānta*, of their founding teachers).

In such association, continues Jīva, one studies the requisite texts associated with that tradition, engaging them in the manner established by Vedānta exegesis (methods of interpretation),[14] deliberating on their import and dispelling doubts and misconceptions as to their Truths. Simultaneously, the aspirant gradually develops faith in the form of *Īśvara* central to that tradition as well as an emotional attachment to that form. Typically, this involves viewing that form as primary among all other forms of *Īśvara* and carefully adopting the ritualistic and meditative *bhakti* practices associated with that form, according to the specifics of that tradition (such as performing *japa*, *mantra* repetition of the name of that form, as one's meditation practice).

Jīva considers this first type of approach an analytical path, which he contrasts with the second approach, which is guided by taste (*anu* 202) that transcends the analytical mind. By "taste" (*ruci*), he intends the natural attraction spontaneously experienced when directing the mind to *Īśvara*, a corollary of *rāga*. While the association of *bhaktas* is the trigger for both types of aspirants, there are those who immediately experience attraction for the narrations of

Īśvara once they hear them; they do not need to cultivate their devotion or analyze it. For this type of *bhakta*, deliberation and study are not requisite ingredients.[15] But here, too, since relishing any kind of taste is the product of past experience recorded in the *citta* (that is, *saṁskāra*), one can surmise that this second type of aspirant who experiences immediate attraction had previously practiced *bhakti* in past lives to reach this stage. Therefore, Jīva suggests that such a fortunate newcomer should worship the form of *Īśvara* to which he or she is already spontaneously attracted (XI.3.48 and XI. 27.7); those preexisting *saṁskāras* are already in place.

Eventually, the person from whom one begins to hear teachings, or someone from the community of such people, becomes the *śikṣā guru*, "instructing teacher," says Jīva (*anu* 202). While a person may have many *śikṣā gurus*, an aspirant generally accepts one of them as the primary guide in the specifics of practice and worship, and this person is known as the *dīkṣā guru*, "initiating *guru*." This *guru* initiates one into the lineage, and one's primary spiritual allegiance is subsequently offered to him or her. This choice of a *guru* is a matter of taste:

> One seeking knowledge of the ultimate welfare should approach a *guru* who is learned in the scripture, absorbed in *Brahman*, and is the abode of peace. Holding the *guru* as his own self and as the Lord, and attending him free from deceit, one should learn the *Bhāgavata dharma*. By this, Hari, the *ātman* [of the universe] and the one who bestows realization of the *ātman*, is pleased. (XI.3.21)

The *bhakta* who takes the role of *guru* is the most important entity to emerge from *satsaṅga*, or the company of the *bhaktas*: "I [Kṛṣṇa] am not as satisfied by worship, [high] birth, austere practices and tranquillity of mind as I am by obedience to the *guru*" (X.80.34). Rūpa lists sixty-four practices that constitute *vaidhī bhakti*, from which he identifies the first three as the most important (*Bhaktirasāmṛtasindhu* II.83), all of them featuring the *guru*: "taking shelter at the feet of the *guru*, accepting initiation (*dīkṣā*) and instruction from the *guru*, and rendering service to the *guru*" (*Bhaktirasāmṛtasindhu* II.74). These are essentially a rewording of the *Gītā*, where seeking the shelter of the *guru* takes the form of rendering service in exchange for receiving guidance: "The learned ones who have seen the Truth can impart that knowledge to you; know that Truth through humble submission, inquiry, and rendering service to them" (VI.34).

Without a *guru*, progress on the spiritual journey is hard going: "Addicted to hundreds of vices, those in this world who neglect the *guru*, and who attempt to control the wild horse of the uncontrolled and very fickle mind through restraint of the breathing and of the senses, become frustrated with their methods. They are like the merchant on the ocean who has not taken a helmsman" (X.87.33). Since the *guru* delivers *Īśvara*, he or she is treated with the greatest respect: "The *guru* is a manifestation of *Bhagavān* Himself, who bestows the light of knowledge. If one thinks of the *guru* as an imperfect human being, all one's scriptural knowledge is wasted, like the bathing of an elephant [who immediately then goes and again rolls around in the sand]" (VII.15.26). And again: "One should consider the *ācārya* (*guru*) to be I Myself [Kṛṣṇa] and never disrespect him or think him to be a common person. The *guru* is the embodiment of all the celestials" (XI.17.27). From the other side, the *guru* too has a responsibility: "One should not be a *guru*, one should not be a relative, one should not be a father, one should not be a mother, one should not be a celestial being, and one should not be a husband, if one cannot liberate [one's dependents] from engagement with the process of death (*saṁsāra*)" (V.5.18).

This might be a good occasion to introduce the first verse from one of Rūpa's other works, the *Upadeśāmṛta*, (*Nectar of Instruction*), which lists six minimal qualifications necessary for anyone who assumes the role of *guru* in guiding others on their spiritual journey: "The person of fixed mind, *dhīra*, who can control the urge (*vega*) to speak, the urges of the mind and of anger, and the urges of the tongue, belly, and genitals, is qualified to teach all over the world" (1). The *guru* can obviously not lead a disciple beyond the impulses of the body and mind to any higher reality that might exist if he or she has not personally surpassed them. Relevant here is Arjuna's question in the *Gītā* pertaining to the characteristics of the *dhīra* (the sage whose mind is fixed on the goals of *yoga*)[16] and Kṛṣṇa's extensive responses, all featuring absence of desire as a central feature (II.54–72).[17]

Detachment and absence of desire are characteristics of the advanced practitioner of all the *mokṣa* traditions. Even Patañjali, in his usual oblique and understated manner, points to the possibility of fixing the mind on a *guru*-like figure but qualifies that such a person must be "free of desire" (*vīta-rāga*, *Yoga Sūtras* I.37).

Given the life of extreme austerity Jīva, the other *Gosvāmīs*, and their fellow radically renounced ascetics were leading in Vṛndāvana in the sixteenth century, in contrast to the spectacle of the extravagant lifestyles and controversial behaviors surrounding many modern-day charismatics, it goes without saying that genuine *bhaktas*, completely enamored with their beloved *Īśvara*, have no attachment to material things. They thus seek no personal gain from their disciples: "O Lord with the lotus navel! Those who associate with Your devotees, whose hearts are enamored by the fragrance of Your lotus feet, forget about this mortal life, sons, friends, households, wealth, and wives" (IV.9.12).

The centrality of *bhakta* association, then, and of the *guru* in particular, simply cannot be overstressed, and Jīva returns to it again and again throughout his work, following the leads of the *Bhāgavata*: "*Saṁsāra* is the continued cycle of ignorance of a living being who in reality is *ātman*. The remedy is supreme *bhakti* to the *guru*" (IV.29.36); "Through service of a topmost *bhāgavata* devotee, the intense experience of love[18] will manifest for the lotus feet of Kṛṣṇa, who removes all vice" (III.7.19); "[Attaining] the celestial realm or liberation is not equal to even half a moment's association with a *bhāgavata* devotee; what then to speak of the blessings of mortal beings?" (IV.24.57[19]); "A sinful person does not purify himself as much through such things as austerity, as one whose life is devoted to Kṛṣṇa does by service to Kṛṣṇa's devotees" (VI.1.16). Association with such *bhāgavatas* overrides all other *bhakti* practices, including the nine standard ones discussed previously, and can award the desired result independently of any other means (although Jīva hastens to add that the other practices should not thereby be discarded! *anu* 283–84):

> By merely *satsaṅga*, the association of saints, in different *yugas* [ages], those whose nature was *rajas* and *tamas*, even demons . . . animals, birds; . . . various kinds of celestial beings; . . . and, among humans, merchants, laborers,

women;[20] and many others, attained My abode. They did not study the Veda, nor serve great *mahātmās*, nor undertake vows or *tapas*, but attained Me through the association of saints. Indeed, merely by their love (*bhāva*) did the *gopī* cowherding women, the cows, deer, and other simpleminded beings such as snakes attain perfection and easily come to Me" (XI.12.3–5).

Some of these remarks about animals and such become clearer in part 3 after reading the narratives of the tenth book, where all the flora and fauna in the entire landscape of Vraj adores Kṛṣṇa, but what should be clear at this point is that this love, *bhāva*, is attained from those who already have *bhāva*: the *satsaṅga* of *bhaktas*. And from among them, the *guru* is particular. And just like *rāga* for Kṛṣṇa Himself, attachment to the *guru* and the *satsaṅga* is a completely different affair from the attachments to the other personages and objects of *prakṛti* that the *bhakta*, just like any other *yogī*, is striving to transcend: "Attachment, when placed in unrighteous people out of ignorance, is the cause of *saṁsāra*; but when placed in the saints, it leads to non-attachment" (III.23.55).

Having said all this, however, and given the seemingly never-ending scandals and controversies associated with many modern-day *gurus* (and past ones, too),[21] we feel obliged to quote Rūpa's cautionary note here that "*bhakti* that is promoted by means of wealth and numerous disciples is discounted, because it loses the highest state through distancing [one from Hari because of these distractions]" (*Bhaktirasāmṛtasindhu* II.259). This statement speaks for itself. Additionally, and related to the same point, students familiar with the non-negotiability of the *yamas* and *niyamas* (moral and ethical restraints and observances)[22] in generic *yoga*—which Patañjali, with uncharacteristic emphasis, stresses are a mandatory and absolute "great vow" irrespective of any criteria such as time, place, circumstance, and condition (II.31)—will soon notice that they do not find a place in the list of the nine main practices of *bhakti*, or even in the much more expansive list of sixty-four practices outlined by Rūpa. This is because the groundwork laid down by texts such as the *Yoga Sūtras* is taken for granted in *bhakti*: "For one absorbed in Kṛṣṇa, the *yamas* and *niyamas* such as cleanliness (*śauca*) and the others are automatically present, hence they are not specifically included under the limbs (*aṅga*) of *bhakti*; qualities such as *ahiṁsā*, etc., are not remarkable: those engaged in *bhakti* to Hari automatically never harm others"[23] (*Bhaktirasāmṛtasindhu* Eastern Quadrant II.261–62). Such basics are so obvious and generic for all mainstream schools of *yoga*, they are assumed by Jīva and Rūpa.

Given the importance of the issue—and the enormous psychological damage caused to the disillusioned disciples of the numerous *guru* figures who have succumbed to scandals—we feel obliged to reiterate that anyone posturing as a *guru* without adhering to the *yamas* and *niyamas*, or who presents some theological or esoteric justification for deviancy from these, is completely at odds with the *Bhāgavata* tradition, Patañjali's *yoga*, and practically all orthodox Indic schools, including the Buddhist and Jain traditions. And, needless to say, genuine saints would never exploit the service rendered them by those seeking guidance on the devotional path: "They are peaceful, impartial, focused on Me, calm, see all beings equally, free of any sense of proprietorship, free of ego, above all dualities, and free of coveting (*aparigraha*)" (XI.26.27). We note that charisma is not a listed ingredient. There is much that could be said here, as the abusive potential of the *guru* disciple relationship is obvious,[24] but such descriptions in the sacred texts at least provide a standard against which the behavior and qualities of *guru* figures can be gauged.

The Varieties of Saints

As will be discussed in some detail from a more philosophical perspective in "The Object of *Bhakti*," there are two basic categories of *mahant*, or great enlightened personalities, recognized by the *Bhāgavata* tradition. There are those absorbed in *Brahman* (that is, their inner *ātman* self) and those absorbed in *Bhagavān*: "The *mahants* are both either the *sādhus* who are equanimous in mind,[25] peaceful, free of anger, and well-wishers to all, or they are those whose goal is to establish affection for Me as Lord" (V.5.2–3). The first of these is considered great, says Jīva, because of awareness of the *ātman*, the other because of awareness of *Bhagavān* (*anu* 186). However, their quality of greatness is not the same: "Even among thousands who are liberated and perfected [that is, who have realized the *ātman*], a peaceful soul who is devoted to Nārāyaṇa [Viṣṇu] is very rare" (VI.14.5). Put more emphatically, "Liberation is not comparable with even a moment of association with *Bhagavān*'s devotees" (I.18.13). The *Gītā* too notes that "from many thousands of people, barely anyone strives for perfection, and from those striving or already perfected, barely one knows Me as I am" (VII.3). Nonetheless, since we will be focusing primarily on the *bhakta* absorbed in *Bhagavān* in this volume, we should take a moment to at least note the extraordinary characteristics of the other type of great personality, the sage absorbed in the nondual awareness of *Brahman* in the form of the *ātman*:

> His consciousness is withdrawn from the external world. He should remain silent, absorbed in the experience of his own inner bliss, free of desire, his thirst extinguished. If, nonetheless, he sometimes still perceives this world, which has been rejected by his intelligence as unreal, as the memory will persist until the end of life, it will not cause any illusion. A perfected being does not perceive whether the perishable body, through which he has realized the true self (*svarūpa*),[26] is seated or arisen, or whether, by chance, it has gone off somewhere, or, under the control of Fate, returned.[27] He is like a person intoxicated by alcohol who does not know if his cloth is still covering him. The body along with the life air will continue, under the control of Fate, for as long as the *karma* that has been activated for that life has not run out.[28] But one who has mastered the state of the *yoga* of *samādhi* does not again participate in the forms of the world, any more than a person upon waking up participates in the objects of a dream. (XI.13.35–37)

The reason such *Brahman* realization is not sought after by *bhaktas*, says Jīva, is that it eliminates the distinction between *Bhagavān* and the *jīva* (or, through Vaiṣṇava perspectives, it is a state in which consciousness is not aware of the eternally distinct *Īśvara* owing to being exclusively absorbed in its own nature of pure consciousness). Without this distinction, there can be no *bhakti* (*anu* 188) and, consequently, no bliss from personal association with *Īśvara*. As we have noted, the *Īśvara*-derived bliss is held to be incomparably greater than the *ātman*-derived one. Hence the many frequent statements throughout the text that the *bhaktas* have no interest in this *Brahman* type of liberation and, indeed, reject it even if offered: "Some *bhāgavatas* do not desire attaining the state of oneness with the *ātman*; they are satisfied with the service of My feet and long for Me. Congregating together, they praise My wonderful deeds" (III.25.34).

The second type of *mahant* is the *bhakta*. Jīva hierarchizes this type into three categories, gleaned, as always, from the *Bhāgavata*: *uttama bhaktas*, highest; *madhyama bhaktas*, intermediate; and *prākṛta bhaktas*, materialistic (*anu* 187–90). From these: "The highest devotee (*bhāgavata-uttamaḥ*) is one who sees the presence of his *Bhagavān* in all beings, and all beings within *Bhagavān*" (XI.2.45). This superlative type of *bhakta* has a universalizing vision similar to that of the *Brahman*-realized *yogī* in the quote above, except that his equanimity is not based just on the ability to perceive the *ātman* in all beings but is bolstered by an awareness that these *ātmans* are in fact manifestations and parts of *Īśvara*. But, more than this, his mind is primarily absorbed in thoughts of the deeds and activities of *Īśvara*, personal *Brahman*, rather than in the passive experience of the *ātman*, nonpersonal *Brahman*. This additional element expresses itself more conspicuously in the behavior of this category of *bhakta* compared with that of the standard *ātman*/*Brahman*-absorbed *yogī*:

> Let him wander around without attachment in this world, hearing about those most auspicious incarnations and deeds of Hari, the bearer of the discus,[29] singing without embarrassment songs and names associated with these. Following this vow, his love awakened and his heart melted while chanting loudly the names of his beloved Lord, he laughs, he weeps, he cries out, he sings, and he dances like a madman, completely indifferent to social norms. With exclusive devotion, he pays respect to the sky, wind, fire, water, earth, stars, living beings, directions, trees and vegetation, rivers, and oceans, and every created thing as the body of Hari. (XI.2.39–42)

While both *Brahman*-realized and *Īśvara*-absorbed *yogīs* are immersed in states of consciousness beyond the *guṇas* of *prakṛti* and are thus behaviorally beyond conventional social norms, the *Bhāgavata* presents the *uttama bhakta* as manifesting intense characteristics of ecstasy that are symptomatically quite different from the peaceful and withdrawn symptoms of the *yogī* immersed in the *ātman*. These states of mind reflect the greater degree of ecstasy experienced from contact with the personal *Īśvara* in comparison with the experience of the bliss inherent in the impersonal *ātman*. Moreover, in this state, the world is perceived everywhere as a manifestation of the Beloved, rather than merely a false or temporary illusory obstacle to be avoided or transcended (similar in some ways to the enlightened perception of the world according to Kaśmir Śaivism).

As we have noted, the *gopīs*, the simplehearted, uneducated, cowherding maidens we will encounter in part 3, are heralded as the highest of all *yogīs* and indeed exhibit the vision noted in the last line of the above quote pertaining to the devotionally surcharged perceptions of the inanimate world. For them, "the trees and creeping plants of the forest seem to be experiencing Viṣṇu in themselves. Richly endowed with fruits and flowers, the trees pour forth streams of honey, their young branches bowing reverentially with their load, and their bodies bristling with the ecstasy of love" (X.35.9). In the *gopīs'* God-intoxicated vision, the entire natural world appears to be worshipping Hari in ecstatic love: "The rivers found their force disrupted by their states of mind after hearing the sound of Mukunda's [Kṛṣṇa's] flute, as could be seen from their whirlpools. Bearing offerings of lotus flowers, the rivers grasped the two feet of Murāri [Kṛṣṇa] and embraced them closely with their arms in the form of waves" (X.21.15).

Before leaving the landscape of Vraj reflected in these verses, where Kṛṣṇa passed His childhood days, to consider the other two types of *bhaktas*—the *madhyama*, intermediate, and *prākṛta*, materialistic devotees—it is worth revisiting the notion of *yogamāyā* and connecting that discussion to the mind-set of the highest *bhaktas*, the *uttamas*: "Whether one knows or does not know who I am—the extent and nature of My being—if someone worships Me with unalloyed devotion, that person is considered an *uttama bhakta*" (XI.11.33). This lack of awareness referred to here of who God actually is, is fundamental to the highest states of *bhakti* that will be encountered in part 3 in the stories from the tenth book—specifically, among Kṛṣṇa's family members and the cowherding community in Vṛndāvana. These simple folks are depicted in the text as having performed *bhakti* for many, many lives before their devotion reached the requisite intensity that earned them a birth in intimate proximity to Kṛṣṇa during His descent, but they are all *uttama bhaktas*: their love is so intense that, aided by *yogamāyā*, it overrides awareness even of Kṛṣṇa's majesty and obliterates even the knowledge that Kṛṣṇa is God. Their devotion has reached such a peak that they can think of Kṛṣṇa only as their lover, friend, child, and the like, depending on their *bhāva*.

The second type of *bhakta mahant* discussed by Jīva is the *madhyama bhakta*, the "middle level" or intermediate *bhakta*. His or her characteristics reflect a schema that was widespread among the soteriological schools (surfacing, for instance, in *Yoga Sūtras* I.33 and as the *brahma-vihāras* in various Buddhist *suttas*),[30] but here with variations in phraseology to reflect the *Bhāgavata*'s devotionality: "The *madhyama* acts with love (*prema*) for *Īśvara*, friendship (*maitrī*) toward those devoted to Him, compassion (*kṛpā*) toward the ignorant, and equanimity (*upekṣā*) toward the envious" (XI.2.46). In this type of awareness characteristic of the *madhyama*, we see judgmental behavior, albeit benevolent, based on the perception of distinctions among living beings, in contrast to the *uttama bhakta*'s feelings of love for all beings as manifestations of *Īśvara* with no sense of differentiation.

The third category of *bhakta mahant*, the materialist (*prākṛta*) devotee, is far more restricted in his or her ability to perceive the omnipresence of *Īśvara*: "One who offers *pūjā* (worship) to Hari in the form of the deity with faith, but not to the *bhaktas* or to other people, is a worldly devotee" (XI.2.47). Such a neophyte practitioner who differentiates, says Jīva, and who does not have reverence for all beings, has not developed love of God. Such a person is either new to the path, or devoid of deep study, or expressing devotion only out of social convention (*anu* 190). Jīva further characterizes such a person (somewhat unflatteringly) with this quote from the *Bhāgavata*: "One who identifies this corpse made of the three elements to be the self, considers his wife and family to be his own, holds the earth to be worthy of worship, understands water to be sacred, but does not accept those who are wise, is truly a donkey or a cow" (X.84.13).

Jīva then considers these three divisions of *bhaktas* from the perspective of the attitude toward *dharma* and social conventions exhibited by each of them, respectively. The worldly (*prākṛta*) devotee performs *bhakti* mixed with other concerns, such as attachment to the performance of *dharma*, as discussed previously in the analysis of "mixed *bhakti*." The *madhyama* (intermediate) *bhakta* renounces *dharma* in his or her complete dedication to the service of *Īśvara* but is still aware of the conventional norms and results pertaining to *dharma* and *adharma*, and so in this minor sense the uninhibited and full immersion of the mind in *bhakti* is mildly delimited. Additionally, the *bhakta*'s devotion is also curtailed by knowledge of God's majesty and omnipotency in this stage. But the *uttama bhakta* is so immersed in love of God that he or she has no awareness of whether his or her behavior conforms to *dharma* whatsoever—indeed, entertains no considerations of *dharma* or social gradations in the first place. And as we have seen with the *rāgātmika bhaktas*, the devotee at this stage often has no awareness of the majesty and supreme ontological status of God Himself even when entering into very intimate relationships with Him.

Before concluding this section on the varieties of *bhaktas*, we can include Rūpa's hierarchization of devotees in his *Upadeśāmṛta*, but here with the purpose of suggesting how one should appropriately interact in a devotional environment with different levels of *bhaktas*:

> One should offer respect in the mind toward one who utters the name "Kṛṣṇa"; one should offer respect with obeisances to one who has taken spiritual initiation into a Vaiṣṇava lineage (*dīkṣā*) and is worshipping *Īśvara*; and one should offer respect by seeking the cherished association of, and serving and hearing from one whose heart is completely cleansed of faults such as criticizing others, and who is mature in full absorption in devotional practices. (5)

Rūpa also cautions us not to judge *bhaktas* by any type of bodily criteria, including caste, social status, or any other such material designations:

> One should not look upon the *prakṛtic* (material) nature of a person who is a *bhakta* here in this world, nor at the visible defects of his or her body which are attained at birth due to

> past-life *karma*. The transcendent (*Brahman*) essence of the waters of the *Gaṅgā* river is lost [if one looks at] the quality of the water, with its bubbles, foam, and mud. (6)

Rūpa makes one further set of relevant comments as to what transpires between *bhaktas* in addition to their discussions about Kṛṣṇa: "The six signs of love [between *bhaktas*] are: giving gifts and receiving them; inquiring confidentially and revealing one's mind confidentially; and offering and accepting foodstuffs" (4). This is not the place to embark on a discussion of the *āśrama* experiences of the various forms of *yoga* transplanted to the West in the 1960s, but without such loving reciprocations and honest exchanges of confidentialities that Rūpa notes, life in communities of practitioners can very easily and quickly become institutionalized, hierarchical, judgmental, spiritually oppressive, and, all too often, abusive.

The Liberated *Bhakta*: Different Types of *Mokṣa* in the *Bhāgavata*

We can conclude this section on the *bhakta* by considering the ultimate destinations that the accomplished and perfected practitioners can attain in the postmortem liberated state. Let us recall that the *Bhāgavata*'s definition of *bhakti* quoted at the outset was that those who perform it were "so free of motive . . . that, without service to [Kṛṣṇa], they do not accept the five types of liberation, even if these are offered. We have made several references to these varying types of liberation and it is now time to discuss them. These are: residing in the same abode as Viṣṇu (*sālokya*), having the same opulence as Him (*sārṣṭi*), being close to Him (*sāmīpya*), having the same form as Him (*sārūpya*), and merging into Him (*ekatvam*)" (III.29.12–14).

In the *Bhāgavata* schema expressed in this verse, the generic goal of conventional *yoga* corresponds to the fifth item on the list, *ekatvam*, "the state of oneness." It is described by Patañjali as "the immersion of the seer [consciousness] within its own nature" (*draṣṭuḥ svarupe 'vasthānam*, I.3). We have been referring to this variously as the experience of *ātman*, realization of *Brahman*, or impersonal realization (and will be referring to it in the next section as the monistic experience). Other terms include *kaivalya*, "oneness";

ātma-jñāna, "awareness of the self"; *nirvāṇa*, literally "blowing out";[31] and the by now familiar synonyms *mokṣa* and *mukti*.

We can briefly note in passing that there are differences in how this "oneness" is understood in certain *jñāna* and *yoga* traditions. In *advaita Vedānta*, for example, there is only one Supreme *Ātman*, which is in fact the nondual *Brahman*, as we will discuss in the next section; so in liberation, when consciousness attains this state, it loses all sense of individuality as well as awareness of the world of duality, which were both illusory in the first place according to *advaita* tenets. In this state consciousness is aware of only "one" experience—its own nature of pure, blissful, eternal consciousness. For the Sāṅkhya and Yoga traditions, the liberated *ātman* maintains individuality and the world remains real, but, absorbed in its own infinite nature, pure consciousness is aware neither of the real world nor of other individual *ātmans* whether liberated or not. We would suggest that although the scholastics of the former school posit that in ultimate reality there is only one infinite *ātman* and no real world, and those of the latter maintain that there is an eternal plurality of infinite *ātmans* and an eternally real world, this is an intellectually constructed issue. From an experiential point of view, their experiences appear identical: an awareness of nothing other than eternal and infinite awareness free from all suffering.[32] Hence, all these traditions can lay claim to terms such as *ekatvam*, "oneness," and its synonym *kaivalya* (as well as the term *jñāna*, "knowing"), to describe this experience. In other words, in this state it is irrelevant if the world is real or not, or if there are other individual *ātmans* simultaneously absorbed in this experience, or if they have all merged into one undifferentiated unity, as the experience of *ekatvam* itself is trans-spatial (infinite) and transtemporal (eternal) and devoid of any notion of "individuality" and "world out there" at all. This is because there is no *buddhi*, intellect, covering the *ātman* deliberating on such things. It is only for the scholastics left behind embedded in their intellect, mind, and senses for which such issues are important and become the basis for debate among schools.

In keeping with these traditions, the *Bhāgavata* recognizes this impersonal experience of oneness, *ekatvam*, as one of the five types of liberation. Like these other schools, it accepts it to be a state in which the *ātman* has no form or qualities and that the experience of the *ātman* in this state is exclusively one of *sat-cit-ānanda* (being, consciousness, and bliss). It accepts everything noted above that *advaita* or Sāṅkhya posit about that state experientially. However, when *bhakti yoga* to *Īśvara* is practiced rather than *jñāna* or *yoga*, the *Bhāgavata* tradition (and Vaiṣṇavism in general) posits that there are four other types of liberation that become available in addition to *ekatvam* and that these bestow divine (*Brahman*) personal transcendent forms and qualities on the individual *ātman* when liberated. We can note in passing that the *Vedānta Sūtras*, in its characteristically minimalistic and truncated way, also recognizes that there is an option in liberation as to whether the released souls attain a liberated body or not (IV.4.11–12), as does the ancient *Mokṣadharma* section of the *Mahābhārata* epic (196.21–22).

God too has a divine bodily form, or more precisely, being unlimited, has unlimited divine forms, and these inhabit divine abodes, also unlimited—the realms within *Brahman* we have touched upon called Vaikuṇṭha. These forms and realms are made not of *prakṛti* stuff—the three *guṇa* qualities we will discuss in the next section—but of *Brahman* stuff, pure consciousness—*sat-cit-ānanda*. There is no inert matter there (in fact, this realm of nonconscious *prakṛti* can be seen as something of a dull and imperfect reflection of those *Brahman* realms). Vaikuṇṭha, to borrow Abrahamic language, is the Kingdom of God. So the liberated *ātman* attains *Brahman*, but not the impersonal, formless, qualityless *Brahman* devoid of active experiences as attained in the *ekatvam* state. Just as the *ātmans* receive *prakṛti* minds, forms, relationships, and situations in this realm of *saṁsāra* that reflect their *guṇas* and *karma*, they receive *Brahman* minds, forms, relationships, and situations in the Vaikuṇṭha realm that reflect the nature of their *bhakti* (their *rāgas*, *bhāvas*, and so forth). With these, they engage in a loving relationship with one of the unlimited divine forms of *Īśvara* corresponding to their preference. This is not anthropomorphism, but theopomorphism (we have noted that Vaiṣṇavas would intuitively resonate with the Abrahamic idea of man being made in the image of God). Embodied beings as effects have forms, qualities, and activities because their cause has form, qualities, and activities (to an unlimited degree). So in Vaikuṇṭha the very realms themselves, as well as the forms of *Īśvara* and of the *bhaktas* that abide there, are made of pure, eternal, blissful consciousness (*sa-guṇa Brahman*). These forms are inconceivable: they cannot be fathomed or conceived of by the rational mind or intellect, which is limited to the spatial, temporal, and physical conditions of *prakṛti*.

Some of these relationships were discussed in *rāgānugā bhakti*, but for our present purposes, the four other liberations listed in this verse in addition to the impersonal one of *ekatvam*, include *sālokya*, residing in the same abode as Viṣṇu (that is, residing in Vaikuṇṭha, the divine realm); *sārṣṭi*, having the same opulence as Viṣṇu (omnipotency);[33] *sāmīpya*, being close to Viṣṇu (a closer and more intimate physical proximity than that of *sālokya*); and *sārūpya*, having the same form as Viṣṇu.[34] In other words, the liberation offered by Yoga, Sāṅkhya, *advaita Vedānta*, and other schools is of no ultimate interest to the *Bhāgavata* tradition not because these are not genuine experiential states, which the text certainly asserts that they are, but because these available options do not allow for the possibility of an eternal personal relationship with *Īśvara*. And it is this desire for eternal relationship in devotion and service that characterizes true *bhakti* in Vaiṣṇavism. Indeed, Jīva and Rūpa note here that in addition to their disinterest in merging into impersonal *Brahman* (*ekatvam*), even one of the personal types of liberation—having the same opulence as Viṣṇu (*sārṣṭi*)—is unacceptable, as both of these are not suitable for service; the others may be accepted if they enhance one's service.[35]

Also, from an ontological point of view, while the *Bhāgavata* describes the experience of the fifth type of liberation, *ekatvam* (also known as *sāyūjya*), in the same way as the other *jñāna* and Yoga traditions, its metaphysical understanding of the state partly differs. In his *Prīti Sandarbha* (*anu* 15), Jīva states that it can indeed denote realizing one's own *ātman* as a part of the infinitely omnipresent *Brahman*,[36] more or less as proposed by the other schools (*brahma-sāyūjya*), but it can also denote merging into Kṛṣṇa's actual body and relishing the bliss of this (*Bhagavat-sāyūjya*).[37] Furthermore, even with regard to the first option, *Brahman* is considered the effulgence of *Īśvara* rather than an independent essence, like the light of the sun, which, even though it can be experienced in its own right, is nonetheless always emanational from the sun itself. Jīva is not partial to either option, as each eliminates the possibility of love being expressed through service. But he nonetheless accepts their realities.

And there are numerous other possible liberated states in the *bhakti* universe. We can very briefly refer to Kaśmir Śaivism, for example, which occupies an interesting place somewhere between *advaita Vedānta*, further discussed in the next section, and Vaiṣṇavism. It holds the world as well as Śiva's form to be eternally real (and vigorously opposes *advaita Vedānta*, which considers the world illusory on this score) but shares the latter's monism with regard to the illusoriness of the individual *ātman*. The liberated *ātman*, in this and related traditions, becomes one with Śiva (hence the *mantra Śivo 'ham*, "I am Śiva"). From this vantage point it need not reject the world of *prakṛti*, which in Kaśmir Śaivism is ultimately not matter but pure emanational consciousness, *citi-śakti*, and enjoy it as Śiva enjoying an expression of Himself. However, unlike in Vaiṣṇavism, the actual form of Śiva is not the ultimate expression of Truth, which, as *parama-Śiva*, is ultimately considered impersonal: *Īśvara*'s form in these Śākta systems is secondary and derivative. But it is nonetheless real and decidedly not illusory.

A different stream of Śiva-centered tradition, Śaiva Siddhānta, in contrast, does hold the *ātman* to be eternally individual and also that it attains a form of liberation that parallels the Vaiṣṇava *sārūpya*—here attaining a divine form similar to *Īśvara*'s rather than merging into Him as with Kaśmir Śaivism—but a form of *Īśvara* as *Śiva*. Liberation therefore entails a union between the liberated soul and a distinct God—a loving union between two individuals; this Śaivite school is not monistic like Kaśmir Śaivism.[38] So in Śaiva Siddhānta there are unlimited Śivas, even as only one is the preeminent *Īśvara* who can create universes, where in Kaśmir Śaivism there is only one Śiva and all souls merge (or realize their oneness) with Him. The Śaiva Siddhānta preference for a relationship of love between a Godhead and the liberated *ātman* in a unity of two distinct individuals is closer to the type of liberation of interest to Jīva's school than the enlightened enjoyment of *prakṛti* in the monistic oneness of Kaśmir Śaivism, even as both types are accepted as true options. So the Śaiva Siddhānta's closest parallel in Vaiṣṇavism is the fourth from the five types of liberation (*sārūpya*), where Kaśmir Śaivism is closer to the fifth, *ekatvam* (*sāyūjya*).

In either case, from the Gauḍīya Vaiṣṇava perspective, Śiva abides in his own transcendent (trans-*prakṛti*) abode, which is a parallel to Viṣṇu's Vaikuṇṭha, where those devoted to him blissfully reside eternally in his company. And this abode and its residents are eternal and not derivative or a secondary manifestation of a higher transpersonal Truth. Thus, in the *Bṛhad Bhāgavatāmṛta*, a transcendental travelogue written by Sanātana, another of the six *Gosvāmīs*, Jīva's other uncle (and brother of Rūpa):

> Maheśa (Śiva), who increases love (*bhāva*) is non-different from beautiful Madana-Gopala [Kṛṣṇa]. . . . In his eternal form, *Bhagavān* Śiva lives in his abode (*loka*). Eternally manifest, he is always visible to his exclusively dedicated devotees, who accept Him as their personal *iṣṭa-devatā*,[39] and are content to live there. He is non-different from Viṣṇu. (II.3.62–65)[40]

In the next section, we will lay great stress on the essential oneness of these two forms of *Īśvara*, Viṣṇu and Śiva (as of the various forms of *Īśvarī*), despite devotional partialities.

And we can here do no more than rather superficially mention that the options continue to expand when one considers the galaxy of Devī (Goddess) traditions and the liberated states offered in those.[41] Add to this that all of these traditions have seemingly never-ending subtraditions and variants, and we are faced with many different possible types of liberation being offered through *bhakti*. Irrespective of the sectarian debates between the various Vedānta and Purāṇa scholastic traditions, the *Bhāgavata*'s acceptance of five primary types of liberation, and its acknowledgment of other Śiva-associated forms of liberation, opens the door to a heterogeneous and, in principle, unlimited array of liberated possibilities reflecting the free will and partialities of the living entities. This might be expected if the Absolute is to be deemed unlimited and all-inclusive.

The possible contribution all this makes to the study of religion will be touched upon in our "Concluding Reflections," but we can note for now that the *Bhāgavata* questions the presupposition that the ultimate, perfected liberated state, if there is one, must be monolithic or one-size-fits-all, an assumption typically made by both believers and nonbelievers of a postmortem perfected existence. This assumption is not supported by the *Bhāgavata*. The contribution it makes to the problem of accounting for the apparent variegation of the ultimate perfected state posited by the different religions of the world is that it opens the door that all, or certainly far more than one claim, could be simultaneously correct. Experientially and ontologically true in accordance with (at least many of) the categories and conditions expressed by the religions themselves, not true in some sort of an accommodating, "politically correct," or metaphoric sort of way. The *Bhāgavata* offers us five "standard" types of liberation (which include monotheistic and monistic possibilities) and contains a multidimensional view of reality that does not preclude unlimited other possibilities, include Śaivite- and Devī-related states of liberation. This is not unique to the *Bhāgavata*: we have noted that the *Vedānta Sūtras* also allows for the possibilities of a liberated state either with form or without, as does the *Mahābhārata*'s *Mokṣadharma*.

And, of course, within *prakṛti*, and prior to attaining the ultimate state, similar variegation is expressed in Patañjali's seven levels of transrational *samādhi* states (only the final state, that of *nirbīja*, is full liberation from all involvement with *prakṛti*) and with the options expressed in the *Gītā*.[42] And while not transcendent destinations, when we factor in various other cosmological dimensionalities within *prakṛti*—the multiple (unlimited) universes emanating from Viṣṇu and the various progressively subtler celestial realms within each one—the postmortem possibilities of a progressive nature are very variegated. Granted there is hierarchy among all these transcendent states, but the Absolute, being infinite and unlimited, must be unlimitedly diverse and multifaceted for the *Bhāgavata*.

But hierarchies are important to those entrusted to preserve and perpetuate specific *bhakti* lineages by bringing them into dialogue with the intellectual currents of their day. And so it is to the theological and philosophical understanding of *Īśvara* in sect-specific contexts that we must next turn our attention. In order to complete our analysis of *bhakti yoga* as a relationship expressed through various practices and mind-sets between a *bhakta* and a form of *Īśvara*, we must now engage a long overdue topic: an analysis of some of the ways *Īśvara* as object of *bhakti* has been construed in some important Hindu theologies.

The Object of *Bhakti*: *Īśvara*, *Bhagavān*, *Brahman*, and Divine Hierarchies

Bhakti and Other Paths of *Yoga*

As a prologue to discussing the nature of *Īśvara*, let us first consider a related topic Jīva raises: What is particular about *bhakti* from the perspective of *yoga* in general? There are numerous *yoga* paths claiming to free one from suffering and lead one to enlightenment; do they not all take one to the same goal? Here, we reiterate that the *Bhāgavata* shares the view common to all the *yoga* and other *mokṣa* (that is, soteriological, liberation-seeking) traditions of ancient India—namely, that ignorance of the true self is the cause of suffering, and it is suffering and frustration that initially prompt one to ponder whether there might be a state beyond suffering and hence consider a *yoga* path in the first place. After all, if one is perfectly content with one's life, why would one wish to change—that is, seek a "path" to go somewhere else? Any *yogic* journey can begin only when there is a realization that all is not well, or at least when one cannot shake off some sort of simmering existential malaise.

This initial starting premise is most succinctly expressed in the sequential nature of the four Truths that became enshrined at the core of Buddhism but were a standard set of perspectives for almost all the *mokṣa* traditions.[1] Here the "path" is the fourth Truth, but it is consequent on realization of the first Truth, *sarvaṁ duḥkham,* everything is suffering, or at least unfulfilling (which is then bolstered by the other two truths: that there is a cause for this suffering—

desire—and subsequently the possibility of a state beyond suffering once the cause is removed).[2] The realization of being unfulfilled lies at the core of the impetus to take up practice in the *Yoga Sūtras* (II.16) and is universally associated with the quest for *mokṣa*, liberation in the soteriological traditions of ancient India. As noted previously, the fourth- to fifth-century *Sāṅkhya Kārikā* comes out and states this plainly in its very first verse; it is precisely because of being subject to unfulfillment/suffering that one seeks knowledge. Indeed, terms such as *mokṣa* and *mukti*, "liberation," denote nothing other than liberation from suffering or frustration—and Nyāya even defines *yoga* as such (I.1.22, IV.2.46), as does the *Gītā* in VI.23.

In terms of the metaphysics of suffering common to all *yoga* schools, when consciousness identifies with its subtle and gross *prakṛtic* coverings of mind and body due to *māyā*/*avidyā* (illusion/ignorance), and consequently sets out to seek happiness through the mind and senses by attempting to fulfill desires associated with these coverings, it experiences frustration, *duḥkha*, instead. This is due to the temporary and ephemeral nature of *prakṛtic* enjoyment and the vulnerability of the body and mind to various mental and physical disturbances, especially disease, old age, and death. It is also due to the fact that, for the Vedic-affiliated[3] schools, the body and mind are not the true self, *ātman*, but inert material coverings.[4] Desires gratify only these external coverings, leaving the innermost self neglected. Moreover, desires are never satiated but demand ever more or morph into some other form. And all actions initiated from a place of ignorance and desire plant seeds, good or bad—the law of *karma*—and these produce reactions. Since one cannot accommodate these reactions in one lifetime—and even if one did, one would simply re-react to them anew, planting a whole new generation of seeds with ever self-multiplying consequences—one must constantly return to receive one's fruits. And this, of course, simply feeds the self-perpetuating process in a never-ending cycle of action, reaction, re-reaction, and so on. *Saṁsāra* is nothing other than this.

This overall pessimistic view of the quest for material enjoyment is broadly accepted by most Indic soteriological traditions, and the tales in part 2 will reinforce for the reader unfamiliar with Indic thought these basic presuppositions shared by the *bhakti* paths with the *jñāna* (knowledge), *karma* (unmotivated duty), *dhyāna* (meditation), and other *yoga* traditions of ancient India.[5] For Jīva, the pursuit of *yoga* practice culminates in direct experience of (what for now we will call) "the Absolute," as is typical of the *yoga* traditions, and it is only by dint of such direct experience that ignorance, desire, and their consequent suffering is fully dispelled. Here, with difference in terminology, he upholds the assumptions of all the *yogic* schools.[6]

So, then, given this common denominator starting premise, what about other *yogas*? Is *bhakti* not just one *yoga* path among many that can lead the living entity out of this entrapment by the senses and the consequent perpetuation of *saṁsāra*? The *Bhāgavata* condenses the various paths of *yoga* into three basic categories:[7]

> Three types of *yoga* have been proclaimed by Me [Kṛṣṇa] out of a desire to bestow welfare on humankind: *jñāna*, *karma*, and *bhakti*; there are no other means anywhere. *Jñāna* is for those people who have become disgusted by actions in this world that are motivated out of personal desire (*karma*), and who have renounced them; *karma yoga* is for those who have desires, and have not yet become disgusted with actions associated with these; and, for that person in whom, by good fortune, faith in the narratives, etc., about Me has arisen, *bhakti yoga* bestows perfection. (XI.20.6–8)

However, as we will see, the *Bhāgavata* promotes *bhakti* as the highest path for everyone, not one among three. First of all (but less important), as is explicit in the *Gītā* (XII.1–6) and hinted at in the *Yoga Sūtras* (II.45), the *Bhāgavata* ubiquitously promotes *bhakti* as the easiest and most expedient *yoga* process. This is for the simple reason that here, as in the *Gītā*, the *ātman*'s veil of ignorance is a power (*māyā-śakti*) of Kṛṣṇa and hence can be removed only by His grace: "This divine *māyā* composed of the three *guṇas*, is Mine and is very hard to surpass, but one who surrenders to Me can cross over it" (*Gītā* VII.4). Because of grace, then, the path of *bhakti* is deemed easy, where other paths are fraught with difficulties (*Gītā* XII.1–6). The *Bhāgavata* too presents Uddhava soliciting "an easy method by which a person can quickly attain perfection, O lotus-eyed Kṛṣṇa, as usually, when trying to control the mind, *yogīs* become exhausted in restraining it, and despondent when they cannot retain concentration" (XI.29.1–2). When exhausted by efforts based on one's own *yogic* prowess in the attempt to still the mind, "one should worship *Īśvara* joyfully . . . as it is by this means that the cause of *saṁsāra*, the cycle of birth and death, ceases" (II.2.6). So as to transcend suffering and attain liberation, the *yogī* turns to *Īśvara*, given that *māyā*, the source of suffering, is *Īśvara*'s power, so it is only *Īśvara* who can effortlessly remove it.

But, more important than this—which, in essence, is nothing other than a practical consideration of ease—there is a more profound hierarchical issue at stake. For Jīva, the cause of suffering is not just ignorance of one's *ātman*, but, more fundamentally still, ignorance of, or aversion to, a higher Supreme *Ātman* (*Paramātman*), *Īśvara*, God. This leads to the second reason *bhakti* differs from other *yogas*: the much more significant difference for the *Bhāgavata* is not ultimately just a prosaic matter of ease between *yoga* systems, but one of metaphysical hierarchy. There are different transcendent levels to the Ultimate Truth. The *ātman* may be the ultimate essence of an individual beyond the categories of body and mind, but *Īśvara* is a still higher Truth beyond the *ātman*. Realizing this, the *bhakta* redirects consciousness to *Īśvara*, rather than striving to direct it to its own inherent nature of objectless consciousness. This, in essence, is *bhakti yoga*. While some can indeed attain the *ātman* (also known as *puruṣa*) through *yogic* virtuosity and meditational prowess based on personal willpower, the attainment of *Īśvara*, a higher and Supreme *Ātman*, and entrance into *Īśvara*'s divine transcendent realm of Vaikuṇṭha, the personal abode of Viṣṇu, the Kingdom of God, is attainable only (but easily) by *bhakti*:

> Those whose minds have become purified by the performance of mature *bhakti* by drinking the nectar of narrations about You, O Lord, attain knowledge, the essence of renunciation, and easily attain the divine realm of Vaikuṇṭha. Others, those who fix their minds . . . by the power of their *yoga-samādhi*, enter into You [in Your partial manifestation] as the *puruṣa*. But theirs is hard work, unlike through the path of service [that is, *bhakti*]. (III.5.45–46; see also IV.22.40)

So in addition to the "hard work" involved, the destination differs: other processes, for Jīva, such as the *jñāna* path of realizing the truths of scripture; *aṣṭāṅga yoga*, the path of stilling the mind; Sāṅkhya, the path of metaphysical analysis; and *karma yoga*, the path of selfless duty, can all awaken detachment and lead one to the *ātman/Brahman* aspect of the Absolute.[8] From the perspective of the *Bhāgavata*, these other traditions provide exactly what they claim to provide: direct experience of the *ātman* beyond the *guṇas* (namely, realization of *Brahman*, the experience of pure, eternal, blissful consciousness devoid of all objects other than consciousness itself). But we will discuss in this section how the *ātman* aspect of the self, while transcendent, is not the ultimate expression of the Absolute Truth in the *Bhāgavata*, but only a part of it. As will become increasingly evident as we proceed, and as with the theistic readings of the *Gītā*,[9] the *Bhāgavata* considers *Īśvara*, the Supreme *Ātman*, to be the highest aspect of *Brahman*. *Īśvara* is distinct, transcendent to, and eternally related as supreme cause to His reflections as the myriad individual *ātmans*. The individual *ātman* is only a part of, but not the entirety of, the Absolute. So *bhakti* is different from other *yogas* hierarchically in *Bhāgavata* theology; it leads to the highest and most complete level of Truth—God, the unlimited, eternal Supreme Being—where other *yogas* reveal only the individual *ātman*, which is a partial and limited expression of Truth (even as it can attain a state of infinity and eternality). In fact, if *yoga* or any spiritual practice does not lead to *Īśvara*, then it has very little ultimate value for the *Bhāgavata*.[10] Jīva defines *bhakti yoga* in general as this basic refocusing of consciousness toward *Īśvara*. To understand *Bhāgavata bhakti*, therefore, we must first understand something more deeply about *Īśvara*.

Let us first briefly recall once more what we have called the "grammar" of *bhakti*. *Bhakti* itself as practice—linguistically a type of action noun—requires a subject or agent of the action—the *bhakta* who performs *bhakti*—and an object or recipient of the action—an *Īśvara*, Supreme Being, who receives the action of *bhakti*. Now, having discussed the former two ingredients, *bhakti* and the *bhakta*, in this section we will devote some focused attention to some of the principal ways *Īśvara* is construed in the various expressions of *bhakti*. This section will be unavoidably more philosophically dense than the previous sections and thus more challenging for the non-specialist. Hence, while Jīva places it first in his work, we have placed it last in the hope that those not familiar with Indian thought will have developed some confidence by this point. But we do need to put some metaphysical building blocks in place in order to discuss the status of *Īśvara* as the object of *bhakti*, which are indispensable for anyone interested in understanding how the *Bhāgavata* understands God, *Īśvara*, the receiver of *bhakti*, in contrast with the philosophical context of other important *Īśvara* or theistic traditions of India. We will need to deal with sectarian differences here. After all, if we are called upon to devote our lives to *bhakti*, and if *bhakti* involves complete devotion to *Īśvara* (which almost always takes place in a sect-specific context), some attention needs to be directed to the philosophical discussions pertaining to the ontological position of *Īśvara* among the different schools even as this discussion will require a little more intellectual rigor and philosophical detail.

Let us begin with a brief definition of terms, which will serve as an initial semantic base whose modalities can then expand as the discussion continues. We will need to nuance the term *Īśvara* vis-à-vis the term *Brahman*, which is the prominent term referring to the Absolute Truth in the Upaniṣads and derivative Vedānta traditions. We will also contrast it with the term *Bhagavān*, which appears in the titles of both the *Bhagavad Gītā* and the *Bhāgavata Purāṇa*. Such issues will occupy us next, and we beg the indulgence of the reader unfamiliar with classical Indian thought, even as we will make every endeavor to present the material accessibly while attempting to maintain the integrity of the intellectual sophistication and subtleties of Vedānta thought. We also trust the reader more familiar with Indic philosophical categories will forgive some purposeful repetition of concepts here, adopted for those unfamiliar with the Indian metaphysical traditions in mind (and such specialists will know well that the *mokṣa* texts themselves can be very repetitive owing to their oral nature precisely with such pedagogical purposes in mind).

Definition of *Īśvara*, *Bhagavān*, and *Brahman*

The *Īśvara* (that is, theistic) element in Indic thought stretches back at least to the late Vedic period, circa 1000 B.C.E.[11] After the emergence of the philosophical traditions, *Īśvara* (feminine, *Īśvarī*) becomes the term preferred in philosophical discourse concerning the existence (or not) of a creator God—somewhat generically conceived (akin to the God of natural theology). As noted previously, ontology is the branch of philosophy that deals with the basic and ultimate categories of reality and their relations—such as, in our case, God, the souls, and the world of matter. So in partial contrast to the term *Bhagavān*, *Īśvara* is often associated more with an ontological or metaphysical category when the term occurs in philosophical contexts rather than with specific and personal Supreme Beings with qualities, such as Viṣṇu, Śiva, and Kṛṣṇa, who all lay claim to the title *Īśvara* in Purāṇic and epic texts. So there were *Īśvara-vāda* (theistic) traditions, which defended the philosophical necessity of a creator God—most of the Vedic-derived traditions (Yoga, Vedānta, Nyāya, Purāṇa, *Itihāsa*, and most Sāṅkhya strains) and *nir-Īśvara-vāda* (nontheistic) traditions, which challenged the philosophical coherence of theistic arguments (Jainism, Buddhism, the Cārvāka materialists, and, from the Vedic traditions, Mīmāṁsā and [debatably] some Sāṅkhya strains[12]). Whether *Īśvara-vāda* or *nir-Īśvara-vāda*, everyone understood the term *Īśvara* to refer to the existence of some type of a Supreme Creator Being (variously construed) and hence raised reason-based arguments for or against the inferential necessity of such a postulate from the point of view of philosophical discourse and debate (*anumāna*).

Now, while this is by no means hard and fast, where the term *Īśvara* often refers to the ontological category of God as first Cause, prime Mover, Creator, Overseer, and so forth, as can be sensed from its etymology (from the root *iś*, to have extraordinary power and sovereignty), the term *Bhagavān* tends to be used when the personal form and qualities of *Īśvara* are referenced. Put simply and simplistically, *Īśvara* would be the term used in more philosophical environments and *Bhagavān* among the faithful, so to speak, in which milieus *Īśvara*, as an accepted entity, would usually be associated with the specifics of a divine form and personality. These more personal and quality-related associations inherent in the title *Bhagavān* can be sensed from the definition of the term in the *Viṣṇu Purāṇa* as the being who possesses the six qualities of knowledge, beauty, renunciation, majesty, potency, and fame in complete fullness (VI.5.73–75[13]).

All theistic traditions accept that *Īśvara* can adopt unlimited forms and exhibit multifarious qualities—Kṛṣṇa, Viṣṇu, Śiva, Rāma, and various Goddess forms being the most commonly encountered—so the terms *Bhagavān* (and feminine *Bhagavatī*) surface most commonly when referring to these specific manifestations, each with unique and wonderful characteristics. A very clumsy parallel to these two terms might be the usage of the title "king," which is a functional or political category, as opposed to the actual person sitting on the throne, with a unique name, form, and set of qualities, even as the two coincide as the same entity. *Īśvara* and *Bhagavān* are synonymous terms, then, referring to God the Supreme Being—the Purāṇic equivalent of Jehovah, Yahweh, Allah, and the like—but while this is by no means hard and fast, the choice of term may, depending on context, invoke these different valences. The special association of the term *Bhagavān* with the specific manifestation of Kṛṣṇa is evident in the titles of texts featuring Him—the *Bhagavad Gītā* and of course the *Bhāgavata Purāṇa* itself[14]—but it is used abundantly for Śiva (for example, IV.29.42), Viṣṇu, and other manifestations of *Īśvara*.[15]

The term *Brahman*, by the time of the Upaniṣads,[16] signifies the Ultimate Truth underlying all reality. It is with this term that things get technical and rather more complicated. While *Brahman* is often described as beyond descriptive categories and conceptuality,[17] the qualities typically associated with it are *sat*, literally "being";[18] *cit*, consciousness; and *ānanda*, bliss.[19] Now in some places in the Upaniṣads, this Truth is depicted in nonpersonal terms as a qualityless and formless but conscious infinite omnipresence[20]—whereas in other places it is depicted in personal terms—as a thinking, willing individual who is the Supreme Creator God.[21] Thus the simple term *Brahman* can refer to either an impersonal/nonpersonal Supreme Truth or a personal Supreme Truth, depending on different Upaniṣads (or, indeed, sections within an Upaniṣad)[22] and, thereafter, on the partialities of the later Vedānta schools derived from them. We can refer to these possibilities as monistic (nonpersonal Absolute) and monotheistic (personal Absolute), respectively, or simply impersonalism and personalism. When the term *Brahman* is used in the latter sense, referring to a Supreme Being who is the God of Creation, it becomes equated and synonymous with *Īśvara*. Thus *Brahman* and *Īśvara* can also be synonyms, especially in the monotheistic traditions such the Vaiṣṇava ones. And in the *Bhagavad Gītā* and *Bhāgavata*, all these terms—*Īśvara*, *Bhagavān*, and *Brahman*—refer to one and the same Kṛṣṇa—as they do to Śiva in the Śaivite traditions and their feminine forms to Devī in the Goddess traditions (the relationship between these divine manifestations—a Purāṇa issue—will occupy us later, once we have our semantic and ontological building blocks—a Vedānta issue—in place).

The term *ātman* is inseparably associated with the term *Brahman* and usually (but by no means always) used when referring to *Brahman* as embodied in the individual micro living entities, where the term *Brahman* is usually used where the ultimate macro source Truth underpinning all reality is intended. The terms are often used interchangeably, however. Depending on the school (which again reflects partiality to differing Upaniṣadic references as we will discuss), *ātman* is either understood as completely identical with *Brahman*, rendering the two terms entirely synonymous, most notably with the "nonpersonal" monist schools such as *advaita Vedānta*;[23] or perceived as a differentiated part of *Brahman*, qualitatively the same insofar as it comprises pure consciousness but nonetheless quantitatively a vastly lesser part or individualized portion of *Brahman* and an eternally distinct part. This latter view is the defining feature of Vaiṣṇavism, the cluster of "personalist," monotheistic schools, such as that of the Vedānta of the twelth-century theologian Rāmānuja, whom we will quote frequently, the theological forerunner to Jīva's own school.[24]

As a point of interest, the Krishnamacarya-derived yoga lineages that have spread the practice of *āsana* and basic *yoga* philosophy so widely in the West have their Vedānta roots in Rāmānuja's Vedānta tradition, the philosophical name for which is *viśiṣṭādvaita Vedānta*. Krishnamacarya was a staunch adherent of this tradition, and his son Desikachar as well as his son-in-law Iyengar maintained their identity with it, even though very few students of these teachers have any awareness of this aspect of their *guru*'s philosophical and spiritual identity, as it was not stressed by them.[25] The other great teacher associated through his disciples with the general spread of *yoga* in the West, Swami Śivānanda, was, in contrast, an adherent of *advaita*. This focus is clearly evident not only in his own writings, but in the teachings of his students Vishnudevananda and Satcitananda (there are, of course, always exceptions to such categorizations: Krishnamacarya's disciple Pattabhi Jois, for example, was a follower of *advaita*).

In any event, for our present purposes, since *Brahman* can take either these personal or nonpersonal semantic inflections, where *Īśvara* is less ambiguous, as it is the term usually used when one specifically wishes to refer to the personal, individual, or, at least, distinct expression of *Brahman* as Creator Deity, *Īśvara* is the term I have primarily used here for God as the recipient of *bhakti*. The term is especially useful when one wishes to underscore the more generic trans-sectarian aspects of *bhakti* that would be recognized by other *Īśvara* traditions such as Śaivism, as opposed to Kṛṣṇa-specific expressions. We have also used the term *Bhagavān* in the same manner, as it is essentially synonymous with *Īśvara*, albeit with heightened personal inflections. The personal Being Kṛṣṇa, as we know, is synonymous with all three of these terms: *Īśvara*, *Bhagavān*, and *Brahman* (as are Śiva and Devī in their respective *bhakti* traditions). Having said all this, the reader must be prepared to encounter slippage and interchangeability among some of these terms but should soon develop an intuitive sense of contextual nuances.

Returning to the role of *Īśvara* as recipient of *bhakti* in Jīva's system, there are a few important questions that need to be addressed if Jīva's analysis of *bhakti* is to be considered systematic and rational rather than dogmatic. The first is the existence or necessity of any sort of *Īśvara* as Creator God in the first place. Second, if this can be established, or at least defended on rational grounds, what is the precise relationship between the personal aspect of *Brahman* as *Īśvara*/*Bhagavān*, a Being distinctive by form and qualities, and the nonpersonal expression of *Brahman*, devoid of form and qualities? And third, given that in Hindu *bhakti*, *Īśvara*, being unlimited, can and does adopt unlimited forms, and given that Hindu *bhakti* is not polytheistic, what is the justification for the *Bhāgavata*'s prioritization of Kṛṣṇa as the ultimate causal *Īśvara*—the source of all other *Īśvara* forms and manifestations—as opposed to other claimants to this position, most specifically Śiva or Viṣṇu? We stress here, on this latter score, that the question is not who is the one true *Īśvara* with the implication that other claimants are somehow "false gods," but who is the *source Īśvara* from whom other *Īśvara* forms emanate or are derived? In other words, given that all Vedānta schools whether monist or monotheist accept a plethora of *Īśvara* forms on some level, whether these are primary expressions of *Brahman* or secondary expressions (we will explain this below), then what is the ontological relationship between all these eternal *Īśvaras*? Hence, although technical, this section is indispensable in gaining a sense of the various ways *bhakti yoga* can be understood and practiced, given that *bhakti* requires an *Īśvara*, howsoever construed, as recipient.

With regard to the first issue raised above, the necessity of positing a creator *Īśvara* in the first place, the history of Indian theistic (and antitheistic) argumentation—frankly as vigorous and inconclusive an intellectual enterprise in ancient India as it has been in the West—understandably takes us far beyond our focus here. We will simply note that Jīva is heir to much of this history, which had long been fine-tuned by predecessor Vedāntins (followers of Vedānta), who defended the theism of the Upaniṣads,[26] prioritizing hermeneutics (scriptural analysis)[27] as method, as well as by Nyāya, the school of logicians, who defended theism on rational grounds, prioritizing inference (*anumāna*).[28] (As a point of interest, Caitanya, the founder of Jīva's lineage, prior to becoming an ecstatic mystic, is said to have been an outstanding teacher of Nyāya in Navadvīpa, the stronghold of the new school of Nyāya that reached its peak in the sixteenth century, when and where he was born.[29]) As is the case in the West, some of the most brilliant intellectual minds of ancient India had used reason and logic in defense of the necessity of an *Īśvara* as the ultimate intelligent cause of reality, on the one hand, and in a refutation of any such postulate on the other. But by the sixteenth century, various forms of theisms had long dominated the intellectual traditions of the subcontinent, and Jīva inherits theistic currents that had been built on long-established philosophical rationales and argumentation (see "The Object of *Bhakti*," note 71, for an example of these).

Nonetheless, with regard to these theistic traditions, we made the claim in the introduction that understanding one expression of *bhakti* provides us with a template, which can usefully be applied to other expressions. This is especially true for many of the practices of *bhakti*, as well as some of the psychological states it engenders, but much less true philosophically, in terms of the ontology of theism, that is, *Īśvara*'s relationship with the ultimate ingredients of reality. There are important and fundamental differences as to whether the Being *Īśvara* is the ultimate causal entity in terms of tracing all effects in reality back to their ultimate causes—the cause of all other causes or final "STOP sign," so to speak—or whether *Īśvara* is a partially Supreme and causal Entity but one who, in turn, is Himself also derived from some higher, nonpersonal, even more ultimate causal Absolute and hence not the final "STOP sign."

So despite the many commonalities in the various *bhakti* traditions, there are significant differences in the ultimacy assigned to *Īśvara*. To be absolutely clear about how we are using our terms, and connecting all this with the term *Brahman*, is *Īśvara*, who as the object of *bhakti* is a distinct supreme sort of personalized *ātman*,[30] the primary and final expression of *Brahman*,[31] or is *Īśvara* a secondary truth who is himself derivative of a higher nonpersonal source, which also lays claim to the term *Brahman* and thus also something that is eventually transcended? And, for that matter, what kind of ultimacy is assigned to the individual *ātman* as *bhakta*—is this individuality also ultimate and eternal or merely an illusory condition of embodiment in *saṁsāra* that dissolves in liberation? These issues have occupied the Vedānta traditions stemming from the ancient Upaniṣads for well over two millennia, with no consensus—Bādarāyaṇa's *Vedānta Sūtras* of the second century C.E. makes reference to differences among predecessor Vedāntins throughout.[32]

These concerns are not merely intellectualism: let us consider the devotional implications of these positions. If the individuality of the *ātman* is eternal, and *Īśvara* is also an eternal Supreme Being and Ultimate Truth, then the relationship between them—*bhakti*—can also be eternal. This would require an eternal trans-*prakṛti Brahman* realm or dimension wherein this relationship can take place and modalities whereby *bhakti* between the *ātman* and *Īśvara* can be expressed—a "Kingdom of God," such as, in Jiva's case, Vaikuṇṭha or Goloka replete with the *rāgātmika* liberated souls. If, on the other hand, the individuality of the *ātman* is contingent on embodiment and ultimately dissolves in liberation, and if the personal *Īśvara* too is ultimately derived from a higher nonpersonal *Brahman* Truth—a lesser manifestation or representation of some more Ultimate Truth—then *bhakti* is not eternal, but merely a temporal practice relevant in *saṁsāra* only as a method for freeing oneself from the ephemeral world of *prakṛti*. It is thus jettisoned upon liberation, a state of transpersonal, formless, and qualityless oneness, where there is no individuality and thus no ontological space for devotional relationships. So the issue deals with not only ultimate categories of reality, but the ultimate status of *bhakti*, and it is certainly relevant to the eternal destiny of the *ātman* and, thus, of considerable import.

Perhaps we can now understand more clearly, given all this, why different schools are going to assign great value and attention to deliberations and debates on these most important of issues and why we must perforce encounter the sectarian nature of the Vedānta or Purāṇa traditions in order to understand some of the various possible modalities of *bhakti* and some of the different ways in which *Īśvara* is conceived in Hinduism. And all this requires technical attention and a modicum of philosophical rigor.

Prakṛti* and the Three *Guṇas*: *Sattva*, *Rajas*, and *Tamas

Before we proceed with this, since we are setting out ubiquitously occurring terms and concepts here, let us interrupt our flow for a moment and take the opportunity to briefly discuss the metaphysics of *prakṛti*, the world of matter, the third entity in the triad of *Īśvara*, *ātman*, and the created world. In fact, this is not unrelated to our overall concerns at this point, as *Īśvara* is commonly conceived in the theistic traditions as the creator of the material world of *prakṛti* (physical reality)[33] and *bhakti* as nothing other than the offering of ingredients of *prakṛti* (including one's *prakṛtic* body and mind) to *Īśvara*. With regard to the essential makeup of *prakṛti*, the *Bhāgavata* accepts the overall schema of the metaphysics of the Sāṅkhya (literally "numeration") system,[34] although it subsumes the evolutes of *prakṛti* as completely subordinate to and derived from *Īśvara*. But bracketing the position of *Īśvara* for a moment, in Sāṅkhya metaphysics, the universe of animate and inanimate entities is perceived as ultimately the product of two ontologically distinct entities coming together. These two entities are *prakṛti*, or the primordial unconscious material matrix of the physical universe,[35] and *puruṣa*, a term synonymous with *ātman*, the innumerable conscious souls or selves embedded within it.

As a result of the interaction between these two entities, the material universe evolves in a series of stages. The actual catalysts in this evolutionary process are the three *guṇas*, literally "strands" or "qualities," which are inherent in *prakṛti*. While it is impossible to translate these terms into a one-word English equivalent, three prominent qualities associated with each of these, respectively, are *sattva*, "tranquillity"; *rajas*, "action"; and *tamas*, "inertia."[36] These *guṇas* are sometimes compared with the threads that underpin the existence of a rope; just as a rope is actually a combination of threads, so all manifest reality actually consists of a combination of the *guṇas*. These *guṇas* are mentioned incessantly throughout the *Bhāgavata*, as are the various evolutes from *prakṛti*, and thus require some attention in order to navigate the frequent references to them in our translations in parts 2 and 3.

Given the meditative focus of the text, the *guṇas* are especially significant to the Yoga tradition in terms of their psychological manifestations; in Yoga, since the mind and therefore all psychological/cognitive dispositions and functions are products of *prakṛti*, they are also made up of the *guṇas*—the only difference between the subtle mind and grosser matter being that the former has a larger preponderance of *sattva* and the latter of *tamas*. Therefore, according to the specific intermixture and proportionality of the *guṇas*, living beings exhibit different types of mind-sets and psychological dispositions. Thus, when *sattva* is predominant in an individual, the qualities of lucidity, tranquillity, wisdom, discrimination, detachment, peacefulness, and happiness manifest; when *rajas* is predominant, hankering, attachment, energetic endeavor, passion, power, restlessness, creative activity, and, ultimately, frustration and unfulfillment result (the term *rāga* comes from the same root); and when *tamas*, the *guṇa* least favorable for Yoga, is predominant, sleep, ignorance, delusion, disinterest, lethargy, depression, destructive behavior, and disinclination toward constructive activity ensue.

Just as there are an unlimited variety of colors stemming from the intermixture of the three primary colors, different hues being simply expressions of the specific proportionality of red, yellow, and blue, so the unlimited psychological dispositions of living creatures (and of physical material forms) stem from the intermixture of the *guṇas*, specific states of mind being the products of the particular proportionality of the intermixture of the three *guṇas*. The *guṇas* are continually interacting and competing with one another, one *guṇa* becoming prominent for a while and overpowering the others, only to be dominated in turn by the increase of one of the other *guṇas* (*Gītā* XIV.10). The Sāṅkhya text, the *Yuktidīpikā*, compares them with the wick, fire, and oil of the lamp, which, while opposed to one another in their nature, come together to produce light (13). Clearly, *sattva* is the *guṇa* most favorable to Yoga in general, and one for which there is no excess, where the other two, in excess, are obstacles (even as some degree of *rajas* and *tamas* is indispensable for embodied existence[37]). Much *yoga* practice in general, then, occupies itself with maximizing *sattva*.

Not only do the *guṇas* underpin the philosophy of mind in Yoga, but the activation and interaction of these *guṇa* qualities result in the production of the entirety of physical forms that also evolve from the primordial material matrix, *prakṛti*, under the same principle.[38] Thus the physical compositions of objects such as air, fire, water, stone, and so on differ because of the differing constitutional makeup of specific *guṇas* underpinning these elements: air contains more of the buoyancy of *sattva*, stones more of the denseness of the *tamas* element, and fire more of the energy of *rajas*. The *guṇas* allow for the infinite plasticity of *prakṛti* and the objects of the world. The process by which the universe evolves from *prakṛti* is usefully compared with the churning of milk: when milk receives a citric catalyst, yogurt, curds, or butter emerge. These immediate products, in turn, can be further manipulated to produce a tertiary series of products—toffee, milk desserts, cheese, and the like.[39] And, again, connecting all this to our present discussion, *prakṛti* with its *guṇas* is a *śakti*, power, of *Īśvara*, and thus all these permutations are the immanent aspect of *Īśvara*, God as world (*Gītā* VII.4–7, 17).

The Nature of *Īśvara* in Vedānta: Primary or Derivative?

With these basic definitions and metaphysical infrastructure in place, we can return to our questions pertaining to the transcendent aspect of *Īśvara* as object of *bhakti* and whether this Being is the ultimate aspect of *Brahman* or not. For our purposes here, we can identify two general spheres of discussion or contention pertaining to the nature of *Īśvara* in the Vedānta and Purāṇa traditions that have spanned two millennia, both with their roots in the Vedic (Upaniṣad) texts and both revolving around issues of cause and effect. One, touched on above, pertains to whether *Īśvara* is the highest feature of *Brahman*, the Ultimate, the personal source from which everything else is manifest, or whether *Īśvara* represents a secondary aspect of *Brahman*, derived from a higher nonpersonal expression of *Brahman* beyond all forms and qualities. Put differently, the question is whether the *ultimate* causal expression of *Brahman* is personal or nonpersonal. This is primarily a Vedāntic issue. The second and subsequent discussion is, irrespective of whether *Īśvara* is primary and causal or whether secondary and derived, which specific Divine Being, *Bhagavān,* is the ultimate causal *Īśvara* from whom all other *Īśvaras* derive or, at least, are sustained? This is more a Purāṇic issue.

We note that almost all traditions stemming from these textual traditions accept that *Brahman*, if it is to be complete (and also to account for the fact that *yogic* practice and experiences attest to two primary modes of encountering the Ultimate), must have both personal and nonpersonal features: almost all followers of the Vedānta and the Purāṇas accept some sort of *Īśvara* as well as some type of nonpersonal aspect to the Absolute.[40] So the first question is whether *Īśvara* is primary and foundational or a secondary-derived manifestation from a higher Truth, and the second question relates to the hierarchical relationship among the various *Īśvara* forms and manifestations. And it is important to reiterate with regard to the second question that the various followers of the Vedānta and the Purāṇas all accept that *Īśvara* takes many different forms, which are all *Īśvara*, so when considering which *Īśvara* is ultimate and causal to the others, there is no implication that the others are not true *Īśvaras*. Put differently, since *bhakti* is embedded in traditions that are either monistic (subscribing to a "nonpersonal" Absolute) or monotheistic (subscribing to a "personal" Absolute),[41] and in both cases rejects the label of polytheism, then there cannot be a plurality of independent and autonomous *Īśvaras*, as is the case with polytheism.[42] In polytheism, the gods—small "g," perhaps better termed demigods (the *devas* in the Indic case, whom we have been calling "celestials")—are more or less equal or, at best, there is a minor hierarchy among them. In Hinduism, such gods, *devas*, are retained, but they are nontranscendent but rather embodied beings, relegated to the temporal celestial spheres of *saṁsāra*, where they too are bound by their (exceptionally good) *karma* and hence retain their positions only temporarily. They are eternally subordinate to the various forms of *Īśvara*. So with polytheism discounted, either the various manifestations of *Īśvara* are all derivative of a higher, qualityless *Brahman* (nonpersonalism or monism), or they are all secondary manifestations from one supreme source *Iśvara* (personalism or monotheism).

On this first question, by the end of the first millennium and thereafter (but with roots in the Upaniṣad texts, *Mahābhārata* epic, and *Gītā*, dating back several centuries prior to the Common Era), the Vedānta tradition broadly split into two major streams with multiple substreams: the *advaita*, or monist tradition, and its offshoots, which consider the highest *Brahman* to be ultimately devoid of form and qualities; and the monotheist Vaiṣṇava traditions, which hold the highest *Brahman* to be the eternal personal *Īśvara* who possesses unlimited forms and qualities. *A-dvaita* means "no duality" (and is thus more or less synonymous with the term "monism"; "a" prefixed to a noun in Sanskrit negates the noun, as in *atheist* in English). According to this Vedānta lineage, there is precisely only the one nonpersonal, formless, qualityless *Brahman*. Indeed, this tradition goes a significant step further than this—anything else is ultimately unreal. There are absolutely no dualities whatsoever in *Brahman*. So the apparently plural and individual *ātmans* are illusory, the product of ignorance; they are, in fact, nothing other than the one undivided *Brahman*.[43] And, more, the world of *prakṛti*, with all its forms and dualities, including the bodies that appear to individualize and differentiate the *ātmans* containing them and the minds that characterize them, are all also false: an illusion. In the language of *advaita*, they are a superimposition (*adhyāsa*) on the one undivided *Brahman*, like an image superimposed upon another in photography or, using the standard *advaita* metaphor, the notion of a snake superimposed because of defective perception upon what is actually a rope lying on the road. Thus, for *advaita*, all manifest forms (that is, all creation), although appearing apparently real, are ultimately illusory, appearing real only because of being superimposed upon the formless *Brahman* by *māyā*, illusion. They are in essence like the forms in a mirage.

For our purposes, consequent on this, if the creation is illusory, then so, ultimately, is the notion of a Creator for *advaita Vedānta*. *Īśvara* is apparently real only to the extent the world of created forms is conventionally real (*vyavahāra*), but from the perspective of the highest reality (*paramārtha*), neither the world nor *Īśvara* ultimately exists. Just as in the world of the mirage, there may appear to be an oasis with water and palm trees, but when correct perception is attained one realizes there is only desert, so the creation, along with its creatures and creator, appears real only in conventional reality, but all are dispelled when awareness of ultimate reality dawns. *Īśvara* thus also proves to be as much a part of the illusory superimposition upon *Brahman* as anything else. In actuality, there is only the nondifferentiated (*advaita*) *Brahman*; any perceived differences or dualities are the product of *avidyā*, ignorance.

Importantly for our purposes, following on these presuppositions, the *bhakti yoga* performed by an embodied *ātman* to *Īśvara*, for *advaita Vedānta*, is useful as a preliminary aid in the pursuit of enlightenment for those still laboring under the grip of the illusion of dualities but eventually becomes discarded along with the very notion of an *Īśvara* once knowledge of the one formless nonindividualized Absolute dawns. Put succinctly, neither *bhakta*, *bhakti yoga*, nor *Īśvara* as object of *bhakti* has a factual existence in the fully enlightened, postmortem liberated state.[44] There are simply no dualities whatsoever in the Supreme reality, hence *a-dvaita*. In sum, although the *advaita* traditions may perform with serious intent and devotional vigor all the processes of *bhakti* that we discussed previously, *bhakti* in these traditions is, at the end of the day, method, not goal.

With one important exception, the Vaiṣṇava traditions such as the *Bhāgavata* (and some Śaivite traditions) also consider themselves to be nondualists, insofar as they accept everything as an expression of the one Truth, but hold that the nonduality of the Absolute nonetheless has real differences inherent within it.[45] This is amply reflected in the name given by Rāmānuja, who was the first Vaiṣṇava theologian to write a commentary on the *Vedānta Sūtras*, to his Vedānta school: *viśiṣṭa-advaita*.[46] Here, the *advaita* signification is retained but prefixed with the term *viśiṣṭa*, "differentiated." *Brahman* is indeed nondual, but there are "differences" inherent within it, distinct components within the oneness of *Brahman*—namely, an ontologically real world with real souls. For the Vaiṣṇavas, while *Brahman* does indeed have nonpersonal qualities and powers (*śaktis*)—such as *prakṛti* and the *guṇas*—in contrast with *advaita*, it is understood, in its highest causal expression, to be personal, *Īśvara*. This Person is Viṣṇu/Nārāyaṇa/Kṛṣṇa. *Īśvara* is a distinct Supreme Being, who, while an individual, is unlimited in names, forms, qualities, and deeds. Hence these traditions can be considered robustly monotheistic (even as this Person can also manifest in other derivative *Īśvara* forms such as Śiva and Devī, as will be explained later).

The *ātmans* are manifestations of *Īśvara* and thus, as parts, are similar to their cause in their inherent makeup as eternal conscious beings. But they are distinct individual entities, even as their constitutional dependence on *Īśvara* requires that they be relationally connected with *Īśvara*. This relationality can manifest either, ideally, in a direct relationship of eternal *bhakti*, previously discussed, or, indirectly and perversely, by being subject to *Īśvara*'s power of ignorance and illusion, *māyā/avidyā*, in *saṁsāra*, embodied life. These options reflect the free will and choices of the *ātman*. And the world, like the *ātmans*, is real and emanated. Within this variegation of the one Absolute, the personal *Īśvara* is the highest expression and the support of all other aspects of reality (that is, of the world and the souls). All of these entities, in contrast with *advaita*, are inherently real; they are not false superimpositions.

Perhaps we can say that Rāmānuja's *Brahman* is "holistic"—where parts and differences exist, but in a holistic harmony—and Śaṅkara's is "homogeneous"—there are no parts.[47] Curiously, this means that, ontologically, in terms of its understanding of the basic ingredients of reality—God, world, souls, with the last distinct from but derived from the first—Vaiṣṇavism is much closer theologically to the Abrahamic monotheistic traditions, despite the geographic, cultural, and textual disparities, than the fellow Vedānta traditions of *advaita*, despite sharing the same locus, religious and cultural ethos and practices, and identical scriptural traditions with the latter. And, as an aside, these Vaiṣṇava (and some Śaivite) traditions undermine the ill-informed and culturally myopic notion that monotheism is a uniquely theological development of the Abrahamic traditions.

Therefore, in Vaiṣṇavism, the divine forms of Kṛṣṇa, Viṣṇu, and Śiva and their feminine consorts and counterparts—Lakṣmī and Parvatī and so on—are not illusory. They are ultimate, transcendent Beings, and it is they who are the source of all nonpersonal powers (*śaktis*) and entities such as *prakṛti* and the *ātmans*. Moreover, since these Beings are eternal and transcendent to *prakṛti*, they occupy non-*prakṛtic* realms within *Brahman*, Vaikuṇṭha—the Kingdom of God, within which, for the Gauḍīya tradition, lies Goloka, the realm exclusive to Kṛṣṇa, and also Śiva-loka. Consequently—connecting all this to the theme of this volume—*bhakti* is not simply a utilitarian process relevant for those embodied in ignorance in this world: it is never discarded but can continue eternally in the postmortem liberated state in these divine realms. Now we have a more grounded philosophical basis to understand our discussion on the *rāgātmikas*: the loving exchanges and interactions and reciprocal service between Kṛṣṇa and His *bhaktas*, when He incarnated into this world as described in the tenth book of the *Bhāgavata* and featured here in part 3, serve as a window into the eternal relationships that can transpire between Kṛṣṇa and the liberated *bhaktas* in the divine realm of Goloka. *Bhakti*, in these traditions, is thus both method and goal.

And there are all sorts of variants. Given our focus on Kṛṣṇa, we again wish to refer, albeit summarily, to Kaśmir Śaivism, by way of an example of non-Vaiṣṇava theism. We can now situate it as occupying an interesting location somewhere between these two Vedānta streams. We should note that Vedānta, whether monist or monotheist, has been primarily a Vaiṣṇava enterprise. But although Śaiva philosophy has not been included in most of the official doxographies (compilations of philosophical schools),[48] the notion of the "six schools of Indian philosophy" that eventually becomes reified as standard is something of an artificiality.[49] For whatever reason, the Śākta/Tantra/Siddha cluster of traditions did not make it into the final list, but these are intellectually rich and metaphysically sophisticated traditions, with very ancient roots,[50] so their exclusion has likely a lot more to do with the partialities and influence of elitist caste-sensitive scholastic traditions than a lack of philosophical coherence and theological vigor on the part of the Śaiva/Śākta traditions.

In any event, Kaśmir Śaivism is monistic, insofar as the ultimate highest Truth (*parama-Śiva*) is transpersonal and the individuality of the *ātman* is illusory. But this tradition does hold the world to be real and not illusory, as also the personal form of Śiva, and strongly rebuts *advaita Vedānta* on that score. All form and individualism are products of *śakti*, vibrational creative consciousness, real but emanating from an ultimate higher nonpersonal expression of Śiva. So these traditions are monistic, but this is not the extreme monism of *advaita Vedānta*. Nonetheless, here too *bhakti*, while usually performed in a much more robust manner than in *advaita* given that the person Śiva, while secondary to a higher impersonal Absolute, is decidedly real and not illusory, is still ultimately made redundant when one realizes one's oneness with the ultimate Supreme aspect of formless Śiva.[51]

This type of qualified monism of Kaśmir Śaivism is in contrast with another Śaiva tradition, the dualist Śaiva Siddhānta, where *bhakti* constitutes the eternal relationship between Śiva and the *ātman*, two individuals united in the oneness of love. The *ātman* does not merge into Śiva and lose its individuality in this tradition. Therefore, as we have noted, Śaiva Siddhānta is thus closer to Vaiṣṇavism on the Vedānta spectrum, as it upholds an eternal distinction between Śiva and His devoted *ātmans*, even as the focus on the forms, qualities, and deeds of *Īśvara* and His *bhaktas* in the liberated state are less evident in Śaiva Siddhānta, if at all.

Let us consider a spectrum between radical nonpersonalism, a *Brahman* completely devoid of all qualities and forms as represented by *advaita* on the one hand,[52] and, on the other, Jīva's Gauḍīya Vedānta tradition, with its full-blown personalism, the ultimate expression of which is Kṛṣṇa and his *rāgātmika bhaktas* in Goloka, a realm of pure consciousness bursting with transcendent forms and qualities. Kaśmir Śaivism might be located somewhere in the center of this spectrum, and Śaiva Siddhānta center right, veering slightly more toward Jīva's modality. Rāmānuja's *viśiṣṭādvaita* school is very close to Jīva's, along with that of the twelth-century theologian Madhva. These schools are both sister (or perhaps more accurately parent) traditions to Jīva's Gauḍīya Vaiṣṇavism, except that in Rāmānuja and Madhva's tradition, Kṛṣṇa is an incarnation of Viṣṇu/Nārāyaṇa, assumed only when the latter wishes to incarnate into the world and not vice versa.[53] It is Viṣṇu and His divine realm of Vaikuṇṭha that are ultimate here.

While, as we have seen, Jīva and Rūpa take great pains to substantiate their understanding of *bhakti* with quotes from the *Bhāgavata*, the notion of Goloka with its *rāgātmikā* modes of love of God is, to all intents and purposes, a new "revelation" imparted by Caitanya to his disciples, who in turn "theologize" it systematically through a massive output of devotional literature in the sixteenth century, as discussed in the introduction. The philosophical name of the Caitanya (Gauḍīya) school is *acintya-bheda-abheda* (inconceivably one and different), *acintya-bheda-abheda* points to the position that the world and the souls are one with Kṛṣṇa (*abheda*) but also different (*bheda*). This relationship is inconceivable (*acintya*) and beyond the capability of human intelligence to comprehend (however, Jīva invests as much philosophical energy as any other Vedāntin in arguing why this must be so). All this is very similar to Rāmānuja's *viśiṣṭādvaita* (qualified nondualism) tradition—differing in terms of its metaphysical basics on technical details of interest only to scholastics. There is no doubt that the Gauḍīya tradition rests its theological superstructure on the substructural foundations established by Rāmānuja, along with the later twelfth-century theistic Vedāntin Madhva, two highly revered predecessors of the tradition.

Madhva, briefly introduced (as the Gauḍīya tradition formally situates itself within this lineage),[54] established a radical dualist school in explicit oppositional contrast with Śaṅkara's *advaita*. Indeed, his school is polemically called *dvaita* (dualist)[55] *Vedānta*. A powerful and provocative philosopher,[56] Madhva argued that there are five eternal fundamental differences among the ultimate "reals,"[57] or ingredients of reality (we use the term "reals," as Madhva vigorously opposes Śaṅkara's illusionism pertaining to the unreality of *prakṛti* and the individuality of the *ātman*).[58] There are eternal differences between Viṣṇu and the world, between Him and the souls, among individual souls themselves, and among the atoms of the world. For our purposes, Madhva differs marginally from the other Vaiṣṇava traditions in that, given the above metaphysics, he deems the world and souls not to emanate from God, but to be eternal coexistents, even as the former requires Viṣṇu as their support, instigator, and enabler in all things. There are other Vaiṣṇava lineages in addition to the ones we have touched upon.[59]

Such fundamental disagreements over the metaphysical location and status of *Īśvara* have been central to Vedānta since certainly the time of Śaṅkara, whose *advaita* commentaries on the Vedānta texts in the eighth to the ninth century made him a figurehead of that tradition. But these issues are referenced throughout the *Vedānta Sūtras* of the second century C.E. and ultimately have their genesis in the Upaniṣads spanning much of the first millennium B.C.E. The roots of the problem, if we can call it such, originate in the fact that the Upaniṣads appear to make conflicting statements. In some places, these texts suggest that the highest *Brahman* is a personal being (for example, see *Śvetāsvatara* III.1ff.), in others that it is nonpersonal (for instance, in *Kena* I.4–5). Likewise, some places imply that the *ātman* and *Brahman* are nondifferent (as in *Chāndogya* VI.8.7ff.), others that they are nondifferent insofar as they are *Brahman* yet simultaneously still separate as individuals and hierarchically distinct (such as in *Chāndogya* VI.2.3; *Śvetāśvatāra* I.6–10). And, again, there are references that can be read to suggest the world is unreal (see *Bṛhadāraṇyaka* IV.4.9), and others that it is real (*Chāndogya* VI.3.2). The debates among the modern representatives of these lineages on such issues continue to the present day and are, indeed, part of the traditional training in the schools. Such debates mostly prioritize and revolve around scriptural exegesis but also engage reason and argument in substantial ways.

For text-critical academic scholars such differences are natural, reflecting the composition of the Upaniṣads over the course of several centuries and thus of different thinkers expressing distinct views that are diachronically as well as synchronically various. An orthodox Vedānta thinker, however, does not perceive the Upaniṣads either as chronologically evolving or as synchronically authored by different humans: as discussed in appendix 1, they are considered *Śruti*, eternal divine revelation not composed by humans (*apauruṣeya*).[60] Consequently, from a traditional perspective, as transcendent scripture, they cannot be contradictory or imperfect in any way, but are a priori consistent (*Vedānta Sūtras* 1.4). Since the vagaries of human historical context and composition are not an option, then any supposed internal contradictions can only be apparently so but in fact must stem from an imperfect understanding or reading of these texts. That being the case, an interpretative lens is required—one that will organize the apparently contradictory or inconsistent statements into meaningful harmony. Hermeneutics refers to the methods applied in scriptural interpretation, and a good deal of traditional Vedānta hermeneutics is nothing other than applying such a lens. In fact, it is with the intention of systematizing the Upaniṣadic statements into a cohesive set of teachings[61] that the *Vedānta Sūtras* (also known as the *Uttara Mīmāṁsā* or *Brahma Sūtras*) was written in the first place and its authorship assigned to our sage Vyāsa (Bādarāyaṇa), whom we will encounter in the tales.

This, however, did not exactly solve the problem, as the *Vedānta Sūtras* are so minimalist in content, frugal in explanatory detail, and cryptic in meaning[62] that they are incomprehensible in their own right without commentaries. They too require clarification. This leads to the requirement of a third tier or layer of what has come to constitute the Vedānta corpus: the commentaries (*bhāṣya*), but now on both the Upaniṣads themselves as well as the Sūtras that were ostensibly written to clarify them. These commentaries, however, further compounded the problem rather than resolving it, but for different reasons. Although, unlike the previous two *Vedānta* strata, the commentaries are extensive, clear, internally consistent, and comprehensible, the new dilemma they introduce is that the interpretative lenses the different schools adopt to clarify the Upaniṣads produce explanations that differ radically from each other on the most fundamental of ontological issues. Put more precisely, what we might call the Vaiṣṇava-associated lineages differ significantly from the *advaita Vedānta*–derived ones,[63] along the lines we have touched upon above.

After all, broadly and simplistically put, much human intellectual endeavor, irrespective of time or place, or whether philosophical, religious, or scientific, is directed toward attempting to understand the nature of the physical world, the nature of life and the living entities within it, and the nature of its cause. Put into Vedānta categories: Is the ultimate cause, *Brahman*, personal or nonpersonal? Is the living entity, *ātman*, unequivocally nondifferent from *Brahman*, or is it individualized and thus distinct in some way? And is the physical world, *prakṛti*, real and actual, or is it an illusory, false superimposition? These are the most basic, essential, primordial, and universal of intellectual issues, yet ones over which the *Vedānta* lineages differ about as radically as it is possible to differ.

Thus, for example, Śaṅkara (following a Buddhist schema[64]) creates harmony from the apparently conflicting statements of the Upaniṣads by organizing them into a two-tiered hierarchy. From this *advaita* perspective, when the Vedānta texts[65] speak of the *ātman* as individual, *Brahman* as personal (*Īśvara/Bhagavān*), and the world as real, they are speaking from the perspective of *vyavahārika*, lower conventional reality. As we know, conventional reality in *advaita* is ultimately false and illusory. On the other hand, the statements indicating *Brahman* to be nonpersonal and nondual, the individualism of the *ātman* illusory, and the world false, are speaking from the perspective of *paramārthika*, higher absolute reality, and thus ultimately true. He can thus accept all the statements in the Vedānta texts as absolute and true (as he is bound to do as an orthodox Vedāntin) by relegating conflicting statements to one or other of his two hierarchical strata, lower and higher.

For Rāmānuja, in stark contrast, the vigorous opponent of Śaṅkara, when the texts speak of *Brahman* as nondual, they intend that everything emanates from the *Brahman* and is thus of one essence. But this does not preclude differences within the oneness (that is, the *viśiṣṭa*, "differentiation," within the *advaita*), and thus the oneness is rather a "holistic" than an absolute, nondifferentiated oneness. Likewise with the individual *ātman*: it may be nondual from *Brahman*, as part to whole, but this does not negate its individuality. Along the same lines, when *Brahman* is spoken of as without qualities, this points to a lack of *prakṛtic* qualities of the three *guṇas*: it does not preclude divine (*Brahman*) qualities and forms.[66] When described as impersonal, *Brahman*'s all-pervasive energies (*śaktis*) are intended (like the light vis-à-vis the sun), and when depicted as personal, *Brahman*'s ultimate feature as Viṣṇu is signified. And the unreality of the world points to its temporality, not its illusionality. Thus, Rāmānuja's interpretative lens also allows him to accept all the apparently conflicting textual statements to be absolute and true. But rather than resolving this through a two-tiered hierarchical model like Śaṅkara—conventional (lower) and ultimate (higher)—he relegates them to different modalities of *Brahman*: some statements refer to *Brahman* as *Īśvara*, some to *Brahman* as the world, and some to *Brahman* as the individual *ātman* in *saṁsāra*.

So the interpretative lenses the traditions apply to harmonize the apparently conflicting statements of the Upaniṣads work well in terms of appearing convincing for those who already subscribe to that lineage (that is, using the language of Yoga psychology, those whose *saṁskāras* have been trained to align with that viewpoint). And certainly an extensive and impressive amount of hermeneutical energy is invested in them. But the fact is, other equally carefully crafted lenses can be, and obviously have been, formulated with their own harmonizing persuasiveness. At the end of the day, the relative merit of these interpretative lenses ends up being evaluated along sectarian lines.

So, in summary, because the Upaniṣads appear contradictory and unsystematic, the *Vedānta Sūtras* cryptic and incomprehensible, and the commentaries, at least of the two streams noted above, conflicting and in radical disagreement among themselves,[67] the various *Vedānta* traditions have engaged in debate for centuries on these basic ontological issues. Indeed, they continue to do so and, in fact, this has become part of their very mandate and preparatory training for lineage initiates (and new Vedānta schools periodically emerge).[68] These debates prioritize and revolve around hermeneutics and exegesis (scriptural interpretation) but engage logic, *nyāya*, in substantial ways. In fact, since Indic philosophy rarely proceeds without a refutation of opposing views, the *pūrva-pakṣa*, the argumentation honed around these issues, has been one of the primary issues defining the various schools, particularly, but by no means exclusively, within Vedānta circles.[69] One need only consider the massive amount of attention the twelth-century theologian Rāmānuja directs against the *advaita* position right at the very outset of his commentary on the *Vedānta Sūtras* (I.1.1), which takes up about a fifth of his bulky commentary on the entire text,[70] to get a sense of how philosophically problematic—and theologically offensive—the Vaiṣṇavas find this attempt to deny ultimate ontological reality to their beloved *Īśvara*.

Jīva is heir to a number of anti-*advaita* arguments, which, along with so much else, we have noted are inherited from the great theologians Rāmānuja and Madhva by the later Vaiṣṇava schools. An exposition of them would be extensive and beyond the scope of our focus.[71] But we hope the reader who has been patient enough to endure the modicum of background philosophical information outlined above has a better sense of some of the different ways of understanding *Īśvara* and their origins. Hopefully it is also clear by now why the status assigned to *Īśvara* will be pivotal to understanding the different ways *bhakti* is understood in these various traditions, keeping in mind our framing of the syntactical nature of *bhakti* as involving an *Īśvara* as distinct object of *bhakti*, a *bhakta* as a distinct agent of *bhakti*, and *bhakti yoga* itself as the performance of devotional acts in a phenomenal world.

In this regard, before proceeding, I suggest that the friction such arguments generate is more than mere standard interschool polemics. For our purposes in understanding Kṛṣṇa *bhakti*, the perennial impulse to defend the ultimacy of *Īśvara* can perhaps also be understood as a reflection of the deep devotion of the Vaiṣṇavas, and the eternality of the loving relationship with *Īśvara* that they envision for themselves forevermore, such that they will vigorously contest any suggestion "that *Īśvara* has been imagined by the *jīva* (*ātman*) under the spell of *avidyā*" (*Bhakti Sandarbha anu* 40). Hence Jīva, after presenting his personalist, individualist, realist, and monotheistic arguments, concludes: "Since the distinction between *Īśvara*, the support of *māyā*, and the *jīva* who is deluded by *māyā*, is established, it can be concluded that devotional activity, *bhajana* (*bhakti*),[72] is the method of attaining perfection" (*anu* 44). Indeed, the main concern of his *Sandarbhas* is to marshal philosophy and hermeneutics in support of *bhakti* as both method and goal.

Finally, and not at all irrelevant to the *Bhāgavata*'s self-perception, as well as its verdict on these differing possible monistic and monotheistic readings of the Vedānta texts, is the fact that it presents itself as being written by the great Vyāsa (also known as Bādarāyaṇa). As noted previously (and discussed further in appendix 1), Vyāsa is the same person whom tradition assigns as author of the *Vedānta Sūtras* itself, the commentary on the Upaniṣads that was intended to clarify all such philosophical differences. We will discover, in the Tale of Vyāsa, that he was despondent after writing the *Vedānta Sūtras*, as well as all his other works, including the Vedas and Upaniṣads, precisely because he had not clearly and unambiguously elaborated on *Īśvara* as the highest eternal reality: "Having compiled the collection of Purāṇas, and composed the *Vedānta Sūtras*, he remained dissatisfied; thus he composed the *Bhāgavata* as the natural commentary on his own *Vedānta Sūtras*" (*Tattva Sandarbha*, 19). In this way, the *Bhāgavata* positions itself as "the essence of all Vedānta," a clarificatory commentarial elaboration on the Vedānta by the same author and thus the last word in regard to all these issues (XII.13.15).

A Three-Tiered Hierarchy of *Brahman*

We now turn to the position of the *Bhāgavata Purāṇa* itself on all this, which will open up a further dimension pertaining to an issue we have skirted repeatedly: the experiential difference between exclusive absorption of the consciousness of the *ātman* in its own nature as pure consciousness and exclusive absorption of the consciousness of the *ātman* in *Īśvara* and, specifically, in the specifics of a personal relationship with Him. In other words, it will probe the hierarchy within the transcendent Absolute Truth itself as argued by the Vaiṣṇava Vedānta theologians (the "differentiation" of Rāmānuja's *viśiṣṭādvaita*). Here we introduce the most important *Bhāgavata* verse dealing with the ontology (the basic categories of existence) of Jīva's Kṛṣṇa tradition:

> Those who know the Truth speak of the knowledge of that nondual Truth (*advaya*)[73] as being known as *Brahman*, *Paramātman*, and *Bhagavān*." (I.2.11)[74]

This verse is essential in understanding this tradition's metaphysics of *bhakti*, because the three terms it contains are not synonyms, but ontological hierarchies. Before commencing the *Bhakti Sandarbha*, Jīva had dedicated the previous four *Sandarbhas* to discussing the differences among these three expressions of the Absolute mentioned in this verse: *Brahman*, *Paramātman*, and *Bhagavān*. This subject is understandably too extensive to detain us in great detail here, but we can partly summarize things by noting that while the Absolute Truth is indeed nondual (*advaya*, more typically referred to as *advaita* or *abheda*), this does not preclude differences within that one reality, as we have encountered with Rāmānuja. There are differences between *Īśvara* and His powers, *śaktis*. Just as, in a favorite Vaiṣṇava simile,[75] the sun and its powers are in one sense nondual—that is, the sun is one with its powers of light and heat—yet they are also in some sense distinct (one is causal, the other derivative, diminished, and secondary), so, likewise, there are differentiations within the nonduality of the Absolute (*Tattva Sandarbha anu* 43). Additionally, says Jīva, continuing the metaphor, just as the individual particles of light rays are always distinct from one another, so is the case with the plurality of eternally individual *ātmans*.

Incidentally, Vaiṣṇavism shares this latter view—the irreducible individuality of the *ātman*—with almost all schools of Hindu philosophy, including all the so-called six classical schools of Hindu philosophy except the *advaita* sub-branch of Vedānta: Yoga, Sāṅkhya, Nyāya, Vaiśeṣiká, Mīmāṁsā, and, from Vedānta, the "Vaiṣṇava" strains noted above all defend the individuality of the *ātman* on philosophical grounds. The *ātman* may be infinite in terms of the potential spread of its awareness, like the light of a solitary lightbulb were there no atmospheric or other blockages, but it is an irreducible and individual spiritual quantum, distinct from other *ātmans*. This holds true even as there is no awareness of any distinctions or "otherness" in pure consciousness when it is immersed in its own nature—there is only an awareness of infinite, eternal, nondual awareness itself. While it is prevalent in both domestic and exported neo-Hindu expressions, the *advaita* sub-branch of Vedānta is not representative from the perspective of the classical schools of premodern Indic philosophy—including Jain and Buddhist thought—in terms of not recognizing the individuality of consciousness (although, as discussed, the Śākta traditions are also monistic when it comes to the individuality of the *ātman*). This is not to say that it did not become a very important school, as is underscored by the fact that all the other later schools had to respond to its tenets in some form or fashion.

Within this tripartite hierarchy of *Bhāgavata* I.2.11 quoted above, for Jīva, the *Brahman* aspect is nonpersonal consciousness—the *ātman/puruṣa* goal of some of the Upaniṣads, the *Yoga Sūtras*, and most other *ātman*-seeking traditions, including *advaita Vedānta*.[76] In the sun metaphor, it can be analogized with the formless, qualityless, all-pervading light: "You are also that *Brahman*, the supreme light, spread out like the ether" (*Bhāgavata* IV.24.60). But the point in this analogy is that light emanates from a higher source, the sun. Nonetheless, within this impersonal effulgence, there are myriad individualized *ātmans* that, like the sun-ray particles, can partake of and "merge into" the greater body of the all-pervading light. Thus, this experience is one of eternality and infinity, devoid of all objects other than blissful consciousness itself. As the light of numerous small autonomous flames can radiate out and coextensively "merge" into one greater generic body of light, while yet remaining the light of multiple individual flames, so the consciousness of myriad *ātmans* can all "merge" into *Brahman*, sharing in one infinite, blissful, eternal experience of pure contentless awareness itself, while yet remaining distinct *ātmans*, according to Vaiṣṇava thought (and, for that matter, the philosophies of Sāṅkhya and Yoga).

The *Bhāgavata* joins other traditions in calling the experience of this aspect of *Brahman* "*jñāna*, the perception of the nondual *ātman*" (XI.19.27). In other words, since the *ātman* is an eternal part of *Brahman*, when it becomes aware of its own nature as pure consciousness, this is tantamount to awareness (*jñāna*) of *Brahman* itself (albeit of only one expression of *Brahman*), hence the synonymity of labeling this experience either *Brahman* awareness or *ātman* awareness (*brahma-jñāna/ātma-jñāna*, or sometimes just *jñāna*). Indeed, there are many passages in the text that focus on this nondual type of experience in very *advaitic* language.[77] But for Vaiṣṇava theologians, this merging of the sun ray into its light does not necessarily lead to an experience of the source of light, the sun itself. Likewise, the *ātman*'s "merging" into the impersonal *Brahman* effulgence does not lead to an experience of *Bhagavān*, as we will see.

We need not concern ourselves here with the second aspect of the Absolute mentioned in the verse, *Paramātman*, to which Jīva has dedicated an entire *Sandarbha*, the *Paramātma Sandarbha* (the third from the six), other than to note that it refers to the plethora of derivative Viṣṇu forms.[78] However, beyond even these, and certainly beyond the nonpersonal, nondual *Brahman/ātman* expression of pure consciousness, in hierarchical turn, is the third item quoted, *Bhagavān*, who is *Īśvara*, the Supreme Person in complete fullness, the source and possessor of all powers, including both the *ātman* and *prakṛti*.[79] In our metaphor, Kṛṣṇa is the source sun, from whom all derivative powers and entities such as *prakṛti* and the *ātmans* emanate and are sustained (*Gītā* VII.4–7). It is this very personal *Bhagavān* abiding in His *Brahman* realm of Goloka that is the object of *bhakti* in the Kṛṣṇa traditions.

The Absolute is thus not monolithic, standardized, or, so to speak, one-size-fits-all. The aspect of the Absolute that appears coherent and appealing to any particular individual is a reflection of that person's presuppositions (which, in *yoga* categories, are nothing other than previously cultivated *saṁskāras*, mental imprints, embedded in the *citta*, quite likely from previous lives). In actuality, one generally simply accepts the theological and metaphysical specifics of the tradition to which one connects, either because of inherited cultural or family reasons or because of being inspired by a charismatic *guru* figure whose lineage one simply adopts out of faith, as noted previously. In any event, the aspect of the Absolute one perceives is a reflection of the perceiver: "Although *Bhagavān* is one, he is approached through different mind-sets and perspectives [of the perceivers] and so perceived variously as the person *Īśvara*, as *Paramātman* or as *Brahman*, pure consciousness" (III.32.26). As with everything else, free will plays a role here: "The sages see [the absolute] differently and in a particular way according to their desire" (*anu* 7). There are choices to be made. One can seek the reimmersion of pure consciousness in its own nature as *ātman*/*Brahman*—the goal of the *Yoga Sūtras* of Patañjali[80] and of Sāṅkhya and, as we know, of *advaita Vedānta*, irrespective of whether it is individualized or not (anyway a scholastic issue, of interest to the *prakṛtic* mind). Or one can seek an eternal loving relationship with a personal God who encompasses but transcends the individual *ātman*—the goal of the *Bhāgavata* and the Vaiṣṇava reading of the *Bhagavad Gītā*.

This highest personal Truth of *Bhagavān*, then, for those selecting this latter option, being supremely independent, cannot be captured by *yoga* virtuosity and diligence, as can the *ātman*, but can be attained only by grace. We can now better appreciate the previous discussion as to why this grace is incurred only by *bhakti*: "Neither Yoga, nor Sāṅkhya, nor *dharma*, nor study (*svādhyāya*), nor austerity (*tapas*), nor renunciation can attain Me, O Uddhava, as can intense *bhakti* to Me" (XI.14.20; see also *Gītā* XI.53–54). These other paths are by no means erroneous or incorrect, but they are deemed partial in the goals they provide according to their own reckonings of these goals. Put differently, in *Bhāgavata* theology, since the *ātman* is only an aspect of the Absolute,[81] one experiencing the *ātman* through other *yoga* systems has experienced that aspect of the Absolute, but not the Supreme Person Himself (*Puruṣa-uttama*[82]). *Īśvara*, *Bhagavān*. *Bhagavān* supports but transcends the *ātman* and thus constitutes the full and complete entirety of the Absolute. We will continue to expand below on all this ontology, but note, for now, that through *bhakti*, realization of the *ātman* (*ātma-jñāna*) is anyway picked up unsolicited along the way:[83] "Because of the insurmountable bliss of *bhakti*, although the *bhaktas* have no interest even in final liberation, which is the supreme goal of life, liberation anyway manifests itself, so all goals are fulfilled by dint of devotion to *Bhagavān*" (V.6.17); "*Bhakti yoga* performed for *Bhagavān* Vāsudeva quickly bestows detachment (*vairāgya*) and causeless knowledge, *jñāna* [of the *ātman*]" (I.2.7). But the *bhakta*, either realizing that this is not the end of the journey, or, as will be exemplified below, encountering fortuitously the narrations of *Īśvara*, keeps going, as his or her interest is the Supreme *Ātman* beyond, *Paramātman*[84] *Bhagavān*, the Godhead who sustains but transcends the individual *ātman*.

The Rejection of *Brahman*

Ultimately, the reason the *bhakta* is interested in *Bhagavān* rather than solely the individual *ātman* boils down to a simple fact: whatever bliss (*ānanda*) is inherent in the *ātman* (*Brahman*) pales in comparison with the bliss experienced when coming in contact with the source of all bliss, *Bhagavān*. Rūpa states that "if the bliss of *Brahman* were multiplied billions of times, it would not equal a drop in the ocean of the happiness of *bhakti*!" (*Bhaktirasāmṛtasindhu* Eastern Quadrant I.1.38). This is a response to the Upaniṣads, where the bliss of *Brahman* is itself billions of times greater than the highest imaginable bliss in the world (*Bṛhadāraṇyaka* IV.3.32–33; *Taittirīya* II.8).

All living beings ultimately seek bliss, *ānanda*, in some form or fashion, but what constitutes bliss is evaluated differently. For those ignorant of the *ātman*, it is determined in accordance with the *guṇas* prominent in the mind. So, following the *Gītā*, for those in *sattva*, happiness comes from tranquillity of mind, and even though cultivating this in the beginning is unpalatable (typically because old *rājasic* and *tāmasic saṁskāras* forcefully protest at the outset as one struggles to break their impulses), it develops into nectar in the end

(XVIII.37).[85] For those in *rajas*, happiness is sought from sensual indulgences, and although this appears like nectar in the beginning, it ends as poison (XVIII.38). Sensual pleasures are temporal, and one becomes frustrated when they come to an end or when they cannot be attained in the first place; moreover, there is always a hidden and unexpected price tag on sensual indulgences. Happiness in *tamas* is sought in sleep, laziness, and intoxication, and these delude the self both in the beginning and in the end (XVIII.39). Thus, while the happiness of *sattva* is deemed to be the highest attainable by the material mind, as Patañjali states, the wise perceive that all happiness produced by the *guṇas* is actually suffering, even that of *sattva*. This is because such happiness is always temporary and subject to change, and it is always afflicted by the inevitable unwelcome intrusions and inconveniences of embodied life (II.15). So all happiness derived from the *guṇas* binds the *ātman* (*Gītā* XIV.5ff.).

For those pursuing knowledge of the self, who reject these types of so-called happiness temporarily produced by the *guṇas* (*Gītā* V.21–22), happiness is identified as lying beyond the mind, as the "infinite bliss" inherent in the *ātman* itself (*Gītā* VI.21–22). The paths of generic *yoga* and *jñāna* strive for this bliss (or, with Nyāya, freedom from suffering[86]). But *bhakti* proposes an even higher state of bliss attainable by the devotionalized mind. First of all, even before attaining its grand finale of a vision of *Bhagavān* and a direct personal relationship with Him, simply initiating the practices of *bhakti yoga* is joyful in comparison with other processes, precisely because of its connection with *Bhagavān*, who is the source of bliss.[87] Compared with this, "even pure knowledge (*jñāna*) [of the *ātman*] is unattractive when devoid of love for Kṛṣṇa" (I.5.12). For the *Bhāgavata*, the path of *jñāna* and nondevotional *yoga* is, in actuality, dry, tedious, frustrating, and seemingly never-ending in comparison: "Those who have rejected *bhakti*, the most beneficial path, toil hard to obtain knowledge [of the *ātman*] exclusively. For them toil itself is the only outcome, nothing else, just like those who thresh the coarse outer husks of grain" (X.14.4).

In fact, the text goes so far as to suggest that those who realize the *ātman* may not in fact even be able to remain in that state if they neglect *bhakti*: "Others, O lotus-eyed One [Kṛṣṇa], consider themselves liberated, but their minds are impure because of turning away from You. They attain the highest destination [realization of the *ātman*] with difficulty, but, since their minds are indifferent to Your lotus feet, they fall back down" (X.2.32). In other words, the latent desires (*kleśas*) of the mind may be in a state of suppression (*nirodhaḥ*) for prolonged periods, but without *bhakti*, they may resurface and compel consciousness back into the realm of *prakṛti*. We note that even Patāñjali includes *Īśvara-praṇidhāna*, devotion to *Īśvara*—which Vyāsa in his commentary glosses as *bhakti viśeṣa*, "a special type of *bhakti*"—as a requisite practice for removing the *kleśas* (II.1–2). This position that even *mokṣa* can be attained only by the grace of *Iśvara* in fact has much earlier precedents (*Śvetāśvatara Upaniṣad* VI.15; *Mokṣadharma* 300.3).

But the *Bhāgavata* takes a significant step further still: some *yogīs* who have already attained the state beyond the *guṇas*—whose minds have been suppressed such that consciousness can be exclusively immersed in its own nature of consciousness, *ātma-jñāna* (in other words, who have attained the goal of classical *yoga*)—relinquish this state and voluntarily *reconnect* with their senses and minds in order to hear, study, and speak about the pastimes (*līlās*) of Kṛṣṇa. The goal of traditions such as that of Patañjali is precisely to *disconnect* from the mind and senses in order to reimmerse consciousness in its own nature.[88] But numerous *ātman*-realized *yogīs* who have actually attained this state, if they somehow encounter *Bhagavān* and consequently become *bhaktas*, opt to reconnect with the very mind and senses they had previously endeavored so arduously to transcend. This is in order to be able to become immersed in thoughts of *Bhagavān*, specifically of His form, qualities, and deeds, for which they need the mind and senses of perception (we will discuss the spiritual *Brahman* mind and senses attained in the postmortem liberated state later). King Parīkṣit, the recipient of the *Bhāgavata*, is confused by sage Śuka's exemplification of this anomaly:

> "Śuka had renounced all worldly activities, and was without attachments, and indifferent to everything, O sage. He was absorbed in the bliss of the *ātman* self. Why did he then study this huge work [the *Bhāgavata*]?"
>
> Sage Saunaka replies:
>
> "Sages who delight in the *ātman* self, who are without

worldly bonds, perform devotion to Hari without any motive, such is the nature of His qualities. Therefore, Śuka, son of Bādarāyaṇa [Vyāsa], whose mind had become captured by the qualities of Hari, studied this great narration." (I.7.9–11)

This is repeated again at the end of the text: "Śuka's consciousness (*ceta*) was fixed in the bliss of his own self and he had cast off all notions of duality. Nonetheless, his fixity was drawn away by the delightful *līlās*, pastimes, of the infallible Ajita [Kṛṣṇa]" (12.12.68). And, indeed, Śuka states this about himself: "Although I was fixed in the state beyond the *guṇas*, my mind was captured by the *līlās* of Kṛṣṇa; and so I learned about His pastimes" (2.1.9). His father, too, the great Vyāsa, "although he was fixed in the bliss of the self and devoid of any other thought, his heart was attracted to the enchanting *līlās* of the infallible Kṛṣṇa; out of kindness [for others], he then composed this *Bhāgavata Purāṇa*" (XII.12.68).

As will be especially encountered in the tenth book, then, the *Bhāgavata*, promotes the bliss of sensual contact with Kṛṣṇa as far superior to any bliss inherent in the *ātman* when immersed in its own nature after uncoupling from the *prakṛtic guṇas*. Such contact with Kṛṣṇa can be attained either directly for those who had accumulated enough merit to have been born during His incarnation or, for those born thereafter, indirectly by means of hearing about His pastimes from the tenth book (or, of course, eternally in the post-liberated realm of Goloka or Vaikuṇṭha). Either way, the bliss received by means of the senses and mind, whether made of *prakṛti* or *Brahman*, from contact with *Īśvara*, including hearing about His activities through the ear, is held to eclipse the bliss of the *ātman*'s self-absorption. We can recall that one of the characteristics of *bhakti* delineated by Rūpa is that it minimizes interest in *mokṣa—Brahman/ātman*-centered liberation. This is a theme repeated again and again in the *Bhāgavata*.[89] The text is simply pervaded with claims to the effect that *mokṣa* is rejected by the *bhaktas* who are fully satisfied serving Kṛṣṇa,[90] or simply hearing or chanting about and meditating on Him,[91] and especially rejected if it means separation from Kṛṣṇa.[92] Put more dramatically, devoid of the presence of the beloved Lord, *mokṣa* is, in fact, equal to hell (VI.17.28). This phenomenon, in turn, leads to another of the six characteristics of *bhakti* identified by

Rūpa—the difficulty of the attainment of real (unmixed) *bhakti*: "Among tens of millions of those perfected beings who have attained *mukti*, liberation, one who is devoted to Nārāyaṇa is very hard to find" (VI.14.5). Here, the *Bhāgavata* is echoing the *Gītā*: "Among thousands of people, hardly any strive for perfection. And of those striving and even from those who have attained perfection, hardly any know Me in truth" (VII.3). The flip side of this is that "until the *yogī* does not become disillusioned with the various other paths of *yoga*, he or she will not develop attraction for the stories of Kṛṣṇa" (IV.23.12).[93]

Who Is the Supreme *Īśvara*?: The Purāṇic Context

Moving on to the second fundamental issue we raised at the beginning of this section concerning *Īśvara* as the object or recipient of *bhakti*, what is the *Bhāgavata*'s justification for identifying the highest expression of *Īśvara* as Kṛṣṇa, as opposed to other claimants to this position, most specifically, Śiva or Viṣṇu? In other words, given that most Hindu traditions, including *advaita Vedānta*, accept *Īśvara* in some sort of sense, then, bracketing the issue touched upon above as to whether *Īśvara* is the ultimate and causal entity or a nonultimate and derivative entity (or, as per *advaita*, a superimposition on the Absolute), since everyone accepts an *Īśvara* at some level, then who is the ultimate *Īśvara*? This discussion plays out more in Purāṇa-related than in Vedānta contexts. At the risk of repetition (given the common misperception of Hinduism as polytheistic), Hindu theists of all *bhakti* schools hold that *Īśvara*, if unlimited, can assume unlimited *Īśvara* forms (irrespective of whether these are ultimately true, as per the Vaiṣṇavas, or only relatively true, as per *advaita*). So the question is not who is the real and true *Īśvara* and who is not, but which of these forms is the source, causal *Īśvara* from whom the other *Īśvaras* emanate—or, in the language of the *Bhāgavata*, the seed from which other *avatāras* emerge (III.9.2)? Readers familiar with the various streams of post-Vedic *bhakti* know that these are not polytheistic, but either monotheistic or monistic. Therefore, these *Īśvara* forms are not independent autonomous equals, as is (more or less) the case with polytheism, but emanate from one source. Either this source is monistic—reflecting the discussion above, where *Īśvara* (whether real or illusory) is held to be nonultimate and derived from a higher Absolute—which in its highest and ultimate expression is a qualityless, nonindividualized Truth, or this source is monotheistic, which requires one original, ultimate, Supreme *Īśvara.* So both monism and monotheism in their very different ways constitute a "mono-source," not a "poly-source." But either way, one still has to account for the relationship among the multifarious *Īśvaras.* Accordingly, most traditions (even, in his own way, Śaṅkara) end up subscribing to one particular form of *Īśvara* as the fountainhead of all other *Īśvara* emanations. And, once again, we are referring exclusively to Kṛṣṇa, Viṣṇu and His incarnations, Śiva, and their consorts (God on high with a capital "G")—not to the lower-level celestials in *saṁsāra* (gods with a small "g"), whose worship in the Vedic period can in fact be seen as constituting a type of polytheism.[94]

We should also note that this is a scholastic issue: the vast majority of Hindus offer devotion to numerous forms and personalities of *Īśvara*, especially in cultural contexts such as participating in the major celebratory days associated with the different forms of *Īśvara*—for example, *janmāṣṭami*, Kṛṣṇa's birthday; *Rāma-navamī*, Rāma's birthday; and *Śivarātrī*, sacred to Śiva.[95] Even though most Hindus, and certainly most who have a serious *bhakti* practice, will orient their own personal and private everyday devotion toward one particular form, the *iṣṭa-devatā*, Lord of the heart (noted, for instance, in *Yoga Sūtras* II.44), the question of which *Īśvara* is primary and ultimate and which derivative and emanational is far more a feature of scholastic and lineage-bearing[96] *bhakti* than the generic *bhakti* encountered on a grassroots level. Nonetheless, emerging traditions needed to establish their credentials and sectarian partialities based on the intellectual and epistemological criteria of the time. This, in Vedānta circles, as we can see with Jīva's defense of the authority of the *Bhāgavata* itself (see appendix 1), meant quoting scripture, the *Śrūti* and *Smṛti.*[97] And this, in turn, required a significant degree of scholasticism.

Before we engage some of the intellectual issues that have been (and remain) important to the theologians of the various *bhakti* sects, let us consider *Īśvara* from a heart (nonscholastic) perspective—one much more reflective of the on-the-ground *bhakti* of the practitioner.

Ultimately, one's preference for a particular *Īśvara* form, the *iṣṭa-devatā* (worshipful Lord) such as Kṛṣṇa or Śiva, over any other should reflect the heart inclination of the devotee and nothing more. There are various ways one can encounter and subsequently develop such an emotional relationship with who becomes one's *iṣṭa-devatā*. Often, for example, this may simply be inherited from one's family tradition, or local culture, and thus reflects one's *karma* in the form of birth (*jati*), and geography (*deśa*), along the lines of *Yoga Sūtras* II.13. For those perhaps more dedicated to pursuing a path less preconditioned by the accidents of familial or regional culture, one's *iṣṭa-devatā* is most often simply inherited from one's *guru*, as discussed previously. In other words, one first becomes attracted by a charismatic individual whose spiritual qualities one wishes to emulate, and then, as this relationship deepens into a *guru*-disciple relationship, one subsequently adopts the *Īśvara* form—and in fact entire edifice of theological and ritual specificities associated with that form—from this *guru*'s lineage. This is by far the most common manner of connecting to a form of *Īśvara* for those stepping outside of their birth traditions, including Westerners. (We see, in the West, the partiality of Neem Karoli Baba's followers to Rāma and Hanumān, for example, Swami Muktānanda's to Śiva, and Bhaktivedānta Swami's to Kṛṣṇa, the disciples typically following the preference or lineage deity of their *guru*.)

Attraction to one's *iṣṭa-devatā* may also be born from reading the stories connected with the various *Īśvara* incarnations and manifestations, as per Patañjali's *svādhyāyād iṣṭa-devatā-samprayogaḥ*, "from study, one encounters one's Lord of the heart" (II.44). Just as in romantic relationships in the human realm (at least in their idealized form), a person looking for love or for a spouse might undertake a dating spree in order to seek opportunities to become acquainted with a suitable person, so in *bhakti* one can seek one's *iṣṭa-devatā* by undertaking a study project of the respective texts associated with the various *Īśvara* options—Kṛṣṇa, Śiva, Rāma, the Goddess, and so on. As in human relationships, from all the available possible romantic partners, an eventual attraction evolves from association and from discovering more and more about the qualities and attributes of one particular person, and this (ideally) develops into love, so, in divine relationships, an attraction to a particular *Īśvara* form can be accomplished by *svādhyāya*, study. One explores the universe of various *Īśvara* forms by immersing oneself in their stories, forms, qualities, deeds, and modes of interaction with their devotees (for instance, by reading the *Bhāgavata*, *Rāmāyaṇa*, and Śiva- and Devī-centered texts), and eventually one's heart becomes naturally especially attracted to one specific manifestation of *Īśvara*. He or She becomes one's *iṣṭa-devatā*. This usually means that one subsequently adopts that manifestation's specific name as one's *japa mantra* and engages in worship of His or Her deity form following the specifics of ritual associated with that form[98]—in other words, one engages the nine processes of *bhakti* (or sectarian variants of them) centered on that form. For most Hindus, it is these types of natural and spontaneous attractions for a particular form of *Īśvara*—always appreciative of and ready to honor and participate in the worship of other forms, but privately devoted to one's own cherished *iṣṭa-devatā*—that lies at the heart of the dedicated *bhakti yoga* of the committed practitioner.

There is a touching story in the *Caitanya Caritāmṛta* underscoring the personal and heart nature of true *bhakti*, where love for an adored form of *Īśvara* transcends all social or cultural legislation and, in this case, even the presence of an enormously powerful *guru* charismatic (indeed, one considered an incarnation of Kṛṣṇa Himself in Jīva's Gauḍīya tradition), *Śrī* Caitanya. Caitanya lovingly recounts the immovable faith of Murāri Gupta in *Śrī* Rāma, despite his testing this by persistently promoting the unsurpassed superexcellence of Kṛṣṇa:

> Once I tried to tempt him again and again, "Most sweet, O Gupta is Vrajendrakumāra [Kṛṣṇa], Bhagavān Himself; . . . His actions are sweet, the *līlā* of Kṛṣṇa is sweet. Worship that Kṛṣṇa, take refuge in that Kṛṣṇa; there is no worship in the heart apart from that Kṛṣṇa." In this way again and again he listened to my words, and because of my praise, his mind was turned a little . . . he went to his home and he reflected, into the night, and he thought anxiously about his abandonment of Raghunātha [Rāma]. "How shall I abandon the feet of Raghunātha? Kill me, O Rāma, tonight!" Thus he wept the whole night; he had no peace of mind, and he was awake all the night. In the morning he came and held my feet, and

weeping he pleaded with me thus. "I have laid my head at the feet of Raghunātha. I cannot take my head away, there is pain in my heart. . . . Tell me what I should do. In this situation, give mercy to me, O you who are full of mercy; let me die before you, let this indecision be over." When I heard this, I was very happy in my mind, and I raised him up and embraced him. "O most perfect Gupta, your faith is very deep; your heart has not been shaken by my words . . . to know the firmness of your *bhāva* (love) I have tempted you again and again. You are a servant of Rāma like the incarnate Hanumān; how could you abandon His lotus feet?" That Murāri Gupta is like my own heart; when I hear of his humility, my heart bursts. (*Caitanya Caritāmṛta, Mādhya līlā* 15.138–57)

The point is, just as in human romantic affairs, although one may personally find the qualities and appearance of one's intimate beloved the most attractive, there is no need to disparage other candidates or seek to lure someone away from his or her heart's different choice. Likewise, one can have an intense relationship with one's *iṣṭa-devatā* without the need for any sectarian exclusivism (or, for that matter, the inclusivistic hierarchization that we will encounter with Jīva that is so typical of Hinduism). This author's own teacher, just as an example of this, despite being a lifelong ascetic *bhakta* of Kṛṣṇa and ultraorthodox *ācārya* lineage bearer of Gauḍīya Vaiṣṇavism, initiates his last published work[99] with the following invocation:

Mādhavomādhavāv īśau sarva-siddhi-vidhāyinau
Vande parasparātmānau paraspara-nati-prīyau

I offer my obeisances to the two *Īśvaras*—Kṛṣṇa, the husband of Mā[100] (Lakṣmī), and Śiva, the husband of Umā (Parvatī), who are the source of all perfection.

They are always united, and filled with mutual love and respect for each other.

Such catholic spirit is not just a cultural matter, and certainly not anything to do with modern notions of political correctness: all schools accept that the different manifestations of *Īśvara* are factually and ontologically the same Supreme Being. Consider the *Bhāgavata* story of sage Atri (IV.1.19–30), who performed intense austerities on one foot (*eka-pāda-āsana*), meditating on "the *Īśvara* of the universe" (*jagad-Īśvara*). Eventually, Viṣṇu, Śiva, and Brahmā all appeared before him. Confused, he told them that he had supplicated "the one *Bhagavān*." Why had three of them come? Smiling, they replied, "We are that one!" This multiplicity-in-oneness is the Vaiṣṇava form of monotheism.

Nonetheless, if one has been entrusted with the *dharma* of safeguarding the parameters of a sect's theological specifics, as is the case with Jīva, one must rise up to establish the bona fides of one's tradition in accordance with the methodologies and epistemologies of one's time, lest it be belittled by opposing schools or ridiculed as emotional foolishness. And the Gauḍīya tradition, while honoring and relishing all the divine manifestations, is entrusted by its founder, *Śrī* Caitanya, with spreading the sweetness of *rāgānugā bhakti* to *Śrī* Kṛṣṇa as the highest expression of personal love of God (a goal deemed not only to be the summum bonum of life and human existence, but the solution to all human problems). Perhaps we can consider this feature of Hindu *bhakti* a type of eclectic sectarianism. Jīva and the other *Gosvāmīs* perceive their dedication to making these teachings of *bhakti* available in accordance with the scholastic and intellectual criteria of their day as the highest welfare work for human well-being. Apart from the belief that the sweetness of Kṛṣṇa *bhakti* produces the highest possible ecstasy attainable by the *ātman*, these *bhakti* teachings are, of course, embedded within the generic *yoga* perspective that the ultimate cause of the suffering of all embodied beings stems from the pursuit of desires pertaining to the body/mind temporal self, as we have discussed. Teaching about such things is their solution to suffering and the human condition. But while Vaiṣṇavas accept the standard *yogic* notion that the only ultimate solution is knowledge of the true *ātman* self, they additionally identify the even more fundamental cause of suffering as aversion toward *Īśvara*. The *Gosvāmīs* are thus entrusted to present these teachings—especially the unparalleled sweetness of Kṛṣṇa *bhakti*—as their contribution to ultimate human welfare. Hence the enormous investment Jīva and Rūpa devoted to their writings and to justifying their prioritization of Kṛṣṇa by recourse to reason and scriptural engagement, where they could easily have followed the life of other *bābās* (ascetics) of their day and simply immersed themselves in their *japa*, *kīrtana*, and *pūjās* in solitude. This is their service.

Before returning to our scholastic and sectarian questions pertaining to the source *Īśvara*, let us linger on this for another moment: from the point of view of theologians like Jīva, scholasticism itself is perceived as a spiritual service to humanity. Even though *Īśvara* is beyond the grasp of the intellect, formulating coherent and systematic theologies is seen as a service for those who need some degree of rationality to underpin their foray into the transrational. Intellectuality, scholasticism, or the articulation of lineage-specific theologies and practices need not be, in and of themselves, spiritually oppressive, limiting, or stifling to spiritual reality, as they are sometimes depicted, or somehow blockages to or overlays over the experience of unfettered Truth. Those intellectually inclined need at least a preliminary rational platform from which to take that leap of faith into a domain beyond reason. This is all the more so since *bhakti* traditions are often condescendingly portrayed as emotional religiosity for the populous masses devoid of any intellectual substance (and this was so even in the sixteenth century in Jīva's time, as in the eleventh century in Rāmānuja's before him).[101] In addition to this, certain scholastics may be entrusted with preserving the logic, rationale, and time-tested value of lineage-specific rituals, practices, and protocols lest these become diluted in the name of eclecticism. All this is the *dharma* of the theologian, which, like any *dharma*, becomes *bhakti* when performed with devotion and offered to *Īśvara*. *Bhakti,* as we know from the *Gītā* (for instance, see IX.27), entails offering whatever one possesses and whatever assets one is endowed with to *Īśvara*. Thus, there are those with intellectual gifts and inclinations, who are moved by their love and devotion to the form of *Īśvara* with which they are enamored to attempt to articulate the superexcellence of their beloved and justify their devotion in accordance with the standard sources of knowledge of the time (such as sense perception, reason, and a consistent interpretation of the sacred texts).[102]

This is what Jīva is doing here and what others have done for other *bhakti* traditions, such as the brilliant scholar-practitioner Abhinavagupta for Kaśmir Śaivism, and Rāmānuja for Śrī Vaiṣṇavism, and so forth. Reason and argument, then, like art, dance, poetry, or anything else—indeed, like the modest leaf, fruit, flower, or water of *Gītā* IX.26—can be offered in devotion to one's beloved *Īśvara* as *bhakti*. With Jīva as our exemplar, then, the following discussion grants us a glimpse at the concerns of one such scholastic practitioner in the sixteenth century, who had been entrusted with articulating a theology centered on Kṛṣṇa *bhakti* that could form the bedrock for the fledgling Gauḍīya Vaiṣṇava tradition that was beginning to define itself after the passing away of *Śrī* Caitanya and thus needed to find scriptural authority to substantiate the tradition's exclusive focus on Kṛṣṇa as Supreme *Īśvara*.

Drawing from sources long predating the Common Era, the Purāṇa tradition develops into two or perhaps three basic streams: those holding Viṣṇu or Kṛṣṇa to be the Ultimate *Īśvara,* the Vaiṣṇavas, and those holding Śiva as Ultimate *Īśvara*, the Śaivites.[103] Overlapping with the latter, and sometimes subsumed within it, a later Śākta stream emerged in literary form (but also with roots in the hoary past), some major expressions of which hold the Goddess to be the Ultimate source Being.[104] We have painted all this with very broad, simplistic strokes here, since our purpose is just to give a flavor of the landscape within which the *Bhāgavata* is negotiating its position. There are all sorts of cross-fertilizing permutations of some of the elements noted above.[105]

The position taken by the various sects on such issues is not assumed but must be substantiated by scriptural reference for a lineage to be taken seriously in the vibrant heterogeneous landscape of the *bhakti* traditions. Summarizing briefly, in his first *Sandarbha*, the *Tattva* (*anu* 17), where he defends the supremacy of Kṛṣṇa over other forms of *Īśvara*, Jīva enlists the support of other Purāṇas, beginning with a sequence of verses in the *Matsya Purāṇa*. In this text, we find the Purāṇa corpus divided according to the *guṇas*, with those glorifying Viṣṇu (Hari) considered to be Purāṇas associated with *sattva*, and those Śiva, with *tamas*.[106] In another Purāṇa, the *Padma* (CCXXXVI. 18–21), the specific names of the eighteen Purāṇas[107] are allocated to their respective *guṇas*, with the *Bhāgavata* and other *Vaiṣṇava* Purāṇas placed in the *sattva* category, and the Śaivite ones placed in the *tamas* one. Part of the reason for these associations, in the larger epic and Purāṇa framework, is that Hari/Viṣṇu/Kṛṣṇa is typically associated with *sattva* and the maintenance of the universe, maintenance being a quality of *sattva*, and Śiva with its destruction, a quality of *tamas*.[108]

Since *sattva* is a prerequisite for knowledge (see, for example, *Gītā* XIV.17), Jīva feels justified in asserting the supremacy of the Purāṇas in the *sattva* category. He can now quote the *sāttvic Bhāgavata* itself with less risk of circularity:

> *Sattva*, *rajas*, and *tamas* are the *guṇas* of *prakṛti*. There is one Supreme Being who directs these for the purpose of creation, maintenance, and destruction of this universe. He is named Hari [Viṣṇu], Viriṇci [Brahmā], and Hara [Śiva]. From these, the ultimate good is derived from the One whose form is *sattva* [that is, Viṣṇu].[109] [Just as, for the performance of Vedic ritual,] smoke is higher than wood, and fire is higher than that, as it lies at the essence of the [rituals prescribed in the] three Vedas,[110] [so] *rajas* is higher than *tamas*, and *sattva* is higher than that, as it bestows the vision of *Brahman*. In the beginning, the sages worshipped *Bhagavān* Viṣṇu, who is pure *sattva* (*viśuddha-sattva*).[111] Those who follow their example are eligible for liberation. (I.2.23–25)

Having argued for the primacy of *Īśvara*, the personal Godhead, over His derivative nonpersonal powers on the basis of Vedānta texts, and then advocated the supremacy of Viṣṇu as ultimate *Īśvara* over other forms of *Īśvara* on the basis of the Purāṇa texts, Jīva had one further step. The Vaiṣṇava schools differ as to whether Viṣṇu is the Ultimate and Supreme *Bhagavān,* who periodically incarnates into the world in various forms, one of which is Kṛṣṇa, or whether Kṛṣṇa is the source Being and Viṣṇu a derivative Being manifest from Him for the purpose of the creation and maintenance of the cosmic order (as the *Paramātman* touched upon previously). Following the opinion of the *Mahābhārata* epic, *Hairivaṃśa*,[112] and *Viṣṇu Purāṇa*, the former position is held by the older Vaiṣṇava sects dominant in the south, noteworthy among which are the tenth- to eleventh-century Rāmānuja and twelfth-century Madhva traditions, whose theologies we know paved the way for and significantly underpin the Gauḍīya one. The latter position, based on the *Bhāgavata Purāṇa* and *Bhagavad Gītā*, surfaces most conspicuously across the north of the subcontinent in the sixteenth century, particularly in the form of Jīva's own school founded by Caitanya, as well as the spiritually cognate tradition stemming from Caitanya's contemporary Vallabha, the founder of the *puṣṭi mārga*.[113] In addition to this identification of Kṛṣṇa as the First Cause of all causes, these latter schools especially stress the unsurpassed nature of Kṛṣṇa's sweetness compared with all other *Īśvara* forms.[114] Once again, all schools ultimately hold both Kṛṣṇa and Viṣṇu—and Śiva—to be manifestations of the same transcendent "One Supreme Being" who has one form but appears in many forms (X.40.7), so in terms of who came first, the difference is something of a plant-and-seed situation and one mostly of scholarly concern.

The crucial verse in the *Bhāgavata* used by the Kṛṣṇa theologians to justify this preeminence of Kṛṣṇa over all other manifestations of the Godhead is I.3.18. Situated after a number of verses listing Viṣṇu's previous incarnations, this verse states: "These [other incarnations] are partial derived incarnations (*aṁśa,* or *kalā*), but Kṛṣṇa is *Bhagavān*, God, Himself (*Kṛṣṇas-tu Bhagavān svayam*)." *Aṁśa* means a "portion" or "partial incarnation." Similar to the relationship between God the Father and God the Son and God the Holy Spirit in the Christian trinity, the sense of the term is that Kṛṣṇa, as the Supreme Godhead, can maintain His own presence, while simultaneously manifesting some aspect of Himself elsewhere in a separate and distinct presence (or any number of presences). Those secondary or derivative manifestations exhibit a part but not the full characteristics or potency of the source Being (the term *kalā* has similar connotations).[115] This concept is very important for understanding the difference between polytheism, where beings are completely separate and more or less equal ontological entities, and the plethora of divine presences in Kṛṣṇa monotheism, which can be thought of as an unlimitedly prolific parallel of the Christian trinity concept: a "multiplicity in one," so to speak.

This verse becomes something of a *mahāvākya,* a "most important expression" or pivotal, foundational statement,[116] for the theology of the Kṛṣṇa sects: all other incarnations are *aṁśas* or *kalās,* partial incarnations, but Kṛṣṇa is *Bhagavān* Himself, the original Being and source of the other incarnations. The importance of I.3.28 for the *Bhāgavata* tradition cannot be overestimated, and it overrides all other conflicting statements: the commentators consider it to be a *paribhāṣā sūtra,* an explanatory assertion that, while occurring in only one verse, illuminates the entire text, like a lamp that, although situated in only one place, illuminates an entire house. And, again relevant here, and just as was the case with the *Vedānta Sūtras*, since all the Purāṇas are deemed compiled by sage Vyāsa, as we will see in his tale, with the *Bhāgavata* as his grand finale, so to speak, it is consequently taken by Jīva as Vyāsa's final word not only on all such issues of personal versus nonpersonal modalities of *Brahman*, but also on the hierarchies among *Īśvaras*. And the *Bhāgavata* promotes Kṛṣṇa as the Supreme causal *Īśvara*.

We must stress once more that while this type of argumentation is clearly sectarian, the *bhakti* traditions are inclusivistic sectarianism, not exclusivistic. The *Bhāgavata*, for example, extols Śiva, using similar categories it elsewhere directs to Viṣṇu:

> I know you, Rudra [Śiva] are the Lord, the undivided *Brahman*, beyond Śiva and Śakti[117] who are the seed and womb of the universe. You are *Bhagavān* who, like a spider with its web, playfully create, maintain, and destroy this universe in the forms of Śiva and Śakti, who are one essence. (IV.6.42–43)

This is typical of Hinduism, and examples are ubiquitous. In the *Mahābhārata* epic, for example, Viṣṇu says to Śiva: "He who knows You, knows Me. He who follows You, follows Me. There is not the slightest difference between Us both. Let there be no judgment otherwise" (*Mokṣadharma* CCCXLII.233). The verse is repeated verbatim earlier, adding: "Their reality (*sattva*) is one, their forms are two" (CCCXLI.16). While the *Bhāgavata* generally does not waver about who is the ultimate source Supreme Being,[118] it allows those devoted to Śiva to perceive and eulogize Śiva as not only the Supreme Being, but even as the source of Viṣṇu (VIII.7.23), the creator, protector, and destroyer of the universe (IV.6.42–43), the originator of the *guṇas* and everything in existence (VIII.7.21–35), whose abode is inaccessible even to Viṣṇu. The eulogy to Śiva of the *prajāpatis*

(VIII.7.21ff.) could have come right out of the Purāṇas that prioritize Śiva—the *Śiva*, *Liṅga*, and *Skandha Purāṇas*. Ultimately, the *Bhāgavata* allows everyone to follow their own devotional inclinations: "One should worship the Supreme Being in accordance with the preference of one's mind" (XI.3.48). And, reciprocally, it allows that the Supreme Being assumes forms not only according to functions (Śiva, as we know, is typically accorded the role of the destroyer in the overall Purāṇic schema), but also in accordance with the particular desires of individual devotees: "You assume whatever form Your devotees meditate upon" (III.9.11); "Whatever forms please Your devotees, are pleasing to You, O Lord" (III.24.31). So this sectarianism is of an eclectic and inclusivistic nature, typical of the *bhakti* of the Purāṇas.

Īśvara, Pure *Bhakti*, and Motivated *Bhakti*

Continuing thematically with the differences among the various *Īśvara* forms, another way of differentiating between the *bhakti* performed for Kṛṣṇa and that performed for some of the other divine manifestations, according to the *Bhāgavata* tradition, is that since Kṛṣṇa is pure *sattva*, those who seek the fulfillment of *prakṛti*-related desires are naturally more likely to approach and offer *bhakti* to those other forms of the Divine, which are associated with the fulfillment of those desires. We know from the *Gītā* (XVIII.9 and 23) that *sattva* is associated with freedom from desire and detachment from the fruit of action; *rajas* with desire and attachment to the fruit of desire (indeed, the word for desire, *rāga*, comes from the same root); and *tamas* with apathy toward the fulfillment of desire in general (XVIII.24–25). In the overall Hindu hierarchization of divine plenitude, different types of beings, not all of whom are divine or even benevolent, become associated with different modes of worship and the attainment of different material goals:

> Those desiring liberation reject the ghastly forms of [other] powerful beings[119] and, free from envy, worship the peaceful manifestations of Nārāyaṇa. Those whose natures and characteristics are *rājasic* and *tāmasic*, desiring offspring, power, and opulence, worship the celestial beings, ancestors, and ghosts, etc. (I.2.26–27)

This principle is illustrated in the *Bhāgavata* in the story of Vṛka. This demon approaches Nārada and, upon asking him which of the great Deities is most easily propitiated, is informed: "Worship Lord Śiva, and you will quickly attain success. He can be easily pleased or easily angered by a small amount of either merit or fault" (X.88.15). Nārada points out that the great demon Rāvaṇa who kidnapped Sītā in the *Rāmāyaṇa* epic attained his power from worshipping Śiva, as did numerous other demons.[120] The point here is that those with *tāmasic* malintentions tend to worship forms of Śiva, who, being highly benevolent and easily gratified, accepts such worship, where Viṣṇu, being pure *sattva*, would not (generally[121]), nor would His worship likely attract those in *tamas*. Vṛka proceeded to worship Śiva through ghastly austerities—offering the flesh from his own limbs and preparing to sever his own head—and did indeed attain a *tāmasic* boon—the ability to kill anyone by merely laying a hand on that person (X.88). Since the preamble to this story narrated by Śuka to Parīkṣit amply illustrates the *Bhāgavata*'s perspective on the differentiation among Divine Beings and their appeal to different types of worshippers, it is worth quoting at length:

> Those among the gods, demons, and mortals who worship the austere Śiva are often wealthy and lead a life of enjoyment. But this is not the case with those who worship Hari even though He is the Lord of Lakṣmī, the Goddess of Fortune. . . . The end results are different for the worshippers of these two Lords, whose personalities are so opposite. . . . Śiva is always associated with His *śakti* powers. He is enveloped by the *guṇas*, with their three characteristics.[122] . . . So anyone having recourse [to Śiva] enjoys the acquisition of all riches. Hari, however, is untouched by the *guṇas*. He is the Supreme Person beyond *prakṛti*. He is the witness, the seer of everything. One who worships Him becomes free from the *guṇas* . . . your grandfather, King Yudhiṣṭhira . . . asked Kṛṣṇa the same question [you, Parīkṣit, have asked]. . . . *Bhagavān* Kṛṣṇa replied as follows . . . "I will deprive the person whom I favor of his wealth. At this, his own family members abandon the person who has become poverty-stricken and afflicted by suffering. When his endeavors come to nothing, and he

becomes despondent in his attempts to [gain] wealth, then I bestow my favor on him, once he has formed friendship with those devoted to Me. . . . But, because I am so hard to worship, people reject Me and worship other gods." (X.88.1–10)

Hopefully the point is clear: the idea that the Supreme *Īśvara* assumes different personae to cater to the different inclinations and desires of humans would be accepted by most *bhakti* sects. The *Bhāgavata* allows Śiva Himself to state that those who have attained equanimity of perception "do not see even a speck of difference between He Himself and Viṣṇu." But those with more intense desires perfectly naturally worship the Being who can most quickly fulfill those desires (as indicated in the *Gītā* IV.12), and Śiva is supremely munificent and easily satisfied, *asutoṣa*.[123] The *Bhāgavata* certainly recognizes that Śiva is the same *Īśvara* who can bestow liberation (VIII.7.22), that there are realized *yogīs* dedicated to Him who are liberated[124] (IV.6.45–46), and that there are "*gurus* delighting in the *ātman* who contemplate Śiva in their hearts" (VIII.7.33). So clearly it does not consider all of His devotees to be motivated by mundane *prakṛtic* needs. But it does associate at least most of His followers with those who still have some level of interest in the enjoyments of *prakṛti*.

We will no more than again cursorily note here that some forms of Śiva devotion, such as the Kaśmir Śaivism of the Siddha tradition, promote a goal of complete identification with and the eventual reimmersion of the *ātman* into its potential and inherent Śiva nature, from which vantage point it can, in fact, enjoy the spectacle of *prakṛti*. After all, in Kaśmir Śaivism, *prakṛti* is the *citi-śākti* energy of the Divine—pure vibrational consciousness—so for this tradition it is not *prakṛti* that should be renounced, but the sense of self as an enjoyer separate from Śiva. Once *prakṛti* is fully and actually realized as non-different from Śiva, what is there to renounce? Such Śākta schools are philosophically rich and coherent traditions, with considerable theological sophistication. Engaging a robust form of Śiva *bhakti* as method, they promote one of their ultimate goals precisely as the enjoyment of the creative spectacle of *prakṛti* once the practitioner has transcended the limitations of personal ego, *ahaṅkāra*, and realized his or her own true Śiva nature (*svarūpa*).

But this is not the goal sought by the Kṛṣṇa *bhaktas* of Jīva's tradition. Of course he does not reject the soteriological possibility of such liberation, as becoming one with Śiva can certainly be accommodated in *Bhāgavata* ontology, given the Vaiṣṇava equivalent in one or two of the five basic types of liberation we have discussed (*ekatvam* with *sārūpya* flavorings). But the reason Jīva deems any form of liberation from the various options discussed previously—or their Śaivite parallels—to be of no interest to true *bhaktas*, even if available, is that they do not facilitate eternal service to *Īśvara*. Service is the sign of true love. And as the other main Śaivite tradition, Śaiva Siddhānta, would agree, eternal service requires an eternal distinction between *Īśvara* as object of *bhakti* and the worshipful *bhakta*. According to the *Bhāgavata*, the worship of the pure forms of Viṣṇu and Kṛṣṇa are attractive to those who are without desire to enjoy *prakṛti* from any vantage point whatsoever (other than by means of offering *prakṛti* in love and devotion to their beloved). Such *bhaktas* aspire for what for them is the ultimate perfection of *bhakti* free from all personal motives of enjoyment. This perfection is service to the beloved that culminates in an eternal relationship with *Bhagavān* assuming the form of their preference in the trans-*prakṛtic* realms within *Brahman* itself, Vaikuṇṭha and Goloka.

Again, this partiality or preference does not imply that Vaiṣṇavas would deny the possibility of the specific type of liberation proposed by Kaśmir Śaivism or any other such tradition, since, as we have discussed, Vaiṣṇavas accept a parallel type of liberation: Kṛṣṇa *bhaktas* too can merge into Kṛṣṇa (as we will see in the Agha story). Why not, then, a parallel option for Śiva *bhaktas*?[125] But since, in the *Bhāgavata*, Śiva is accepted as an eternal transcendent Being abiding in His own abode with His liberated *bhaktas*, Jīva's form of *bhakti* finds a closer Śaivite spiritual cognate with Śaiva Siddhānta, since the equivalent of *sārūpya* liberation in that tradition is a state where the liberated *ātman* attains a divine form and qualities identical to Śiva's but distinct from His. Their relationship is both a dualism—as here the soul retains its individuality—and a oneness, since it is inseparably united with Śiva with the bond of love.[126] It is such love shared between an individual soul and an eternal *Īśvara* that Kṛṣṇa *bhaktas* seek.

Having said all this, we have applied a Kṛṣṇa-centered lens for our case study to exemplify with some depth one expression of *bhakti*, but we must in fairness note that other Purāṇas express different hierarchies and relationships on such issues: certainly the three main Śaivite Purāṇas, the *Śiva* and the *Liṅga*, especially, and also the *Skanda*, all promote Śiva's ultimate supremacy over Viṣṇu in various passages,[127] as does the *Devī Bhāgavata Purāṇa* on behalf of the Goddess.[128] Much of this type of sectarian rhetoric from all sides, Vaiṣṇava and Śaivite, is not likely to appeal to those who are not already deeply committed to a specific sect. But, by way of a conclusion to all this, the various Purāṇic sects do accept and respect all forms of *Īśvara*. The sectarian hierarchization among the various *Īśvara* forms that becomes important to the scholastic theologians of the various traditions can be seen as expressions of their intense devotion, *bhakti*, for their own *iṣṭa-devatā*. It also reflects their duties as lineage bearers to justify this devotion according to the standard epistemological methodologies of their day for the sake of their followers and for the intellectual dignity of their traditions. But most of all, from a *bhakti* perspective, all this can perhaps be best relished as something of a *līlā*, divine play, among the traditions reflecting the playful exchanges among the divinities themselves described in the various stories of the different Purāṇas as manifestations of what all agree is the one Supreme Being. The bottom line is that *Īśvara* will bestow faith in whatever form is attractive to the *bhakta* (*Gītā* VII.21), and ultimately, if that faith becomes pure, unflinching, and all-consuming, *Īśvara* will appear to the faithful *bhakta* in that form: "You appear in that very form in which they contemplate You, O glorious One" (*Bhāgavata* III.9.11).

Materialistic Religiosity

Given the division of the Purāṇas according to the three *guṇas* noted in the *Matsya* and *Padma Purāṇas* discussed above, the question could now be raised as to why the various Purāṇas and, we can add, Vedic sacred texts bother to prescribe forms of *bhakti* religiosity to cater to fulfilling the desires of those in *rajas* and *tamas* in the first place. Isn't this sending mixed messages? As with any *yoga* worldview, and indeed (almost) all Indic soteriological systems, the very cause of bondage is desire,[129] and thus desire must be renounced for liberation to become possible.[130] So don't scriptural prescriptions catering to fulfilling desire counter the spiritual well-being of those following them and, even worse, do so insidiously since they are embedded in sacred texts and thus claim the aura of being sacrosanct (as Nārada suggests in the Tale of Vyāsa within)? We can also mention here that in addition to the various *bhakti* paths associated with different forms of *Īśvara* in the Purāṇas, the older Vedic texts are laden with prescriptions for rites to the celestial beings (*devas*)[131] promoting various material boons. These rites are also focused on fulfilling desire and require a type of *bhakti* to the *devas* for their fulfillment. Here too the same basic question remains: Since Kṛṣṇa is the *Vedas* (*Gītā* IX.17), and their knower (XV.15), and seems to condone Vedic sacrifice (III.10–14), why did He bother to compose them, only to then urge Arjuna to renounce their "flowery words" (II.42–43)?[132]

The *Bhāgavata* takes the view that full renunciation of self-centered desire is not (except in occasional grace-related contexts) instantaneous. One needs to gradually progress through the *guṇas* by discipline and sacrifice. As the *Gītā* informs us, this usually takes lifetimes (VI.45). People cannot be expected to renounce desire overnight (*Gītā* III.26). Thus, the religious rites and boons associated with non-*sattva* modes of *bhakti* may indeed be legitimizing the fulfillment of desires, but they nonetheless do so embedded in disciplinary regimens that prescribe the worship of a form of *Īśvara*, or at least of some higher celestial power, and that require some form of discipline and austerity for their accomplishment. We know from the *Yoga Sūtras* that from the performance of discipline (*tapas*), and surrender to *Īśvara* (*praṇidhāna*), the *kleśas,* impurities—including desire—are weakened (II.1–2). By offering various desire-related boons that nonetheless come with this type of discreet price tag, these texts thereby entice those in the lower *guṇas* to at least begin this process of discipline and ("mixed") *bhakti* to some entity higher than themselves, as this will eventually lead toward purification and consequent ultimate well-being. In the words of the *Bhāgavata*:

> The Vedic utterances conceal their meaning. They prescribe ritual activity (*karma*) for the purpose of becoming free from *karma* just as medicine [is covered by something sweet] for the healing of children. If an ignorant person with uncontrolled senses does not follow the injunctions of the Vedas, he attains death after death [in *saṁsāra*] because of the

> *adharma* incurred from forbidden actions. The material fruits offered in the Vedas are for the purpose of attracting [people to prescribed actions]. And if one [eventually] follows the prescriptions of the Vedas without attachment, and offers them to *Īśvara*, that person [eventually] attains the perfection of being free from *karma*. (XI.3.44)

This, then, can perhaps be considered a form of *upāya*, skillful means: the promise of *prakṛti*-related boons coaxes embodied beings toward *dharma*, righteous actions, that are regulated and connected to higher beings. Thus, one is enticed away from non-*dharma* that will simply perpetuate the lower destinations of *saṁsāra* (even if, as with Vṛka, one starts from a place of *adharma* and deepest *tamas*). Satisfying desires under these regulated conditions, rather than observing no restrictions whatsoever, one begins one's ascent through the *guṇas*. In time, as one approaches *sattva*, and thus its qualities of insight and wisdom, one eventually realizes one is seeking to overcome suffering by fulfilling desires, but it is actually those very desires themselves that are the *cause* of suffering and bondage (*Gītā* V.22, XIV.17; *Yoga Sūtras* II.15ff.). At this point, renunciation from desire becomes obvious and liberating.

To conclude this section on *Īśvara*, in terms of the most suitable object of *bhakti*, then, the culmination of all these lines of reasoning for the *Bhāgavata* tradition is that "one desiring freedom from fear, should hear about, glorify, and remember Hari, who is *Bhagavān*, *Īśvara,* the soul of everything" (II.1.5). It is Kṛṣṇa, as Ultimate Being, who is ultimately both the source and goal of all religious activity:

> Vāsudeva [Kṛṣṇa] is the ultimate goal of the Veda, Vāsudeva is the ultimate goal of ritual sacrifices, Vāsudeva is the ultimate goal of *yoga*, Vāsudeva is the ultimate goal of actions. Vāsudeva is the ultimate goal of knowledge, Vāsudeva is the ultimate goal of austerity (*tapas*), Vāsudeva is the ultimate goal of *dharma*, Vāsudeva is the ultimate goal. (I.2.28–29)[133]

Or, in the words of the *Gītā*: "After many births, a wise person takes refuge in Me, knowing that 'Vāsudeva is everything.' Such a great soul is very rare indeed" (VII.19).

Concluding Reflections

Some Academic Considerations

Readers unfamiliar with Hindu devotion will be struck by how personal the processes of *bhakti* are. That is to say, just as in worldly love affairs in the realm of *prakṛti*, the lover first encounters and feels a seed of attraction for and then ultimately falls in love with the beauty, qualities, acts, personality, and so forth of the beloved, such is the case with *bhakti*. The encounter in the case of *bhakti yoga* occurs between the devoted seeker and one of the multifarious manifestations and activities of *Īśvara* as depicted in the two epics and the vast Purāṇa corpus and its derivative literatures. And this, in Jīva's case, means Kṛṣṇa as encountered in the narratives of His incarnation recorded in the *Bhāgavata*.

A related issue this presents to those unfamiliar with the great Hindu divinities is a corollary of such personal specificity. Western readers, whether with theistic or nontheistic orientations, will in either case usually be responding to Abrahamic notions when envisioning the ultimate nature of God—the portrayals in the monotheistic traditions of Judaism, Christianity, and Islam. Jahweh/Jehovah is often construed as a personal but distant and opaque Father-like figure beyond human categories and comprehension (we speak of God the Father here: of course, Jesus, depicted as the son of God, is extremely personal and approachable for Christians). There are references in the Old Testament to prophets who were awarded a personal vision of

God the Father,[1] juxtaposed with other references suggesting that God cannot be perceived by humans,[2] but we are afforded few detailed visuals co-relatable with much that is humanly describable (visions typically using the language of fire and splendor, as in Ezekiel 1.1). God remains transcendent to the limitations of human senses and hence concise description (other than through absolutist characteristics such as "almighty," "all-knowing," and the like).

There are, in fact, parallels to this in Hinduism. The same tension between special souls being awarded a vision of God and less qualified souls overwhelmed by His majesty being unable to perceive Him even while in His presence occurs in, for example, the *Mokṣa-dharma* section of the *Mahābhārata* epic (*śānti parva* 336–38).[3] Yet whether any individual person is eligible to perceive God or not, the Purāṇas and epics are replete with detailed imagery as to what many of the forms of *Īśvara* and *Īśvarī* are held to look like when manifest to human vision. Indeed, to a great extent these texts owe their own literary raison d'être precisely to encoding and preserving the narratives of their incarnations in the world and other such personal involvement with human affairs.

When encountering such Purāṇic and epic depictions of God, which are highly visual and descriptive in language and conceptual structures familiar to the human mind, the default interpretative category most Western readers have at their disposal, and so reflexively draw from so as to make sense of these descriptions, is that of anthropomorphic myth. In other words, the characteristics associated with the various *Īśvara* forms in the Purāṇas are understandably held to constitute a projection of human qualities and activities onto the Supreme Being who is in actuality beyond human comprehension, with some superhuman flourishes to indicate this supremacy. This is all the more so since the cosmographical context of these texts—for example, the world of lower celestials with whom humans interact in various ways—is, in fact, cognate with the Greek, Roman, Celtic, Germanic, and other Indo-European pantheons, as indeed are the gods themselves—whom we have thus far referred to as celestials (*devas* in Sanskrit).[4]

With the spread of monotheistic Christianity, the preexisting Indo-European religions of Europe—including the cognate stories from the Greek, Roman, Germanic, and similarly derived epics, sagas, and other such classical sources—have long been overwhelmed and relegated to the category of classical myth (with some selective appropriations[5]). We are thus challenged, in the *Bhāgavata*, to comprehend the emergence of a theistic tradition, which retains rather than eradicates the cognate theophanies and cosmologies of the old Indo-European world that remain preserved in India and combines these with the manifestation of a monotheistic transcendent Deity. As God the Father Kṛṣṇa claims primal causal dominion and supremacy over everything, a dominion extending most especially over what becomes relegated to lower-level (Indo-European) gods. Indra and the hosts of *devas* do not get brushed aside as "false gods" in Hinduism (or Buddhism, for that matter), but they are relegated to the dimensions of *svarga*, the higher celestial realms of *prakṛti*, although still subject to its laws of *karma* and the temporality of material embodiment. They too are *ātmans* playing out their (exceptionally good) *karma* in the more subtle dimensions of *saṁsāra*.[6] Their nearest Christian trans-human parallels might be the angels, seraphims, and cherubims (indeed, the winged and musically skilled celestial *gandharvas* are similar in this regard[7]). *Īśvara* is transcendent to these dimensions and their inhabitants,[8] abiding in what corresponds to the Kingdom of God in the Purāṇas—the transcendent realms of Goloka for Kṛṣṇa, Vaikuṇṭha for Viṣṇu, Śiva-loka for Śiva, and Devī-loka for the Goddess.[9] This is why the transcendent forms of *Īśvara* should not be confounded with the great Indo-European celestials (gods with a small "g") or with notions of polytheism, any more than God and His angels express polytheism in the Abrahamic traditions, and why we have stressed that Hinduism's dominant—by which I intend transregional and pan-Hindu—expressions (other than in the very earliest literary period[10]) are either monotheistic (personal) or monistic (nonpersonal).

But most important of all, a further essential feature to keep in mind if one is to understand the power of *bhakti* is that these transcendent manifestations of *Īśvara* are considered real and actual by their devotees. These Beings are supreme personalities with forms, qualities, and activities eternally existent beyond the realm of physically accessible *prakṛti*. Likewise, the accounts of Their interactions with Their *bhaktas* and incarnations into the world are also not deemed mythological. Myth means not historically true. The stories pertaining to Kṛṣṇa are presented as historically real, not myth by the *Bhāgavata*—as is the case with the *Īśvara* manifestations in the other Purāṇas—and accepted as such by their *bhaktas*. While, as in Christianity, *Īśvara* may send a representative to the world (usually conceived of as an *aṁśa* or *kalā*, "partial incarnation," such as Vyāsa,[11] rather than as a son figure), God the Father, whom it should be clear by now is identified in the *Bhāgavata* as Viṣṇu/Kṛṣṇa, Śiva, and, in terms of God the Mother, forms of Devī, the Goddess, can also personally directly appear in the world. This occurs either by these divinities bestowing visions—in the literal sense of manifesting before Their *bhaktas* as visually perceivable presence—as we will find in the Tale of Prince Dhruva—or by assuming forms and entering into the world for prolonged periods resembling a conventional lifetime. This is the *avatāra*, literally "one who descends" (a term problematically translated as "incarnation").[12] It is the deeds and activities of these *avatāras* performed in the world as recorded in the two epics and the Purāṇas that underpin the devotional practices of most of the major *bhakti* traditions and the bulk of its literary corpus.

So, as we prepare to read parts 2 and 3 of this volume, our main challenge when striving to understand *bhakti* on its own terms is to keep in mind that these stories are not considered myth in premodern India, but sacred history. Purāṇa means "that which occurred in the past," and, likewise, *itihāsa*, epic, translates as "this is what happened." Modern theorizing on the study of religion has either imposed reductionistic categories of interpretation on religious narratives of this sort or sought some kind of perennial core. Reductionism entails rejecting the face-value claims made by a tradition, which are seen as expressions of prerational, prescientific, mythological thinking, and instead strives to impose some modern rational explanation for why religions exist, make the historical claims they do, and wield the power they exert. Their essence is thus "reduced" to some sort of natural, rationally explainable—as opposed to supernatural—cause. Perennialism also rejects the surface-level claims and stories of religious traditions but makes an effort to retain a supernatural element in the form of a common transcultural hidden spiritual core. Like a perennial flower that reappears consistently every year, this core is deemed to surface consistently—"perennially"—across traditions, once one digs behind the clutter of superimposed mythological trappings.

So, for example, in a reductionist approach, a claimed vision of Kṛṣṇa might be interpreted as nothing other than some psychological projections from the subconscious (as with Freud), or the influence of mundane social forces on the psyche (Durkheim and Weber), or concocted by social elite groups to preserve political or economic power over other social groups (Marx). For such theorists, religions are consciously or unconsciously "invented" by humans, created to serve social, political, or psychological purposes or other such mundane needs in the real world.[13] Perennialism, in contrast, which is prepared to allow a spiritual core to religious phenomenon and resists such materialistic reductionism, ends up imposing a reductionism of its own. Although committed to acknowledging some transcendent element to religion, perennialists typically jettison all surface-layer narratives (such as the stories of the activities of *Īśvara*'s incarnations) in the quest of some perennial core buried beneath them. This core is deemed to emerge consistently across religions, irrespective of time and place, once excavated by the perennialist savant. It is typically construed as some form of a monistic essence—understandably, as monism is the most conveniently appropriated metaphysics for anyone seeking a baseline generic commonality from the comparison of religions. The stories themselves are deemed later accretions added as concessions for the unenlightened superstitious masses, or are at best accepted as metaphor, symbol, or archetype of some higher Truth.[14] All this is an enormous domain in its own right, foundational to, and indeed constitutive of, the academic study of religion, but for our present purposes, both these types of treatments violate the claims such texts make about themselves, albeit in very different ways and underpinned by opposing intentions. (Strenski, 2006, likes to call the "perennialists" "caretakers of religion," and reductionists "undertakers of religion"!)

In any event, as something of a reaction against such interpretative impositions from the elite ivory towers of Western scholarship on non-Western traditions, with many of these theories reflecting the Eurocentric, Christian, colonial, and racist attitudes of their times,[15] an academic approach to the study of religion, called "phenomenology," emerged among certain intellectuals. Despite meaning different things to different scholars in the history of the term, phenomenology typically strives to refrain from imposing Western post-Enlightenment so-called rational modes of interpretation on the truth claims of other traditions, often far distant in space, time, and context, and strives, rather, to consider them on their own terms. This approach does not entail necessarily accepting traditional claims as historically or scientifically true, but it does entail making at least a serious commitment to bracketing one's own beliefs and presuppositions (even as this is impossible). It attempts to suspend judgments of veracity or falsity and refrains from evaluating traditions based on their compatibility with modern categories of knowledge. This is intended to allow the traditions to narrate their own tale and speak in their own voice through their own categories as "phenomena" in their own right. This is the approach I have adopted throughout, as outlined in the introduction.

If we wish to gain any level of empathy, phenomenological or other, as to the power of *bhakti*, it is useful to keep in mind that nowhere in the sixteen thousand verses of the *Bhāgavata* does the text claim to be myth, metaphor, or symbol. Nor is any such suggestion made in the approximately four hundred thousand verses of the entire Purāṇa corpus, the one-hundred-thousand-verse *Mahābhārata*, and the twenty-four-thousand-verse *Rāmāyaṇa*. In fact, when metaphoric readings are intended, they are clearly indicated, as we will see in the Allegory of the Forest and the Allegory of King Purañjana in part 2.[16] Thanks to the intellectual conditionings we have inherited from post-Enlightenment presuppositions (another vast and interminable topic in its own right), we would do well to be aware of our own cultural presuppositions and intellectual embeddedness and bear in mind that most modern heirs to the Western Enlightenment do not read these stories in the same way the tradition-sensitive *bhaktas* do.

Ultimately, this is an epistemological issue. Epistemology deals with the sources and means through which knowledge is acquired. Briefly stated, prior to the Enlightenment, the Christian Bible had been deemed the ultimate source of knowledge in most mainstream contexts in Christendom for the best part of a millennium and a half (despite its many dissenters). The Enlightenment displaced scripture in favor of human reason as the highest source of knowledge. The "light" of reason was deemed epistemologically paramount. Despite dissenters here too, we now inhabit an intellectual world where the claims of scripture are subject to the scrutiny of reason and empirical data, at least in most scholarly circles. Even as most thinkers in academic circles are fully aware of the myth of objectivity and the limitations of reason and the empirical method, they are still considered the de facto safest epistemological methods. Few are willing to countenance a return to what most would consider a faith-based, nondemonstrable, magical, superstitious, mythological worldview inhabited by invisible beings and controlled by supernatural forces. (Although, increasingly, with some scientists talking of parallel universes and other such phenomena, the Purāṇic cosmography can sometimes seem a little less "mythic" in comparison!)

Where the modern West has prioritized reason and empiricism[17] as the highest reliable source of knowledge since its "enlightenment," other cultures such as those of India have not had the same conflict between religion and science and the tension inherited from the subsequent separation of these two domains, at least historically. Let us keep in mind that the Christian context that triggered this separation was a European affair. The Western Enlightenment assumption that the ultimacy of reason is a universal and absolute given will be challenged by anyone open to understanding most *mokṣa* traditions of India on their own terms, and certainly the *Bhāgavata* tradition. While developing a rich array of highly sophisticated reason-based intellectual systems,[18] these traditions have often marshaled these in support of transrational and supraempirical realities. And the existence of these realities frequently rests on the authority of sacred texts (see the *Vedānta Sūtras* I.1.3) and/or on the accounts of rugged *yogī* exemplars. The authoritativeness of such *yogīs*, in turn, rests on their own claims to direct personal experience that is "transempirical" (*para-pratyakṣa*).[19] *Yoga*'s very definition is to experience states of consciousness beyond the intellect, announced by Patañjali in the very opening verses of his *sūtras* (I.1–4).

Thus the practices and appeal of *bhakti* will make no sense—or at least no sense recognizable to traditional Vaiṣṇavas—unless we recognize the fact that these texts locate themselves as sacred history—records of the superhuman deeds and arrangements enacted by the supreme *Īśvara* when He broke into human time and space or, in the opening words of the tenth book, "the deeds performed by the Almighty Lord, the Creator of the Universe, when He incarnated" (I.2–3). We can take this or leave it: our task, established at the onset, is simply to present the Truth claims of the *Bhāgavata* tradition in its own terms to the best of our abilities, not to attempt to influence how the reader chooses to make sense of them. We trust it is eminently clear by now that the central feature of those claims is that—to once again borrow some phraseology in order to stress the universalism as opposed to the "Hindu-ness" of the claim—Kṛṣṇa is God the Father for the *Bhāgavata Purāṇa*. And the text's tenth book we will encounter in part 3 claims to be a record of His deeds when He descended on earth.

So, as we have seen from the nine processes of *bhakti yoga*, in essence, *bhakti* is nothing other than becoming attracted to these deeds, hearing them, remembering them, reciting them, enacting them in drama and festivals, commemorating them at the times of year they occurred, undertaking pilgrimage to the places made holy by their activities, worshipping them through temple mediums, and other such immersive ritual practices. In advanced stages, one becomes so absorbed and enamored by these stories that one loses interest in everything else—that is, everything pertaining to *prakṛti* (as with the ultimate stage of detachment of *Yoga Sūtras* I.16).[20] The same holds true for the other *bhakti* traditions based on other manifestations of *Īśvara*. So there we have it: when all is said and done, this is what *bhakti yoga* is, not just in Jīva's tradition, but in almost all premodern *bhakti* traditions. The metaphysical differences and variants outlined in the previous section notwithstanding, most forms of *bhakti* are predicated on accepting some sort of reality to a form of *Īśvara* or *Īśvarī* and commemorating His or Her associated qualities and deeds.

In sum, while the historicity of Kṛṣṇa might be the glaring anomaly in all of this from a rationalist point of view (the elephant in the room, so to speak), to understand the appeal of *bhakti* to its followers, it serves to keep in mind that these stories are not considered myth. They are as true to the *bhaktas* as the narratives of the Old Testament, New Testament, and Koran are to the faithful of the various Abrahamic monotheistic traditions. For the *bhaktas*, if there is an almighty *Īśvara*, then that *Īśvara* can surely enter into the world and manipulate *prakṛti* to perform astonishing deeds irrespective of what our finite minds and limited knowledge systems might care to say about it. For the *Bhāgavata*, what else is the meaning of words such as "infinite," "unlimited," and "almighty"? In fact, such confounding of our human rational capabilities to comprehend these deeds or pigeonhole them into familiar human empirically based epistemic categories is not only self-evident, but a source of great relish for the devotee: "Just as an ignorant person does not understand the behavior of an actor, so no creature of limited intelligence can understand through words, mind, or cleverness, the pastimes of the Supreme Creator when He exhibits His names and forms" (I.3.37).

Having said all that, I would venture to speculate that even for most modern educated *bhaktas*, schooled in the intellectual currents flowing from Western post-Enlightenment thought, whether or not the fabulous events pertaining to Kṛṣṇa's incarnation *actually* happened in verifiable historical time and space is less important than relishing the meditation that if *Īśvara* is unlimited and omnipotent, as all theists hold Him to be, then any or all events featuring Him such as those we will encounter in part 3 certainly *could* have happened simply as an expression of His divine will. While one cannot renegotiate the fact that the text clearly presents itself as passing down historical records of *Īśvara*'s divine descents, it nonetheless identifies its main purpose in its very opening verses as conveying *rasa*, love of God. It is the experience of this *rasa* that is of interest to *bhaktas*, not the laborious minutiae of historical reconstruction:

> The literature, which reveals the qualities of *Bhagavān*, is literature that is true, that is auspicious, that is purifying. It is such literature, which is pleasing and charming and which always provides an ever-fresh joyful experience for the mind. It is such literature which dries up the ocean of despair for all people—the literature wherein the glories of Kṛṣṇa are recited . . . *even if there are errors in every line.* (XII.12.48–51, my italics)

The *Bhāgavata* is signing on to being a venue for transmitting a beautiful vision of God as its ultimate raison d'être. The insistence on historicality that can be empirically verified via archaeology, linguistics, numismatics, text criticism, and so forth has emerged since the European Enlightenment as a response to intellectual dynamics, tensions, and developments in Christendom in response to the historical claims of its textual traditions.[21] That these methods and ways of thinking have been exported and seemingly universalized is a feature of past European colonialism and present Western economic and political power,[22] but they may not always be so relevant or share the same importance with what is central to the *bhakta*'s experience.[23]

But the fact is, post-Enlightenment modes and methods of evaluating sacred histories have been exported and they have been made de facto normative, at least in academic centers of learning. And it is also a fact that the monotheistic traditions of Hindu *bhakti* such as Gauḍīya Vaiṣṇavism, centered on the historicality of Kṛṣṇa's incarnation (as that of Rāma and the other *avatāras*), have much more of a challenge engaging modern scientific methods of historical reconstruction than the monistic traditions. It was the incompatibility of biblical chronology and the Genesis narratives of the Old Testament with the emerging historical methods of geology, archaeology, linguistics, and text criticism (as well as the encounter with non-European civilizations) that lay at the heart of the Enlightenment and spawned the academic study of religion in the first place. Monistic traditions such as *advaita Vedānta*, while nonetheless certainly accepting the Purāṇa accounts as historical and literally true in the realm of conventional reality discussed previously (*vyavahārika*—that is, true to the same extent pots, pans, mountains, stars in the sky, and any other perceivable phenomenon are true and real), consider them ultimately all illusory, *māyā*, on the level of absolute reality (*pāramārthika*). There is a bit less at stake here. Monotheistic Kṛṣṇa *bhakti*, as we know, revolves around the deeds performed by a real *Īśvara* in real human space and time, just as normative Christianity depends on the reality of a historical Christ. Such centrality of the historical dimension is much less negotiable and so is much more challenged by modernity.[24]

Pertinent here is that centuries before the challenges introduced by the Western juxtaposition of myth versus history during the colonial period impacted Hindu intellectuals, Jīva had outlined in his *Kṛṣṇa Sandarbha* that Kṛṣṇa's *līlā* has a divine counterpart, which is eternally enacted in a trans-*prakṛtic Brahman* dimension. This *Brahman* realm, Goloka, coexists with this earthly realm but is inaccessible to sensual perception and rational thought (*anu* 106, 110–16,

153, 172).[25] It can, however, be accessed by advanced *bhāgavatas* in deep states of *samādhi* (as we encountered in the passages from Caitanya's life). So while Kṛṣṇa's *līlā* is certainly held to be a historical event in the *Bhāgavata*, Jīva also finds ground in the text itself to suggest that the *līlās* are simultaneously always transpiring in this eternal, coexisting, non-*prakṛtic* counterpart. While Goloka is beyond the range of empiricism and human reason, it is nonetheless a realm that is coextensive with this realm of *prakṛti* and hence can be experienced in this world in *bhakti samādhi*, as we have seen.

Indeed, while Hindu responses to modernity are an enormous topic in their own right, we can briefly note that a much later representative of Gauḍīya Vaiṣṇavism, Bhaktivinoda Thakur, in the nineteenth century, availed himself of this alternative spiritual reality when confronted with the empirical methods of historical reconstruction reaching the Hindu intelligentsia of his time from the West.[26] As a high court judge in colonial India and very much an early apologist for the Kṛṣṇa tradition responding to the challenges of modernity, Bhaktivinoda separated what he called the *ādhunika-vāda*, "modern approach" to the study of scripture, from its *paramārtha-prada*,[27] "transcendent aspect." The sphere of historical authority of the *ādhunika-vāda* pertains to the text's references to space and historical time, which could be subject to the scrutiny of empirical methodologies and consequently tinkered with and, if necessary, readily adjusted in response to modern historical methods. The *paramārtha-prada*, on the other hand, is the divine dimension of Kṛṣṇa's *līlā*, beyond *prakṛti*, and hence immune to the intellect and senses, but, following Jīva, a realm experientially accessible by deep *bhakti*. In this way, Bhaktivinoda strove to safeguard the claims of the *bhakta* mystics from the threatening deconstructive dismantling of Western methodologies of historical reconstruction (unlike some of his contemporaries and successors who were much more willing to completely jettison the *Bhāgavata* Kṛṣṇa and the Purāṇas in general in their determination to find modes of monotheism in Hinduism that could pass—and surpass—the standards set by Western moral and rational discourse[28]).

In fact, revisionist readings of older texts go back to the middle Vedic period. Already in the *Brāhmaṇas*, *Āraṇyakas*, and Upaniṣads, mystical interpretations of the Vedic rites become increasingly evident (see, for example, *Bṛhadāraṇyaka Upaniṣad* I.1), as do naturalistic interpretation of Vedic myths.[29] Commenting on the oldest Vedic material, the twelfth-century theologian Madhva identified his own three different ways of reading the *Ṛg-Veda*: the historical, the mystical, and the transcendent.[30] Jīva himself notes that the *Bhāgavata* can instruct in three different moods: either as a master, or as friend, or as the beloved (*Tattva Sandarbha* XXVI.2). A later exegete of the same school, Viśvanātha, uses another triple lens: the *Bhāgavata* contains three progressive levels of content. On a generic level, it is like the light, shining knowledge on the soul, in accordance with the older *ātman* traditions; beyond this, it is like the sun (a greater source of light), illuminating the superexcellence of Kṛṣṇa as the Ultimate Truth; and, highest of all, it is the ripe fruit of bliss. While this highest third phase breaks the luminosity metaphor, it surpasses the other two ways of reading the text insofar as it deals with experience rather than just providing knowledge.[31] In fact, it is to promote this experience of love of God that is the ultimate goal of the *Bhāgavata*.

While these traditional theologians mean rather different things by their respective schemas, present-day readers may thus find themselves following a well-worn path of tripartite hermeneutics. Most modern lenses may also very well view the text as containing three distinct levels that correspond to our own intellectual milieu: a historical core preserving records of royal dynasties and kingdoms; a mythological overlay involving a world of various levels of divine beings and superhuman mortals and their fabulous deeds; and a theological one representing the emergence of a powerful monotheistic tradition drawing from a *yogic* backdrop and centered on the worship of *Śrī* Kṛṣṇa that was to sweep across the subcontinent. In any event, clearly the *Bhāgavata* offers profound insights into the human condition that transcend time, place, and the vicissitudes of the ever-changing empirical and rational knowledge systems pertaining to material reality. For those interested in the wisdom traditions for their insights into the nature of the mind and its workings, or guidance into what might constitute the higher goals of life, one is perfectly entitled to extract the *yoga* teachings of the *Bhāgavata* from their larger social, scientific, historical, cosmological, and related contexts, just as one does with insights of the great Greek philosophers, who, after all, navigated within the contours of a cognate cosmography. In fact, those familiar with the *Bhāgavata* may notice we have favored precisely such *yogic/jñāna* (wisdom) narratives in our selections in part 2. The tales and teachings here can certainly be read from the point of view of the psychological, philosophical, and soteriological messages they impart over and beyond the surface narratives.

In fact, there are numerous instances of premodern Indian thinkers proposing alternative or nonliteral readings of sections or elements in the Purāṇas without rejecting them as authoritative texts. The later astronomers come to mind, who accepted the observation-based data of the later *Sūrya Siddhānta* (astronomical) traditions without overtly rejecting the very different cosmological accounts in the much older Purāṇas. Likewise, and of great relevance here, strains of the Sanskrit literary tradition theorized about when indirect signification is to be applied to a passage where a literal reading is rendered impossible by other knowledge systems.[32]

In fact, one can find instances of the *Bhāgavata* itself offering opportunities for nonliteral readings. In the twelfth book, for example, Viṣṇu's *kaustubha* gem is said to represent the *ātman*; his flower garland, the *guṇas*; his yellow garment, the Vedic meter; his sacred thread, the syllable *oṁ*; his club, *prāṇa*, the life airs; the various implements he holds in his hands, the elements; his bow, Time; and so on for a number of verses (XII.11.10–20). All this is not to say that the text is renegotiating the ontological reality of these items, but, rather, that it does not appear to be threatened by nonliteral readings for those conditioned by and subject to rational modes of thinking. Along similar lines, after describing the various realms of the universe in book 5, the text concludes by specifying that these cosmographic descriptions are intended to bring the mind to contemplating *Īśvara* through His "material" perceivable form of creation. This is the God of natural theology. Once the mind has become proficient in this, and purified simply by dint of contemplating *Īśvara* in whatever mode this takes in accordance with the mental predisposition of a person, then one "should lead the mind to the subtle form of *Bhagavān*" (V.26.38–40; see also II.2.14). In other words, contemplating the wondrous realms of the universe as God's body is first and foremost a method to develop *bhakti*. In the same way, the descriptions of king lineages "have been narrated with the intention of expressing detachment from and insight into [the temporal nature of material grandeur].

They are just a display of rhetoric, they are not the Ultimate Truth" (XII.3.14–15). It is not the minutiae of dates, historicality, geography, or cosmology, etc., that interests the *Bhāgavata* but revealing the fleeting nature of even the grandest material accomplishments and conquests. The text's central claim and raison d'être is that if one absorbs one's mind in the stories pertaining to Kṛṣṇa and His amazing deeds, one will speedily and easily attain the generic qualifications of *yoga* (dispassion toward the world of sense objects and the like) and develop an experience of love of God. What the rational mind may make of the stories is secondary to this effect.

So although the *Bhāgavata* from its opening verses on unambiguously situates itself as simultaneously sacred and temporal history, it does not demand that one is required to accept this claim for the stories to perform their function. In fact, as was discussed in "Meditation in Hate and Lust," the text takes some pains to describe how various individuals who could never accept the transcendent factuality of Kṛṣṇa as claimed by the *Bhāgavata* tradition nonetheless attained the goals of *bhakti* by dint of immersing their minds in thoughts of Him, some in hatred and with violent intent.[33] The stories ultimately seek to implant a seed of *rāga*, love of God, embedded in the larger generic *yoga* context of stressing the futility of pursuing any other self-centered *prakṛtic rāga*. If one attains this *bhakti rāga*, irrespective of how one interprets the stories—literally, metaphorically, symbolically, or, as with Bhaktivinoda, esoterically—then the *Bhāgavata* has attained its ultimate goals.

In any event, returning to the ontological status of these forms of *Īśvara* and *Īśvarī*, to perhaps underscore the fact that acceptance of their reality is not part of some classical mythic traditions of the premodern past but very much part of a living tradition, we might just mention in passing that a number of modern-day *gurus* have claimed (or were recorded by their disciples as claiming) to have had visions of all forms of *Īśvara*. Focusing just on claims pertaining to Kṛṣṇa, and from Hindu figures well-known in the West, the hagiography of Rāmakrishna, Vivekānanda's *guru*, records his visions of Kṛṣṇa.[34] One of the most influential *gurus* of modern India (and, through his disciples, in the West), Śivānanda, writes in the first line of his autobiography of his vision of Kṛṣṇa.[35] His disciple, too, Vishnudevananda, who established the Śivānanda Organization in his *guru*'s name, claimed to have had a vision of Rādhā-Kṛṣṇa in a place that he consequently purchased as a result and developed as the organization's Grass Valley, California, *āśrama*.[36] Aurobindo, the remarkable freedom fighter turned mystic, had a vision of Kṛṣṇa while imprisoned.[37] Iyengar, whose influence in the spread of *āsana*, modern postural *yoga*, has been immense (but, as we have noted, who still maintains identification with Rāmānuja's Śrī Vaiṣṇava Vedānta lineage), when young and struggling to maintain his family in the days before *yoga* became a global phenomenon told his disciples that Viṣṇu appeared to him in a dream and told him that he should continue with his commitment to this path and that all his difficulties would be resolved.[38] Amma, "the Hugging Mother" (Mata Amritanandamayi), had visions of Kṛṣṇa in her youth.[39] Yogananda Paramahamsa reports a vision of Kṛṣṇa in his autobiography.[40] We can also note that while not identifying this being as Kṛṣṇa (but rather as Śiva), but along similar lines, Muktānanda describes a vision of a blue boy in his remarkable autobiography (along with a prior vision of a form of *Īśvarī*).[41]

These are just samples of claims to visions of Kṛṣṇa from very recent famous *guru* figures who became well-known in the West. There are countless other claims to visions of other forms of *Īśvara* (for example, the famous mathematician Śrīnivāsa Rāmāṇujan claimed not only to have had visions of a form of the Goddess Nāmagiri Tāyār, but to have received many complex equations from her). Obviously they are all anecdotal and hagiographical, but whatever we may choose to make of them, and whatever alternative (typically post-Freudian) explanations we may prefer to adopt in order to fit them into our intellectual comfort zones, claims to visions of all the various forms of *Īśvara* and *Īśvarī* are ubiquitous throughout the history of Indian culture from the late Vedic age till the present. In short, *bhakti* texts all claim that *Īśvara* can be seen by the sincere and fully dedicated devotee (see *Gītā* XI.54 for an example of this), and however we in the so-called rational West may opt to interpret these assertions, and whatever reductionistic interpretations we may prefer to impose on them, the point we are making here is simply that *bhakti yoga* very much remains a living tradition and, as with other mystical traditions, one that lays its claims to verification in direct personal experience. Our Western "enlightenment" and the historical factors that triggered its intellectual trajectory are clearly drawing from a very different set of epistemological experiences and presuppositions from the "enlightened" traditions long current in India.

Be all this as it may, our own methodological approach in this volume has been phenomenological—allowing the *Bhāgavata* to tell its own story and make its own truth claims both in its own voice and through the lenses applied to it by the later tradition represented by Jīva and Rūpa. We have avoided imposing any external modern interpretative models upon its meanings and significance; our task, established immediately and clearly at the beginning of the introduction, has been to offer the interested reader a glimpse into one universe of traditional *bhakti* prior to its encounter with modernity, not to attempt to influence how the modern reader should make sense of it all. Of course, from the perspective of *bhakti* practitioners, it remains to be seen what forms transplanted *bhakti yoga* will take among the various *yoga* communities in the West. We have seen what has happened to the radical world/body/mind-renouncing asceticism of Patañjalian Yoga in its appropriation by and commodification into what has better been called "modern postural *yoga*" in many expressions of practice laying claim to that tradition, at least in name.[42] Even then, for those who do in fact engage classical *yoga* philosophy on its own terms, the basic conceptual commitment it requires—that consciousness can be removed from all objects and withdrawn into its own nature (I.3)—is a lot less demanding than the leap of faith central to the *Bhāgavata*. Although the dualism of, say, Plato and normative Christianity is different from that of Yoga,[43] some sort of a mind/body dualism has remained if not hegemonic, certainly the dominant view in most Western intellectual traditions throughout recorded history. And even as a neurological view of consciousness now has a strong following among some communities of scientists, and the Cartesian variant of dualism has long faced various philosophical challenges, the notion of consciousness being distinct from the body is still very much a defensible and certainly a culturally familiar belief.

The point here is that a non-*bhakta* can engage (much of[44]) the *Yoga Sūtras* and still feel connected to familiar cultural, theological, and intellectual landmarks. The *Bhāgavata*, if taken on its own terms—that the forms and manifestations of *Īśvara* are real transcendent Beings and their wonderful deeds factually enacted in human time and space—is clearly demanding a much more drastic conceptual leap of faith from the perspective of reality as construed not only by our modern intellectual and scientific traditions, but by the Western world's historically religious ones. This is a leap that, from the point of view of the Western literary tradition, finds its closest cognate in a Greco-Roman past that has been long eclipsed and relegated to the realm of myth. Such a leap is obviously expecting a lot.

There is thus every reason to suppose that in its efforts to establish roots on the landscape of transplanted Eastern spirituality, *bhakti* will develop even more radically reconfigured meanings and expressions from its traditional genealogies than generic *yoga* has done. And it, too, while hopefully still attracting practitioners committed to the worldview of the traditional sources, will in all likelihood continue to be seen as another source of Eastern material that provides further ingredients for the pick-and-choose, mix-and-match approach typical of modern watered-down Western spiritualities. (By "watered-down," I partly intend that the *tapas,* austerity/discipline, so central to all Indic *mokṣa* traditions tends to get, if not jettisoned, significantly diluted in the New Age alternative religious landscape.) Even if this is so, independent of the cosmological, historical, and social context within which it situates itself, and the *Īśvara*-centered theism that is its all-pervading raison d'être, it is hard to deny that at its most basic level in terms of generic *yoga* teachings, the *Bhāgavata* offers powerful insights into the human condition and the nature of the mind that will always remain perennially relevant to human beings of any time and place.

Whatever future awaits them, the stories of Kṛṣṇa and the other forms of *Īśvara* have a power of their own that, as we know from the preceding discussions, can plant a seed of attraction for this mischievous figure, but one that does not always sit comfortably with the rational mind. On a personal note, as an academic committed to the ideals of objective intellectual rigor and integrity, who has nonetheless devoted his life to this tradition, I can attest that these tensions are irresolvable, as perhaps they should be. The dance between reason and the heart is never-ending—sometimes causing one to sway and veer toward one modality, sometimes the other. One can remain in a state of dissonance about this, or one can simply become comfortable wearing different hats appropriate to the different *dharmas*, or domains: the *dharma* of objective, historical, contextual analysis as required by academia, and the *dharma* as defined by the *Bhāgavata* discussed previously—the subjective, ahistorical, and transcontextual devotion to a Supreme Being. These *dharmic* spheres require different theoretical languages, vocabularies, conceptual structures, methodologies, and associations of participants. One can navigate between them without needing to resolve their tensions and disjunctions—and, indeed, recognize the impossibility of ever doing so. By definition, transrational transempirical states and experiences are metaphysically and epistemologically incompatible with rational methods of empirical analysis and verification—a very well-worn and persistent topic in the study of religion. The *Bhāgavata* repeatedly claims that Kṛṣṇa's attractive qualities supersede and flout all intellectual, social, cultural, and similar considerations.

However, apologetics can go only so far: at the end of the day, for the *bhakti* traditions to remain living worldviews with positive relevance to the intellectual communities of their times, especially in their transplanted forms outside of India, they will increasingly have to engage the challenges of modernity, even given the epistemological disjunction noted above, just as Christian thinkers have done for almost two centuries. Vaiṣṇava theologians have historically invested great intellectual energy in presenting their theologies in as rational and philosophically rigorous a manner as possible—and in dialogue with the scholarly currents of their day and age (as is the theologian's *dharma* in any time and place). They have addressed opposing viewpoints incompatible with their essential premises (the *pūrvapakṣa*) with integrity and confidence. Continuing that process has barely begun, given the still very recently transplanted nature of *bhakti* in the West, and it remains to be seen what forms this might take. These traditions have only just begun to produce public intellectuals adequately equipped academically to engage in scholarly dialogue—in conversation both with other monotheisms in particular as well as the broader comparative field of religion on one side and with modern science and the scientific method on the other.[45] There is good reason (see Edelmann 2014) to suppose these fledgling but very commendable efforts will continue and increase. And one would like to hope that the orthodox *paṇḍits* and *ācāryas*, the bearers of the traditional Vaiṣṇava, Śaiva, and Śākta *saṁpradāyas* (lineages), will also be inspired to engage the intellectual currents of their present time in a more active and public manner than has hitherto been the case, either personally or by inspiring their followers who have the requisite scholarly credentials to do so. In doing so, they would thereby follow in the footsteps of their predecessors who have always stalwartly risen to the occasion over the centuries—indeed, over the two millennia—before them.[46]

But, ultimately, when everything is said and done, *bhakti* is about love of God, and that is a matter of the heart[47] that lays claim to a transrational domain. This may not always be reconcilable with what constitutes reality as reconstructed by the intellect using the methods of empiricism and human reason. In the end, one's interpretative partialities and modes of making sense of what is going on with these stories reflect how comfortable one is with this dichotomy and what one accepts as one's ultimate source of epistemological authority (which is a matter of faith, whatever episteme ones prioritizes). And, perhaps more ultimate still from a *bhakti* perspective, one might even suggest that one's position on such things in turn reflects the depth, or absence, of one's personal *bhakti rāga* and nothing else.

Hierarchies of Bliss

Let us now, by way of conclusion, return to the frames of reference and categories of the *Bhagavata* itself, which has been our commitment in this project all along, and summarize the implications of everything we have discussed from the perspective of *yoga* in general. As we have seen, one of the main subtexts of the *Bhāgavata* and its derivative literature such as the *Sandarbhas* is to repeatedly contrast the bliss of a personal relationship between *Īśvara* and the *bhakta* with the experience of impersonal, nonrelational *ātman/Brahman* immersion. We have used the language of monotheism and monism for these modalities—but we should mention that they will often be encountered in theological texts as *saguṇa Brahman*, the Absolute Truth with personality, form, and qualities, and *nirguṇa Brahman*, formless and qualityless Truth (as in III.32.36). We have discussed how, according to *Bhāgavata* ontology (and mainstream

Hinduism in general), *prakṛti* is an active dynamic, sensual, personalized, and object-focused realm of reality, in which the *ātman* is embedded. Beyond this is the passive, nondynamic, trans-sensual, impersonal, and subject-centered[48] dimension of reality, consisting of the experience of the *ātman*, a state synonymous with *Brahman* immersion, where consciousness is absorbed in its own nature. Beyond this again, there is another active, dynamic, sensual, personal, and object-focused realm of reality, but in this case made not of temporal unconscious *prakṛti* stuff, but of eternal conscious *Brahman* stuff, the realms of Vaikuṇṭha and Goloka. The liberated *ātmans* attaining these realms again become reembodied, but this time not in a *prakṛtic* form in which suffering is constitutional and endemic, but in an eternal body made of pure *sat-cit-ānanda Brahman*—a divine form made of being and consciousness in which bliss is inherent and ever-expanding.

Therefore, given that in the Vedānta and Purāṇa traditions, from the earliest Upaniṣads and through practically the entire history of late Vedic-derived literature onward, there is little disagreement that the *ātman* is eternal and conscious[49] (with the partial exception of the Nyāya and Vaiśeṣiká traditions),[50] one's options, therefore, are merely of what it is that one ends up being conscious or aware. In other words, since it can never be not conscious or not aware, owing to its eternal unchanging nature, the *ātman*'s essential inherent constitution requires that it be conscious of something for all eternity, so what is it that awareness ends up being aware of? For as long as we are embodied, the instrument utilized by consciousness when seeking any object of awareness is the mind, so, put differently, what is it that we are going to do with this mind, as it is never inactive in the waking state (other than in the states of *samādhi*)?

In embodied existence, fueled by objects of desire, awareness is focused primarily on the sensations produced by these objects through the instruments of the mind and sense organs, all provided by *prakṛti* in accordance with those desires.[51] Upon realizing that it is this very quest for sensual pleasure that is itself the fundamental cause of suffering, one may seek to renounce desire, transcend its *karmic* consequences and hence suffering, and realize the true source of consciousness freed from its ensnarement with *prakṛti* and all objects.[52] Gaining success in this, one attains *nirbīja samādhi*, a passive state of self-awareness[53]—that is to say, the object of awareness becomes awareness itself, although, put more precisely, the subject/object duality evaporates and pure objectless consciousness is all that remains. But if, as described earlier, one encounters and becomes attracted to the object of consciousness called *Īśvara*—that is if, while embodied, one happens to hear about *Īśvara*'s names, qualities, forms, deeds, and so on by having the good fortune to encounter the *Bhāgavata* or the *bhāgavatas*—one might become attracted to developing a relationship with this Being. For this, awareness again needs the instruments of mind and senses—whether made of *prakṛti* in this world or of *Brahman* stuff in the Goloka realm—in order to see, hear, think about, and interact with Kṛṣṇa. Thus, as we have discussed, after hearing about Kṛṣṇa, even *jñānis* who have realized their own *ātman* may decide to reconnect with the psychophysical mechanism of the mind and senses so as to dive into the ocean of Hari's *līlās*.

So for the *Bhāgavata*, consciousness has three basic options: to be absorbed in *prakṛti*, to be absorbed in itself, or to be absorbed in devotional thoughts and loving service of *Īśvara*. We might wish to note here that any process of *yoga* is taking place in the mind. The mind is nothing other than a storage container (*āsaya*) for *saṁskāras*. Both *bhoga* (*prakṛtic* enjoyment) and all forms of *yoga* are ultimately enacted by the *saṁskāras* of the mind. In conventional life in the world, when ignorant of the self, the prominent *saṁskāra* in the mind is *prakṛtic rāga*, desire; the goal of life is *bhoga*, pleasure; and everything else is processed in terms of its value to the fulfillment of *rāga*. The *jñāna yoga* path for those frustrated with *bhoga* involves fixing the mind on the teachings of the Upaniṣads or other such knowledge texts pertaining to the ultimacy of the *ātman* and the temporality of *prakṛti*. This boils down to keeping the *ātman saṁskāra* as the dominant *saṁskāra* or presence in the mind, which monitors all other *saṁskāras*, ensuring they are in line with thoughts pertaining to *mokṣa*, the ultimate goal of *jñāna*. *Dhyāna yoga* (Patañjalian-type *yoga*) involves the ultimate suppression of all states of mind whatsoever, so the practice here is to keep the *nirodha* (suppressing) *saṁskāra* reigning supreme and suppressing any other *saṁskāra* that might try to make its presence felt (I.50–51). And *bhakti* involves keeping thoughts of one's beloved *Īśvara* foremost in the mind, and of one's *vaidhī* or *rāgānugā* relationship with Him, hence the *Īśvara saṁskāra* is dominant in this practice. But whether one is cultivating the *prakṛtic rāga saṁskāra*, the *ātman saṁskāra*, the *nirodha saṁskāra*, or the *Īśvara saṁskāra*, these are all *saṁskāras* and therefore all states of mind. Bottom line: We get to choose which set of *saṁskāras* we wish to pursue in life.

In ultimate postmortem liberation, as I trust is clear by now, the *bhakta* seeks to replace the mind made of *prakṛti* stuff with one made of *Brahman* stuff, but in any circumstance one still needs a mind to perform *bhakti*, and mind is not inherent in the *ātman*, it is an external covering (*Gītā* VII.4). So until attaining a *Brahman* mind (and senses) in Vaikuṇṭha or Goloka in the postmortem state, for as long as *bhaktas* remain embodied in *prakṛti*, they choose to retain the mind and senses made of *prakṛti* so as to contemplate and actively serve their beloved *Īśvara*, rather than uncouple from the mind and remain in a state of pure but passive consciousness, as per standard Patañjalian-type *yoga* practice. Ultimately, why some *yogīs* would abandon the state of *ātman* immersion, promoted as enormously blissful in the Upaniṣads,[54] and hence the goal of so many *jñāna* and *yoga* traditions, so as to again reconnect with their minds, after so much hard work detaching themselves from these very minds as the source of suffering, is very simple. Channeling consciousness through the mind, intellect, and senses onto *Īśvara* is simply incomparably more blissful than any other experience in existence, including that of the bliss, *ānanda*, inherent in the *ātman*: "The pleasure [experienced] by embodied beings from meditating on Your lotus feet or from hearing about Your deeds from Your devotees does not exist in *Brahman*, even though that is also a part of Your own majesty, O Lord" (IV.9.10).

Therefore, in all this, we find a difference among the various Hindu soteriological (*mokṣa*) traditions with regard to liberation—even as all agree that this is a state beyond suffering. Let us compare some of them in this regard (leaving aside the Cārvāka/Lokāyata-grouped materialist schools that do not accept any postmortem liberation).[55] The Nyāya and Vaiśeṣiká schools hold that the liberated state, which they also accept as uncoupling the *ātman* from the mind (*manas*), is simply one of *sat*, being.[56] For these schools, there is not even consciousness, *cit*, in *mokṣa*, as this is a quality that emerges only when the *ātman* is connected with the instrumentality of the mind in *saṁsāra*. Nor, certainly, is there *ānanda*; there is just unconscious being. The soteriological goal of *yoga* here, *mokṣa*, is freedom from suffering (*Nyāya Sūtras* I.1.2, 9, 22), not some beatific state of bliss, and this freedom is attained by not activating the presence of consciousness altogether in the liberated state.

Sāṅkhya and classical Yoga, in their attempt to attain a state beyond suffering, go a step further: while these schools accept that the liberated state consists of *sat*, being,[57] they differ from Nyāya in also assigning *cit*, consciousness, to *mokṣa*. Thus, Sāṅkhya posits a liberated state of conscious being, *sat* and *cit*.[58] Since this consciousness in liberation remains immersed in its own being or essence, it is free from the suffering inherent in immersion in the temporal experiences of *prakṛti* (*Yoga Sūtras* II.16), but here, too (at least for Sāṅkhya), this is not deemed a blissful experience. It is contentless consciousness.[59] Thus, the common denominator of all these traditions' view of *yoga* and *mokṣa* so far is primarily one of freedom from pain.

Vedānta goes a step further than just freedom from suffering and ascribes a positive experience of bliss, *ānanda*, to the liberated *ātman*, since it considers *Brahman/ātman* to be constitutionally "made of bliss" *ānandamayo 'bhyāsāt* (*Vedānta Sūtras* I.1.12). The *Taittirīya Upaniṣad* (II.8) and *Bṛhadāraṇyaka Upaniṣad* (IV.3.37) consider this bliss countless times greater than the temporal pleasures of *prakṛti*. When consciousness is redirected to its source, *ātman*, it reexperiences this bliss inherent in its own being. Thus, for Vedānta, the experience of *mokṣa* is certainly one of *sat* and *cit*, but also of *ānanda* as well.

The *Bhāgavata* takes the graded notion of bliss much further still, since, as we know, those who encounter the *līlās* of Hari find the bliss of *Brahman/ātman* inconsequential in comparison (IV.9.10). We can recall that right at the outset of his treatise, Rūpa describes *bhakti* as minimizing *mokṣa*, and thereby any associated bliss inherent in the *ātman*, but he also contrasts this with the "special intense bliss" of *bhakti* (Eastern Quadrant I.17).[60] In fact, he goes on to state that "if the bliss of *Brahman* were multiplied billionfold, it would not equal an atom in the ocean of bliss of *bhakti*." In fact, *Brahman* bliss is no greater than the "water in the footprint of a calf for one swimming in the ocean of bliss after attaining a vision of Kṛṣṇa" (Eastern Quadrant I.38–39). Just as the *Taittirīya Upaniṣad* takes the bliss of *ātman* to be billions of times greater than the greatest bliss of *prakṛti*, so do Kṛṣṇa practitioners take the bliss of *bhakti* to be billions of times greater than the bliss of *ātman*. Rhetoric aside, *Īśvara*, after all, is the whole, and the *ātman* His part, *aṁśa*, so the bliss ensuing from the infinite whole eclipses anything inherent in its infinitesimal part. In sum, as Rūpa notes: "There are three kinds of happiness: from the senses, from *Brahman*, and from *Īśvara*" (Eastern Quadrant I.130).

Not only do the *bhaktas* eschew liberation, they would rather remain embodied in *prakṛti* if this means they can have senses to hear, speak about, and serve their beloved Lord, even if this means remaining eternally in *saṁsāra*. Indeed, they would prefer to have thousands of senses simultaneously all the more to be able to immerse their minds in thoughts of their beloved Kṛṣṇa: "Please grant me this boon: let me have 10,000 ears [to hear about You]" (IV.20.24). Of course, Hari frees them from this dilemma and awards them a divine *Brahman* body and senses and His personal association for all eternity in His realm of Goloka in accordance with their *bhāva*. But *bhaktas* seek a body with sense organs and a mind of one sort or another, whether made of *prakṛti* or *Brahman*, rather than conventional *mokṣa*, so that they can relate for all eternity to the qualities and pastimes of *Īśvara* by which they have become enamored. Because for them, this is the bliss that has no substitute.

Rūpa concludes the first "wave" of his *Ocean of the Nectar of the Experience of* Bhakti with the truism common to *yoga* traditions in general[61] that the only proof is simply the experience itself. In the case of *bhakti*: "From just a tiny taste of *bhakti*, an experience of its nature occurs; but this does not occur from just rational thought" (Eastern Quadrant I.45). In the words of the *Bhāgavata*: "*Bhakti*, experience of the Supreme, and detachment from all other things, these three things manifest simultaneously for one who is surrendered to Kṛṣṇa, just as satisfaction, nourishment, and the removal of hunger manifest with every mouthful for one who is eating" (XI.2.42). Without tasting its bliss, one cannot claim to have had experience of *bhakti*: "Where is *bhakti* without the hairs standing on end in ecstasy, without the heart melting, and without tears of joy? . . . One absorbed in *bhakti* to Me [Kṛṣṇa], whose voice is choked up, whose heart melts, who sometimes cries incessantly and sometimes laughs, who cries out without embarrassment and dances, purifies the world" (XI.14.23–24). Such claims cannot be rationalized, and one's inspiration to seek such experiences or not to do so reflects one's faith in the words of the *Bhāgavata* or *bhāgavatas* or not.

With regard to rational thought and human reason, continues Rūpa (as anyone who has studied the history of philosophy—Indic or Western—might concur), "a position established diligently by a skillful philosopher, is demonstrated to be inadequate by someone else, who follows a different view" (*Bhaktirasāmṛtasindhu* Eastern Quadrant 54–46). Or, as the *Nārada Bhakti Sūtras* we will encounter in part 5 puts it: "Philosophical debate should not be relied upon, because it is inconclusive, and because there are so many points of view" (74–75). One is reminded here, too, of a verse in the *Mahābhārata*: "Logic is unreliable, the *śrutis* (sacred texts) express divergent viewpoints, and there is no *ṛṣi* (sage) who does not have a different philosophy [from other sages]. The essence of *dharma* is hidden in the innermost recesses of the hearts of realized souls; one should therefore follow the path traversed by an enlightened soul."[62] And, earlier still, in a delightful verse from the Upaniṣads: "Therefore a *brāhmaṇa* should give up scholarship and remain childlike; when he has given up being a scholar as well as being a child, he becomes wise; and when he has ceased to be both wise and unswise, he becomes a [real] *brāhmaṇa*. . . . All else is frustration" (*Bṛhadāraṇyaka Upaniṣad* III.5). Thus, reflecting the *Bhāgavata*,[63] one of Rūpa's sixty-four principles of *bhakti* is "renouncing [the study] of many books" (Eastern Quadrant II.79).[64]

In conclusion, there are thus choices to be made in human life in the worldview of the *Bhāgavata*. In conjunction with the other *jñāna* and *yoga* traditions of its day,[65] the text conceives of the purpose or raison d'être of the infinite realm of *prakṛti* as existing simply to indulge those who choose to pursue material desires stemming from ignorance of their true selves. It does this by providing those in ignorance with a psychophysical mechanism with which to experience the objects of desire, as well as an unlimited array of sense objects. In fact, *prakṛti* provides vast numbers of bodily forms[66] in multiple dimensions, including celestial realms, for souls to attempt to enjoy.[67] One can wander through them indefinitely, seeking to fulfill these unfulfillable and insatiable desires (*Gītā* III.39) by sampling this or that flavor of sensual indulgence and offering of *prakṛti* through the widely varying sense organs of these bodily forms. *Saṁsāra* as a dynamic, active realm is nothing other than this. But: "One whose mind is attached to possessions, spouse, and offspring in the duties of the household, does not find higher Truth, but wanders on the many paths of *saṁsāra*" (IV.25.6). Material desires always fail to fulfill. And there is a price tag on this option: the laws of *karma*. Every action performed in the pursuit of *prakṛtic* happiness breeds a corresponding reaction, which binds and delimits the *ātman*'s freedom in pursuing its future desires (*Yoga Sūtras* II.14).

After becoming exhausted with failing to find ultimate fulfillment through the mind and senses given the temporality of any enjoyment they can provide, and after repeatedly experiencing frustration instead, insight dawns in an occasional person.[68] This insight recognizes that it is embodied life itself that is essentially suffering, and it is desire itself that is its ultimate cause (*Gītā* III.37–41; *Yoga Sūtras* II.15ff.). For the Vedic-derived traditions, this leads to the option of renouncing desire and undertaking a quest for *mokṣa*, freedom from suffering, by seeking the true *ātman* self. This is accomplished by dedication to a *yoga* path—which can be defined, in its lowest common denominator, as nothing other than freedom from this suffering.[69] For such seekers, given that suffering seems encoded and endemic in all activities of *prakṛti* experienced by embodied beings, any end to suffering appears logically to be the opposite—inactive, passive, and static.[70] Stripped of all *prakṛtic* overlays, such a state naturally appears to consist of just eternal consciousness,[71] and this indeed is the experience of *ātman* when its awareness is redirected to itself as object (*Yoga Sūtras* I.3).[72]

From the ranks of such seekers, a few may come in contact with *Īśvara* and undertake a *bhakti* practice: "From thousands of people, just one may aspire for perfection, and from those who have attained perfection, hardly one knows Me in Truth" (*Gītā* VII.3; see also *Bhāgavata* VI.14.5). Here, the *Bhāgavata* still keeps company with many but not all *jñāna* and *yoga* traditions.[73] But as discussed previously, for some of these theistic traditions, *Īśvara*'s role is only relevant and even delimited to His function as the bestower of realization of the self[74]—that is, the *yogī* can attain *mokṣa* from *saṁsāra* by *Īśvara*'s grace. In other words, in such schools, the relationship with *Īśvara* and any performance of *bhakti* is practical and one might even say mercantile: the *yogī* essentially utilizes this *Īśvara* Being to ultimately attain freedom from suffering—not out of a deeper permanent commitment to or interest in *Īśvara* Himself.

This functionalist relationship with *Īśvara* is also recognized in the *Bhāgavata*—although less enthusiastically, as we have seen (the mixed *bhakti* discussed previously). But where the *Bhāgavata* and Vaiṣṇava traditions differ from these *mokṣa*-oriented *Īśvara* traditions is that some *yogīs*, irrespective of any initial spiritually mercantile motivation, become so completely enraptured with *Īśvara* once encountered that they prefer to perpetuate this devotional relationship for all eternity. From those who do develop such an attraction, some such *yogīs* recognize *Īśvara* to be the Supreme *Ātman* (*Paramātman*) greater than their own *ātman* (see *Gītā* XIV.18–19), and others are simply enamored by this wondrous Being without necessarily understanding His ontological majesty or caring to do so. For those pursuing this attraction (*rāga*) devoid of any functionalist or recompensatory motivations (the "cheating religions" mentioned in the very first verses of the *Bhāgavata*), these traditions offer the option of liberated postmortem reembodiment, but now in an eternal *Brahman* form and in an eternal *Brahman* locus, beyond *prakṛtic* time and space in a realm comprising *sat-cit-ānanda* rather than the three *guṇas*. For the *Bhāgavata*, *Brahman* includes a dynamic sensual dimension of pure consciousness with forms and qualities—a possibility also hinted at in the *Vedānta Sūtras* and *Mahābhārata*.[75] These are the realms of Vaikuṇṭha and Goloka, as well as that of Śiva; beyond both the dynamic sensual realm of *prakṛti*—including its variegated celestial dimensions—where form and quality are temporal, vulnerable, ephemeral, and painful—and beyond, too, the passive, trans-sensual, inactive realm of *ātman*/*Brahman* devoid of forms and qualities, that also transcends *prakṛti*. Until one attains a higher *rasa*, so to speak, this latter passive experience of *ātman* naturally appears the best option: "The seeker does not become disinclined toward the practices of *yoga* until he or she has developed an attraction for the stories of Kṛṣṇa."

For the *Bhāgavata*, from all the forms of *Īśvara*, including that of Viṣṇu and Śiva, Kṛṣṇa is simply the most attractive[76] (indeed, one of the etymologies of the verbal root *kṛṣ* is "to attract"). Kṛṣṇa's *bhaktas*, the *bhāgavatas*, become so enamored by this flute-playing, mischievous blue boy that all the above options and considerations become redundant—indeed, barely even intrude upon their frame of reference: "The *Bhāgavata* is proclaimed as the essence of all Vedānta; one who is satisfied with the nectar of its *rasa* has no interest in anything else" (XII.13, 15). As so many of the quotes presented previously have indicated, and as the ensuing tales and teachings will stress repeatedly, all that such *bhaktas* wish to do is fill their minds with the thoughts, and their ears, tongues, eyes, and other senses with relishing the qualities, of their beloved *Iśvara*. In this state, one loses "all concern for scriptural prescriptions or logical thought" (*Bhaktirasāmṛtasindhu* II.292). This is not anti-intellectualism: Jīva, Rūpa, and the other *Gosvāmīs* were intellectual giants of their times, thoroughly schooled in and in dialogue with the scholastic conversations of their day. It is love of God, transrational intoxication that recognizes the limitations of empirical sensual observation and inferential rational thought and has attained blissful experience that bypasses and eclipses these epistemic sources of knowledge (*pramāṇa*). These ecstatic experiences produce a mind-set that seeks only opportunities to love and therefore serve this wondrous Being, irrespective of any locus or dimensionality, whether of embodied life in *prakṛti* or in the divine realm of Goloka—provided, of course, it is not a state of *mokṣa*. The *bhāgavata* would rather remain embodied than attain *mokṣa*. Once again, this is because in conventional *mokṣa* one is deprived of mind and senses with which to focus awareness on *Īśvara*, that is, "because in that state there is no nectar about Your lotus feet, which flows out of the depths of the hearts and through the mouths of the great souls" (IV.20.24). Other than this, anything and everything else, material or spiritual, becomes irrelevant. As the *gopīs* will exemplify within, in advanced stages of *bhakti* one becomes insanely intoxicated with Kṛṣṇa and can think of nothing else.

Indeed, both at the beginning and at the end of the *Tattva Sandarbha*, Jīva actually discourages anyone not interested in worshipping Kṛṣṇa from reading his work.[77] Likewise, Rūpa cautions the unwary of the consequences of engaging with the very text that takes up part 3 of this volume. This is because the tenth book is nothing other than the literary embodiment of Kṛṣṇa, this mysterious, mischievous stealer of hearts, the etymology of whose very name points to the ultimate seducer and enchanter of souls.[78] The *Bhāgavata* was written precisely to entice beings away from the attachments and consequent sufferings of *saṁsāra* toward the possibility of an eternal, blissful relationship with the playful, lotus-eyed blue Lord:

Hey friends!
If you have any attachment to the company of your family members
Do not gaze upon the form of Hari, who goes by the name of Govinda
Standing here near the banks of the sacred Keśi ghaṭ
Smiling
Poised with three curves
Radiant with the eye of a peacock feather
His wide eyes casting sidelong glances
And bud-like lips resting on His flute
Hey ho, you are very naive!
I presume that the sounds
Produced by the verses of the tenth book of the *Bhāgavata*
Have become like travellers along the pathways of your ears
Just see, it is because of this
That you are now dismissive of the material goals of life:
Duty, material well-being and the fulfillment of desires (*dharma*, *artha*, *kāma*),
Which bestow the highest well-being
And you are even rejecting liberation (*mokṣa*)
Whose essence is happiness.
(Eastern Quadrant IV.239–40)

PART II

Tales and Teachings from the *Bhāgavata Purāṇa*

Book I

Invocation and Glories of the *Śrīmad Bhāgavata Purāṇa*

Yoga Blueprint

Authors of sacred text typically begin with an invocation to their beloved deities and then announce the nature of their work. In the first three verses below, the author establishes Kṛṣṇa as the Supreme Deity and the Bhāgavata *as the supreme scripture.*

The first verse is philosophically dense, as it sets out to establish the credentials of the text. We noted in the chapter "The Object of Bhakti: Īśvara, Bhagavān, Brahman, *and Divine Hierarchies" that the* Bhāgavata *is responding to both Vedānta and Purāṇa currents. Thus, the first phrase replicates the second verse of the* Vedānta Sūtras, *thereby underscoring the claim that the* Bhāgavata *is a commentary by Vyāsa, the reputed author of the* Vedānta Sūtras, *on his own work. Likewise verses 2–3 seek to present the* Bhāgavata Purāṇa *as the ultimate text in the Purāṇa genre and final word on all things Vedic. These opening verses need not detain the reader with no interest in such things.*

Book I, Chapter 1

Oṁ Namo Bhāgavate Vāsudevāya

(I offer obeisance to Lord Kṛṣṇa, son of Vasudeva.)*

*In this section, I have used parentheses for both Sanskrit-to-English and English-to-Sanskrit translations; I have used brackets when I have added some wording into the text for clarification purposes and when giving a common name for a lesser-known one.

1. I meditate on the Supreme Truth. From Him come the creation, maintenance, and destruction of this universe.[1] He is the self-independent ruler, and knower of all things. He is omniscient due to his immanence in and transcendence beyond all things. By Him was the Veda revealed to Brahmā,[2] the first sage, through the heart. Even the wise are bewildered about the meaning of the Veda. In Him, the threefold creation [of *sattva*, *rajas*, and *tamas*[3]] appears to be real, like the mutual [illusory] appearance of fire, water, and earth in each other [such as the mirage of water on land]. By His potency, illusion is always dispelled.

2. For the righteous, who are free of envy, the highest *dharma* is to be found in the *Śrīmad Bhāgavata*, in which all dishonesty has been rejected.[4] Composed by the great sage [Vyāsa], only the real object of knowledge is revealed here, which bestows auspiciousness and uproots the threefold miseries.[5] Is *Īśvara* immediately captured in the heart by anything else? In this text, He is captured in an instant by the virtuous who desire to hear.

3. It is the succulent ripened fruit of the desire tree[6] of the Vedic scriptures. It is permeated with the nectar flowing from the mouth of sage Śuka.[7] *Aho!*[8] O connoisseurs of poetic experience (*rasa*) and experts of poetic moods (*bhāva*),[9] while in this world drink continuously the spiritual flavors (*rasa*) of the *Bhāgavata* to your full satisfaction.

The Setting of the *Bhāgavata*

Yoga Blueprint

The first chapters in the text establish the frame narrative for the story, which is in fact a frame within a frame, as Sūta is relaying to the sages of Naimiṣa what he had previously heard Śuka narrate to the king (just as the Bhagavad Gītā *is actually Sañjaya relaying to king Dhṛtarāṣṭra what Kṛṣṇa had narrated to Arjuna). So the various chapters in the* Bhāgavata *can switch from one frame to the other.*

The following three chapters essentially establish what the goal of life and the purpose of human existence are, according to the Bhāgavata*—what questions should be asked for those interested in ultimate truths, in short, what one should do with the ever active mind. This section contains some of the key verses fundamental to the Kṛṣṇa-specific theology discussed in the chapter "The Object* *of* Bhakti: Īśvara, Bhagavān, Brahman, *and Divine Hierarchies": the three levels of* Brahman, *the supremacy of Kṛṣṇa over all other* Īśvara *incarnations, and the radical reinterpretation of* dharma. *Most important, too, is that the text situates itself as a literary substitute for Kṛṣṇa for those born after His incarnation.*

Book I, Chapter 1

4. Once, in Naimiṣa, a place sacred to Lord Viṣṇu, the sages, headed by Śaunaka, were performing a thousand-year sacrifice for the purpose of attaining Viṣṇu's divine realm.[10]
5. One day, those sages, when they had completed their morning oblations into the sacred fire, respectfully posed these questions to the sage Sūta, who had been comfortably given a seat with due hospitality.
6. The sages asked:
"O faultless Sūta: it is said that you have not only deeply studied but also explained the Purāṇas, ancient legendary accounts; the *Itihāsa*, epic traditions; as well as the texts on *dharma*, codes of conduct.[11]
7. O Sūta! These are all understood by the great Vyāsa,[12] the highest authority on the Veda, as well as by other sages, knowers of the higher and lower truths.[13]
8. By their grace, you know all those sacred texts perfectly, O gentle sage! Teachers speak of even the most intimate things to their affectionate students.
9. O long-lived one! Please explain to us the single-most highest good for a person, as far as you have ascertained this from all these various sources.
10. O noble one! People in this age of *Kali*[14] are generally short-lived, lazy, dull-witted, ill-fated, and oppressed.
11. There are a multitude of scriptures with varied sections prescribing a wide variety of activities. Therefore, O saint, for the benefit of living entities, kindly extract the essence from them with your insight and express that to us, so that the mind can become peaceful.
12. O Sūta, may all good fortune be with you! You know with what intention *Bhagavān*, the Lord of the Sātvatas, took birth from Vasudeva in the womb of Devakī.
13. You should kindly describe this to us, dear Sūta: we are eager to hear about Kṛṣṇa's incarnation (*avatāra*) for the happiness and welfare of living beings.

14. A helpless person fallen into this terrifying *saṁsāra* (cycle of birth and death) is immediately liberated from it upon taking His Name. Fear itself fears Him.
15. The peaceful sages who have taken shelter of His feet purify instantly when others come in contact with them, whereas the waters of the *Gaṅgā* purify only through repeated service [such as ritual bathing].[15]
16. What person, desiring to become pure, would not listen to the wonders of *Bhagavān*—His deeds are praised in verses that purify the mind and destroy the impurities of the age of *Kali*.[16]
17. His amazing deeds are recounted by the wise. He is continually assuming incarnations playfully. Tell us about Him; we have faith.
18. Narrate to us the auspicious stories of the incarnations (*avatāra*) of Hari, O wise Sūta. *Īśvara* engages in *līlā*[17] pastimes out of His free will, by means of His own *māyā*[18] potency.
19. We never become satiated by the deeds of Kṛṣṇa (Uttamaśloka),[19] they manifest increasing sweetness at every step for the connoisseurs of *rasa*[20] who listen to them.
20. *Bhagavān*, Kṛṣṇa (Keśava) performed superhuman activities along with Balarāma,[21] concealed in the guise of a human being.
21. After realizing that the *Kali* age has arrived, we are seated here in this place for [the performance of] this long sacrifice; we have plenty of time for narrations about Hari.
22. Like the helmsman of a boat on an ocean, You have been brought to us by Providence. We are eager to traverse the ocean of the age of *Kali*, which destroys the good qualities (*sattva*) of people and is difficult to surpass.
23. Kṛṣṇa is the Lord of Yoga (*Yogeśvara*) and protector of the *brāhmaṇas* and sacred texts. Now that He has returned to his own [transcendent] abode, please tell us: Where has *dharma* gone for safekeeping?"

Book I, Chapter 2

1. Vyāsa said:
"Sūta, the son of Romaharṣaṇa, was very pleased with the questions of the *brāhmaṇas*. After honoring their words, he set about replying."
2. Sūta said:
"When Śuka gave up all duties and was leaving home without undergoing his education, his father, Dvaipāyana Vyāsa,[22] pained by feelings of separation, called after him: 'O son!' But only the trees, who

were absorbed in the same mood as Śuka, echoed in response. I bow to that sage (Śuka), who is the well-wisher of all living beings.
3. I accept that son of Vyāsa, the *guru* of the sages, as my guide. Out of compassion for those in *saṁsāra*, he spoke, from his own personal realization, the most intimate of the Purāṇas (the *Bhāgavata*).[23] It is the essence of all the revealed scriptures, and the only spiritual light for those seeking to cross beyond deep darkness (*tamas*).
4. One should recite the *Bhāgavata* after offering respects to Nara and Nārāyaṇa, the best of men;[24] to Sarasvatī, the Goddess of learning; and to Vyāsa.
5. O sages! You have posed the perfect questions to me about the welfare of the world. It is through questions about Kṛṣṇa that the mind becomes completely satisfied.
6. The highest *dharma* is that through which *bhakti* for Kṛṣṇa (Adhokṣaja) [is born].[25] And it is through *bhakti*—performed without motive and uninterrupted—that the mind becomes completely satisfied.
7. *Bhakti yoga* performed for *Bhagavān* Vāsudeva quickly bestows detachment (*vairāgya*) and causeless knowledge.
8. If *dharma*, howsoever perfectly performed, does not produce attraction for the stories of Kṛṣṇa (Viṣvaksena), then it is simply brute labor.
9. The goal of the *dharma* that leads to liberation is completely different from the *dharma* performed for the goal of material gain.[26] The goal of the *dharma* that is devoted to the One Supreme Being is not presented in the sacred texts as being desire for material gain.
10. The purpose of desire is not to fulfill the gratification of the senses, but to fulfill only as much as is necessary to sustain life. And the purpose of life in this world is to inquire into Truth, not to engage in actions dedicated to material gain (*karma*).
11. Those who know the Truth say that knowledge of that Truth is nondual (*advaya*).[27] It is named *Brahman*, *Paramātman*, and *Bhagavān*.[28]
12. The sages who have faith in this, and who are endowed with knowledge and detachment, perceive the *ātman* within themselves through the practice of *bhakti* presented in the sacred texts.
13. Thus, O best of the twice-born *brāhmaṇas*,[29] the ultimate perfection of *dharma*, performed diligently by people according to the divisions of the *varṇas* and *āśramas*,[30] is the satisfaction of Hari.
14. Therefore, it is *Bhagavān*, the Lord of the Sātvatas, whom one should constantly hear about, glorify, meditate upon, and worship with a concentrated mind.

15. Equipped with the sword of meditation, the wise sever the bondage of the knot of *karma*. Who would not develop an attraction for narrations about *Bhagavān*?
16. For one who is faithful and desires to hear, attraction to the stories of Vāsudeva [Kṛṣṇa] develops by means of service to the sages, assisting great saints, and dwelling in holy places.
17. To those who hear his narratives, Kṛṣṇa, who is the friend of the Truthful and is situated within the heart, cleanses inauspicious things. Hearing about Him and performing His *kīrtana*[31] are purifying.
18. When almost all inauspicious things are destroyed by means of constant service to the *bhāgavatas*, then unshakable *bhakti* for *Bhagavān*, Kṛṣṇa (Uttamaśloka), manifests.
19. Then, the mind, situated in *sattva* and not being agitated by states of *rajas* and *tamas*,[32] nor by lust, greed, and so on, becomes content.
20. For one whose mind is content and who is free from attachment [to all material things] by the practice of *bhakti yoga* in this way, realization of the Truth of *Bhagavān* is born.
21. When *Īśvara* is seen within oneself,[33] the knot in the heart is broken, all doubts are destroyed, and *karma* is weakened for that person.
22. Therefore, the poet-sages always engage in great ecstasy in *bhakti* for *Bhagavān* Vāsudeva, which satisfies the mind.
23. *Sattva*, *rajas*, and *tamas* are the *guṇas* of *prakṛti*. There is one Supreme Being who directs these for the purpose of creation, maintenance, and destruction of this universe. He is named Hari [Viṣṇu], Viriñci [Brahmā], and Hara [Śiva]. From these, the highest good is derived from the One whose form is *sattva*.[34]
24. [Just as, for the performance of Vedic ritual,] smoke is higher than wood, and fire is higher than that, as it is the essential element for the [rituals prescribed in the] three Vedas,[35] [so] *rajas* is higher than *tamas*, and *sattva* is higher than that, as it bestows the vision of *Brahman*.
25. In the beginning, the sages worshipped *Bhagavān* Viṣṇu, who is pure *sattva*. Those who follow their example are eligible for liberation.
26. Those desiring liberation reject the ghastly forms of [other] Lords of beings[36] and, free from envy, worship the peaceful manifestations of Nārāyaṇa.

27. Those whose natures and characteristics are *rājasic* and *tāmasic*, desiring offspring, power, and opulence, worship such entities as the ancestors, ghosts, and celestial beings.
28. Vāsudeva [Kṛṣṇa] is the ultimate goal of the Veda, Vāsudeva is the ultimate goal of ritual sacrifices, Vāsudeva is the ultimate goal of *yoga*, Vāsudeva is the ultimate goal of actions.
29. Vāsudeva is the ultimate goal of knowledge, Vāsudeva is the ultimate goal of austerity (*tapas*), Vāsudeva is the ultimate goal of *dharma*, Vāsudeva is the ultimate goal.
30. In the beginning, it was *Bhagavān* who, through His own *māyā*, which consists of the *guṇas* and takes the form of cause and effect, created this world, even though He Himself is all-pervading and beyond the *guṇas*.
31. Radiating wisdom, He enters into these *guṇas* that have been manifest by *māyā*, and thus He appears as if endowed with the *guṇas*.
32. Just as fire is one, but manifests as many when placed into pieces of wood, which are its sources, so does the Supreme Person, the Soul of the Universe, manifest as many in the living entities.
33. He enters into the living entities created by Himself and then experiences the *guṇas* through the mind, senses, and gross and subtle elements, which are themselves the creations of the *guṇas*.
34. The Creator of the worlds maintains the worlds through *sattva*. He is fond of assuming incarnations for play (*līlā-avatāra*) among beings such as the celestials, men, and animals."

Book I, Chapter 3

[*A list of some of the previous primary incarnations prior to Kṛṣṇa's descent precedes.*]
26. O *brāhmaṇas*! Just as many thousands of small channels flow from an inexhaustible lake, so are the *avatāras* of Hari, the abode of *sattva*, innumerable.
27. The sages, Manus,[37] celestials, and sons of Manu, who are extremely powerful, are all only partial manifestations of Hari; so are those who are known as the procreators of species (*prajā-patis*).
28. All these [other incarnations] are secondary and derivative manifestations of the Supreme Being.[38] Kṛṣṇa is *Bhagavān* the Supreme Being Himself [that is, the source of all other divine manifestations].[39]

These incarnations bestow their grace on the world when it is troubled by the enemies of Indra.[40]

29. A person who recounts the mysterious birth of *Bhagavān* with devotion in the morning and evening is freed from all sorts of suffering.

30. The form [the body] has been created by the *guṇas*, which are the *māyā* of *Bhagavān*, who has no material form. It is imposed on the *ātman* as intelligence and on the other layers as *prakṛti*.

31. Just as hosts of clouds exist in the sky, and earthly particles in the wind, so the nature of the seen is imposed upon the seer by those who are not intelligent.[41]

32. Beyond [the gross perceivable body] is a higher body which, because it cannot be seen or heard, is subtle. This is [formed] from the *guṇas* prior to their evolution into solid matter.[42] It is because of this subtle body that the *jīva* (embodied soul), is born again.

33. When these two forms—one cause and one effect[43]—which have been imposed on the *ātman* by ignorance (*avidyā*), are removed by realization, then the vision of *Brahman* manifests.

34. [The sages] know that if this skillful divine illusion (*devī-māyā*) ceases, then knowledge arises. When this occurs, the perfected [soul] becomes glorious in its own majesty.

35. For this reason, the poet-sages describe the births and actions of the One who is Unborn and does not act, the Lord of the heart. These activities are not revealed in the Vedas.[44]

36. His *līlās* are irresistible. He creates, sustains, and then devours this universe, but He is not attached to it. Self-dependent and situated within all beings, the Lord of six qualities,[45] experiences the six senses [as the nose experiences] fragrances.[46]

37. Just as an ignorant person does not understand the behavior of an actor, so no creature of limited intelligence can understand through words, mind, or cleverness the pastimes of the Supreme Creator when He exhibits His names and forms.

38. The person who knows the ways of the unlimitedly powerful Supreme Creator, wielder of the disc weapon (*cakra*),[47] is one who uninterruptedly and devoid of any deceit worships the fragrance of His lotus feet.[48]

39. Therefore, fortunate are the great souls who dedicate their whole heart and soul to Vāsudeva the Lord of all the worlds in this way; they do not experience the terrible rounds of rebirth in this world.

40. The great sage Vyāsa composed this Purāṇa, called the *Bhāgavata*, about the activities of Kṛṣṇa (Uttamaśloka), for the ultimate welfare of people. It is equal to the Vedas, bestows good fortune, and is supremely auspicious.
41. Then he taught it to his son [Śuka], the most preeminent of those who have realized the *ātman*. It is the cream extracted from the cream of all the Vedas and sacred histories.[49]
42. Śuka then narrated it to the great king Parīkṣit, who was seated on the banks of the *Gaṅgā* fasting to death, surrounded by the great sages.
43. Since Kṛṣṇa had departed to his personal divine abode along with knowledge and *dharma*, etc., this Purāṇa has now arisen like the sun for those who have lost their sight due to [the darkness of] the age of *Kali*.
44. I arrived there at that place as the greatly effulgent *brāhmaṇa* sage Śuka was reciting the *Bhāgavata*, O *brāhmaṇas*, and, by his kindness, I sat down there. I will retell it to you, to the best of my understanding and reflection.[50]

Book I, Chapter 4

1. Vyāsa said:
"Śaunaka was the senior leader of the assembly of sages who were performing that long sacrifice, and he was well-versed in the Vedas. He first honored Sūta who was speaking in this way, and then spoke."
2. Śaunaka said:
"Sūta, O greatly fortunate Sūta! Recount to us, O eminent speaker, that pure narration about *Bhagavān* that was spoken by the noble Śuka.
3. In which age, in which place, with what motive, and inspired by what did the sage Vyāsa compose this scripture?
4. His son, Śuka, is a great *yogī* who is beyond dualities and sees all equally [as *Brahman*]. He has overcome sleep, and goes around [with his greatness] concealed, like a half-wit, his mind fixed exclusively on Truth.
5. When maidens [who were bathing] saw Vyāsa following his son they covered themselves with clothes out of modesty, even though Vyāsa was not naked; but they did not do so for the son [even though Śuka was naked]. When he saw this puzzling behavior, the sage inquired about it. The maidens replied: 'The discernment of male and

female sexual differences exists in you, but there is no such distinction in the perception of your son.'[51]

6. How was he recognized by the citizens, when he arrived in the jungle areas of the Kuru kingdom? He was wandering around the city called Hastināpura[52] like a deranged, dumb half-wit.

7. How did the conversation between the sage-king of the Pāṇḍu dynasty (Parīkṣit) and sage Śuka take place? It was from this conversation that this scripture sacred to Kṛṣṇa was produced.

8. That great soul Śuka waits at the houses of householders only for as long as it takes to milk a cow, and even then he does so only to transform that residence into a sacred place [by dint of his purity and not for the purpose of begging milk].[53]

9. O Sūta! They say that Parīkṣit, the son of Abhimanyu, is a preeminent devotee (*bhāgavata*).[54] Please relate to us the account of his extraordinary birth and deeds.

10. He was the supreme monarch, who increased the pride of the Pāṇḍu family. For what reason did he renounce the opulence of the emperorship and sit fasting to death on the banks of the *Gaṅgā*?

11. After bringing him tribute, his enemies offered homage to his footstool for their own protection. How did that hero, O dear Sūta, while in the prime of life, give up opulence, which is so hard to renounce, along with his own life?

12. Those people who are devoted to Uttamaśloka [Kṛṣṇa] live for the protection, well-being, and prosperity of living beings, not for their own gain. Why did that king renounce his body, which provided shelter to others, and abandon it?

13. Please relate everything to us that we have inquired about. I regard you as versed in all topics other than that related to the Vedic hymns."[55]

The Tale of Vyāsa: Existential Malaise

Yoga Blueprint

This tale outlines the traditional Purāṇa narrative pertaining to the origin of the compilation of the Vedic corpus (the Śruti *and* Smṛti*). The* yogic *message imparted here is that even though Vyāsa had mastered and compiled all manner of scriptures relating to the various goals of life, he remained unfulfilled since he had not described the* līlās *of* Bhagavān. *For the* Bhāgavata, *it is only when the mind is absorbed in thoughts of Kṛṣṇa that it can attain the level of deep,* *ultimate, and permanent fulfillment that it seeks. This is further underscored by the text noting that even sages who have fully realized the* ātman, *like Vyāsa's son Śuka, nonetheless find their minds captured by the* līlās *of* Bhagavān. *As we know, this minimization of conventional* mokṣa, *liberation, is a major subtheme of the* Bhāgavata *and of Vaiṣṇavism in general.*

Other noteworthy features in this narrative include the fact that Vyāsa has a vision of Kṛṣṇa in his meditations. Like all yoga *traditions, the goal of* bhakti *is direct experience, in this case direct perception of the form of Kṛṣṇa.*

Book 1, Chapter 4

14. During the period of the *Dvāpara Yuga*, toward the end of this third of the ages, sage Vyāsa, a partial incarnation of Vishnu, was born of Parāśara and Vāsavī.

15. Once, as the sun's orb was rising, Vyāsa took a bath in the pure waters of the *Sarasvatī* river and sat down alone in a secluded place.

16. The sage, who could see past and future, perceived that behavior contrary to the *dharma* of the age (*yuga*) had begun to manifest. This decline occurs on earth every *yuga*[56] owing to the imperceptible force of Time.

17.–18. The sage saw with his divine vision[57] the decrease in ability (*śakti*) in both body and mind wrought by this change. He saw the wretched state of people: their life spans had become reduced, their intelligence decreased, and they lacked faith and potency. So that sage of perfect vision began to contemplate the welfare of all the stages and professions of life (*varṇāśrama*).

19. He saw that the Vedic rituals performed by the four specialist priests (*hotṛs*)[58] were purifying for people, and so, for the propagation of sacrificial performance, he divided the one Veda into four.

20. The four Vedas—*Ṛg*, *Sāman*, *Yajus*, and *Atharvan*—were extracted [from the one original], and the epics and Purāṇas were named the fifth Veda.

21. From these, Paila became responsible for the *Ṛg-Veda*, sage Jaimini became the chanter of the *Sāma-Veda*, while Vaiśampāyana alone became expert in the *Yajur-Veda*.

22. The intense sage Sumantu was given the *Atharva-Veda*, which is associated with the Aṅgiras, and my father, Romaharṣaṇa, the epics and Purāṇas.

23. Those sages each divided up their own respective Veda into several through their disciples, grand-disciples, and their subsequent students, so those Vedas developed many branches.
24. *Bhagavān Vyāsa*[59] is compassionate to the less capable and thus made those Vedas easy to memorize for people of less intelligence.[60]
25. Women, *śūdras* (the laborer caste), and fallen *brāhmaṇas* are ineligible for Vedic study.[61] For the benefit of those who have no access to knowledge about how to act in the world in a way that leads to their ultimate welfare, the great story of Bhārata (the *Mahābhārata* epic) was composed by the sage.
26. Despite this, the heart of the sage, devoted as he was to the welfare of living beings by all possible means, was still not satisfied, O twice-born sage.
27. His heart dissatisfied, that expert in *dharma*, sitting alone on the pure banks of the *Sarasvatī* deliberating over this, uttered these words:
28. "Upholding my vows, I have respected the sacred chants, *gurus*, and ritual fire, and I have upheld the sacred teachings.
29. And the ancient doctrines have been disclosed in the form of the *Mahābhārata* epic, through which this *dharma* has been made accessible to women, *śūdras*, and others.
30. Unfortunately, despite all this, and despite the fact that I am the most preeminent of all the *brāhmaṇas*, my embodied *ātman*, which has attained perfection, appears to be unfulfilled.
31. Perhaps this is because the *bhāgavata dharmas*[62] have barely been disclosed. They are dear to the infallible lord Kṛṣṇa, and dear to the *paramahaṁsa* perfected beings."[63]
32. As Vyāsa was lamenting and reflecting on his inadequacies in this manner, Nārada arrived at his *āśrama*,[64] which was described previously.
33. When he realized that Nārada, who is honored by the celestials, had arrived, the sage immediately arose and honored him according to due protocol.

Book 1, Chapter 5

1. Sūta said:
"When he was comfortably seated, his *vīṇā* stringed instrument in hand, the celebrated celestial sage spoke to Vyāsa, who had sat down nearby."

2. Nārada said:
"O greatly fortunate son of Parāśara, are you self-satisfied in body and mind?
3. Everything you desired to know has been fully accounted for: you compiled the wonderful epic of the Bhāratas, which is replete with all the *arthas* (the goals of human life).[65]
4. And you understood whatever you desired to know about that eternal *Brahman*. Yet, despite all this, You lament your situation, as if your goals had not been attained, O master!"
5. Vyāsa said:
"I attained everything you just described, yet still my mind is not content. So may I ask you about the underlying cause of this? You have profound intelligence, and are the son of Brahmā [the most intelligent being in the universe].
6. That primordial Person is the controller of the great and the small. He has no attachments, yet He creates the universe from His mind, and then maintains and destroys it by means of the *guṇas*. Because you have worshipped Him, your honor knows all hidden things.
7. Traveling around, you move about within the three worlds like the sun, and like the wind, you are the witness of the mind. Reveal to me the cause of my malaise—even though I am initiated into knowledge of the higher and lower *Brahman* [matter and spirit] according to the traditional teachings."[66]
8. *Śrī* Nārada said:
"Sir, for the most part,[67] you have not described the pure glory of *Bhāgavan*. I consider any philosophy which does not satisfy the Lord to be barren.
9. You have not described the greatness of Vāsudeva [Kṛṣṇa] to the same extent that you have glorified the four [mundane] goals of life—*dharma*, righteous conduct; *artha*, material well-being; *kāma*, satisfaction of desires; and *mokṣa*, liberation.
10. The glory of Hari purifies the world. Those who dwell in the lovely abode [of Kṛṣṇa *bhakti*] do not find those words which do not describe the glory of Hari attractive, even if they are replete with literary embellishments—just as the swans from the celestial Mānasa lake do not dwell in the ponds frequented by crows.
11. But that composition that contains [the sacred] names denoting the glory of the unlimited Lord destroys the sins of the people, even

if every verse is improperly composed. Saints hear, recite, and glorify these names.

12. Even pure knowledge of the *ātman* free of desire does not illuminate if devoid of love for Acyuta, the infallible Lord—what then to speak of *karma,* action, which is always inauspicious, even if it is free of self-centered motive.

13. O great soul, you have infallible vision, your reputation is spotless, you adhere to truth, and you are true to your vows. Recall, by means of *samādhi* vision, the activities of Kṛṣṇa, who frees one from all bondage.

14. Unfortunately, desiring to speak of other unrelated things, your focus became distracted away [from Kṛṣṇa]. But your mind, distracted by names and forms (*nāma-rūpa*),[68] can never gain tranquillity by any other means whatsoever; it becomes like a boat swept away by the wind.

15. You have made a serious oversight in teaching things in the name of *dharma* that are detrimental to people who are by nature inclined to fulfilling desires. Most people will think: 'That which has been uttered [by Vyāsa] is authorized *dharma.*' They will not pay heed to any other point of view.[69]

16. A wise sage, who is detached from actions, is qualified to understand the blissful nature of the unlimited Supreme Lord. But for those whose minds are attached to actions and who are ignorant of their *ātman* because of the influence of the *guṇas*, you, dear sir, should disclose the activities of the Lord.

17. If a neophyte, after renouncing conventional duties (*dharma*) falls down [from the standards] while worshipping the lotus feet of Hari, what harm is there in that for him? On the other hand, what [ultimate] benefit is attained for one following his duties without such worship?

18. Therefore, a wise person should strive for that objective, which is transcendent to [mundane] happiness, and so which is not attainable by wandering about in the higher and lower [realms of the universe]. After all, mundane happiness, just like distress, is available everywhere in the due course of relentless Time.

19. A person who serves Mukunda [Kṛṣṇa] will certainly never again return to *saṁsāra*, dear Vyāsa. A person who has experienced the nectar (*rasa*) of remembering the embrace of the feet of Mukunda will never wish to relinquish them again.

20. This entire universe is *Bhagavān*, in one sense, but also different. From Him creation, maintenance, and dissolution of the universe

occurs. You, of course, know this, but, still, I have indicated just this much as an illustration [for what you must now describe].
21. O infallible seer, you should describe in detail the wonderful glories of the Supreme Being! You yourself know that you are a partial incarnation (*kalā*)[70] of the Supreme Person and highest soul (*parama-ātman*). Although unborn, He has taken birth for the welfare of the world.
22. It is this, the description of the qualities of the Lord, that has been described by poet-sages as the eternal goal of a person's charity, knowledge, recital of Vedic hymns, performance of ritual sacrifice, hearing from sacred texts, and austerities. His glories are supreme."

Book I, Chapter 7

[*Here follows the Tale of Sage Nārada.*]
1. Śaunaka said:
"After Nārada had departed, O Sūta, what did the great esteemed Bādarāyaṇa (Vyāsa) do, after hearing his suggestion?"
2. Sūta said:
"On the West bank of the *Sarasvatī*, the river sacred to the *brāhmaṇas*, there is a hermitage (*āśrama*) known as Śamyāprāsa, which is a conducive place for the sages to perform sacrifices.
3. Vyāsa seated himself there, in his *āśrama* surrounded by a grove of *jujube* trees, consecrated himself with water, and began to concentrate his mind.
4. His mind had been completely purified by the practice of *bhakti yoga*. When it was in a state of full concentration, Vyāsa had a vision of Kṛṣṇa, the perfect Person, along with His *māyā* power, which is His assistant.
5. Although the *jīva* is transcendent, he is bewildered by that *māyā*, and considers himself to be a product of the three *guṇas*. As a result, he falls victim to the undesirable consequences resulting from this [*saṁsāra*].
6. The learned Vyāsa then composed the *Bhāgavata Purāṇa* for the mass of people who do not know that *bhakti yoga* dedicated to Adhokṣaja [Kṛṣṇa], directly mitigates suffering.
7. Indeed, *bhakti* for Kṛṣṇa, the Supreme Being (*parama-puruṣa*), removes sorrow, illusion, and fear from people. It is awakened by hearing the *Bhāgavata Purāṇa*.

8. After writing and arranging this scripture dedicated to *Bhagavān*, the sage instructed it to his son, Śuka, who was absorbed in renunciation."

9. Śaunaka said:

"The sage Śuka was absorbed in renunciation and indifferent to everything else; He was immersed in the bliss of his own *ātman*. So why would he have undertaken the study of this huge literature?"

10. Sage Śaunaka replied:

"The fact that sages, who are without worldly bonds and delight in the *ātman* self, perform devotion to Hari free from all motive is because of the nature of Hari's qualities.

11. This is why Śuka, son of Bādarāyaṇa, studied this great narration, which is dear to the devotees of Viṣṇu: his mind had become captured by the qualities of Hari.

12. Now I will speak to you about the birth, deeds, and death of King Parīkṣit, and about the death of the sons of Pāṇḍu, since these will create an opportunity to recount narrations about Kṛṣṇa."

The Tale of Sage Nārada: The Maidservant's Son

Yoga Blueprint

We see from the section on his previous birth that even Nārada, the greatest sage of them all, was once a lusty, arrogant person, just like anybody else. Moreover, despite being born in a situation not considered particularly conducive to yoga *practice, he nonetheless found opportunity to pursue the goals of life outlined in the* Bhāgavata, *which he not only attained, but in which he became preeminent—Nārada is considered one of the twelve* mahājānas, *great* bhāgavatas, *who alone fully understand* bhakti.[71] *The* yogic *message here is that in accordance with the* Gitā *(IX.30–32), no one is disqualified by caste, race, gender, or past behaviors from attaining the supreme goal of life; social demarcations are irrelevant to* bhakti yoga.

The other main teaching imparted in this narrative is the importance of association with and service to the great bhaktas *for the beginning impetus of an individual's devotional journey (see "The First Step in* Bhakti*: Association with a* Bhakta*"). The first seeds of* bhakti *are planted by association with and service to those who already have attained an attraction for the stories of Kṛṣṇa. It was by the* *blessings of the ascetic sages that Nārada's own seed of* bhakti *was planted.*

Additionally, we see in 5.38 the idea of sonic incarnation. Mantras, *such as the one we encounter in 5.37, are not symbols or signifiers, but divine presences—transubstantiated sounds. Also, we see in this narrative, as elsewhere, that the practice of* bhakti *leads to a direct vision of God (6.16). Finally, we find a reference in I.6.28 to the spiritual body—made of* Brahman *stuff, rather than* prakṛti, *bestowed on* bhaktas *upon gaining the realm of Vaikuṇṭha.*

Book VII, Chapter 15[72]

[*Nārada's previous birth. Note: We briefly interrupt the sequencing of the* Bhāgavata *here to present Nārada's lives in chronological order.*]

69. Nārada said:

"In a previous existence, in an age long past, I was a certain *gandharva* celestial[73] known as Upabarhaṇa. I was highly regarded among the *gandharvas*.

70. I was handsome, attractive, perfumed, pleasing to look at, and very appealing to the ladies. I was always intoxicated and engaged in satisfying my lust in my own city.

71. Once, the hosts of celestial *gandharvas* and *apsarās*[74] were invited by the *Prajāpatis* (celestial progenitors) to a ritual sacrifice conducted by the gods, for chanting the glories of Hari.

72. Learning of this, I too went along there, surrounded by women and singing. Considering that an offense, the progenitors cursed me by dint of their ascetic power: 'Because you have committed an offense, you will lose your beauty and immediately enter into the state of a *śūdra*.'

73. As a result, I was born in the womb of a servant lady. But, even in that life, through the association and service of those conversant with Vedic knowledge, I attained the state of being the son of Brahmā."

Book I, Chapter 5

[*Nārada relates his subsequent birth to Vyāsa.*]

23. Nārada said:

"As for me, O sage, in a previous age, I was born of a certain maidservant to sages learned in the Vedas. Although I was only a boy, I was appointed to serve the *yogīs*, since they were planning to live together during the rainy season.[75]

24. Although those sages looked upon everyone impartially, they bestowed their kindness upon me, a young boy. I was free of all fickleness, disciplined, obedient, not interested in playing games, and I spoke sparingly.

25. I was permitted by the sages to eat the remnants of whatever food they had left over, and ate this once daily. From doing so, all my sins were destroyed.[76] Engaged in this manner, my mind became purified, and a strong personal interest in their religion grew in me.

26. As a result of this, thanks to their kindness, I kept on listening to the captivating narrations of Kṛṣṇa's pastimes that they were reciting. Listening attentively to every word of those narrations with faith, an attraction for Kṛṣṇa arose in me. Hearing about Him is so pleasing to the heart.

27. Consequently, once I had developed this attraction, my mind became firmly fixed in Kṛṣṇa; narratives about Him are so satisfying, O great sages! As a result of this, I could perceive that due to my illusion, I had imagined this gross and subtle reality [of the body and mind] to be the real me. But I am actually the Supreme *Brahman*.[77]

28. In this manner, *bhakti*, which diminishes *rajas* and *tamas*, grew within me, as I constantly listened to the pure glories of Hari that were being recited by the great-souled sages over the course of the rainy season and the autumn season.

29.–30. I was their servant—a boy who was attached to them, humble, free from sin, faithful, and disciplined—and they were compassionate on the less fortunate. So, as they were about to depart, those sages, out of kindness instructed me in that intimate knowledge of *bhakti* by which God Himself is revealed.

31. I came to understand the potency of Vāsudeva from that knowledge. He is *Bhagavān*, the Creator. By this knowledge, people can attain His divine abode.

32. O *brāhmaṇas*! *Bhagavān* is *Īśvara—Brahman*. It has been stated [in the sacred texts] that whatever act is performed for Him is the medicine for the threefold miseries of embodied existence.[78]

33. O sages who always uphold your vows! That which causes disease for living beings cannot [under normal circumstances] be the remedy for that very disease. But it can cure when used as medicine.

34. In the same way, the performance of all actions, which normally are the causes of bondage for people, become capable of destroying themselves, when performed for the Supreme.[79]
35. The knowledge associated with *bhakti yoga* is clearly based on those kinds of actions in this world, which are performed for the satisfaction of *Bhagavān*.
36. Wherever people are always performing actions according to the teachings of the *Bhāgavata*, they absorb themselves in the names and qualities of Kṛṣṇa and remember Him constantly.
37. *Oṁ namo Bhagavate Vāsudevāya* ('Reverences to you, *Bhagavān* Vāsudeva'). Reverences to Pradyumna, Aniruddha, and Saṅkarṣaṇa.[80]
38. The Lord of worship (sacrifice) is without material form, but He takes the form of *mantras*. By worshipping Him by means of the forms of these names, a person becomes a sage and his or her perception becomes perfect.
39. O *brāhmaṇa*! Seeing that I was following the instructions of His scriptures, Keśava [Kṛṣṇa] bestowed upon me knowledge, mystic powers, and devotion for Him.
40. O master! Your learning is vast. You should also impart these teachings. They satiate the desire of the wise to seek knowledge! For those who seek to remove the sorrows from all those constantly tormented by suffering, there is no other means."

Book I, Chapter 6

1. After he had heard about the birth and actions of Nārada, the sage of the celestials, the powerful Vyāsa, son of Satyavatī, asked him more questions, O *brāhmaṇa*.
2. Vyāsa said:
"After those mendicants who instructed you in spiritual knowledge had departed, what did you then do, sir, being still at that early age of life?
3. O son of the self-manifest Brahmā,[81] how did you live your later life? How did you give up your body, when the Time came?
4. O best of the sages, Time erases all things! How is it that it did not cover your memory of these events which were from a previous world age?"
5. Nārada replied:

"This is what happened after the mendicants who had instructed me in spiritual knowledge had departed. I was still a child at the time.

6. My mother was a maidservant and knew nothing of spiritual truths, and I was her only son. She bound me with bonds of affection, as I was her son and had no other shelter.

7. She was not self-sufficient and so, although she wished to do so, she was not able to provide for my maintenance. After all, people are under the control of God, like wooden dolls.

8. As a boy of five years, I had no sense of time, place, or direction, and lived in that dwelling of the *brāhmaṇas* bracing for what was to come.

9. One day, instigated by the force of Time, a snake on the path bit the poor woman, touched by her foot when she went out of the house at night to milk the cow.

10. So, accepting this as the mercy of God, who is always desiring the well-being of his devotees, I then set out toward the northern direction.[82]

11. On my way, I passed through prosperous countries, cities, villages, cattle-herding communities, mines, agricultural villages, hill villages, forests, and groves.

12. [I saw] wonderful mountains replete with various minerals, trees with their branches broken by elephants, and reservoirs of water. There were lotus ponds of pure water that were frequented by celestials and beautified by buzzing bees and the charming sounds of birds.

13. Traveling alone in this way, I saw a great forest. It had caves, hollow bamboos and other types of bamboos, *kuśa* grass, clumps of reeds, and *nala* grasses. It was terrifying and dangerous—the stalking grounds of jackals, owls, and snakes.

14. I was exhausted in body and mind, afflicted by thirst, and hungry. I bathed and then drank from the lake of a river. After sipping water, my fatigue dissipated.

15. That forest was unfrequented by humans. I took shelter of a *pippala* tree within it and sat beneath it. I concentrated my mind on the Supreme Soul who was within me, as I had heard [from the instructions of the sages].

16. As I was meditating on His lotus feet, with my mind overwhelmed with love, and my eyes flooded with tears of longing, Hari gradually appeared in my heart.

17. The hair on my body stood on end due to being overwhelmed with excessive love. I was utterly satiated, O sage. Immersed in a flood of ecstasy, I was unable to perceive both [myself and Hari] at the same time.
18. That form of God, *Bhagavān*, is most pleasing to the mind, and removes all sorrows. When I could no longer perceive it, I rose up, my mind thrown into despondency over this loss.
19. Desiring to see that form, I again concentrated my mind in my heart. Although I was focused, I could not see it again, and so despaired, like a distressed person.
20. The Lord, who is beyond the range of the senses, spoke these words to me as I was struggling in that desolate place. His voice was deep but gentle, as if to assuage my grief:
21. 'I'm afraid that in this life, you are not ready to see me again. A vision of Me is difficult to attain by imperfect *yogīs* whose impurities have not been cleansed.
22. That form which was revealed to you once by My grace, O sinless one, was for the purpose [of increasing] your desire. Desire for me most certainly frees one from all material desires lying latent in the heart.
23. By dint of your lengthy service to the saints, your heart became fixed on Me. Therefore, when you leave this world of ignorance, you will proceed to become My associate [in Vaikuṇṭha].[83]
24. Your mind which has been absorbed in Me will never deviate. By My grace, you will retain your memory, despite the cycles of creation and destruction.'
25. Having said this, that great Being fell silent. He is *Īśvara*, God, [the Creator of] the manifest and unmanifest *prakṛti*, the sky, and all elements. I offered my obeisance to Him, the greatest of the great, by bowing my head to the ground. I had been blessed.
26. My distraught state of mind evaporated. After that, I wandered around the earth awaiting Time in the form of Death, while reciting the names of the Infinite Lord, and contemplating His mysterious and wonderful deeds. My mind was satisfied, all my desires were gone, and I was freed from all pride and envy.
27. In this way, with my intelligence fixed on Kṛṣṇa, O *brāhmaṇa*, with pure mind and free of all attachments, Death in the form of Time appeared at its allotted time, like a flash of *Saudāmanī* lightning.[84]

28. As I was attaining a pure *Bhāgavata* body,[85] my gross body made of the five elements fell away, its accumulated *karma* extinguished.
29. Then, through his breath, I entered Brahmā, who desired to lie down with Lord Viṣṇu. He did this at the end of that particular *kalpa* world cycle, as Viṣṇu lay on the waters of the *Kāraṇa* ocean after withdrawing this universe within Himself.[86]
30. At the end of a thousand *yuga* ages, Brahmā awoke, desiring to create. I along with various sages such as Marīci, was then born from his breath.
31. Without ever breaking my vows, I wandered around both within and beyond the three worlds. By the grace of Lord Viṣṇu, my movements were unimpeded.[87]
32. I wander about singing of the deeds of Hari and playing on this *vīṇā* stringed instrument bestowed on me by the Lord, which is distinctive by emitting the sound of *Brahman* (*oṁ*).
33. The Lord, whose feet are holy places of pilgrimage,[88] and whose great deeds are relishable, suddenly appeared in my mind, as if He had been called.
34. It is well-known that describing the activities of Hari is the boat for crossing over the ocean of *saṁsāra* for those whose minds are constantly afflicted by desire for material enjoyment.
35. The mind, which is constantly assailed by lust and greed, is not as pacified by the paths of *yoga* consisting of the *yamas*, etc., as it is by service to Mukunda [Kṛṣṇa].
36. O sinless one! Whatever your honor asked me about the mysteries of my birth and activities, I have completely recounted to your mind's satisfaction."
37. Sūta said:
"After speaking this to Vyāsa, the son of Satyavatī, the great sage Nārada bade him farewell and then departed, spreading joy with his *vīṇā*. He had no personal goals to fulfill.
38. *Aho!*[89] How blessed is this sage of the celestials! While singing the glories of Viṣṇu, whose bow is made from horn, and experiencing bliss himself, he also gives delight to this afflicted world with his stringed instrument.

The Tale of Dhṛtarāṣṭra: The Blind Emperor's Final Days

Yoga Blueprint

This narrative pertains to events connected to the great Mahābhārata *war. We can recall Vyāsa composes the* Bhāgavata *after he had finished compiling the epic pertaining to the developments surrounding this. The* Bhāgavata *does, on occasion, refer back to events in the epic, but only insofar as they are relevant to narrations concerning to Kṛṣṇa* bhakti, *as per the mandate it sets for itself.*

The main yogic *message of this passage is that irrespective of whether one has led a compromised life, as certainly was the case with King Dhṛtarāṣṭra, and irrespective of how old and infirm one is, it is imperative that, at least at the end of life, one renounce all attachments and fix the mind on Kṛṣṇa before death strips one of this opportunity and the goal of human life.*

Book I, Chapter 13

1. Sūta said:
"After Vidura had received knowledge about the destination of the *ātman* from Maitreya while he was traveling to places of pilgrimage, he arrived at the city of Hastināpura.[90] He had received what he had desired to know.
2. Although while Maitreya was with him Vidura had posed questions to him, he later desisted from asking them once exclusive devotion to Govinda became manifest [in his heart].
3.–5. When they saw Vidura arriving, O *brāhmaṇa*, Yudhiṣṭhira, the son of Dharma, along with his brothers, Dhṛtarāṣṭra, Yuyutsu, Sañjaya, and Kṛpa, as well as Kuntī, Gāndhārī, Draupadī, Subhadrā, Uttarā, Kṛpī, and the rest of the womenfolk of the Pāṇḍava clan accompanied by other women with their children and in the company of relatives, all joyfully surged forth toward him, like a body when its life airs return. They approached him and embraced him in accordance with the appropriate protocol.
6. They shed abundant tears of love, as they had suffered in his absence due to missing him. After Vidura had accepted the seat arranged for him, King Yudhiṣṭhira honored him.
7. After Vidura had enjoyed food, rested, and taken a seat on a comfortable couch, the king, his head bowed with respect, questioned him while everyone was listening.

8. Yudhiṣṭhira said:
'Do you still remember us, who used to prosper under the shelter of your protection? We were saved along with our mothers from a host of dangers such as poison and fire, etc.[91]
9. When the main holy places of the world were graced by your good self traveling about the earth [on pilgrimage], how did you sustain yourself?
10. Devotees such as you have themselves become places of pilgrimage, O master. With Lord Viṣṇu, the holder of the club, situated within your heart, it is you who make holy places holy.
11. Did you see our well-wishers, O dear Vidura, and our relatives, whose Lord is Kṛṣṇa? And did you see whether the Yādavas are residing happily in their city?'
12. After he had been addressed in this way by Yudhiṣṭhira, king of Dharma, Vidura described everything that he had experienced, step by step—everything except for the news about the destruction of the Yadu dynasty.
13. Vidura was kind, and could not bear to see them distressed—after all, unpalatable and undesirable events appear of their own accord for human beings.
14. Vidura then resided there happily for a period of time, well treated like a god. He bestowed the highest good on his elder brother Dhṛitarāṣṭra, and brought happiness to everyone.
15. For the duration of the one hundred years that Yama had to endure the state of being [born] a *śūdra* [as Vidura] because of a curse, Aryamā wielded the rod of punishment on those who performed misdeeds [in his place].[92]
16. Yudhiṣṭhira, the sovereign of the kingdom, witnessed [the birth of] his grandson, Parīkṣit, who was to perpetuate the dynasty. He enjoyed unparalleled opulence with his brothers, the guardians of all the directions.
17. In this manner, insurmountable Time, unnoticed, overtakes those who are attached to their households, and deluded by their desire to enjoy them.
18. Noticing this, Vidura spoke to Dhṛtarāṣṭhra: 'O king, you must depart immediately. Just see the fear [of Time in the form of imminent death] that is approaching!
19. There is no remedial measure through any means from any quarter against this Time, O master. It is God himself and arrives for us all!

20. When overpowered by Time, people are immediately separated from their very life airs, which are their dearest possession—what to speak of other possessions, such as wealth, etc.!
21. Your father, brother, friends, and sons are dead, and your own life span has expired. Your body has been grasped by old age, and you live in someone else's home.
22. You are blind from birth,[93] you are now deaf, and your intellect is feeble. Your teeth are loose, your digestive fire is weak, and you cough up mucus noisily.
23. *Aho!* Just see how strong is the hope for life of living beings like you, sir![94] You are accepting the remnants discarded by Bhīma, like a household dog.[95]
24. What is the worth of a life given in charity by those very people whom you doused with fire, to whom you administered poison, whose wife you violated, and whose property and wealth you seized?[96]
25. Even though you desire to live, this body of a miserly person like you will perish against your will, worn out by old age, like a set of clothes.
26. One is said to be wise when, unattached and free from the bondage of *karma*, one gives up this body in a secluded place after it has become useless for the attainment of one's goals.
27. One in control of the self due to the awakening of detachment, either as a result of one's own efforts or [the guidance of] others, who leaves the household and wanders forth after fixing Hari in the heart, is eminent among people.
28. Therefore, sir, leave for the northern direction[97] without disclosing your destination to your relatives. Inviolable Time, which is now approaching, strips away the qualities of men.'
29. Enlightened in this way by his younger brother Vidura, the king, descendant of Ajamīḍha,[98] whose intellect served as his eyes [since he was blind], severed the bonds of affection for his relatives, and resolutely set forth on the path indicated by his brother.
30. Gāndhārī, the daughter of Subala, a true wife faithful to her husband, followed her husband as he was departing for the Himālayas. These mountains give pleasure to those who have taken up the staff of the renounced order,[99] just like a good battle gives pleasure to the brave.[100]
31. Meanwhile, Yudhiṣṭhira, who was without enemies, performed prayers to the sun and offered oblations to the fire. After honoring

the *brāhmaṇas* with gifts of sesame, cows, land, and gold, he entered his house to offer respects to his *guru*. But he did not find his uncles or Gāndhārī there.
32. His mind became full of concern, and he inquired from Sañjaya, who was sitting there: 'O son of Gavalgaṇa, where is our beloved uncle? He is old and bereft of sight.
33. And our aunt, who is desolate because of her slain sons?[101] And where has our well-wisher, Uncle Vidura, gone? He is distressed on account of his relatives being slain. Has he, fearing harm from a fool like me, thrown himself into the *Gaṅgā* river along with his wife?
34. When our father, Pāṇḍu, died, our two uncles protected all of us small children, their relatives, from dangers. Where have they gone now?' "
35. Sūta said:
"Sañjaya, not finding his master, became distraught due to separation from them, and overwhelmed with affection and compassion. He was so disturbed that he could not answer.
36. Wiping his tears with his hands as he thought of the feet of his master, Dhṛtarāṣṭra, he finally replied to Yudhiṣṭhira, controlling his mind with his intelligence.
37. 'I do not know the decision made by your uncles, O delight of the dynasty, nor of Gāndhārī. I have been deceived by those two great souls, O mighty armed one.'
38. At that moment, the great sage Nārada arrived, accompanied by the sage Tumburu. After arising from their seats, and worshipping him along with his younger brothers, Yudhiṣṭhira said:
39. 'I do not know the whereabouts of my uncles, O sage: where have they gone? And my austere aunt who was distraught by the death of her sons: where has she gone?
40. You are the captain of the ship, O Lord, which can convey us to the other side of the ocean (of grief).'[102] At this, sage Nārada, the best of the sages, replied:
41. 'O king, do not grieve for anything: the world is under the control of *Īśvara*. He is the Controller. All these worlds with their guardian deities offer worship to Him, as it is He who unites and separates living creatures.
42. Just as cows are pierced through the nose by a cord, and then bound together by ropes, so, bound by cords in the form of the

words of the Vedic injunctions, beings conduct worship to the Controller.
43. Just as in this world the bringing together and separating of game pieces might take place through the will of the player, so in the same way the bringing together and separating of human beings takes place through the will of the Lord.
44. Whether you consider beings to be eternal, non-eternal, or both, they should not be mourned in any circumstance. To do so is the result of attachment born of ignorance.
45. Therefore, my son, give up your distress. It is caused by ignorance of the *ātman*, and it is because of this that you are thinking: "But they are helpless and without protection: How can they survive without me?!"
46. This body, made of the five elements, is itself subject to the *guṇas*, *karma*, and Time. How can it, then, protect others any more than one grasped by a python can protect others?
47. One living being is the means of sustenance for another: those without hands, for those with hands; those without feet, for those with four feet; and the weak for the strong.
48. This universe is *Bhagavān*, the sole *ātman* among *ātmans*, O king. He is self-manifest—manifesting both within and without [of all things]. Know that it is only on account of His *māyā* power of illusion that He appears to be manifold.
49. O great king, He, the Creator of all beings, is none other than this *Bhagavān* [Kṛṣṇa]. He has incarnated into this world in the form of Time for the destruction of the enemies of the celestials.
50. *Īśvara* has accomplished that which was to be done on behalf of the celestials, and is expecting [to complete] whatever remains.[103] As long as he remains on this earth, you should witness [his activities].
51. Dhṛtarāṣṭra, accompanied by his brother and his wife, Gāndhārī, has gone to the *āśrama* of the sages, on the south side of the Himālayas.
52. The place is called Sapta-śrota (Seven Rivers), because the *Gaṅgā* divided sevenfold into seven rivers for the satisfaction of the seven different sages.[104]
53. Observing a fast of only drinking water, he bathes three times a day, offers oblations into the sacred fire according to the prescribed rules, and remains there with a peaceful mind, free of desires.

54. He has mastered posture (*āsana*) and breath control, withdrawn consciousness (*pratyāhāra*) from the six senses, and overcome the taints of *rajas*, *sattva*, and *tamas* by his absorption in Hari.
55. He has merged the mind into intelligence, merged that into the *jīva* (*kṣetra-jña*[105]), and then merged that into *Brahman*, the substratum [of everything], just like the air in a pot merges into the totality of air.
56. He has destroyed all the effects of the *guṇas* of *māyā*, restrained his mind and senses, abstained from all food, and is sitting motionless like a pillar. Do not try to hold him back—he has renounced all activities.
57. In fact, on the fifth day from today, O king, he will abandon his body, and burn it into ash.
58. While the body of her husband is burning along with the thatched hermitage, his chaste wife, standing outside, will enter into that fire.
59. After hearing about this amazing thing, O joy of the Kuru dynasty, Vidura, feeling both joy and sorrow, will depart on a pilgrimage of holy places.'
60. Then, having said all this, Nārada, along with his *tumburu* stringed instrument, ascended to the celestial realms. Taking his words to heart, Yudhiṣṭhira gave up his sorrow."

The Tale of King Parīkṣit: Cursed to Die in Seven Days

Yoga Blueprint

The yogic *message imparted by this tale is that, like Parīkṣit, all embodied beings face death. Parīkṣit's question, then, pertaining to the ultimate duty, purpose, and goal of human existence, what it is that one should do in the world at every moment—in essence, what one should do with one's mind—sets the stage for the entire text to impart its teachings. Of additional interest is the text's illustration of the state of* samādhi *by Śamīka. In* nirbīja samādhi *(*Yoga Sūtras *I.47ff.), consciousness is exclusively immersed in its own nature and has no awareness of any external stimulation.*

Book 1, Chapter 18

24. Once, after taking up his bow, King Parīkṣit set out to the forest to hunt. While he was pursuing a deer, he became extremely tired, hungry, and thirsty.

25. Not finding any body of water, he entered into Śamīka's [renowned] hermitage, and saw the sage sitting peacefully, his eyes closed.
26. Śamīka had attained the state beyond the three states of consciousness—waking, dream, and deep sleep[106]—and so was completely inactive, his senses, *prāṇa* life airs, mind, and intelligence restrained.
27. His dreadlocks were disheveled, and he was draped in a deerskin. The king, whose throat was dry, requested water from the sage, who was in that state.
28. Upon not receiving a straw seat, and not being offered sweet words or a hospitable beverage, or indeed anything at all, the king, feeling that he had been disrespected, became angry.
29. O *brāhmaṇa* (Śaunaka), the king's anger and resentment suddenly erupted against the *brāhmaṇa*. This had never happened before to the king, but he had become compromised by hunger and thirst.
30. So, as he was leaving, the king placed a dead snake with the tip of his bow on the shoulder of the *brāhmaṇa* sage out of anger, and returned to his city.
31. [The king wondered:] "Were his eyes closed because he had closed down his senses? Or was it rather really a feigned state of *samādhi* because of [not wishing to interact with me], a lowly member of the *kṣatriya* warrior caste?"
32. While this had been taking place, the *brāhmaṇa*'s son had been out playing with other young children. Although he was but a boy, he was very powerful. When he heard that his beloved father had been subject to an offense by the king, he uttered these words then and there:
33. "Just see the irreligiousness of the rulers, who are like crows who have grown fat from eating the oblations meant for sacrifice! This is an offense against their masters by servants who are doorkeepers, like dogs.
34. A lowly *kṣatriya* is clearly ordained to be the doorkeeper of the *brāhmaṇa* caste. How does one, who is supposed to stand at the door of the house, deserve to eat from the same dish [as the master]?
35. Since Lord Kṛṣṇa, the punisher of the miscreants, has left the world, I myself will today punish the transgressors of the law. Just witness my power!"

36. After uttering this to his companions, the sage's son, his eyes red with anger, touched the water of the *Kauśikī* river, and released a verbal thunderbolt in the form of a curse.
37. "Unleashed by me, the snake-bird Takṣaka will bite that destroyer of his family's reputation. He has transgressed the limits of the law and insulted my beloved father," he said.
38. Having done this, the boy returned to the *āśrama* hermitage and saw his father with the corpse of the snake on his shoulder. Overwhelmed with pain, he cried out aloud.
39. The father, a descendant of sage Aṅgirā, heard the cry of his son. Slowly opening his eyes, he saw the dead snake on his shoulder, O *brāhmaṇa*.
40. He threw aside the snake, and then inquired: "My son, why do you wail? Who has wronged you?" Addressed in this way, the son informed him about what had happened.
41. When he heard the account, the father did not approve of his son's curse upon the king, who had not deserved such a thing: "*Aho! Aho!* You have done a grave thing today; you have inflicted an enormous punishment for a minor offense.
42. You should never equate the king with ordinary men, you foolish boy. He is declared [in the sacred texts] to be preeminent. Through his formidable power, the citizens are protected without fearing anything and live in well-being.
43. The king, lord of men [is equal to] Lord Viṣṇu, the wielder of the discus. If he does not oversee [the kingdom], O son, then, in an instant, the world, unprotected and filled with thieves, becomes destroyed, like a herd of sheep.
44. People, many of whom are thieves, will curse, kill, and rob cattle, women, and wealth from each other. [Because of your deed], we will today incur the sin committed by the plunderers of wealth in those places where the king has been destroyed, even though that sin was not directly performed by us.
45. Without a king, the righteous codes of the Āryas—the injunctions of the four *varṇas*, castes, and *āśramas* (stages of life), outlined in the three Vedas—will vanish from society. As a consequence, when people become absorbed in lust and profit, the mixing of the castes will ensue.[107] People will then behave like monkeys and dogs [that is, with few regulations].

46. The king is the protector of *dharma*. He is the Lord of men, a sovereign of wide renown. He is the performer of horse sacrifices,[108] a sage-king, and a great devotee in person. The poor man was beset by hunger, thirst, and fatigue; he did not deserve to be cursed by us in that manner.
47. *Bhagavān*, the soul of all, should please forgive the sin performed by this young immature boy against His sinless servant, the king.
48. The Lord's devotees, even though certainly capable of doing so, do not retaliate when abused, insulted, cursed, dishonored, or even when struck."
49. In this way, even though he had been disrespected by the king, the great sage did not consider this to be an offense, but rather was distressed by the offense made by his son.
50. Generally, saintly persons, when made to encounter the dualities of the world,[109] are neither disturbed nor elated by [the actions of] others.[110] This is because [they have realized] the *ātman*, situated beyond the *guṇas*.

Book 1, Chapter 19

1. Sūta continued:
"Meanwhile, the great king, thinking about the offense that he had done, was extremely troubled in mind: '*Aho!* I performed a despicable deed, as if I were a non-Āryan, against an innocent *brāhmaṇa*, whose *yogic* power is retained concealed.
2. Therefore it is certain that a terrible calamity will very soon befall me because of the offense I performed against this divine being. Let this freely occur to absolve me of sin so that I never commit such acts again.
3. Since I am so wretched, let the fire of the *brāhmaṇa*'s rage even today consume my kingdom, strength, wealth, and treasury such that I never again harbor a sinful attitude toward the twice-born *brāhmaṇas*, gods, or cows.'
4. As he was thinking in this manner, the king heard about his impending doom looming in the form of [the snake-bird] Takṣaka, invoked by the son of the sage. He considered this to be fitting: he was attached [to worldly life] and the fire of Takṣaka would soon be the means of his detachment.

5. Parīkṣit gave up [any desire for] this world and the celestial one—he had anyway long determined that they should be renounced, considering service to the lotus feet of Kṛṣṇa to be superior. He then sat down to fast to death on the bank of the *Gaṅgā* river.
6. What person, who is about to die, would not worship the *Gaṅgā*? She brings water made divine from the dust of the feet of Kṛṣṇa[111] mixed with the beautiful *tulasī* plant.[112] She purifies both worlds (earthly and celestial), along with their celestial lords.
7. Having made this resolve to sit on the banks of the *Gaṅgā* to fast until death, Parīkṣit, the descendant of the Pāṇḍavas, firm in the vows of a sage, and free from all attachments, concentrated on the feet of Mukunda [Kṛṣṇa] with undivided attention.
8. At this, the great, realized sages, who can purify the worlds, arrived there along with their disciples. The saints, under the pretext of performing pilgrimage, actually themselves purify a pilgrimage place.[113]
9. They were: Atri, Vasiṣṭha, Cyavana, Śaradvān, Ariṣṭanemi, Bhṛgu, Aṅgirā, Parāśara, the son of Gādhi (Viśvāmitra), Rāma, Utathya, Indrapramada, Idhmavāha.
10. Medhātithi, Devala, Ārṣṭiṣeṇa, Bhāradvāja, Gautama, Pippalāda, Maitreya, Aurva, Kavaṣa, Kumbhayoni, Dvaipāyana, and the great Nārada.
11. And other great sages and eminent *brāhmaṇas* arrived also, as well as prominent kings like Aruṇa, etc. The king honored the eminent sages from various lineages that had gathered there, and paid obeisance by bowing his head [to their feet].
12. When they were seated comfortably and he had once again offered homage to them, the king stood before them with hands folded in supplication, his mind completely detached from worldly affairs, and informed them of his intentions.
13. The king said:
'*Aho!* The dynasty of kings is actually contemptible, and deserves to be discarded far from the place where the water used for washing the feet of the *brāhmaṇas* is found.[114] But nonetheless, because of this, we kings are actually the most fortunate among men, since this character of ours makes us eligible for the compassion of magnanimous souls.
14. I am a sinful member of such a dynasty, and my mind is always attached to household affairs. The Supreme Lord of all has manifested

in the form of a *brāhmaṇa*'s curse, and in this manner has thereby become the trigger for my detachment from worldly affairs. Because of such a curse, people who are attached to worldly affairs would normally be immediately thrown into a state of fear.
15. May the sages and Mother *Gaṅgā* accept me as someone who has turned to the Lord, and whose mind is fixed on Him. Let Takṣaka, or whatever magical thing was discharged by the *brāhmaṇa*, bite me as is fitting. And may you all please sing the glories of Viṣṇu.
16. May fellowship with those who have taken shelter of the unlimited Lord, as well as affection for them, be bestowed upon me in whatever be the next birth I may obtain in this material world, and may I be a friend to all. I offer homage to the *brāhmaṇas*.'
17. The king, who had handed over his responsibilities to his son, was determined and resolved in mind. On the southern side of the *Gaṅgā* facing north, he sat down on *kuśa* grass with its roots facing east.[115]
18. When the king of kings was seated on that seat and awaiting death in this manner, the hosts of celestial beings in the heavens joyfully praised him, showered flowers on the earth, and played kettledrums continuously.
19. The great sages who had assembled there also praised him with joyful hearts: 'Well done!' Their nature is to bestow blessings on living beings, and so they spoke to him about the pleasing qualities of Lord Viṣṇu, whose glories are supreme:
20. 'O best of sage-kings, from among those who are devoted to Kṛṣṇa, there is nothing surprising about the fact that the ones who desire to become personal associates of *Bhagavān* renounce the royal throne, which is honored by the helmets of other kings.[116]
21. So now we will all remain here until this foremost of *Bhagavān*'s devotees relinquishes his material body and departs to the supreme realm, Vaikuṇṭha, which is free from sorrow and hankering.'[117]
22. Those assembled sages were fixed in *yoga*, and their words were impartial, full of sweetness, profound, and true. After listening to them, Parīkṣit, desiring to hear about the deeds of Viṣṇu, offered the sages his respects and addressed them:
23. 'You have all assembled here from all the corners of the world—just as the Vedas which are beyond the three worlds manifest divine bodily forms.[118] One whose nature is to bestow grace on others has

no other purpose whatsoever, either in this world, or in the next, other than to do this.

24. Therefore, with full faith in you, O learned ones, I submit to you this most worthy query: From all those duties that are to be performed by everyone, which is the optimum duty that should be performed specifically by those about to die? Please give this your full consideration.'

25. At that moment, by chance, the son of Vyāsa, the great Śuka, happened to arrive there. He was wandering around the earth in the guise of an ascetic renunciant, completely unattached to anything, as he was satisfied by the realization of his *ātman*, the inner self. Surrounded by young boys, his elevated characteristics lay concealed.

26. He was sixteen years of age, with handsome and youthful feet, hands, thighs, arms, shoulders, cheeks, and body. His face had beautiful wide eyes, a stately nose, symmetrical ears, and attractive eyebrows. His fine neck was like a conch shell.

27. His collarbones were concealed, and he had a broad, attractive chest. His navel was like a whirlpool, and his stomach had beautiful lines. He was naked, and his hair was scattered about his face. His arms were long, and he was as attractive as the best of the celestials.

28. He was dark complexioned and displayed an attractive, youthful appearance. He was captivating to women because of his charming smile. All those sages could recognize his [saintly] characteristics even though his luster was covered over, and so they rose up from their seats.

29. Thereupon, Parīkṣit, beloved of Viṣṇu, offered respect by bowing his head to Śuka, who had arrived as an unexpected guest. At this, all the simple folk, women and children [who were following him], departed. Honored in this way, Śuka sat on an elevated seat.

30. Surrounded by *brāhmaṇa* sages, kingly sages, and celestial sages, the divine Śuka, a great soul among great souls, shone forth in that place like the moon surrounded by the multitude of planets, constellations and stars.

31. Śuka was acutely intelligent. The king, devotee of Viṣṇu, approached the sage, who was sitting peacefully. Parīkṣit bowed his head to him, and attentively offered him respects with joined hands. Then he inquired from him with joyful words.

32. Parīkṣit said:

'*Aho!* By your lordship arriving here unexpectedly out of kindness, we, who are mere *kṣatriyas*, members of the warrior caste, have today become worthy of being served by saints, O *brāhmana*; we have been transformed into pilgrimage places by your presence.
33. By simply remembering such persons [as yourself], our houses become purified. What then to speak about seeing and touching you, washing your feet, and offering you a seat, and so forth?
34. From being in your presence, O great *yogī*, even the greatest of sins are immediately destroyed, just like the enemies of the celestials are destroyed in the presence of Viṣṇu.
35. *Bhagavān* Kṛṣṇa, who is dear to the sons of Pāṇḍu, is surely pleased with me: so as to please his paternal aunt's sons, the Pāṇḍavas,[119] he has accepted the descendants of their lineage.
36. Otherwise, how is it possible for me to be blessed by seeing you? You are perfect and compassionate, but your ways are concealed to humankind—especially to those who are about to die.
37. Therefore I ask of you, the most eminent of *gurus* among *yogīs*: What is the means to perfection? What should be done at every moment by a person in this world about to die?
38. What should be heard? What *mantra* should be chanted (*japyam*[120])? What actions should be performed by men, O master? What should be remembered? And what should be worshipped? And also please tell me what should be avoided.
39. Indeed, O *brāhmaṇa*, it is known that your honor never lingers in the homes of those attached to their households for more than even the brief time taken to milk a cow.' "[121]
40. Sūta said:
"Addressed and questioned in this way with those sincere words, the great Śuka, son of Bādarāyaṇa (Vyāsa) and knower of *dharma*, responded to the king."

[*Continued in the next tale.*]

Book II

The Teachings of Sage Śuka: The Wandering Enlightened Sage

Yoga Blueprint

We notice in verses I.7 and I.9 that sages who are already enlightened, and consequently have completely lost attraction for all things related to the guṇas *from having attained realization of the* ātman, *nonetheless are attracted to the narratives of Kṛṣṇa. Here again we find one of the main subthemes of the* Bhāgavata. *The text thus indicates that Kṛṣṇa's nature and qualities are not only transcendent to* prakṛti, *but higher than the individual* ātman. *His form and characteristics are the highest and most blissful expression of* Brahman, *and a vision of Him is the ultimate spiritual experience. In this regard, we see here, as elsewhere, the repetition of a fairly detailed description of the form of Viṣṇu. This recurs frequently throughout the* Bhāgavata *in order to fully ingrain the details of this form in the practitioner's mind, such that it can be recalled during meditation along the lines indicted in 2.9–14.*

Other noteworthy points are the equivalence of sacred texts with Brahman *in I.8 (the sixteenth-century theologian Vallabha considered the* Bhāgavata *a type of literary* avatāra*). This section also includes a technical and esoteric passage on the subtle physiology that is of particular interest to the Śākta traditions (II.19–32). The somewhat technical practice outlined here involves an involution of the Sāṅkhya categories of the body from their grossest to progressively* *subtler forms until one arrives at the* ātman. *However, the ultimate goal of all and any practice is to remember Nārāyaṇa at the end of life (II.1.6).*

Book II, Chapter 1

1. *Śrī* Śuka said:
"This question of yours, posed for the welfare of people, is excellent, O king. It is appreciated by those who know the *ātman*, and, from everything that is useful for people to hear, it is the most worthwhile topic.
2. For those people who have not seen the truth of the *ātman* and are attached to their homes and households, there are thousands of things that seem worth hearing, O king.
3. The prime of life is carried away by sexual intercourse and sleep during the night, O king, and, through striving for wealth and maintaining one's family during the day.
4. Obsessed with one's body, children, and wife, etc., which are like illusory soldiers [subject to death at any moment], one does not perceive their demise, even while actually perceiving it.
5. Therefore, O son of Bhārata, one desiring freedom from fear should hear about, glorify, and remember Hari. He is *Bhagavān*, *Īśvara*, the soul of everything.
6. Indeed, the perfection of life for a person, whether through the paths of Sāṅkhya or Yoga, through performance of duty, or through knowledge, is to remember Nārāyaṇa at the end of life.
7. Usually, O king, sages who have desisted from [mundane ritualistic] rules and regulations, and are situated in the state beyond the *guṇas*—i.e., have attained *Brahman*—relish the qualities and stories of Hari.
8. This *Bhāgavata Purāṇa* is nondifferent from *Brahman*. I learned it from my father, Vyāsa, at the end of the *Dvāpara yuga*, the third world age.
9. Although I had attained perfection and was situated in the state beyond the *guṇas*, my mind was captured by the pastimes of Kṛṣṇa; hence I studied this history, O sagely king.
10. I will narrate that Purāṇa to you; you are a great soul, sir. Devotion for Mukunda [Kṛṣṇa] is awakened in those who have faith in it.
11. The chanting of the name of Hari has been prescribed for those *yogīs* who are disinterested [in material enjoyment] and who desire freedom from fear.

12. What is the use of many years squandered mindlessly by a deluded person? Let it be known that it is better for one hour to be spent striving for one's ultimate welfare.
13. After the sage-king by name of Khaṭvaṅga found out what remained of his life in this world, he renounced everything in an instant, and dedicated himself to Hari, who bestows fearlessness.[1]
14. There is a limit also, O Kaurava, to your life span: seven days. Take all steps necessary to prepare for death during this time.
15. When the end comes, a person should sever desire for this body and all that is associated with it [family, possessions, and the like] with the weapon of detachment, free from fear.
16. With mind fixed, one should leave home alone, wash in the waters of a sacred place, and then sit on a seat prepared according to the prescriptions.
17. One should concentrate on the three constituent phonemes of *oṁ* [*a-u-m*], the great and pure *Brahman* in the form of sound. One should restrain one's mind and control one's breathing, keeping one's mind fixed on that seed of *Brahman* [*oṁ*].
18. With the intelligence as the driver,[2] one should remove the senses from the sense objects by means of the mind. If one's mind becomes disturbed by agitation, one should focus it on the desired object, Lord Kṛṣṇa, by means of the intelligence.
19. Then, one should meditate on one limb of the Lord, with uninterrupted mind. After controlling the mind and removing it from sense objects, one should not think of anything else. The mind should take pleasure there alone: the Supreme destination of Viṣṇu.
20. Normally, one's mind is harassed by *rajas* and deluded by *tamas*. A wise person should control it by concentration (*dhāraṇā*) and destroy all the impurities created by it.
21. While this concentration on the refuge [of Lord Viṣṇu] is being practiced, the symptoms of *bhakti*, devotion, appear in the *yogī*. This *yoga*, which is most auspicious [that is, *bhakti*], quickly manifests."

Book II, Chapter 2

1. *Śrī* Śuka said:
[. . .]
2. "The path of the Vedic scriptures is such that one's intelligence puzzles over the meaningless words. Wandering here and there in the

world of *māyā*, illusion [in pursuance of the Vedic injunctions], one does not attain one's goals,[3] just like a sleeping person [does not attain his goals] through dreams, which are made of memory imprints.[4]

3. Therefore, a sage, who is not deluded, but whose intelligence is fixed [on the self], should accept whatever things are necessary for accomplishing this purpose and no more; one should not struggle [for anything more] than this, realizing that doing so would simply be labor [for nothing].

4. When the ground is there, what is the use of endeavoring for beds? When two arms belong to oneself by nature, what is the use of pillows? When there are two hands, what is the use of a variety of implements for food? And when nakedness or the bark of trees[5] is available, what is the use of clothes?

5. Are there no torn clothes discarded on the road? Do the trees, who maintain others, no longer give alms? Have the rivers dried up? Are the caves closed? Does the almighty Hari not protect his devotees? Why should wise people serve those who are blinded by the pride of wealth?

6. It is the *ātman* that is the cherished goal. It is [a part of] the unlimited *Bhagavān*. It is self-manifest and perfect and lies within one's heart. This *ātman* is the goal that one should fix in mind and worship contentedly. It is in this way that the cause of *saṁsāra* is brought to an end.

7. Upon seeing people fallen into the *Vaitaraṇī* river [on the way to hell][6] and experiencing the suffering generated by their *karma*, who other than a beast would neglect contemplating on the Supreme and instead engage in immoral behavior?

8. Some people contemplate with concentration on the Supreme Being as situated in the inner space of the heart within their own bodies. The size of the span of a hand,[7] He has four arms bearing lotus, disc, conch, and club.

9. He has a smiling face and eyes large as lotuses. His cloth is yellowish like the filament of a *kadamba* flower. He has ornaments brilliant with precious jewels and gold, and earrings and a headpiece glittering with great gems.

10. His tender budlike feet are placed by the masters of *yogīs* into the receptacle of their hearts, which are like the pericarp of full-blown lotuses. He is marked with the sign of Śrī, the Goddess of

Prosperity [the *śrīvatsa*, a curl of hair on His chest]. He wears the *kaustubha* jewel around His neck, and is covered by a garland of forest flowers of unfading beauty.

11. He is adorned with a belt, and with very valuable rings, anklets, and bracelets. His beautiful smiling face is delightful with lustrous, clean, curly, bluish locks.

12. His abundant grace is evident from the play of His eyebrows and the brightness of His happy, playful, smiling eyes. The *yogī* should gaze at this mental image of *Īśvara*, which is pieced together by the mind, for as long as the mind can remain fixed in concentration.

13. With one's mind one should focus on each limb consecutively, from the feet up to the smiling face of Kṛṣṇa, the bearer of the club. As one's intelligence becomes progressively purified, one should move on from the previous lower part [of the Lord's anatomy] and fix one's mind on the next higher part.

14. Until *bhakti yoga* is awakened by this form of the universal *Īśvara*, the Supreme Seer, then one should instead contemplate the grosser form of the Supreme Person after the completion of one's daily religious practices.[8]

15. When the ascetic becomes desirous of abandoning this world, dear king, he should establish himself on a comfortable stable seat (*sthira-sukham āsanam*),[9] and, with his breath mastered, control his *prāṇa*. His mind should not become attached to time and place.[10]

16. After controlling the mind by means of his pure intelligence, the *yogī* should merge it into the subtle body (*kṣetra-jña*),[11] and the latter into the *ātman*. The wise person should then absorb the *ātman* into the Supreme *ātman*. Upon attaining complete peace, one should desist from all activity.

17. In that state there is no Time, which is the controller of even the celestials, what to speak of the influence of the higher gods who are controllers over the universe. Neither *sattva*, nor *rajas*, nor *tamas* exists there, nor does ego, intellect, or primordial matter.

18. The *yogīs* long for the supreme abode of Viṣṇu. Desiring to abandon all that is illusory by the process of elimination (*neti neti*[12]), they give up misidentification with the body, and embrace His adorable feet in their hearts with exclusive devotion at every moment.

19. The sage who is situated [in *Brahman*], who is vigorous, whose mind is controlled, and who has gained wisdom from the sacred texts,

should leave his body in the following manner: he should block the anus with his heel, and then energetically raise the life air (*prāṇa*) up through the six locations [the *cakras*].[13]

20. He should raise the air situated in the navel [*maṇipūraka cakra*] to the heart [*anāhata cakra*]; from there, by means of the motion of the upward-moving (*udāna*) life air, the sage should lead it to the breast [*viśuddhi cakra*], and from there the concentrating sage should aim with his intelligence for the root of the palate and slowly lead the life air upward to that place.

21. From there, he should raise it up to between the eyebrows, indifferent [to all desires] and with all the seven outlets of the body [eyes, nostrils, ears and mouth] closed off. After holding the life air there without effort with his gaze fixed, he should eject it through the crown of the head [*sahasrāra cakra*], abandon his body, and attain the supreme.

22. But if, O king, he should wish to reach the abode of Brahmā; or, indeed, the pleasure grounds of the celestial beings who can travel through the air; or achieve the eight mystic powers over anything made of the *guṇas*, then he should retain his mind and senses [in the subtle body] so as to achieve these.

23. They say that the masters of *yoga*, who practice the cultivation of knowledge, austerities, *yoga*, *samādhi*, and devotion, and who have [subtle] bodies that [can travel] through the air, can attain destinations anywhere within or beyond the three worlds. Such destinations are not available for those who engage in *karma*, mundane ritualistic activities.[14]

24. Once he has passed through the pure *suṣumṇā* pathway[15] leading to Brahmā's realm, he reaches the abode of Agni, the god of fire. Thereafter, when all his impurities have been cleansed, he proceeds higher, O king, to the *śaiśumāra*, the whorl in the heavens resembling an alligator, presided over by Lord Viṣṇu.

25. Then, alone, in the pure subtle body, manifesting the *aṇimā* mystic power of becoming smaller than the smallest, the *yogī* proceeds beyond the navel of the universe of Lord Viṣṇu.[16] He thereafter attains the realms adored by the knowers of *Brahman*, where the celestials who live for a *kalpa* aeon[17] enjoy themselves.

26. Then, after witnessing the entire universe being consumed by the fire issuing forth from the mouth of Ananta (Śeṣa[18]), he emerges at Brahmā's highest abode of Satya-loka, which endures for Brahmā's

entire life, a period of two *parārdhas.*[19] This is the realm enjoyed by the masters of the perfected beings.
27. In that realm there is no sorrow, no old age, no disease, no death, and no afflictions. Nor are there any concerns—except sometimes the mind feels compassion from witnessing the terrible sufferings and births and deaths of those who do not know all this.
28. Then, with his mind, the *yogī* fearlessly returns [his body] to the elements: earth to water, and then, without haste, after manifesting an effulgent form, to fire. After merging this into air, in turn, by his mind, he eventually also dissolves this into ether, the great subtle covering of the *ātman*.
29. The *yogī* attains the quality [*tanmātra*] of smell by means of the nose; taste, by means of the tongue; sight, by means of the eye; touch, by means of the skin; and sound, the special quality of the sky, by means of the ear. He accomplishes this goal by manipulating the *prāṇa* life air.
30. Then he attains the *ahaṅkāra* (ego) where the senses, sense objects, mind, and their presiding deities are merged. Then, along with the *ahaṅkāra*, the *yogī* attains *buddhi* (*mahat*, intelligence), and then *prakṛti*, where the *guṇas* are quiescent.[20]
31. Along with *prakṛti* his *ātman* finally attains the supreme soul [Viṣṇu], who is peaceful and blissful. Attaining his blissful nature in that final goal, the *yogī* enters the divine state, and is never again interested in this world, my dear king.
32. These two paths about which you inquired, O king, are eternal, and are described in the Vedas.[21] Actually, *Bhagavān* Vāsudeva had previously spoken about them, after He had become satisfied from being worshipped by Brahmā.
33. There is no path more auspicious than this, for one who is immersed in *saṁsāra*, because by following it *bhakti yoga* for *Bhagavān* Vāsudeva is developed.
34. After applying his intelligence to studying the entire three Vedas, Lord Brahmā, the highest being, determined the means whereby love for the Supreme is attained.
35. *Bhagavān* Hari is perceived in all living beings by means of His presence as the *ātman*. There [must exist] a seer on account of the existence of [instruments of sight] such as the intelligence, etc., as well as the existence of objects of sight; it is by these characteristics that the existence of the *ātman* (the seer) can be inferred.[22]

36. Therefore, O king, it is *Bhagavān*, Hari, who should be heard, recited, and remembered about by people with all their hearts, in all places and all times.
37. *Bhagavān* is the soul of the saintly persons. Those who drink the nectar of stories about Him attained through the vessels of the ears, purify the heart from the contamination of sense objects and attain His lotus feet as their destination."

Book II, Chapter 3

1. *Śrī* Śuka said:
"In this way, the question your highness posed to me has been answered on behalf of all wise people in human society who are about to die.
[. . .]
10. Irrespective of whether one is free of desire, full of all desires, or desirous of liberation, *mokṣa*, one should intensely worship the Supreme Person through the practice of *bhakti yoga*, if one is intelligent.
11. The attainment of the highest good, even for those who worship the celestial beings,[23] is this: unflinching devotion to *Bhagavān*, attained from association with the devotees of *Bhagavān*.
12. Knowledge causes the whirlpool of the waves of the *guṇas* to abate. From that comes satisfaction in the self and disinterest in the *guṇas*. Thereafter comes *bhakti yoga*, which is the best path to liberation. Who, contented by the narrations of Hari, would not develop attraction for these narrations?"
13. Sage Śaunaka said:
"After hearing all these teachings that had been imparted to him, what else did the foremost king of the Bharatas further inquire from the seer sage Śuka, son of Vyāsa?
14. You should kindly relate these to us, O learned Sūta, we are eager to hear. Discussions which culminate in narratives about Hari are surely most fitting in an assembly of saintly people.
15. That very Pāṇḍava king Parīkṣit, the great charioteer, [in his childhood] imitated the pastimes of Hari while he was still playing with toys.
16. Śuka, that great son of Vyāsa, was devoted exclusively to Vāsudeva [Kṛṣṇa]. It is certain that the enlivening qualities of Viṣṇu,

whose glories are broadcast widely, would have been expressed in that gathering of saints.

17. The rising and setting of the sun in the heavens takes away the life of all men here on earth, except for that person whose every moment is spent in talking about the glorious Viṣṇu.

18. Do not the trees also live? Do not bellows breathe? Do not the other animals in the village eat and mate?

19. That person whose ears have never heard the name of Kṛṣṇa, the elder brother of Balarāma, is considered to be a beast, like the donkeys, camels, pigs, and dogs.

20. The cavities in the ears of a person who does not listen to the deeds of the glorious Viṣṇu (Urukrama), are just like empty holes, and the tongue that does not recite the verses about Viṣṇu (Urugāya) is useless, like that of a frog's.

21. The head, even though adorned with a crown or turban, is simply a large burden, if it does not offer obeisance to Mukunda [Kṛṣṇa]. And the hands, even though bedecked with shining golden bracelets, are like those of a corpse if they do not offer worship to Hari.

22. The eyes of men that do not gaze on the forms of Viṣṇu are like the eyes of a peacock's plumage, and the feet that do not travel to the pilgrimage places of Hari are like [the roots] of the tree species.

23. A person who does not obtain the dust from the feet of *Bhagavān* is like a corpse, even though living, and a human being who has not experienced the smell of the *tulasī* plant from the feet of Viṣṇu is likewise a corpse even though capable of smelling.

24. That heart is made of stone, which, when hearing the name of Hari, does not produce bodily transformations such as tears in the eyes and the hair standing erect on the body.

25. Speak to us, dear Sūta, it is pleasing to the mind. Śuka, son of Vyāsa, is expert in the knowledge of the *ātman* and foremost of devotees. Tell us what he related to the king, when being questioned by him in such an exemplary fashion."

Book II, Chapter 4

1. Sūta said:

"After hearing the words of Śuka, which contained clear truths about ultimate reality, Parīkṣit, son of Uttarā, fixed his undivided intelligence on Kṛṣṇa.

2. He abandoned the insidious attachment to his kingdom, which was being well managed, and to his friends, wealth, livestock, residence, wife, and his own body.
3. That high-minded one had faith in hearing about the activities of Kṛṣṇa, and asked this very same question that you have asked, O great saints.
4. After coming to know of his impending death, Parīkṣit renounced the threefold pursuits (*dharma*, duty; *artha*, prosperity; and *kāma*, enjoyment), and entered into a state of devotional absorption in *Bhagavān* Vāsudeva."
5. The king said:
"You are an omniscient being, and your words are true, O *brāhmaṇa*. My ignorance is being dispelled as you narrate the stories of Hari.
6. I wish to know once again about how *Bhagavān* creates this universe by His personal *māyā*, which is so difficult to comprehend, even by the great lords of the celestials.
7. How does He maintain it and then again destroy it? How does that Supreme omnipresent Being, who possesses all power, harness His power, and then playfully engage in creation Himself, as well as enhance His creation through the play of others [such as Brahmā]?
8. There is no doubt, O *brāhmaṇa,* that the wondrous deeds of *Bhagavān* Hari appear difficult to comprehend, even by the sage poets. His feats are amazing,
9. How does He uphold the *guṇas* of *prakṛti*, both simultaneously and sequentially? Although He is One, He engages in activity through manifold incarnations.
10. Since your holiness is well-versed in the Vedic literature and in the Absolute Truth, please address this confusion that I have."

[*Here follows one of the* Bhāgavata*'s several sections on creation.*]

The Tale and Teachings of Lord Brahmā: The Primordial *Yogī*

Yoga Blueprint

Brahmā is the creator of the universe, but a secondary creator, more like an engineer: he does not create the primordial matrix of prakṛti, *which as we know is a* śakti *power of Kṛṣṇa, but is designated to create the forms of the universe from this preexisting stuff. He too is a mortal being with a finite life span. Known also as Hiraṇyagarbha, Brahmā is of interest for a number of reasons, one of which is that he is considered the primeval founder of* yoga *according to tradition,*[24] *the primordial* yogī. *In this, he is associated with first imparting the practices in the original teachings known as the Hiraṇyagarbha Treatise (which is no longer extant but referred to in various texts).*

The narrative here makes several important points. One important yogic message is that even Brahmā, the most intelligent being in the universe, is utterly incapable of perceiving or even understanding Viṣṇu. The limitations of even the most powerful intellect in understanding God is thereby delineated. It is only after he has performed the requisite austerities that Viṣṇu reveals Himself as well as Vaikuṇṭha, the Kingdom of God. The subtext here as everywhere else in the text, is that such a vision can never be attained by one's own intellectual or even yogic *prowess, but only by devotion (see also* Gītā *11.54). However, while devotion is paramount and autonomous, Brahmā nonetheless had to perform intense austerities in order to gain this vision.* Tapas, *austerity, the first element in Patañjali's* kriyā yoga *(II.1), is by no means jettisoned in* bhakti.

This tale patches together two different narratives pertaining to Brahmā's vision from two different books of the Bhāgavata.

Book II, Chapter 5

1. Nārada said:
"Homage to you, Brahmā, lord of the celestials! You are the firstborn being, and the progenitor of all other beings. Kindly explain to me the knowledge through which the *ātman* is revealed.
2. Please disclose the truth about this material reality. What is its form? What is its support? From what is it created, O master? On what is it resting? And what is beyond it?
3. After all, your Lordship knows everything, past, present, and future. You know this universe through direct realization, as if it were an *āmalaka* fruit in the palm of your hand, O master.
4. Through your own *māyā* power, you alone create the embodied living beings by means of the physical elements. But what is beyond

you? What is your support? What is your true nature? And what is the source of your perception?

5. Like a spider, you create those beings without fatigue, but you yourself are not created by anyone else; you rest on your own potency.

6. I do not know from where else anything that has form and is nameable[25] can be created, O master, whether it is an entity that is high or low, gross or subtle, or in between.

7. But yet you undertook that severe austerity (*tapas*) with extremely concentrated mind. Because of that you confuse us: you raise a great doubt in our minds as to whether you are in fact the Supreme Being.[26]

8. O omniscient lord of everything! Kindly explain everything that I have asked about so that I may understand by your instruction."

9. Brahmā said:

"This inquiry of yours could not be better, O son! You are blessing me since I am now inspired to explain the glories of *Bhagavān*, O gentle one!

10. What you have said is correct, my child. Since your knowledge about me is limited, you do not know He who is greater than I.

11. I do illuminate the universe, but it has already been illuminated by His effulgence, just as the sun, fire, the moon, the constellations, the planets, and the stars are illuminated by Him.

12. Reverence to *Bhagavān* Vāsudeva [Kṛṣṇa]. It is because of His insurmountable *māyā* illusion that people call me the *guru* of the world; but the fact is that I myself meditate on Him.

13. People with less intelligence, who are bewildered by that *māyā*, think in terms of 'I' and 'my.'[27] But *māyā* herself is ashamed of presenting herself before Him.

14. There is no other thing in reality apart from Vāsudeva, O *brāhmaṇa*,[28] whether in the form of substance, activity, Time, nature, or soul.[29]

15. The celestials are born from Nārāyaṇa's body. The Vedas accept Nārāyaṇa as the supreme, the various worlds accept Nārāyaṇa as supreme, ritual sacrifices are offered to Nārāyaṇa as supreme.

16. Yoga is dedicated to Nārāyaṇa as supreme, *tapas* is devoted to Nārāyaṇa as supreme, knowledge accepts Nārāyaṇa as supreme, and the final destination of life is Nārāyaṇa as supreme.

17. I myself am created by Him, and then, directed by His glance, create the creation. He is the Seer, the Lord, the highest Truth, and the *ātman* of all.
18. Although He is transcendent to the *guṇas*, by His *māyā* potency, He has adopted the forms of the three *guṇas—sattva*, *rajas*, and *tamas*—for the purpose of maintenance, creation, and destruction, O great one.
19. The *guṇas*, which are the basis of material substances, knowledge, and action, continually bind the *puruṣa* in cause, effect, and agency.[30] Although he is free, the *puruṣa* is subject to illusion.
20. He, *Bhagavān* Adhokṣaja [Lord Viṣṇu], is imperceptible because of these three *guṇas*. But he is my *Īśvara* as well as the *Īśvara* of all others, O *brahmaṇa*."

[*An account of creation follows, involving the Sāṅkhya metaphysical categories*.]

Book II, Chapter 6

[*A discussion of the Virāṭ Puruṣa opens this chapter. This involves a meditational form of Viṣṇu associating the limbs of God with various natural phenomenon such as the sun and moon*.]
30. This universe is situated in *Bhagavān* Nārāyaṇa. Although He is beyond the *guṇas* (qualities) of *prakṛti*, He utilizes His own *māyā* for the creation, maintenance, and destruction of the universe. His qualities are wondrous.
31. It is under His appointment that I create the world, and it is under His control that Hara, Śiva, destroys it. He, the controller of the three *guṇas,* maintains it in the form of the great *Puruṣa*, Viṣṇu.
32. Thus I have explained to you, O son, about that which you inquired. There is no existent, moving or non-moving, other than *Bhagavān*.
33. Because I keep Hari fixed in my heart with great intensity, my words have never proved to be false, my dear Nārada, nor has any falsity ever entered my mind, nor have my senses ever fallen into unrighteous ways.
34. Although I am the keeper of sacred lore, and the embodiment of austerity (*tapas*), and although I am honored as the Lord of the progenitors (*prajāpatis*), and although I am immersed in the practice of *yoga* and have fully mastered that practice, yet I do not understand He from whom I myself am generated.

35. I offer homage to His feet—they are all auspicious, destroy *saṁsāra*, and bring all blessings to those who seek them. Even He cannot fathom the omnipotency of His own *māyā*—just like the sky cannot understand its own limit—so how can anyone else understand Him?!

36. Neither I, nor you, nor Śiva understands His real nature, what to speak of other celestials knowing it. Those of us whose intelligence is bewildered by His *māyā* perceive the composition of this world in accordance with our own perspectives.

37. We all glorify the deeds of His *avatāras*, but we do not understand Him in truth. Obeisance to Him, *Bhagavān*.

38. He is the original unborn *Puruṣa*. Every age (*kalpa*) he creates, maintains, and destroys Himself within Himself through Himself.[31]

39. He is pure autonomous knowledge, pervading everything completely. He is the complete Truth, nondual, transcendent to the *guṇas*, eternal, without beginning or end.

40. O sage! Whereas the wise, whose minds, senses, and body are controlled, realize Him, He becomes distorted by perverse argumentation, and disappears.

41. The first *avatāra* of the Supreme is the *Puruṣa*. He is Time, nature, the mind, cause and effect, material substance, the evolutes of *prakṛti*, the qualities of things, the senses, the Cosmic Being (*Virāṭ*[32]), self-luminous, and the aggregate of all moving and non-moving entities.

42.–44. I myself; Śiva; Viṣṇu; Dakṣa, and all the progenitors of created beings; others such as yourself; the rulers of the celestial realms; the rulers of the realms of accomplished *siddhas* who travel through the ether;[33] the rulers of the realm of mortals; as well as those of the lower realms; the lords of the celestial *gandharvas, vidyādharas*, and *cāraṇas*;[34] the lords of the *yakṣas*, *rākṣasas*, serpents, and *nāga* divine snakes;[35] the best among the *ṛṣi* sages and forefathers; the chiefs among the *daityas*, *dānavas*, and *siddhas*; and others who are the foremost among the deceased spirits (*pretas*), evil beings (*piśācas*), ghosts, *kūṣmāṇḍas*, large aquatics, deer, and birds; in short, whatever in this world possesses supernormal qualities (*bhaga*),[36] greatness, potency, fortitude, strength, compassion, beauty, modesty, power, intelligence, amazing color, with form or shapeless, is nothing other than that Ultimate Truth.

45. O sage! The scriptures describe the principal *līlā-avatāras* of the *Puruṣa*, who is the ground of all beings. I will narrate them to you.

Relish them—they are wonderful, and evaporate all the impurities of the ears.

[*A narration of the principal incarnations ensues.*]

Brahmā's Vision of God

Book II, Chapter 9

1. *Śrī* Śuka said:
"O king! No actual connection can exist between the objects of the world and the conscious transcendent soul. It is only because of *māyā* (illusion) cast over the soul that this appears to occur. This is just like one who sees objects in a dream; [there is no actual connection between these objects and the dreamer].
2. The *ātman* appears to have many forms, by dint of *māyā* assuming many forms. Enjoying itself in the *guṇas* of *māyā*, it thinks: 'I am' and 'This belongs to me.'
3. When, on the other hand, its illusion is dissipated, and the soul revels in its own magnificence, which is transcendent to Time and *māyā*, it is then able to renounce both Time and *māyā* and exist in its own autonomy.
4. Worshipped by Brahmā's sincere vows, *Bhagavān* revealed His form to him. He then imparted divine Truth to him so as to remove all doubts about the reality of the *ātman*.
5. Brahmā, the first of the celestial gods and the foremost teacher of the world, sat on his seat and, with a desire to create, reflected [on how he might do so]. But he could not figure out the necessary means for creating the manifest universe.
6. One day, as he was deliberating in this way, the great Lord Brahmā heard a voice from the water below, which twice uttered two syllables. They consisted of the sixteenth (*ta*) and twenty-first (*pa*) letters of the Sanskrit alphabet: (i.e., *tapas*, austerity). This word is the wealth of the ascetics.
7. Upon hearing this, Brahmā looked all around, striving to see the speaker. Upon not seeing anyone else there, he got up from his seat, and decided that the voice had been for his benefit. So, taking this as if it were an instruction to perform *tapas*, he concentrated his mind.

8. Brahmā's intuition was correct. With his breath and mind under control, and with both sets of senses[37] restrained, he performed *tapas* for a thousand years. Brahmā, the greatest performer of *tapas* from all those who perform *tapas*, engaged in *tapas*, illuminating all the worlds.
9. Worshipped in this manner, *Bhagavān* revealed His personal abode to Brahmā. Extolled by men who have realized their own true selves, Vaikuṇṭha is the supreme place. There is nothing higher that exists. It is free of all suffering, illusion, and fear.
10. *Rajas* and *tamas* do not prevail there, nor *sattva* tinged by either of them. Time has no sway there, nor *māyā*—what then to speak of anything else! The attendants of Hari there are worshipped by both gods and demons.
11. These attendants have brilliant dark hues and lotus-petal eyes. They wear yellowish garments and have extremely attractive and beautiful forms. They are effulgent and decorated with the choicest ornaments and medallions of brilliant flawless gems. Their complexions are of coral, gems, or lotus fiber. They wear dazzling necklaces, crowns, and garlands.
12. Just as the sky is illuminated by rows of clouds filled with lightning, so Vaikuṇṭha shone forth, filled with rows of brilliant sparkling flying vehicles belonging to the great liberated souls accompanied by their lustrous female consorts.
13. There, the beautiful Goddess of Fortune, Śrī, offers devotion at the feet of Viṣṇu in various ways through Her potencies, as She reclines on a swing. She is singing of the deeds of Her beloved, as She Herself is glorified by the bees, the followers of Spring.
14. In Vaikuṇṭha, Brahmā saw Viṣṇu, Lord of the devotees, Lord of Śrī, Lord of sacrificial rituals, and Lord of the Universe. Viṣṇu, God Almighty, was being attended to by the most prominent of His associates: Sunanda, Nanda, Prabala, Arhaṇa, and others.
15. Viṣṇu was favoring His servants with kindness, and His glances were like intoxicating nectar. His face had reddish eyes, and bore a charming smile. He had four arms, and wore a helmet and earrings. He wore yellow garments, and bore the mark on His chest of Śrī, the Goddess of Fortune.[38]
16. The Supreme Being was seated on an invaluable throne, surrounded by His four, sixteen, and five *śakti* powers.[39] He was endowed

with His inherent opulences,[40] which are only found in temporary form elsewhere. He was none other than *Īśvara* Himself, enjoying His divine abode.

17. Brahmā, the (secondary) creator of the universe, was overwhelmed inside with bliss at that sight. His body experienced ecstasy, and his eyes were brimming with tears of love. He offered obeisances to the lotus feet of Viṣṇu, in accordance with the practice followed by the great *paramahaṁsa* saints.[41]

18. The beloved Lord felt love toward His cherished Brahmā, who had approached Him expressing such loving feelings, and touched him with His hand, smiling gently. Brahmā was worthy of His personal direction in the creation of the species, and so Viṣṇu spoke with illuminating words to the great seer.

19. *Śrī Bhagavān* said:

'O Brahmā, source of the Vedas! I am hardly satisfied by the *tapas* of false *yogīs*,[42] but I am fully satisfied by your *tapas*, which you have performed for a long time with the desire to create.

20. Blessings upon you! Choose any desired boon from Me, the Lord of boons, O Brahmā! The perfection of human austerities culminates in a vision of Me.

21. After hearing that [voice], you performed *tapas* for a long time, so I wanted you to have a vision of My divine abode.

22. When you were bewildered as to how to perform your work, it was I who inspired you how to do so. *Tapas* is my heart, and I personally am the soul of *tapas*, O sinless one.

23. *Tapas* is very hard to perform! I create this universe by *tapas*, and then consume it again by *tapas*. I maintain the universe by *tapas*. My potency lies in *tapas*.'

24. Brahmā said:

'O *Bhagavān*! You are seated in the heart (cave)[43] of all beings, and are the supervisor of all beings. So You certainly see their desires with clear insight.

25. Therefore, O Lord, since I am a supplicant, please grant me that which I seek: I wish to know about both Your higher and lower forms, even though You are devoid of form![44]

26. Invigorated by Your various potencies and through Your own *yogamāyā*, You create, support and destroy this universe in Your own self by means of Your self.

27. Your will is infallible. Like a spider [with its web], You surround Yourself [with Your powers].[45] So please give me the intelligence to accomplish this matter [of creation], O Mādhava [Kṛṣṇa]!
28. Instructed by You, *Bhagavān*, I will act without laziness. By Your grace, although endeavoring in the act of creating the species, I will not be bound by the law of *karma*.[46]
29. You have treated me as a friend to another friend, O Lord! When I undertake the creation of species, I will divide creatures without any confusion, fixed in Your service. But, since I am renowned as "the unborn one," let the madness of pride not arise within me.'
30. *Śri Bhagavān* replied:
'Follow this knowledge that I have disclosed, along with its accessories (*aṅga*[47]), which bestows direct realization of the Truth. It is mystical and intimate knowledge.'
31. By My grace, I bestow upon you realized (perceived) knowledge of Truth, namely, My own self as I am, My states of being, and My forms, qualities, and activities.

[*The following four verses are considered by certain commentators to contain the essential philosophy of the entire* Bhāgavata Purāṇa *and are known as the* Catuḥ Ślokī, *"four verses."*]

32. In the beginning [before creation], I alone existed—there was nothing else beyond, neither cause nor effect. After [creation], whatever exists is I, and after [annihilation] whatever remains is I.
33. One should know that things which have no objectivity are revealed or obscured within My own nature because of My *māyā*, just like light and darkness reveal and obscure things.
34. Just as the great elements [ether, air, fire, water, and earth] have both entered and not entered all beings, so I have also entered and not entered all beings.[48]
35. At least this much should be the object of inquiry concerning the *ātman* by means of reason and argument[49] by a seeker of Truth: that it always exists everywhere.
36. Remain fixed in this knowledge by practicing the highest *samādhi*, and your good self will never be subject to illusion, age after age."
37. *Śrī* Śuka said:
"After the immortal Lord Hari imparted these instructions to Brahmā,

the most eminent among mortals, He withdrew His form, before Brahmā's very eyes.

38. Brahmā offered his folded hands in homage to Hari, the object of the senses, who had disappeared. Being the repository of all living entities, Brahmā then engaged in the creation of this universe, as he had previously.

39. Once, Brahmā, the overseer of creation and of *dharma,* desiring the well-being of created beings, observed the *yamas* and *niyamas*,[50] principles of *yoga*, with a desire to accomplish his purpose.

40.–41. O king! Nārada, always true to his vows, was the most beloved of Brahmā's inheritors, and served him with his good disposition, humility, and discipline. Desiring to hear about the *māyā* of Viṣṇu, the Lord of *māyā*, the great *bhāgavata* sage pleased his father Brahmā.

42. When he saw that Brahmā, the great grandfather of all the worlds, was satisfied, Nārada, the celestial sage, inquired from him the same thing you are asking me.

43. Since Brahmā, the creator of beings, was pleased, he recited to his son Nārada this *Bhāgavata Purāṇa*, distinguished by ten defining characteristics.[51] It had previously been spoken to him by *Bhagavān*.

44. Nārada recounted it to the supremely powerful sage Vyāsa on the banks of the *Sarasvatī* river, O king, as he was meditating on the supreme *Brahman*.

45. Since you have asked about how this world came from the cosmic *Puruṣa*, I will now thoroughly recount how this took place, along with answering other questions."

Book III

The Tale and Teachings of Lord Brahmā, Version II

Book III, Chapter 8

10. At that time, this universe was immersed in water. Viṣṇu had closed His eyes—although His ability to perceive is never obscured—and was lying alone [upon the waters] on the bed of the king of serpents (Śeṣa), without exertion. He was waiting for the right time, and absorbed in the bliss of His own self.
11. With the subtle elements withdrawn within His body,[1] Viṣṇu aroused His power (*śakti*) of Time, and remained upon those waters, His resting place, just like a fire concealed within wood, its potency remaining latent.
12. After sleeping on the waters for a thousand cycles of the four *yugas*, the blueprint for creation was revealed by His own power called Time, which had been stirred to action by Him. Then, Viṣṇu gazed on all the worlds dissolved in His body.
13. This matter within Him was agitated by the *guṇa* of *rajas*, which, in turn, had been activated by Time [in the form] of Viṣṇu's glance permeating subtle matter. After it had been stirred, it manifested forth from the area of His navel.
14. Through the instigation of Time, which awakens *karma*, this matter sprang up suddenly in the form of a self-manifested calyx of a lotus, illuminating that vast expanse of water, like the sun.
15. Viṣṇu then entered that lotus. It was a manifestation of all the *guṇas*, and [contained] the universes. Within it, the one they call

Svayambhū (Brahmā, the self-manifest one), the creator and the Veda personified, was manifest.

16. Seated on that lotus stem but not being able to see the worlds within it, Brahmā moved [his neck] around in space with strained eyes. As a result of this, he obtained four heads, one for each of the directions.

17. The lotus was surrounded by the waters buffeted by waves agitated by the winds which bring about the end of the cosmic cycles (*yugas*). Mounted upon it, that first among the celestials could not understand the nature of the worlds, nor even of his own self:

18. "Who am I, this person situated on the top of this lotus? And from where has this solitary lotus on the water come? There must be something existing here beneath it upon which it is resting."

19. Deliberating in this way, the unborn Brahmā entered the waters through the fibers in the stalk of the lotus. Then he went down the rough lotus stalk, seeking its source, but could not find it.

20. As the unborn one was seeking his source in the absolute darkness, a long time passed by. Time is the weapon that generates fear in embodied beings and wastes away their life spans, O Vidura.

21. When his endeavor proved unsuccessful, the god desisted from this, and returned back to his resting place. He sat down, slowly controlled his breath, stilled his mind, and undertook the practice of the *yoga* of *samādhi*.[2]

22. After performing the practice of *yoga* for a period corresponding to a person's life span, wisdom eventually dawned in Brahmā.[3] Then, he saw in his heart the appearance of something that he had never seen before.

23. Brahmā saw a solitary Being lying in the waters [that fill up the universe] at the end of the *yuga* cosmic cycle on a couch made up of the coils of the vast cosmic serpent Śeṣa.[4] Śeṣa was white as the lotus fiber, dispelling the darkness with the radiance from the jewels of his myriad hoods.

24. This Being surpassed the beautiful appearance of an emerald mountain with vast golden peaks; with garments of evening clouds; filled with flowers, herbs, waterfalls, and gems; garlanded by forest flowers, and with trees as feet and bamboos as arms.

25. His body, which enveloped the three worlds, could only be compared to itself in breadth and extension. The [beauty] of His various

divine ornaments and garments was enhanced by [the beauty] of His bodily appearance.[5]
26. Out of grace, He displayed His feet, which were like lotuses, their charming leaflike toes separated by the luster of their moonlike nails. These feet fulfill all desires, and are worshipped through various practices by those people seeking to fulfill personal desires.
27. His face was welcoming, its smile removing the afflictions of the world. It was decorated with gleaming earrings, reddened by the reflection of His *bimba*–fruit colored lips, and had a beautiful nose and eyebrows.
28. He was beautifully adorned, with a garment golden as the filament of a *kadamba* flower, and with a belt around His waist, dear Vidura. He wore a priceless necklace and His beloved *śrīvatsa*[6] on His chest.
29. He was like the most majestic of trees in creation, with roots in *brahman*,[7] and branches in the form of His thousand arms covered by the choicest gems and valuable armlets, and in the form of shoots enveloped by the coils of the great serpent Śeṣa.
30. *Bhagavān* was like a great mountain, the abode of moving and non-moving entities. He was the companion of Śeṣa, who was immersed in the water, His thousand heads appearing like golden peaks of the mountain. The *kaustubha* gem that He wore was like a jewel from the mountain's mines.
31. Hari was bedecked by a garland of forest flowers, which was made of His own glories, and which was beautified by the utterances of the Vedas in the form of swarms of bees. He could not be approached even by the celestial gods of the sun, moon, wind, and fire, and was unassailable, being encircled throughout the three worlds by His weapons.
32. At that same moment, lord Brahmā, the [future] creator of the universe, who had the know-how to create the worlds, also saw the lotus growing from the pond of Viṣṇu's navel, along with his own self, the waters, the wind, the sky, and nothing else.
33. Influenced by *rajas,* the seed of action, Brahmā desired to create offspring, but he could only see the aforementioned things to be in existance. So, inclined toward the act of creation, he fixed his mind on *Bhagavān*, whose ways are mysterious, and glorified the Lord, who is praiseworthy.

Book III, Chapter 9

1. Brahmā said:
"I have realized you today, after a long period [of *tapas*]. It is lamentable that this Your nature, *Bhagavān*, is not known by embodied beings. Actually, there is nothing other than You—anything else is false. You appear to be manifold because of the mixture of the *guṇas* of *māyā*.
2. This form of Yours was manifest in the beginning out of compassion for the saintly, so as to reveal its nature as pure consciousness. It is eternally free from *tamas*, and it is the seed from which hundreds of *avatāras* manifest. I myself manifest from the lotus growing out of the navel region of this form.
3. O Supreme Being! I do not see anything higher than this form (*svarūpa*) of Yours; it is pure bliss, inconceivable, and of infinite radiance. It is the cause of the senses and sense objects, and the source of the universe, yet it transcends the universe. I take refuge in You.
4. You are the source of auspiciousness for the world! Perhaps this form was manifest in meditation (*dhyāna*) to bless we who are Your worshippers. Obeisance to You, *Bhagavān*! I submit to You! This form is spurned by the unrighteous who live a hellish life.
5. But You never depart from the lotus of the hearts of those people who imbibe through the channels of their ears the fragrance of Your lotus feet carried by the wind of the sacred texts.[8] They cling to Your lotus feet with the highest *bhakti*.
6. For as long as people do not accept Your lotus feet, which bestow fearlessness, they are afflicted by greed, humiliation, unlimited desire, and lamentation caused by family, body, and possessions. They are also afflicted by the false notion of possessiveness, the root of all sorrow.
7. Those misfortunate people whose senses are averse to contact with Your Lordship, which removes all inauspiciousness, are worthy of compassion. Their minds overwhelmed by greed, they engage in deeds for some petty pleasure, which only lasts for a fleeting moment, and which always ends up being counterproductive.
8. O Viṣṇu! My mind becomes despondent upon observing beings incessantly tormented by hunger, thirst, and the three humors,[9] as well as by winter, summer, wind, and rain. They are also tormented by their mutual dealings among themselves because of the fire of lust, as well as anger, which is so difficult to bear, O Acyuta.

9. O Lord. As long as a person, due to the power of *Bhagavān's māyā*, sees this body as existing for the purpose of sensual indulgence and as separate from You, he or she will not surpass this *saṁsāra*. Although it is ephemeral, *saṁsāra* causes abundant suffering as the fruit of action.
10. Even sages in this world are caught up in the cycle of *saṁsāra*, O Lord, because of being averse to connecting with You, and their endeavors are destroyed by Fate. Their minds filled with various desires, they engage their senses in the day with great frustration, and experience insomnia at night, their sleep interrupted constantly.
11. O Lord! The path to You for people is from the connection attained through hearing about You. You reside in the lotus hearts that are pervaded by *bhakti yoga*. Out of compassion for Your devotees, You appear in whatever form they meditate upon.
12. Out of compassion for all beings, although One entity, the Lord is situated as the internal *ātman* within all the various entities,[10] although He cannot be attained by the unrighteous. But He is not pleased by the celestial hosts, whose hearts are bound up with material desires, even when worshipped with elaborate paraphernalia.
13. It is the adoration of You, *Bhagavān* that is the real purpose of acts by people, whether by means of worship, severe austerities, charity, ritual sacrifice, or other various deeds. *Dharma* which is offered to You is never vanquished.
14. I offer obeisance to You, O Supreme *Īśvara*! Your enjoyment and pastime (*līlā-rāsa*) is the cause of the creation, maintenance, and dissolution of this universe.[11] You are the wisdom of intelligence by which the illusion of differences is evaporated. Your wonderful form (*svarūpa*) is eternal.
15. I revere Him, the unborn One. Those who recite His names, and the deeds and qualities of His *avatāras*, which resemble those of humans, at the moment of death, even if they do so unintentionally,[12] immediately throw off the impurities of many lives and attain the fullness of immortality."

[*Brahmā continues to glorify Hari.*]

26. Maitreya said:
"After having seen the source of his own self, by means of his austerity, wisdom, and *samādhi*, and after having glorified Him

as far as words and thought can allow, Brahmā fell silent, as if exhausted."

The Tale of Queen Devahūti: The Mystic Powers of *Yoga*

Yoga Blueprint

The story of sage Kardama and Queen Devahūti is noteworthy in its illustration of the mystic powers that accrue from intense meditational practices (a subject matter that occupies almost a quarter of the Yoga Sūtras*). These powers are associated with asceticism throughout the entire history of Indic literature, Hindu, Buddhist, and Jain, from the earliest Vedic textual sources right into the ongoing hagiographies of modern mystics. The classic eight mystic powers include* prākāmya, *the ability to fulfill one's will, and* īsitṛtva, *the ability to control and rearrange the elements, which we see in this story in Kardama's ability to create an aerial palace at will and fill it with desirable objects. Among other supernormal feats, he then expands himself into nine different forms (see* Yoga Sūtras *IV.4–5).*

[*Prologue*: *Kardama, a forest-dwelling ascetic, was offered the hand of Princess Devahūti, who had long been in love with him. He agreed to the marriage on the condition that as soon as she would beget a child, if she so wished, he would leave and take the vow of* sannyāsa, *the fourth stage of life as a wandering ascetic. Devahūti agreed to this condition.*]

Book III, Chapter 23

1. Maitreya said:
"After her parents had departed, the chaste Devahūti, who was expert in reading the moods of her husband, served him constantly with love, just like Bhavānī (Pārvatī) served her husband, Lord Śiva.
2.–3. Dedicated and attentive, O Vidura, and renouncing desire, deceit, aversion, greed, sinfulness, and pride, Devahūti continuously satisfied her noble husband through her affection, service, and loving words offered with intimacy, purity of heart, respectfulness, and self-control.
4.–5. She was submissive and emaciated by observing vows over a long period, and was expecting great blessings from her husband who

was more powerful than Destiny. From his side, with a voice trembling with love, and overwhelmed with affection, Kardama, foremost of the divine sages, spoke to Devahūti, the daughter of Manu, who had been so devoted.

6. Kardama said:

'O daughter of Manu, now I have become pleased by your exceptional service and complete devotion. This body is very dear to embodied beings, but you have neglected it in renunciation for my sake. You have been very dedicated.

7. I now bestow upon you divine vision. See how I, dedicated to the pursuit of the goal of life, have obtained the Lord's blessings by dint of my *yogic* practice, learning, *samādhi*,[13] and austerities (*tapas*).[14] You have attained those same blessings, through your service to me. These blessings lift one beyond fear and lamentation.

8. What is the use of other material achievements, which are repeatedly destroyed by the raising of the eyebrows of Lord Viṣṇu[15] [that is, by Time]? You have attained perfection. Enjoy the divine fortunes you have earned from the performance of your *dharma*. These are hard to achieve by those types of men who have the perverse ambition of becoming kings.'

9. Kapila was versed in all the spiritual knowledge systems, and when Devahūti observed him speaking in this way, she became free of anxiety. Her smiling face beaming with bashful glances, she replied with her voice slightly choked with love and modesty.

10. Devahūti said:

'Lord, best of the twice-born *brāhmaṇas*, naturally I already know that [all] this has been achieved by you, the master of mystic powers (*yogamāyā*). But offspring are a more precious gift to women who have been virtuous [than mystic powers]. Moreover, you once made the promise that one day we would unite intimately.

11. My mind is overwhelmed with love incited by you, but my body, which is full of sexual desire, is wasted and emaciated. Please make suitable arrangements in accordance with the scriptures[16] so that it can be made attractive. And please create a suitable place [for our sexual union], my Lord.' "

12. Maitreya said:

"Then, O Vidura, Kardama, desiring the satisfaction of his beloved, situated himself in *yogic* meditation, and [with his *yogic*

powers] created a flying palace that could travel according to one's wish.[17]
13. It was a celestial palace that fulfilled all desires. It was replete with all kinds of gems, adorned with pillars of jewels, and generated all types of wealth and prosperity.
14.–15. It was filled with celestial paraphernalia, and was pleasant in all seasons. It was decorated with a variety of ribbons and banners; resplendent with fabrics, assorted linens, silks, and fine cloth; and there were bees inside buzzing about beautiful wreaths and exotic garlands.
16. It was constructed with different levels placed one on top of the other. The place was delightful, with seats, fans, couches, and beds placed here and there.
17. It was adorned with various types of artwork placed all about, and was magnificent with emerald floors and coral daises.
18. Resplendent with doors inset with diamonds and with coral thresholds at the entranceway, the palace was crowned with golden urns on its sapphire turrets.
19. It was designed with very valuable arched doorways of gold, and had assorted canopies built into the walls. These walls were inset with diamonds and rubies that looked like eyes.
20. It echoed here and there with the cooing of flocks of pigeons and swans. These kept flying up again and again, mistaking artificial [birds] to be their own kind.
21. Kardama was himself astonished by its pleasure grounds, resting places, bedchambers, courtyards, and patios, all designed to delight!
22. Kardama, who knew the minds of all creatures,[18] addressed himself to his wife, who was staring at this spectacular house, her mind ill at ease.
23. 'Bathe in this lake, O timid Devahūti, and then ascend into this palace. It is a sacred place created by Viṣṇu and fulfills the wishes of human beings.'
24. The lotus-eyed Devahūti, who was wearing dusty clothes and whose hair was matted, accepted the words of her husband.
25. Her body was covered with dirt and her breasts were speckled with grime. She entered the sacred pure waters of the *Sarasvatī* river.
26. Within a building inside the lake, she saw ten thousand young girls who were all youthful and as fragrant as lotuses.

27. When they saw Devahūti, the women immediately rose up and addressed her with folded hands: 'We are your maidservants. Instruct us as to what we can do for you.'
28. The respectful women bathed the wise Devahūti with costly bathing paraphernalia, and offered her new, spotless, fine-quality cloth.
29. They gave her exquisite, valuable shiny ornaments. They fed her with foodstuffs of every flavor, and gave her an inebriating nectar drink.
30. After this, Devahūti saw herself [in a mirror]: she was clean, wearing spotless garments and a garland, receiving great honor from the maidservants, and blessed by the gods.
31. Bathed and with washed hair, she was decorated with all kinds of ornaments, bracelets, tinkling golden ankle bells, and a golden necklace.
32. She was adorned with a golden girdle decorated with jewels placed over her hips, a pearl necklace, and golden ornaments of great value.
33. She had beautiful teeth and eyebrows, and her eyes, which rivaled the lotus, had slightly moist corners. Her face was glowing with bluish curls.
34. As soon as she thought of her beloved husband, the best of sages, she immediately found herself with her thousand maidservants in the very place where Kardama was to be found.
35. Upon observing her husband before her and the thousand maidservants accompanying her, Devahūti fell into a state of confusion from witnessing his display of *yogic* power.
36. Devahūti had been bathed clean, and her lovely breasts covered. Unlike her previous condition, she now appeared effulgent, revealing her original beauty.
37. She was beautifully dressed and was being served by the thousand celestial females. Love arose in the benevolent Kardama, and he brought Devahūti to the palace.
38. Kardama's [*yogic*] glory was not dissipated in that palace, even though he was devoted to his beloved and received personal service from the celestial damsels.[19] He was as effulgent as the beautiful moon, lord of the rows of blooming night lotuses, surrounded by stars in the sky.
39. Praised by the *siddhas*, perfected beings,[20] he enjoyed for a long time in that palace in the valleys of Meru, king of the mountains.

Delightful with breezes, which are the friends of Cupid, and the auspicious sounds of the *Gaṅgā* river's descent,[21] these valleys were the pleasure grounds of the celestial guardians of the eight directions. Surrounded by groups of damsels, Kardama resembled Kuvera, treasurer of the celestials.

40. Fully satisfied, he enjoyed with his wife in the celestial gardens of Vaiśrambhaka, Surasana, Nandana, Puṣpabhadraka, Caitrarathya, and in the celestial Mānasa lake.

41. Moving like the wind through the realms of the universe in that magnificent and resplendent palace, which could travel at his will, Kardama outdid the celestials in their vehicles.

42. What is there that is difficult to attain for those people whose minds are controlled? They take shelter at Kṛṣṇa's feet, which remove distress.

43. After showing his wife the extent of the wondrous sphere of the universe with all its manifestations, the great *yogī* returned to his *āśrama*.

44. Kardama divided his body into nine forms and gave sexual pleasure to his beautiful wife, the daughter of Manu, who was eager for sexual pleasure. They enjoyed for many years; but these passed as if in an instant.

45. Reclining in that palace in the company of her very handsome husband on a magnificent bed, which enhanced sexual pleasure, Devahūti was not aware of the passing of Time.

46. In this manner, through the power of *yoga*, one hundred years went by in the twinkling of an eye for the couple who were enjoying themselves, eager for sexual pleasure.

47. The powerful Kardama, knower of the *ātman* and knower of everyone's desires, considered Devahūti as his other half. He divided himself into nine personal forms and deposited his semen in Devahūti.

48. Consequently, Devahūti gave birth that very day to nine female babies. They were delightful in every limb, and as fragrant as the red lotus.

49. Seeing her husband setting out to leave home [as per their agreement[22]], Devahūti, who desired [a son] was smiling externally, but inside her heart was agitated with distress.

50. Her face downcast, she scratched the ground with her foot, with its beautiful jewel-like nails, and spoke sweetly with her charming voice, holding back her tears.

51. Devahūti said:
'Everything that you promised me, my Lord, I have received. Nonetheless, dedicated as I am to you, kindly provide me with security.
52. O *brāhmaṇa*, your daughters will find suitable husbands for themselves. But there should be someone to free me from anxiety when you set out for the forest.
53. Enough of wasting so much of my time in attachment to sense indulgence. [On account of this], I had given up [seeking] the Supreme Soul, my lord.
54. Attached to you, I indulged in sense gratification, ignorant of your higher nature. Despite this, please bestow fearlessness upon me.
55. Attachment, when placed in unrighteous people out of ignorance, is the cause of *saṁsāra*; but when placed in the righteous, it leads to nonattachment.[23]
56. A person whose work in this world does not lead to *dharma*, or to detachment, or to the service of Viṣṇu, is actually as good as dead, even though living.
57. I am surely such a person: I have been utterly deceived by the Lord's illusion (*māyā*) because, despite obtaining you, the giver of liberation, I did not desire liberation from bondage.' "

Book III, Chapter 24

1. Maitreya said:
"The compassionate sage, remembering what had previously been declared by Viṣṇu,[24] replied to the praiseworthy daughter of Manu, who was speaking despondently in this way.
2. The sage said:
'Do not torment yourself in this manner, O princess: you are blameless. The infallible Lord will shortly enter your womb.
3. May you be blessed: you have been firm in your vows. Worship *Īśvara* with faith, charity, wealth, austerities, moral observances (*niyama*),[25] and sense control.
4. Viṣṇu, as your son, will spread my fame. Worshipped by you, [He will impart to you] teachings on the subject of *Brahman* and cut the knot in your heart.' "[26]
5. Maitreya said:
"With great respect, Devahūti fully trusted the advice of Kardama,

who was one of the *prajāpatis*.[27] She worshipped the Supreme Soul (*puruṣa*), who is the most worthy of worship.
6. After the passing of many moons, the Lord, Madhusūdana [Viṣṇu][28] entered into the seed of Kardama and took birth from Devahūti, like fire from wood.
7. At that time, hosts of clouds and musical instruments resounded in the sky. Celestial *gandharvas* sang and *apsarās* danced joyfully.[29]
8. Divine flowers fell, thrown by celestials traveling in the heavens,[30] and everything became pure: the directions, the waters, and people's minds.
9. Brahmā, along with sages such as Marīci,[31] arrived at the location of Kardama's *āśrama*, which was encircled by the *Sarasvatī* river.
10. Brahmā, who is unborn and self-manifest,[32] knew that the Supreme Godhead had taken birth through His pure partial manifestation.[33]
11. Offering homage to Lord Viṣṇu with pure mind, his spirits enlivened because of that which the Lord intended to do [teach the truths of Sāṅkhya], Brahmā spoke as follows to Kardama.
12. Brahmā said:
'I have been fully honored by you without offense, my dear Kardama. You are respectful to others and have respected my instruction that I previously imparted to you.
13. Sons should perform service to the father in exactly this manner. One should accept the words of the *guru* with gravity, saying: "This will definitely be done."
14. These chaste daughters of yours with beautiful waists, dear Kardama, will certainly increase this creation manifold with their own progeny.
15. Therefore, bestow your daughters in marriage today, according to their wishes and personalities, to the best of the sages, and thereby spread your fame throughout the world.
16. O sage, I know that the original Person [Viṣṇu] has incarnated by His own power and assumed a body as Kapila, a treasure trove for all beings.
17. He has golden hair, lotus eyes, and lotus feet marked with the lotus.[34] By means of *yoga*, wisdom, and knowledge, He will pull out the roots of action performed in ignorance.[35]
18. He, Viṣṇu, the destroyer of the demon Kaitabha,[36] has entered your womb, O Devahūti, daughter of Manu. After cutting your knot of doubt and illusion, He will wander over the earth.

19. This son will be known in the world as Kapila, and will be highly esteemed by the great teachers of the Sāṅkhya knowledge system.[37] He will wander about spreading your fame.' "
20. Maitreya said:
"After encouraging the couple, Brahmā, 'the Swan,'[38] the creator of the Universe, returned on his swan carrier back to his abode, the highest place in the three realms,[39] accompanied by the four Kumāras[40] along with Nārada.[41]
21. O Vidura, Kardama, who received instructions from Brahmā in this way, did as had been instructed. After Brahmā had departed, he bestowed his daughters to the progenitors of the universe.[42]
[. . .]
26. When Kardama understood that Viṣṇu, chief of the gods, had incarnated, he approached Him in private, offered Him homage, and addressed Him:
27. 'At last, after a long time the gods are definitely pleased with those who are burning in hell due to their own misdeeds.[43]
28. Ascetics in secluded places strive to see God's feet by means of pure concentration (*samādhi*) in undeviating *yoga* practice that has matured over many births.[44]
29. That same Supreme *Bhagavān* has today taken birth in the homes of vulgar folk such as us. Disregarding our offenses, He nourishes the aspirations of His devotees.
30. *Bhagavān* broadcasts the fame of His devotees. You have incarnated in my house desiring to establish the knowledge [of Sāṅkhya philosophy] and fulfill Your promise truthfully.
31. [Although] You are without [material] forms, whatever forms please Your devotees are pleasing to You, O *Bhagavān*![45]
32. I offer homage to You. Even Your footstool[46] is always worthy of worship by sages desiring to understand the Truth. You possess complete beauty, potency, knowledge, fame, renunciation, and power.[47]
33. I offer respects to You, Kapila. Your power manifests simply by dint of Your own will. You are the maintainer of the worlds, and You are the three *guṇas*.[48] Through Your intelligence You absorb the material manifestation back into Your own self. You are the Supreme Person, the creation, cosmic Intelligence, Time, and the wise Seer of Truth.
34. Today I am submitting a request to You, O Lord of beings: following the path of the roaming ascetics, I wish to wander forth, free

from sorrow, connected to You in my heart. All my obligations have been erased by You, and all my desires fulfilled.'

35. The Lord said:

'Whatever is spoken by Me in worldly or spiritual matters is authoritative for people in the world. This is the reason for My taking birth in your family: to fulfill what I previously told you, O sage.

36. This birth of Mine in this world is to reestablish the teachings of Sāṅkhya—the analysis of the ingredients of material reality. This knowledge in the matter of self-realization is highly esteemed by those desiring liberation from the subtle body.[49]

37. This path toward realization of the soul is difficult to understand, and so had disappeared, lost due to the passing of the ages. Please know that I have assumed this body in order to reestablish it.[50]

38. Go as you please, with My approval. Overcome Death, which is so hard to overcome, by dedicating all your actions to Me; worship Me to [attain] the state of immortality.

39. I am self-luminous, the hidden refuge within all beings. Without anxieties, you will perceive Me, the [Supreme] *Ātman*, in [your own] *ātman* through the *ātman*.[51] At that time you will attain the state of fearlessness.

40. I will impart spiritual knowledge, which puts an end to all *karma*, to My mother. By this knowledge, she will overcome fear.' "

41. Maitreya said:

"Kardama, the progenitor of species (*prajāpati*), addressed in this way by Kapila, circumambulated Him,[52] and joyfully set out for the forest.

42. The sage, fixed in the vow of silence and absorbed in the *ātman*, wandered forth over the earth, without any company, without residence, and neglecting the sacred ritualistic fire.[53]

43. He fixed his mind on *Brahman*, which is beyond the real and unreal.[54] Although it itself is devoid of the *guṇa* qualities (*sattva*, *rajas*, *tamas*), yet it is through *Brahman* that the *guṇas* are manifest.[55] It can be experienced only by exclusive devotion.[56]

44. Kardama was without ego, without sense of ownership, beyond all dualities,[57] perceiving all beings equally, and the seer of his own inner self. He was fixed, his mind peacefully turned inward, like an ocean whose waves are calm.[58]

45. Freed from the bonds of (*saṁsāra*), he realized his own self by means of the highest devotion to God, Vāsudeva, the omniscient inner Soul.

46. He saw God, *Bhagavān*, as the Supreme Soul situated within all beings, and all beings within *Bhagavān*, the Supreme Soul.
47. With his mind free from desire and aversion, and seeing everything equally, Kardama attained the divine destination by engaging in devotion to God."

The Teachings of Lord Kapila: Sāṅkhya *Yoga*

Yoga Blueprint

The result of the union between Kardama and Devahūti is the birth of Kapila, an incarnation of Viṣṇu. Kṛṣṇa informs us in the Bhagavad Gītā *(IV.7–8) that He descends into the world, among other reasons, to reestablish* dharma. *This is the* bhakti *notion of* avatāra, *the incarnating of Viṣṇu into the world in times of need. Of particular relevance to Yoga, however, is that tradition recognizes Kapila as the original expounder of the Sāṅkhya system of philosophy.*[59] *Yoga operates within the metaphysical contours provided by the Sāṅkhya principles—indeed, while later tradition pairs Sāṅkhya and Yoga as "sister schools," earlier sources, including the* Gītā *(V.4–5) consider them one and the same—Sāṅkhya providing the metaphysics, and Yoga the practices relevant to liberating the soul,* ātman/puruṣa, *from the world of matter,* prakṛti.[60]

Kapila's instructions to his mother represent classic Yoga teachings embedded in the highly devotionalized context of bhakti. *This section contains some of the most important core teachings of the* Bhāgavata*: many of the verses illustrating the teachings of* bhakti *in part 1 are found in these instructions. Particularly noteworthy are the teachings on the experience of birth, as well as on the process of dying and the fate awaiting those who have squandered their human life after the moment of death.*

Book III, Chapter 25

1. Śaunaka spoke:
"Although He Himself is actually unborn, Kapila, who is *Bhagavān* in person, took birth through His spiritual potency as the expounder of Sāṅkhya philosophy, so as to impart knowledge of the *ātman* to mankind.
2. My life force[61] is never satiated from repeatedly hearing about the Lord of the Vedas.[62] He is the best of men, and the foremost of all *yogīs*.

3. Please narrate to me whatever deeds the Lord performed through His own potency and out of His inherent free will. I am a faithful soul, and these deeds are praiseworthy."

4. Sūta replied:

"At this, feeling pleased at being requested in this way about metaphysical subjects, the noble Maitreya, the friend of Vyāsa, proceeded to speak the following words to Vidura."

5. Maitreya said:

"After His father had set out for the forest, Lord Kapila resided there in that forest of Bindusara, desiring to please His mother, Devahūti.

6. One day, remembering the words of Brahmā, the creator, Devahūti asked her son, when He was sitting leisurely, to disclose the highest path to Truth."

7. Devahūti said:

"I am completely disgusted with the illusory thirst for sense pleasure, O Lord. I have fallen into a state of darkest ignorance, O Master.

8. You are the guide over that dense darkness of ignorance (*tamas*), which is so difficult to overcome. By Your grace, today, after many births, I have gained my eye of Truth.

9. Your Lordship is truly the Primeval God, the Supreme *Īśvara* of humankind. You are the eye of the world, which is blinded by ignorance (*tamas*). You are like the risen sun [which dispels darkness].

10. This impediment in this life—the notion of 'I,' 'me,' and 'mine' [the ego]—was created by You.[63] Therefore, it is You, O Lord, who should dispel my illusion.

11. I offer homage to You. You are the supreme Knower of the real goal of life. I desire to know about [the relationship between] *puruṣa* and *prakṛti* (spirit and matter). I have submitted myself to You for refuge, because You are worthy of refuge. You are the axe [that cuts] the tree of *saṁsāra* for Your dependents."

12. Maitreya said:

"Kapila, His handsome face gently smiling, listened to the faultless request of His mother, and welcomed it in His mind. A request such as this advances the goal of liberation for saintly people who are self-controlled."

13. The Lord said:

"I hold the Yoga system directed toward the *ātman* to be the highest goal for humankind. From this comes the ultimate detachment from happiness and distress.

14. Today, I will explain to you that same Yoga system that I imparted of old,[64] O sinless lady, inclusive of all its limbs (*sarva-aṅga*).[65] This is the *yoga* of the sages who are eager to hear.

15. Consciousness is considered to be [inclined] toward either bondage or liberation. Attached to the *guṇas* [it experiences] bondage; on the other hand, devoted to the Supreme Person, [it experiences] liberation.[66]

16. When the mind is freed from the impurities of desire and greed, etc., which are produced from the false notion of 'I,' 'me,' and 'mine,' it becomes pure, equipoised, and transcends happiness and distress.

17. When this occurs, a person [realizes] the soul as autonomous, transcendent to *prakṛti*, eternal, self-effulgent, minute, and indivisible.

18. When consciousness is immersed in knowledge and renunciation as well as devotion, one realizes that *prakṛti* acts with indifference;[67] through this realization, its power is dispelled.

19. There is no auspicious path for *yogīs* to attain *Brahman* that is comparable to the practice of *bhakti* to *Bhagavān*, who is the Universal Soul.

20. The sages know that it is attachment that is the ever-present snare of the soul. Yet, when directed to the *sādhus* (ascetics), attachment opens the door to liberation.[68]

21. The virtues[69] of a *sādhu* are tolerance, compassion, friendship toward all beings, holding no enemies, and peacefulness.

22. *Sādhus* perform staunch *bhakti* to Me with undeviating minds. For My sake, they have abandoned all actions, and they have renounced family and friends.

23. Fully absorbed in Me, they hear and narrate the relishable narratives of My activities. The various sufferings [of the world] do not afflict them, since their consciousness is absorbed in Me.

24. These *sādhus*, O virtuous lady, are free of all attachments—indeed, they themselves remove the faults of attachment [from others]. So you should aspire for their association.

25. From association with saints, the realization of My power arises. These narratives of My activities become pleasing to the ears and the heart. By enjoying them, faith, love, and devotion quickly manifest consecutively on the path to liberation.

26. By means of *bhakti* and the contemplation of My creations, a person experiences the arising of detachment from sensual pleasure—whether pleasure experienced in the past or heard about in scripture.[70] Engaged on the path of *yoga*, and intent on the control of the mind, such a person will persevere with correct *yogic* practices.

27. Such a person, through not dedicating himself or herself to the *guṇas* of *prakṛti*, but rather through dedication to knowledge, the cultivation of detachment, *yoga* focused on Me, and *bhakti*, attains Me, while still in this world. I am the innermost Soul."

28. Devahūti said:

"What type of *bhakti* to You is optimal, and what should my sense activity be, by means of which I can easily attain Your abode, *nirvāṇa*?[71]

29. O You who are the essence of *nirvāṇa*, what is the nature of that Yoga centered on *Bhagavān* that You previously spoke about?[72] How many limbs of *yoga* (*yoga-aṅgas*) are there, by which [one attains] an understanding of Truth?

30. Explain those to me, a woman,[73] O Lord, such that I can easily understand that which is difficult to understand by your grace. My understanding of such things is limited."

31. Maitreya said:

"After understanding the intention of His mother in this way, Kapila felt love for her—He had, after all, taken birth from her body. So He spoke to her about the knowledge of Truth transmitted down [through the ages] that they call Sāṅkhya, as well as about the *yoga* of the various forms of *bhakti*."

32.–33. The Lord said:

"*Bhakti* to *Bhagavān* has no cause. It consists of *sattva* in the activities of the senses[74] and it includes the performance of action prescribed by scripture. It is the natural state of the mind when it is fixed [on God], and is more profound than [conventional] liberation. *Bhakti* dissolves the subtle body quickly,[75] just like the digestive fire burns food that has been eaten.

34. The *bhāgavata* devotees associate among each other and celebrate My deeds [when I incarnate in the world]. Their endeavors are devoted to Me, and they are satisfied in serving My feet.[76] Some of them do not desire to attain oneness with Me.[77]

35. These saints, O mother, perceive My beautiful Divine forms, with their reddish eyes[78] and smiling faces, and they converse with them with pleasing words. These forms bestow blessings.
36. *Bhakti* leads those whose hearts and life forces have been captivated by those forms to My subtle abode,[79] even if they did not desire this. These forms have captivating limbs, sweet words, smiling glances, and perform wondrous pastimes.
37. I am the Lord of *māyā*, but these saints do not desire My majesty, nor Godly opulence,[80] nor the power that ensues from the eight-limbed path of *yoga*,[81] nor the beauty of the Supreme.[82] They nonetheless attain all these in My abode.[83]
38. O mother, you are the embodiment of peacefulness. Those who place Me as the Supreme will never perish, and My weapon, the ever-vigilant Time, does not destroy them. For such people, I am their intimate soul, the son, friend, teacher, well-wisher, and beloved deity.
39.–40. They have renounced this world, as well as that world beyond [the celestial realms],[84] and the [subtle] body that travels between both of them. In this world they have renounced everything—friends and family, wealth, livestock, and household—and they worship Me alone, the all-observing Godhead, with exclusive devotion. I take these devotees to the place beyond death.
41. The oppressing fear [of death] cannot be removed by any means other than by I Myself, *Bhagavān*, the *Īśvara* of *puruṣa* and *prakṛti*, and Supreme *Ātman* of all beings.
42. Out of fear of Me, the wind blows, out of fear of Me, the sun burns, and out of fear of Me, Indra[85] makes the rain pour and Death perform its task.
43. Immersed in knowledge and renunciation and engaged in *bhakti yoga*, the *yogīs* fearlessly take shelter of My feet for deliverance.
44. The mind fixed on Me through the ardent practice of *bhakti yoga* becomes steady. It is only in this manner that ultimate perfection manifests in people in this world."

Book III, Chapter 26

[*We have omitted this chapter as it includes a highly technical and theistic rendition of the evolution of the Sāṅkhya metaphysical categories.*]

Book III, Chapter 27

1. The Lord said:
"Although situated in *prakṛti*, the soul is not affected by the *guṇas* of *prakṛti*. This is because it is unchanging, is not an agent, and is transcendent to the *guṇas*. It is like the sun [reflected] on the water[86] [which remains unchanged although its reflection in the water may appear to change].
2. When this soul is absorbed in the *guṇas* of *prakṛti*, deluded by the ego,[87] it thinks: 'I am the doer.'
3. Because of this, one enters the state of *saṁsāra* against one's will, and is frustrated. As a result of becoming entangled with the negative consequences of action,[88] one [finds himself] in good, bad, or mixed births.
4. Although the objects do not actually exist[89]—just like the appearance of misfortunes in a dream—*saṁsāra* nonetheless does not cease for one who contemplates the objects of the senses.
5. Therefore, by the intense practice of *bhakti yoga*, one should gradually make the mind, which has been attached to the path of illusion, indifferent [to the objects of the senses], and bring it under control.
6. Endowed with faith, one should [bring the mind under control] by practicing the principles of *yoga*—the *yamas* (moral precepts), etc.,[90] and listening to narratives about Me with real affection for Me.
7. Detached, [one should control the mind] by equanimity to all creatures, by being hostile to none, by celibacy, by silence, and by the performance of one's duty which has become more powerful [by being offered to God].
8. The sage is satisfied with whatever comes spontaneously. He is measured in eating, dwells in a solitary place, and is peaceful, friendly, compassionate, and self-possessed.
9. By dint of knowledge and perceiving the reality of *prakṛti* and *puruṣa*, he does not create false attachments to this body and its relationships.
10. Transcending the states of the intelligence[91] and renouncing all other conceptions, the seer of the self realizes the self by means of the self,[92] as clearly as one sees the sun with one's eyes.
11. He perceives it as distinct from the subtle body, a reflection of the real in the unreal.[93] It is the true existent, the friend, the perceiver

of that which is nonreal and nondual, and it is that which pervades all reality.
12. This is just like when one's reflection in water is seen by one standing on land. It is like the sun which is perceived through its reflection situated in a body of water although it itself is situated in the heavens.
13. In this way, the threefold ego [in *sattva*, *rajas*, and *tamas*] is characterized by its reflections made of the mind, senses, and physical body. It is through this ego, which contains the reflection of the truth, that the *ātman*, the seer, is realized.[94]
14. When the gross and subtle elements, mind, and intelligence, etc., are merged in *prakṛti* during sleep, the seer remains awake, free of ego.
15. At the time of deep sleep, when the ego has ceased to function, the seer falsely thinks that the self has ceased to be, although it has not ceased to be, just like a person who is afflicted when his or her wealth has been lost.
16. Contemplating this, one realizes that the one who is the support and animator of all things including the ego, is the *ātman*."
17. Devahūti said:
"O *brāhmaṇa*, *prakṛti* can never free the *puruṣa*, because of the mutual interdependence of the two of them since beginningless time.
18. Just as the existence of smell can never be separate from the element of earth, or taste from water, so in the same way the intelligence (*buddhi*) can never be separated from the higher self, the *ātman*.
19. How can liberation occur while the *guṇas* are still active? The bondage of *karma* envelops the passive *puruṣa* within them.
20. Sometimes, through contemplation on the true nature of reality, the great fear [of *saṁsāra*] can be curbed somewhat. But because its cause has not ceased, it again reappears."
21.–23. *Śrī Bhagavān* said:
"By performing one's *dharma* with a pure mind without attachment to the results; by intense *bhakti* to Me over a long period of time nourished with hearing about Me; by knowledge, which perceives the true nature of the world; by strong detachment; by the practices of *yoga* performed with austerity (*tapas*); and by intense concentration on the *ātman*, *prakṛti*, which engulfs the *puruṣa* day and night, gradually disappears, just like the wooden kindling stick that produces fire becomes consumed [by the fire].

24. *Prakṛti*'s imperfections have been experienced so many times, and she has been renounced in the past after her sensual pleasures (*bhoga*) have been exhausted. At this point, she can no longer create imperfections for the *ātman*, which is now situated in its own glory.
25. This is just like a dream, which brings many inauspicious images to a sleeping mind, yet is not able to cause delusion for one who is awake.
26. In the same way, *prakṛti* can never cause harm for one who has seen the nature of reality, whose mind is fixed on Me, and who delights in the *ātman*.
27. After a period of many lifetimes, the sage who delights in his own *ātman* in this manner is completely detached from everything up to the highest celestial realm of Brahmā.
28.–29. My *bhakta*, awakened to his true purpose, easily attains by My abundant grace his own ultimate nature, perfection, known as liberation (*kaivalya*) even while still in this world. When he has become detached from the subtle body, the *yogī* is fixed and his doubts are destroyed by dint of directly perceiving his true nature. After attaining this, he never returns [to the world of *saṁsāra*].
30. When the mind of the perfected *yogī* is not attracted by the powers accumulated from *yoga* practice, which is the only way of acquiring them, then he attains My ultimate destination, My dear mother, and death can no longer gloat."

Book III, Chapter 28

1. *Śrī Bhagavān* said:
"I will describe to you the characteristics of *sabīja yoga*, O princess [when the mind is fixed undeviating on an object].[95] By this practice, the mind becomes joyful, and undoubtedly attains the path to Truth.
2. It includes: performing one's duties (*dharma*) to the best of one's capabilities, refraining from unrighteousness, contentment with what is obtained by Providence, worshipping the feet of those who know the *ātman*.[96]
3. Giving up mundane *dharma* and attraction to the *dharma* of liberation,[97] the moderate intake of pure foodstuffs, and living always in a solitary peaceful place.
4. One should practice nonviolence (*ahiṁsā*), truthfulness (*satya*), non-stealing (*asteya*), and adopt only as many possessions as required (*yāvadartha-parigrahaḥ*). One should practice celibacy

(*brahmacarya*), austerity (*tapaḥ*), cleanliness (*śauca*), study (*svādyāya*), and worship the Supreme Being (*Puruṣārcana*).[98]

5. Observing silence, one should become fixed [in a sitting posture] by mastering the appropriate *āsanas*, gradually mastering breath control (*prāṇa-jaya*), and practicing withdrawal of the senses from sense objects (*pratyāhāra*), with the mind fixed on the heart.

6. One should fix the breath on one of the *cakras* (subtle energy centers)[99] of the body with one's mind. One should contemplate the activities of Lord Viṣṇu and become absorbed (*samādhāna*) in that way.

7. By these and other processes, alert, and with controlled breath, one should gradually fix one's mind, which is prone to corrupt and unspiritual ways, with one's intelligence.

8. Once one has mastered *āsana* one should establish a seat (*āsana*)[100] in a clean place, and, sitting comfortably with the body erect, one should perform practice.

9. One should cleanse the passageway of the air by performing *pūra-kumbhaka-recaka* breath restraints[101] or by the reverse processes, such that the mind (*citta*) can become fixed and undistracted.

10. The mind of the *yogī* whose breath is controlled should soon become purified, just as iron, [melted by] fire and fanned by wind, releases its impurities.

11. By *prāṇāyāma* one can burn imperfections;[102] by *dhāraṇā*, one's sins; by *pratyāhāra*, contact with sense objects; and by *dhyāna*, ungodly tendencies.

12. When one's mind is perfectly controlled by the practice of *yoga*, with one's gaze fixed on the tip of the nose,[103] one should meditate on the form of *Bhagavān*.

13. He has pleasing lotuslike features, with reddish eyes like the interior of a lotus, and is dark like the petals of the blue lotus. He bears a conch, discus, and club.

14. His shiny silken garments are yellow like the filament of a lotus, the *kaustubha* jewel adorns His neck, and the mark of *śrīvatsa* His chest.[104]

15. His neck is encircled by a forest garland with intoxicated humming bees swarming about it, and He is adorned by a magnificent necklace, bracelets, helmet, armlets, and anklets.

16. His hips are adorned with a brilliantly shining girdle, and He is seated in the lotus of the heart. His countenance is serene and He has the most beautiful appearance, gladdening the eyes and the mind.

17. He is eternally gorgeous to behold, and is worshipped by the entire universe. He has the youthful vigor of the prime of youth, and is anxious to bestow His blessings upon His devotees.
18. The glories of this exalted person are worthy of recitation in hymns, and bring renown to pious people [who glorify Him]. One should perform meditation (*dhyāna*) upon the entire form of the Lord, until the mind no longer deviates.
19. The activities of the Lord are always attractive. Therefore, with the mind full of pure love, one should meditate upon Him in the core of one's heart as standing, walking, sitting, or lying down.
20. When the mind has attained fixed concentration focused on all His limbs together, the sage should then visualize and fix the mind on *Bhagavān*'s respective limbs, one by one."

[*A detailed visualization of each of* Bhagavān*'s limbs follows here.*]

34. A person, at this point, with heart flowing with love for the Lord, Hari, *Bhagavān*; with hair standing on end from ecstasy; and constantly overwhelmed with streams of tears from intense love, gradually withdraws the hook of the *citta*.[105]
35. At this stage, the mind suddenly attains liberation (*nirvāṇa*), and enters the state of freedom, detached and without objects, like the flame of a lamp [when it is extinguished]. Freed from the flow of the *guṇas*, one now perceives the *ātman*, fully manifest and autonomous.
36. The *yogī*, as a result of this supreme dissolution of the mind, becomes situated in the wonders of the *ātman*. Attaining the nature of the higher self, the *yogī* realizes that the cause of the experiences of pleasure and pain (*duḥkha*) that one had previously attributed to one's own self, were actually occurring in the *ahaṅkāra*, which has no ultimate and enduring reality.
37. The highest *yogī*, who has realized his or her own true nature as *ātman*, is not aware of whether the body is sitting or standing, or whether, by chance, it has reached somewhere or else departed under the control of Fate, just like one who is blinded by intoxication is not aware of whether one is covered by clothing or not.
38. The body along with its life airs remains under the control of Fate for as long as its *karma*, which has already been activated, has not expired.[106] But the *yogī* who has attained *samādhi* and awakened to

the reality of things does not again accept it or its expansions as real, but rather as just a dream.

39. Just as a mortal being is seen as different from sons and wealth, even though they are considered to be one's own, so is the case with the *puruṣa*, which is seen as different from the body and its extensions.

40.–41. Just as fire is different from the firebrand and the sparks and smoke produced from it—it is in fact different even from the very firebrand that is considered identical to it, so the *ātman*, who is the seer, is different from the sense objects, senses, and internal organ. And *Bhagavān*, who is known as *Brahman*, is different both from *prakṛti* and from that which is called *jīva*.

42. One should see all beings in the *ātman* and the *ātman* in all beings, by dint of the fact that all beings have the same nature within the material elements.

43. Just as fire, although one, appears different according to its sources, so the *ātman* situated in *prakṛti* appears different due to the diversity in its embodiments [but is one].

44. Therefore, after transcending one's own *prakṛti*, which is divine and very hard to comprehend, and which has the nature of cause and effect, one becomes situated in one's own true nature.

Book III, Chapter 29

1.–2. Devahūti said:

"You have described the characteristics of *mahat* (cosmic intelligence)[107] etc., and of *prakṛti* and *puruṣa* and the higher nature of these two as outlined in the Sāṅkhya traditions. Now please tell me about their root, the path of *bhakti yoga*. Describe this to me in detail, O Lord.

3. Narrate the various destinations in *saṁsāra* of the embodied *jīvas*. From hearing about these complete detachment can arise in the *puruṣa*, O Lord.

4. Please tell me about that manifestation of *Īśvara* called Time, which is the controller of even the higher celestials. It is because of [the fear of] Time that people perform pious activities.

5. You have appeared as the shining light of *yoga* for those people who are spiritually blind due to false understanding and who have have been sleeping under the false security of *tamas* for such a long

time. They are exhausted because their minds are devoted to activities performed for the satisfaction of desire."

6. Maitreya said:

"The great sage welcomed these gentle words of his mother, O best of the Kurus. Pleased and overwhelmed with compassion, He replied to her."

7. *Śri Bhagavān* said:

"*Bhakti yoga* has many different forms, which manifest in different ways, O noble lady! These ways are differentiated in accordance with their natural *guṇas*. And the mental states of people are distinguished in accordance to these ways.

8. A person considering himself different from others, who performs *bhakti* to Me out of a motive involving violence, pride, or envy, is one in *tamas*, full of anger.

9. A person considering himself different from others, who engages in acts of worshipping the deity with a motive involving desire for sense objects, fame, or power, is in *rajas*.

10. A person considering himself different from others, who engages in worship for the purpose of eliminating *karma*, or as an offering to the Supreme, or because worship is something that ought to be done, is in *sattva*.

11.–12. The characteristic of *bhakti yoga* that transcends the *guṇas* (*nirguṇa*) is described as when the mind flows without cessation toward Me, simply from hearing about My qualities. I am the most intimate refuge. This *bhakti* toward *Puruṣottama*, the Supreme Being, is uninterrupted and free of all motives (*ahaitukī*).

13. Devotees do not accept the five types of liberation—*salokya*, living on the same realm as Me; *sārṣṭi*, having the same opulence as Me; *sāmīpya*, living in My association; *sārūpya*, having the same form as Me; and *ekatvam*, undifferentiated oneness with Me—even when these are awarded, if they are devoid of My service.[108]

14. It is this latter which has been described as the highest type of what goes by the name *bhakti yoga*. By this one transcends the three *guṇas* and attains My abode.

15.–19. Through worship and through performing one's duty without attachment to the results; through regular lavish acts of ritual worship which do not involve any violence; through seeing, touching, offering *pūjā* (ritual worship) and praise, and honoring My deities; through

considering Me to be in all living entities; through *sattva*; through detachment; through offering respect to the great saints; through compassion to the less fortunate; through friendship with those who are one's equals and through following the *yamas* and *niyamas* (moral virtues); by hearing spiritual discourses; by chanting My name congregationally (*nama-saṅkīrtana*); through uprightness and association with noble people; through abandoning ego; through these qualities the mind of a person dedicated to Me becomes purified. Then he or she easily draws close to Me, simply by hearing of My qualities.
20. Just as the flow of wind delivers a smell from its source to the nose, so the mind devoted to *yoga* is carried to the Supreme.
21. I am always present in the *ātmans* of all beings.[109] A person disregarding this performs deity worship in the temple that is hypocritical.
22. One who worships Me in the form of the Deity, but, out of ignorance, disregards Me as *Īśvara* in the form of the *ātman* residing in all beings, offers only ashes.
23. The mind of a person who does not see others as equal, honoring Me but hating other entities, who is fixed in hostility with other beings, does not attain peace.
24. O sinless lady, I am not satisfied when I am worshipped in the Deity through the performance of rituals conducted with all sorts of paraphernalia by a person who is disrespectful of other living beings.
25. One should worship Me as *Īśvara* through deity worship and such things, performing one's duty, until one sees Me in one's own heart, and situated in the hearts of all beings.
26. To one who makes a distinction between his own belly and that of others, I inflict great fear in the form of Death. Such a person does not see all beings as equal.
27. Therefore, by means of charity, respect, and friendship, and with equanimity, one should honor Me as residing as the embodied *ātman* in all beings.
28. Living entities are superior to nonliving entities, O pious lady, and among them, those that have life airs (*prāṇa*) are higher. From these, those that have developed minds (*citta*) are higher, and from these in turn, those with sense perception are higher still.
29. Even among these, those that have the sense of taste are higher than those who have the sense of touch, and higher than these are

those with the sense of smell, while those with the sense of hearing are superior.

30. Entities who can distinguish forms are higher than these, and from these those with teeth in two jaws. From these, many-legged creatures are higher, from which the quadrupeds are best, and the two-legged beings higher still.

31. From these, those who respect the fourfold caste division of society are better, and from these, the *brāhmaṇas* are best. From among the *brāhmaṇas*, the knower of the Veda is higher, and better than him, the one who knows the true meaning of the Vedas.

32. One who can remove all doubts is better still, and one who performs his or her *dharma* superior again. Higher still than this is the performance of *dharma* free of all attachments, without seeking any benefit for oneself.

33. From all these, the soul who has completely dedicated his or her wealth and works to Me is best of all. I do not consider any living entity superior to a person whose soul is dedicated to Me, who has renounced all works to Me, who realizes he or she is not the ultimate doer of action,[110] and who sees all beings equally.

34. One should honor all these living beings with one's mind, considering that it is *Īśvara*, *Bhagavān*, who has entered them in the form of his partial manifestation,[111] the *jīva* (embodied *ātman*).

35. My dear lady, I have explained to you both *bhakti yoga* and the eight-limbed path of generic *yoga*. By means of either one of these, a person may attain the *puruṣa*.

36. This *puruṣa* is transcendent to *prakṛti*. It is a form of *Bhagavān*, who is *Brahman*, the *Paramātman*, and Destiny, the force behind *karma*.

37. That which is the source of the changes in the forms of all matter from *mahat* (*buddhi*, the macro cosmic intelligence),[112] to the microatoms of Sāṅkhya, is known as divine Time. It is because of Time that those who do not see the oneness behind all things[113] experience fear.

38. The one who enters all entities, who is the sustainer of everything, and who annihilates them through other entities is known as Viṣṇu. He is Time, the Master of all rulers. He is the Lord of sacrifice.

39. No one is dear to Him, no one an enemy, and no one a friend. Ever vigilant, He approaches in the form of Death those people who are forgetful.

40. It is out of fear of Him that the wind blows, it is out of fear of Him that the sun shines, it is out of fear of Him that the god Indra showers rain, and it is out of fear of Him that the host of stars shine.
41. It is because of Him that the trees along with the plants and creepers bear their fruits and flowers at their appropriate times.
42. It is because of Him that the frightened rivers flow, that the ocean does not rise up beyond its bounds, that fire blazes, and the earth along with its mountains does not collapse.
43. It is under the control of Him that the sky provides space for all breathing creatures, and the first macro-evolute of *prakṛti*, the *mahat*, expands its body into the universe, covered by its seven sheaths.[114]
44. It is out of fear of Him that the divinities, who oversee the functions of the *guṇas*,[115] and in whose power lie all moving and non-moving entities, perpetuate creation, maintenance, and destruction in every *yuga*, age.
45. Time is the eternal destroyer. It has no beginning but is the cause of all beginnings. It causes the birth and destruction of people through other people. It brings death even to the celestial Yama, the Lord of death."

Book III, Chapter 30

1. Kapila said:
"People do not realize the mighty power of this Time. They are like a row of clouds, impelled forward by a powerful wind.
2. Whatever object a person attains after great difficulty for the purpose of finding happiness, *Bhagavān* destroys. The person then laments when this happens.
3. It is because of illusion that a person believes the household, property, and possessions of this vulnerable body, along with its relationships, to be stable.
4. Irrespective of whatever womb one transmigrates into in this worldly existence, once there, one finds satisfaction in that species; one never becomes averse to it.
5. Bewildered by the divine *māyā*, even when situated in hell, one does not wish to relinquish even that birth, as one finds one's pleasure in hellish experiences.
6. A person whose heart has been deeply captivated by friends, wealth, livestock, homestead, offspring, wife, and body thinks himself great.

7. With every limb of his body burning with anxiety created by these, an evil-minded fool engages in never-ending sins.
8. His senses and mind are stolen by the enchantment of unchaste women in the form of sweet words conducted in secret encounters, and by the sweet babblings of his young children.
9. Ever committed to the false *dharma* of the household which only produces unhappiness, the householder thinks himself happy when working to counteract the suffering.
10. He maintains his family with wealth secured by means of great violence from here or there. Although he himself ends up consuming only whatever remnants are left over, it is he who attains lower births because of his [methods of] maintaining them.
11. When his means of livelihood fails, he tries again and again. Overpowered by greed, and becoming feeble, he covets the possessions of others.
12. Unsuccessful in maintaining his family, bereft of wealth, and with all his efforts in vain, the poor unfortunate fellow sighs as he broods on his situation, his intelligence bewildered.
13. Because he is unable to support his family, his wife and other dependents cease to offer him the respect they had previously, just like a farmer does to a worn-out bull.
14. Even then in this situation detachment does not awaken in him. Deformed due to the onset of old age, and himself now maintained by his own dependents, he faces death in his own home.
15. He lives neglected like this, his digestion weak, eating little, and with limited energy, eating whatever is placed before him contemptuously like a dog.
16. His eyes dilate from the air flowing up, and his windpipe is blocked by mucus. His breathing becomes asthmatic and he makes a rasping sound in his throat.
17. Lying on his bed surrounded by his relatives who are grieving, he cannot reply when addressed by them, as he has succumbed to the control of the noose of death.
18. In this way, a person whose senses were uncontrolled, and who had been absorbed in family responsibility, dies, his mind overwhelmed by great pain, while his relatives weep.
19. At that moment, two agents of Yama, Lord of death, arrive. They are terrifying, with ferocious eyes. Upon seeing them, his heart is petrified, and he releases stool and urine.

20. They enclose him in a body suitable for inflicting suffering, and bind his neck forcibly with nooses. Then they lead him down a long road, just like the king's soldiers lead a criminal for punishment.
21. Overwhelmed by trembling due to their threats, his heart is terrified by those two, and he is savaged by dogs along the path. Overwrought, he remembers his own past sins.
22. Afflicted by hunger and thirst on that path of burning sand, and without water or shelter, he is scorched by the sun, forest conflagrations, and wind. He is lashed severely on his back with a whip as he walks, even though he is barely capable of doing so.
23. Fainting and collapsing periodically out of exhaustion, he gets up on his feet again and again, and is led forcibly along that awful road to the abode of Yama, Lord of death.
24. He is dragged along this road, ninety-nine thousand *yojanas*[116] long, in two or three hours, and receives his punishments.
25. His limbs are burned after piling firebrands around them. Then his body is devoured—and this is performed sometimes by his own self, sometimes by others.
26. In the abode of Yama, his entrails are pulled out by dogs and vultures while he is still alive, and his body is punctured by the bites of snakes and scorpions.
27. His limbs are torn off one by one, and he is trampled by elephants. He is thrown off the peaks of mountains, and he is enclosed in caves filled with water.
28. Whether man or woman, he experiences the punishments of the hellish realms of *Tāmisra*, *Andhatāmisra*, and *Raurava*,[117] merited due to their mutual sexual indulgences.
29. Even here on earth, dear mother, heaven and hell are perceived; hellish punishments are visible here, too.
30. In this manner, one who only maintains his family or fills his own belly in this world, after leaving these behind and going to the next world, experiences the appropriate fruits of his actions.
31. He alone is the one who attains darkness after giving up this physical body, which he had maintained by means of enmity to other beings. His own inauspicious deeds are his only provisions for the journey.
32. In hell, a person experiences his *karmic* reactions for maintaining his family, which accrue to him by destiny, just like a person who becomes afflicted upon losing his wealth.

33. A soul eager to maintain his family solely through unrighteous means (*adharma*) goes to the hell called *Andhatāmisra*, the deepest destination in *tamas*.
34. From the lower hellish realms, after experiencing the appropriate number of punishments in due order, he can then return again to this realm, purified."

Book III, Chapter 31

1. *Śrī Bhagavān* said:
"A person, encased in a drop of semen, attains the womb of a woman and enters the fetus of an offspring in accordance with his or her *karma* under the direction of Providence.
2. After the first night, he reaches the embryonic stage; after five nights, a bubble; in ten days, the size of a jujube berry; and after that he becomes flesh or an egg.
3. Within a month, a head is formed; within two months, the forms of arms, feet, and other organs; and within three months, the appearance of nails, hair, bones, skin, genitals, and bodily apertures.
4. By four months the seven *dhātus*[118] are formed; within five, hunger and thirst arise. By the fifth month, he moves to the right side of the womb, impelled by the outer skin membrane.
5. The *dhātus* increase by the mother's imbibing of food and drink, etc. He lies in a disagreeable enclosure with stool and urine, a breeding ground of microorganisms.
6. He is bitten all over his body every moment by organisms, and, experiencing great pain because of his softness, he swoons. And he is frequently afflicted by hunger.
7. He is affected by the mother's eating of food that is excessively bitter, spicy, hot, salty, dry, or sour, etc., and pain spreads through all his limbs.
8. Enveloped in the embryo within, and in the intestines beyond that, he lies there, his head pushed toward his stomach, and his neck and back bent.
9. Unable to move his limbs, he is like a bird in a cage. In that situation, by the grace of Providence, he regains his memory of the past hundred births. Remembering these for a long time, he sighs. What happiness can he attain in such a state?
10. After attaining the seventh month, he gains consciousness. He is shaken by the winds of birth and cannot remain in one place, like the other organisms sharing the womb.

11. The wise soul, embedded within the seven layers [of the *dhātus*], frightened and seeking help with prayers, folds his hands in supplication and invokes with faltering words the one who has placed him in the womb:
12. The living entity says:
'I seek shelter in the One who banishes fear, who adopts various bodily incarnations, whose lotus feet wander on the earth out of a desire to protect it and who is worshipped by it. It is due to Him that I have attained this condition, which is befitting me, as I am unworthy and unrighteous.
13. This *ātman* appears bound here, enveloped by its *karma*. It has entered a state of *māyā*, consisting of the bodily elements, senses, and mind. I offer homage to Him who dwells within my suffering heart. He is pure, unchanging, and of absolute knowledge.
14. The *ātman* exists as a distinct entity in this body made of the five elements. I have been covered by Him, but I, the *ātman*, am not the senses, *guṇas*, sense objects, or mind. I offer homage to that sage Supreme Being who is beyond *prakṛti* and *puruṣa*. His greatness has no bounds.
15. Because of His *māyā*, I am wandering on this path of *saṁsāra*, bound by my *karma* and these formidable *guṇas*. Because of this, my [spiritual] memory is lost out of exhaustion. By what means can I discover again that abode [the *ātman*] without the blessings of the great saints?
16. Which other Lord can bestow such knowledge of the past, present, and future? We, who follow the path of *karma* for the *jīvas*, worship him for the cessation of the threefold miseries.[119] By his partial incarnation,[120] he pervades all moving and non-moving beings.
17. The embodied *ātman* has fallen into this pit of stool, urine, and blood, in an enclosure that is inside the body of someone else. Desiring to escape while counting the remaining months, his body is scorched by gastric fire. When will this pitiful-minded one be released, O *Bhagavān*?
18. The *ātman* has been constrained in this situation for ten months by the great kindness of your Lordship, O God. He, the Master of the fallen, should be pleased by His own actions. What else can one do other than to offer Him homage with folded hands?
19. In a body capable of sense control, this *jīva* in the body enveloped by the seven *dhātus* perceives according to intelligence; others

[in nonhuman forms] perceive according to the abilities of their bodies. I perceive that primordial supreme Being revealed both inside and outside, just like the individual soul is revealed.
20. Although I am living in a dwelling place of extreme suffering, O Lord, I do not wish to leave the womb to go into the blind well of the outside world. One who emerges out there encounters the Lord's *māyā*, attains a bewildered intelligence, and enters the cycle of *saṁsāra*.
21. Therefore, free of all concerns, I will quickly extricate myself from *tamas* with the help of my mind which has been devoted to the lotus feet of Viṣṇu, and so has become my friend. By this means, I hope I will never again enter this condition of being in a body with its various outlets.' "[121]
22. Kapila said:
"Having attained wisdom in this way while offering worship, the wise entity of ten months is suddenly propelled downward by the birth airs for delivery.
23. Propelled by that wind, his head is turned downward suddenly and painfully, and he emerges with difficulty, breathless. But his memory becomes erased.
24. Fallen on the ground mixed with blood, he struggles like a worm in excrement, and wails loudly. His knowledge is gone, and he has ended up in the opposite situation [to that for which he had aspired in the womb].
25. He is offered nourishment by people who cannot understand his actual desires, and so when he is offered some unwanted thing, he has no power to refuse it.
26. Lying on a soiled bed, the newborn child is troubled by insects. He is not able to scratch his own limbs, nor sit, stand up, or move.
27. Mosquitoes, bugs, and gnats bite his soft skin as he wails, deprived of the wisdom he had gained, just like worms bite smaller worms.
28. After experiencing the frustrations of infancy and childhood in this way, he later becomes angry out of ignorance, as his desires are unfulfilled. He then becomes immersed in lamentation.
29. His frustration and pride grow as his body grows, and, full of desires, he creates enmity with other lusty people, and brings about his own destruction.
30. Lacking knowledge, the foolish embodied being dwelling in this body made of the five elements, is constantly absorbed in the illusion of 'I' and 'mine.'

31. He performs activities for the sake of his body, but, bound by the reactions of those acts, he ends up perpetuating *saṁsāra*. Bound by those actions that were performed in ignorance, another body follows him, also causing suffering.
32. If, on the path of *saṁsāra*, the person again follows unrighteous people whose energy is devoted to satisfying the stomach and genitals, and he or she enjoys in this way, that person once again enters a state of *tamas*, just as before.
33. From such association, truthfulness, cleanliness, compassion, gravity, intelligence, wealth, modesty, fame, forgiveness, tolerance, self-control, and good fortune become destroyed.
34. One should not associate with such agitated unrighteous ignorant people, who have destroyed their *ātman*. They are like pet deer under the control of women, and pitiable.
35. There is no other bewilderment, entrapment, or other type of attachment as powerful as the attachment to a woman or those attached to women.
36. Brahmā (*Prajāpati*), after seeing his own daughter, became overpowered by her beauty. When she assumed the form of a doe, he shamelessly pursued her in the form of a stag.
37. Among created beings, and beings created by them, and by those created by the latter in turn, what person is there in existence who does not have his mind disturbed by *māyā* in the form of a woman—other than the sage Nārāyaṇa?
38. Just see the power of My *māyā* in the form of a woman: just by the movements of her eyebrows, she makes the conquerors of all the quarters follow at her heels!
39. One who desires to attain the final goal of *yoga*, who seeks the *ātman*, and who has attained the Supreme by service to Me, should never associate with women. The sages say she is the doorway to hell for such aspirants.
40. *Māyā*, created by the gods in the shape of a woman, approaches enticingly. You should regard her as your death, like a well, covered over by grass.
41. Similarly, out of illusion, a woman thinks of a man as her husband, thinking of him as the provider of wealth, children, and homestead, but he is actually also My *māyā*. She attained the state of being a woman due to attachment to women [in a past life as a man].

42. A woman should likewise perceive a man as her death in the form of husband, children, and household sent to her by Fate, just like the singing [of the hunter is death] to a deer.
43. While a person wanders from realm to realm in the subtle body enjoying, he or she performs actions continually.
44. The subtle body follows the *ātman*. The gross body is made of the gross elements and the senses: when it is overwhelmed, death takes place, when it is manifest, birth.[122]
45. Death is when the body, the location from which objects are experienced, becomes incapable of perceiving objects, and birth is when the perception of objects arise from a sense of 'I-ness.'
46. This is just as when the eyes lose their ability to perceive the parts of an object, the power of sight does so, too, and so the seer (*ātman*) becomes incapable of engaging in the function of perception by means of either.
47. Because of all this, a wise person should not be miserly, bewildered, or fearful of life. After understanding the nature of the *jīva*, one should go about in this world free of attachments.
48. Situated in this body, one should go about in this world created by *māyā*, endowed with full insight, intelligence, and detachment gained from the practice of *yoga*."

Book III, Chapter 32

22. Therefore, with all your heart, worship the Supreme with devotion because of His qualities. His lotus feet are worthy of worship.
23. *Bhakti yoga* directed to *Bhagavān*, Vāsudeva, quickly produces detachment (*vairāgya*). The knowledge ensuing from this causes the direct perception of *Brahman*.
24. The mind of such a person does not perceive differences in the form of pleasant and unpleasant caused by the agitation of the senses toward sense objects. Sense objects are in fact, neutral [neither pleasant nor unpleasant], in and of themselves.
25. In this state, one becomes free of attachments, and one's perception become equanimous. One thus perceives the *ātman* by means of the *ātman*.[123] At this stage, one has transcended all notions of acceptance and rejection, and attained the supreme destination.

26. The being *Īśvara* is the Supreme *Ātman* (*Paramātman*), pure consciousness. Although *Bhagavān* is one, He is approached differently according to different perceptions and states of mind.
27. Therefore, complete detachment is the cherished goal that is to be attained by a *yogī* through any and all of the processes of *yoga*.
28. *Brahman* is consciousness. It is unitary and transcendent to the senses. Due to illusion, it appears through the outward flowing senses in forms other than its own and hence it appears as being endowed with qualities of sound, etc. (i.e., the material world).
29. Just as the *mahat* appears as the *ahaṅkāra* (cosmic ego) in its three expressions [*sattva*, *rajas*, and *tamas*] and as the five [gross elements] and also the eleven divisions [mind and ten working and perceiving senses], so the *jīva* has the universe as its body.[124]
30. The controlled mind, free of attachment, can perceive Truth by means of constant faith, *bhakti*, *yoga* practice, and detachment.
31. So that knowledge leading to the perception of *Brahman* has been explained to you, dear mother! Through this knowledge, one can understand the Truths of *prakṛti* and *puruṣa*.
32. *Jñāna yoga* is transcendent to the *guṇas*, while *yoga* is characterized by *bhakti* devoted to Me. Although two, their goal is actually one: He who is known by the word *Bhagavān*.
33. Just as one object containing many qualities is perceived variously by the different senses, so, in the same way, *Bhagavān* although one, is perceived variously by the different paths outlined in the scriptures.
34.–36. By work, sacrifices, charity, austerity, study, and deliberation; by the control of the mind and senses; by the renunciation of deeds performed out of desire; by the practice of *yoga* with its various limbs—and of course especially *bhakti yoga*—by the performance of *dharma* characterized by both desire for the fruits of actions and disinterest in the fruits; by insight into the Truth of the *ātman*; and by firm detachment, by all these means, the self-manifest *Bhagavān* is perceived variously either with qualities or without (*saguṇa* or *nirguṇa*) [depending on the means chosen].
37. I have spoken to you about the four types of *bhakti* [in each of the three *guṇas* as well as that transcendent to the *guṇas*, *nirguṇa*]. I have also spoken to you about Time, the ways of which are unknown, and which lies concealed among living beings.

38. There are many forms of *saṁsāra* for the *jīvas* all created by ignorance and actions. Entering into these, O mother, the *ātman* cannot even understand its own situation.
39. These teachings should never be imparted to rascals, the ill-mannered, fools, transgressors, or those who make a show of religion.
40. It should not be taught to those who are avaricious, nor to those whose minds are attached to their households, nor to non-devotees, and certainly not to those who despise My *bhaktas*.
41.–42. It should be imparted to the faithful, the *bhaktas*, the cultured, those who are not envious, those who have developed friendship for all living entities, those who are dedicated to serving, those who are detached from external things, those whose minds are peaceful, those who are humble, those who are free of ego, those who are pure, and those for whom I am the most precious of precious things.
43. A person who hears this with faith, O mother, and who imparts it with mind fixed on Me, attains My abode immediately.

Book III, Chapter 33

1. After hearing all these words from Kapila, His mother, Devahūti, beloved of Kardama, had the veil of ignorance dispelled. She honored Kapila, the founder of the perfect knowledge characterized by the subject matter of the evolutes from *prakṛti* (*tattvas*), and pleased Him.
2. Devahūti said:
"Only the unborn Brahmā himself, who was born from the lotus growing from Your stomach, could meditate on Your form, lying in the cosmic waters. It is composed of the elements, senses, and sense objects, contains the flow of the *guṇas*, and is the seed for all reality.
3. Your Lordship brings about the creation, maintenance, and destruction of this universe by means of Your own power, which is divided by the flow of the *guṇas*, even though You Yourself have no desires to fulfill. You are the *Īśvara* of the *ātman*, with unlimited powers, and Your will is infallible. You are beyond human comprehension.
4. How is it possible, O Lord, that He in whose stomach this entire universe is situated was born from my womb? He lies alone as a baby on a banyan leaf at the end of the cosmic age (*yuga*) sucking His big toe![125]
5. The purpose of Your assuming a body is to quell the sinful and bestow prosperity on those who follow Your directions. Just as was

the case with Your other *avatāras* such as the boar,[126] so too now You have come to reveal the knowledge of the *ātman*.
6. By hearing and chanting the sacred names, bowing to Him or even just remembering Him occasionally, even a dog-eater immediately becomes qualified to perform the Vedic ritual of pressing the *soma* juice,[127] not to mention seeing You, O *Bhagavān*!
7. *Aho!* My son, even one who cooks dogs becomes honorable if he takes Your name on the tip of his tongue! Those who recite Your name have thereby become *Āryas*, performed austerities, undertaken Vedic rites, taken sacred bath, and studied the Vedas.
8. I offer my respects to You, Kapila. You are *Bhagavān*. You are Viṣṇu, the Supreme Person, *Brahman*, the source of the Vedas. You can be understood by the mind which has reversed the flow of the senses [from outward to inward]. The flow of the *guṇas* is destroyed by Your potency."
9. Maitreya said:
"The Supreme Person, *Bhagavān*, under the name of Kapila, was adored by His mother. Honored in this way, He then spoke to her as follows, with a choked-up voice:
10. Kapila said:
'This path which I have explained to you, O mother, is very easily performed. By following it, you will quickly attain the highest goal.
11. Have faith in these teachings of Mine; they are relished by the knowers of *Brahman*. By following them, you will attain fearlessness. Those who do not know them attain rebirth.' "
12. Maitreya said:
"After Kapila had revealed the path to the *ātman* to that pious lady, He took leave from her, His mother, who had come to realize *Brahman*, and set forth.
13. Then Kuntī became fixed in *yoga* through the instructions on *yoga* that had been spoken by her son. There, in that *āśrama*, the crown of the *Sarasvatī* river, she concentrated her mind.
14. Her curly locks of hair became matted and tawny from repeated bathing. Her body became emaciated from severe austerities, and she wore the bark garments of the ascetics.
15. Her household had been materialized by the *yoga* austerity of her husband, *Prajāpati* Kardama. It was incomparable and envied even by the denizens of the celestial realms.

16. It had couches of ivory resembling the foam of milk gilded in gold, and golden seats with the softest covers.
17. Jeweled lamps shone on pure crystal walls with huge emeralds, and the women were decorated with gems.
18. The gardens of the house were beautified with flowers and celestial trees, and replete with the warbling of pairs of birds, and the humming of intoxicated black bees.
19. The celestials used to sing when Devahūti, caressed by Kardama, entered the pond, fragrant with lotuses.
20. But she was downcast in appearance, desolate due to separation from her son. Then, she renounced this most desirable location, which was envied even by Indra's lady folk.
21. Her husband had already departed for the forest, and now Devahūti became desolate due to separation from her son. Although she had realized the truth of Sāṅkhya, she was affectionate toward Him, like a cow on the loss of her calf.
22. Meditating on her son, Lord Kapila, who is Hari, she quickly became detached from such a residence, O son.
23. As her son had instructed, she meditated on the form of *Bhagavān* with its smiling face as the object of meditation through concentrating on both the entirety of the form and also limb by limb.
24.–25. By means of the force of *bhakti yoga*, by powerful renunciation, by knowledge born from the adherence to the appropriate vows, which is the cause of [knowing] *Brahman*, Devahūti saw the all-pervading Supreme Truth in her purified mind, through direct personal realization. The dualities caused by *māyā* and the *guṇas* then disappeared.
26. Her mind became fixed on *Brahman*, who is *Bhagavān*, the refuge of the *ātman*. Once her impurities had been purified, she attained bliss and her embodied condition as a *jīva* drew to an end.
27. Because of her constant immersion in the state of *samādhi*, all bewilderment caused by the *guṇas* was dispelled. Then she forgot about her body, just as, upon arising, one forgets whatever was seen in one's dream.
28. She was covered with grime, like a fire covered with smoke. But, since she was free of all cares, her body was nourished by others, and did not become emaciated.
29. Her mind was completely absorbed in Vāsudeva, and so she was no longer aware of her own body, which was dedicated to austerity

and *yoga*. Her clothes had fallen off and her hair was in disarray, but her body was now protected by Providence.

30. In this manner, Devahūti followed the path taught by Kapila and attained [the stage known variously as] *nirvāṇa*, *ātman*, *Brahman*, and *Bhagavān*.

31. O hero Vidūra! That place where she attained perfection became a most sacred place. It became celebrated throughout the three worlds under the name of Siddhapada ('the Place of Perfection').

32. Her mortal body, purified by such practice of *yoga*, became a river, O gentle Vidūra. It became a preeminent river, worshipped by perfected beings, as it bestowed perfection.

33. The great *yogī Bhagavān* Kapila then took permission from His mother and also departed from His father's *āśrama*. He set forth for the northeast.

34. Honored by the celestial *siddhas*, *cāraṇas*, *gandharvas*, *apsaras*, and sages, He was provided a dwelling place as an offering by the personified ocean.

35. He remains there, revered by the Sāṅkhya masters, fixed in the practice of *yoga*, absorbed in meditation for the peace of the three worlds.

36. O sinless Vidūra! I have recounted to you whatever you asked of me about the pure discussion between Kapila and Devahūti.

37. Whoever hears this esoteric teaching of *yoga* imparted by sage Kapila, with mind fixed on *Bhagavān*, whose emblem is Garuḍa,[128] will attain the lotus feet of *Bhagavān*."

Book IV

The Tale of Prince Dhruva:[1] The Five-Year-Old *Yogī* Prodigy

Yoga Blueprint

Prince Dhruva's story illustrates a number of important devotional themes. First, as the Gītā *informs us (IX.30–32), there are no gender, caste, class, background, or age disqualifications in the ability to attain success in* bhakti*: Dhruva was a mere five-year-old child. But he exhibited an unstoppable determination and undeviating focus, which are requisites for success in* yoga. *Where Dhruva's tale departs from many of the other stories in the* Bhāgavata *is that his initial motive in his* yogic *practice was purely materialistic—the "mixed* bhakti" *discussed in* "Bhakti *Mixed with Attachment to* Dharma *and* Jñāna." *However, because he was fortunate enough to fix his mind on Viṣṇu in his quest for realizing his ambition, Dhruva's mind was purified of all desires, and he nonetheless attained a divine vision by the grace of Viṣṇu. That* Īśvara *can award liberation on the* yogī *who selects Him as a devotional object of meditation is a theme stressed ubiquitously in all devotional traditions,[2] irrespective, in some cases, of one's initial motivations for undertaking such meditation.*

Dhruva's story also touches on a number of other important themes in yoga*: the need for a* guru *to oversee one's* yogic *practice is illustrated by the appearance of the famous sage Nārada in the story (see* "Satsaṅga *and the* Guru"*). Nārada imparts the* mantra *to the child and provides him with further instructions on the specifics* *of practice. Sacred sound as* mantra *has been foundational to Hinduism from its earliest Vedic origins to the present day. In the devotional traditions, God manifests in the form of sound, that is, the names of Viṣṇu are nondifferent from Viṣṇu in person. Fixing the mind on the* mantra, *then, not only provides a support upon which the mind can rest in meditative states, but affords the mind an opportunity to bathe in the actual and immediate presence of God in sonic form. As was the case with Dhruva, the mind thereby becomes purified of all impurities.*

Another means by which divinity can manifest in the physical world, prakṛti, *is through a deity made of some form of matter—usually stone or metal. This is perhaps the most dominant and ubiquitously visible expression of Hinduism, which, for most Hindus, involves some sort of relationship with a temple and its deities. As discussed in "*Arcana *(Worship)," this is not considered a limitation of God's omnipresence—on the contrary, denying God the ability to manifest in such forms would be a limitation of God's omnipotency (nor is God depleted or minimized thereby, as He personally can manifest in unlimited forms and still maintain a separate presence). Nārada instructs Dhruva to make such a form and worship it according to time and place. The Dhruva story thus exemplifies five distinct experiences of the divine presence: initially in the form of his* guru, *then through the* mantra *and the deity, and finally through direct perception, first as an internal vision, then as an external one. Dhruva's story thus illustrates various forms of divine epiphany.*

Other than this, the Dhruva story illustrates the practice of saṁyama *(*Yoga Sūtras *III.4ff.). By concentrating with the utmost intensity upon an object the mind becomes one with that object and manifests the qualities of that object—a mystic power touched upon in the* anubhūti *chapter of the* Yoga Sūtras *(see III.23, 24). Since Dhruva had fixed his mind on Viṣṇu, who can be seen as having the universe as His body, he became as if one with the universe. Therefore, Dhruva's bodily state of breath restraint was felt by all creatures in the universe owing to this merging of micro and macro realities by intense mental absorption. As the* Yoga Sūtras *makes clear, however, mystic powers are considered attainments only by those still unenlightened as to the true nature of the self owing to the influence of ignorance. Dhruva's embarrassment at his foolish* *initial motives are poignant instructions for those approaching* yoga *with material goals in mind.*

Book IV, Chapter 8

8. Sunīti and Suruci were the two wives of King Uttānapāda. Suruci was dearer to her husband than his other wife, Sunīti, who was the mother of Dhruva.
9. Once, the king lifted Uttama, the son of Suruci, onto his lap, caressing him. But he did not welcome Dhruva, who also wished to climb up.
10. As Dhruva, the son of her co-wife, was trying to do this, the arrogant Suruci enviously said as follows in the hearing of the king:
11. "Dear child, you should not try to climb up on the lap of your father, because, although you are the son of the king, you were not conceived by me in my womb.
12. You are only a child, but nonetheless you should now know that unfortunately you were born from the womb of another woman, not from me. Therefore, you cannot fulfill your wish.
13. If you desire the throne of the king, worship God, the Supreme Being, and attain my womb [in your next life] by His grace."
14. Maitreya said:
"Dhruva's father looked on without saying a word. Pierced by the harsh words of his stepmother, Dhruva went weeping to his own mother, breathing with anger, like a snake struck by a stick.
15. Sunīti lifted the boy onto her lap. His upper and lower lips were trembling, and he was short of breath. After hearing [what had happened] at length from the mouths of the other residents of the palace, she became agitated at what had been said by her co-wife.
16. Losing her composure, the woman, her face beautiful as a lotus, lamented with the burning fire of grief, like twine in a fire. Thinking of the words spoken by her co-wife, his mother spoke, her words choked up with tears.
17. Breathing heavily, the woman, who was unable to see the means of overcoming this intrigue, said: 'Do not wish harm on others, O son. A person who inflicts harm on others himself experiences the same.
18. Suruci spoke the truth: I am an unfortunate woman and you were born in my womb, and reared on my breast. The king, Lord of the earth, is ashamed to keep me, or even think of me as his wife.

19. Accept without hostility whatever your stepmother told you, my son, since it is the truth. If you wish to take a seat like Uttama [on your father's throne], then you should worship the lotus feet of the lotus-eyed Lord [Viṣṇu].
20. It is Viṣṇu who controls the *guṇas* for the purpose of maintaining the universe. Indeed, Brahmā himself, the unborn one, worshipped His feet. As a result of this, Brahmā assumed the supreme post [in the universe] which is honored by the *yogīs* who have controlled their mind through breath restraints.
21. Likewise, the most honorable Manu, your own grandfather, worshipped Viṣṇu with concentrated mind through abundant sacrifices and charity. He consequently gained worldly and celestial happiness, followed by liberation, which is difficult to attain by other means.
22. Take shelter of Viṣṇu, child: He is affectionate to His devotees. His lotus feet are the path [of liberation] sought for by those desiring liberation. Firm in the performance of your personal duty (*dharma*), fix that Supreme Person in your mind and devote yourself to Him exclusively.
23. I cannot find anyone else to remove your frustration other than Lord Viṣṇu with the lotus-petal eyes. Other people seek the Goddess of Fortune, who holds a lotus in her hand, but She herself seeks Him.' "
24. Maitreya said:
"These words spoken by his mother were intended for his welfare. After hearing them, Dhruva controlled his mind with the mind,[3] and set out from his father's city.
25. The sage Nārada overheard all this, and understood Dhruva's intentions. Astonished, he touched Dhruva on the head with his hand, which can remove all sins, and spoke:
26. '*Aho!* Just see the potency of the warrior caste (*kṣatriyas*)—they cannot bear a slight on their pride! Even though this one is a mere child, he has taken the unjust words of his stepmother to heart.'
27. Nārada said:
'My son: I still cannot fathom how notions of honor and dishonor can exist in a young boy like you who is attached to playful games and such things.
28. Even if the distinction [between honor and dishonor] has already made its presence felt in your life, there is no cause for anyone to

be frustrated, other than because of ignorance. People have different lots in life according to their personal *karma*.
29. Therefore an intelligent person should be satisfied with just whatever has been bestowed by Providence, O child. One should understand this as the way to reach *Īśvara*.
30. You now wish to gain His favor by following the *yoga* instructed by your mother. In my opinion, God is definitely not solicited easily by people.
31. Even sages do not find the path that leads to Him, despite searching for many births free from attachments through intense *yoga* practices and states of *samādhi*.
32. Therefore you had better give up this useless endeavor of yours. You can attempt it later, when a better occasion presents itself.
33. An embodied being, who is self-content in whatever situation of happiness and distress has been ordained by destiny, attains the state beyond darkness (*tamas*).
34. If one is overwhelmed with happiness for someone with higher qualities and sympathy toward one with lower qualities, and seeks friendship with one with equal qualities, one is never overcome by difficulties.'[4]
35. Dhruva replied:
'This equilibrium of mind[5] that you have taught out of compassion for people who are afflicted by happiness and distress, good sir, is difficult to realize for the likes of me.
36. I am an uncouth soul and have inherited a fierce warrior nature. Therefore [your instruction] does not take root in my heart, which was pierced by the arrows of Suruci's harsh words.
37. I desire to attain a domain that is the highest in the three worlds, one that has not been ruled over even by our grandfathers, nor by anyone else.[6] Please instruct me about the right path to achieve this goal, O *brāhmaṇa*!
38. Indeed, you, sir, are the son of Lord Brahmā, highest of the celestial beings. Like the sun, you travel about for the welfare of the universe, plucking your *vīṇā* instrument.' "[7]
39. Maitreya said:
"When he heard this response, the honorable sage Nārada was impressed. He replied to the boy kindly, with words of truth.

40. Nārada said:
'The path of Lord Vāsudeva [Kṛṣṇa] taught by your mother will lead you to the ultimate goal. Worship Vāsudeva with your soul dedicated to Him.
41. For one who desires the best for oneself—namely, righteous duty, prosperity, fulfillment of desire, and liberation [the four goals of life][8]—there is only one source for these: service to the feet of Hari [Kṛṣṇa].
42. I wish you good fortune in this, my son. Go to Madhu forest, a holy place on the banks of the *Yamunā* river. The presence of Hari is always in that place.
43. After bathing there constantly in the auspicious waters of the *Kālindī* (*Yamunā*) river, and performing the rites appropriate for you [given your age], dedicate your time there on a suitable seat, *āsana* [for practicing *yoga*].
44. First, cast off, gradually, the impurities of the mind, senses, and life airs (*prāṇa*) by means of the three forms of breath control (*prāṇāyāma*),[9] then you should meditate on Viṣṇu, the [Supreme] *guru* with a fixed mind.[10]
45. He is always mercifully inclined, and His eyes and face are always benevolent. His nose and eyebrows are gorgeous, and His cheeks are delightful. He far surpasses the celestials in beauty.
46. He is youthful and His limbs are attractive. His eyes and lower lip are reddish in color. He is the refuge of His devotees, and the worthy shelter for all humanity. He is an ocean of mercy.
47. He is a personal Being. His color is dark blue, He wears a garland of forest flowers, and He is characterized by the *śrīvatsa* tuft of hair.[11] He has four arms, each one distinct [in holding] a conch, discus, club, and lotus, respectively.
48. He wears earrings and an ornate headdress, and is endowed with armlets and bracelets. His neck is adorned with the *kaustubha* gem, and He wears a yellow silk garment.
49. Girded with a belt of bells, and wearing shining golden anklets, He is the most beautiful sight of everything that is worth beholding. He is peaceful, and enlivening to the eyes and the mind.
50. One should worship His feet, resplendent with the brilliance of His ruby-like toenails. He is situated in the *ātman*. His seat is the pericarp of the lotus in the heart.[12]

51. He is the ultimate bestower of boons. With concentrated mind, one should constantly contemplate Him smiling and casting affectionate glances.
52. When the mind is meditating on the auspicious form of the Lord in this way, it is quickly immersed in supreme bliss and never ceases to be so.
53. Now hear the highest and most intimate sacred sound recitation, *japa*.[13] A person reciting this aloud for seven nights will be able to see the mystic beings who travel through the air,[14] O prince:
54. *"Oṁ namo bhagavate Vāsudevāya."* [Reciting] this *mantra*, one who is wise and understands how to adjust to context, should make a physical form (deity) of the Lord and worship it with various paraphernalia according to time and place.[15]
55. One should worship the Lord with pure water, garlands of forest flowers, roots, and fruits, etc., freshly cut sprouts and stems, and with the *tulasī* plant, which is dear to the Lord.[16]
56. Alternatively, the sage, who is peaceful, whose mind is fixed and speech controlled, and who subsists by frugally eating the produce of the forest, can worship a physical form of the Lord made from earth or water, etc.[17]
57. By means of His inconceivable personal powers, the Lord (*Uttamaśloka*[18]) will perform deeds in the form of the pure activities of His incarnations. One should contemplate those deeds.
58. These acts of worship to God were practiced by the ancients to the best of their abilities. One should concentrate on the Lord by [chanting] the *mantra* in the heart. The Lord manifests in the form of the *mantra*.
59.–60. The Lord increases the loving feelings [of his devotees]. Being worshipped in this way by devotional acts of worship through body, mind, and words by people worshipping free from guile, He bestows welfare such as *dharma*, etc.,[19] to the living entities, according to their desires.
61. Detached from the pleasures of the senses by means of practicing *bhakti yoga* with great seriousness and with mind always absorbed in the Lord, one should worship in this way in order to attain liberation.'
62. Addressed in this way, the prince offered obeisances to Nārada and circumambulated him.[20] Then he entered the holy Madhu forest, which is imprinted by the footprints of Hari.

63. As Dhruva was entering the forest to perform penance, Nārada entered the king's inner palace. He was welcomed with due respect by the king, and after he was comfortably seated the sage addressed him.
64. Nārada said:
'O king, why are you pining with a withered face? Is there something lacking in your pursuit of righteousness, gratification, and material well-being?'[21]
65. The king replied:
'O wise Nārada, my son, a boy of five years, along with his mother, has been banished by me. I am a cruel soul who is under the control of a woman, O great sage.
66. O *brāhmaṇa*, he is without a guardian: may the wolves not have devoured the boy, his lotus face faded, while he was resting, or sleeping.
67. Oh, woe is me! You should consider me to be a cruel-hearted person. I did not welcome Dhruva, who was desiring to climb up onto my lap out of love. I am the lowest of rascals.'
68. Nārada said:
'Don't worry, don't worry! Your son is protected by the gods, O Lord of men. You are unaware of his power: his fame will spread all over the world.
69. He will perform an exceedingly difficult deed even for kings to perform, O master. He will return after a short period of time, O king, and spread your fame far and wide.' "
70. Maitreya said:
"After hearing these words spoken by the celestial sage, the king, Lord of the Earth, ceased paying any attention to the fortunes of the kingdom, and immersed his mind solely in thoughts of his son.
71. Meanwhile, in the forest, Dhruva took a bath, and fasted that night attentively. Then he worshipped the Supreme Being devotedly, according to the instructions of the sage.
72. He passed one month worshipping Hari while eating only wood apple and *jujube* fruits after every three nights and then only as much as was needed to sustain himself.
73. Then, for the second month, as he worshipped the Lord, the boy took for his food withered leaves and grass once every six days.
74. The boy spent the third month with his mind fixed in unbroken concentration (*samādhi*), on the Lord, who is praised in the best of verses, while consuming water only every nine days.

75. He underwent the fourth month meditating on the Lord with his breath under control while subsisting only on air inhaled once every twelve days.
76. When the fifth month arrived, the son of the king stood on one foot as immobile as a pillar while meditating on *Brahman*, with his breath controlled.
77. He withdrew his mind, which is the support of the senses and sense objects, from all objects, and, meditating on the form of *Bhagavān* in his heart, gave up awareness of anything else.
78. Because Dhruva was concentrating on *Īśvara*, the primeval Lord, *Brahman*, who is the support of the entire material manifestation, the three worlds began to tremble.
79. When the boy prince stood on one leg, the earth, being pressed by his toe, inclined on one side, just as a boat, mounted by a tusker elephant, lurches to the left and right at each of its steps.
80. By dint of his undeviating concentration on the Soul of the Universe, Dhruva blocked the pathways of air in the universe as he was meditating.[22] At this, the [denizens of the] other realms, along with their rulers, feeling greatly afflicted on account of their own breathing being blocked, approached Hari for help.
81. The celestials said:
'O Lord, we do not understand the cause of this suppression of air, which is affecting the condition of all beings, moving and non-moving. Therefore please free us from this distress. We have approached You for shelter, since You can bestow shelter.'
82. The Lord, *Śrī Bhagavān*, said:
'Do not fear! I will restrain the boy from his extreme austerities. Return to your abodes. The son of king Uttānapāda has absorbed himself in Me. It is because of this that your breath has been choked!' "

Book IV, Chapter 9

1. Maitreya said:
"Their fear dispelled by these words, the gods offered their respects to Lord Viṣṇu (Urukrama[23]) and set out to their abodes throughout the three worlds. Then, Viṣṇu (the thousand-headed One[24]) also went to Madhuvan (the sweet forest) on Garuḍa, His eagle carrier,[25] with the desire of seeing His servant Dhruva.

2. Viṣṇu, on account of the intensity of Dhruva's mature *yoga* practice, appeared in the lotus of Dhruva's heart, effulgent as lightning. Dhruva beheld Him. Then Viṣṇu suddenly disappeared. [Opening his eyes] Dhruva saw Him standing outside in the same position.
3. Seeing that vision, Dhruva was thrown into confusion. He prostrated his body on the ground like a stick[26] and offered obeisance. Beholding Lord Viṣṇu, the boy was as if drinking Him with his eyes, kissing Him with his mouth, and embracing Him with his arms.
4. Hari is situated in Dhruva's heart—as well as in everything—and understood that Dhruva, who was standing with hands folded in supplication, was intensely desiring to speak, but did not know how to do so. Out of compassion, He touched the boy on the cheek with his conch shell, made of *Brahman*.[27]
5. At this, Dhruva understood the will of the Supreme Being, whose glories are widespread. Absorbed in devotional feelings, he slowly offered to the Lord in praise the divine words that had been bestowed upon him with which to do so. Dhruva's [future] abode, the polestar, would remain permanent[28] [see IV.9.19–20 below].
6. Dhruva said:
'You, the possessor of all power, have entered within me and, with Your own power, have animated these words of mine from their state of dormancy, as well as my other [faculties]—hands, feet, ears, skin, etc.—and my life airs, too. Obeisance to You, *Bhagavān*, the Supreme Being.
7. O *Bhagavān*, You are the one Supreme Person. Through Your personal powers, You create all the primordial material ingredients of this world, which consists of the vast *guṇas* and is known as *māyā*.[29] You then enter the ever-changing *guṇas* and illuminate them, like fire lighting up an assortment of wood.
8. Lord Brahmā was completely surrendered to You, O Lord, and so perceived the universe by means of the wisdom bestowed by You, like a person awakening from sleep.[30] Your lotus feet were the refuge for Brahmā when he was seeking liberation—what learned person would forget them? You are the friend of the downtrodden.
9. You are a wish-fulfilling tree.[31] You bestow birth, death, and liberation. Certainly those who desire the gratification of this body, which is like a corpse, and worship You for other things [apart from liberation] are people whose intelligence has been stolen by Your

illusory power (*māyā*). Such sense pleasure is available even for people in hell.

10. The pleasure [experienced] by embodied beings from meditating on Your lotus feet or from hearing about Your deeds from Your devotees does not exist in *Brahman*, even though that is also a part of Your own majesty, O Lord.[32] What to speak, then, [of the lesser pleasure experienced by the residents of the celestial realms], who fall from their celestial air-vehicles,[33] when struck by the sword of Death.

11. Let me always have the association of those great pure-hearted devotees, who are constantly immersed in devotion to You, O unlimited One. With this, I will become intoxicated with drinking the nectar of the narrations about You, and easily cross over the ocean of material existence, brimming with grave dangers.[34]

12. O Lord with the lotus navel! Your devotees' hearts are enamored by the fragrance of Your lotus feet. Those who associate with them forget about this mortal life, sons, friends, households, wealth, and wives.' "

[. . .]

18. Maitreya said:

"Upon being glorified in this way by the intelligent and noble-hearted Dhruva, the Lord, who is affectionate to His devotees, greeted him kindly, and spoke as follows.

19. The Lord said:

'I know the resolve in your heart, O prince. Your have upheld your vow, so I will grant you that boon [which you desired], even though it is one that is hard to attain.

20. My dear boy, one place that has never been ruled over by anyone else is the polestar, an effulgent unmoving realm. The circuit of the luminaries, stars, constellations, and planets revolves around it.

[. . .]

25. After this life, you will go to My abode [Vaikuṇṭha[35]]. It is beyond [the realms] of the sages, and worshipped by all the realms.' "

26. Maitreya said:

"Thus, the Lord, who had been worshipped in this way, bestowed His personal abode on Dhruva. Then *Bhagavān*, whose banner bears the emblem of Garuḍa,[36] returned to His abode while the boy was watching.

27. Dhruva returned to the city. Although he had fulfilled his wish and attained the fulfillment of his resolve by serving the feet of Viṣṇu, the boy was not very happy in mind."
28. Vidūra spoke:
"How is it that Dhruva considered his own personal goal to be unfulfilled? He understands the goals of human life.[37] In just one life, he obtained the supreme abode, which is achieved by worshipping the feet of Hari, the possessor of *māyā*!"
29. Maitreya said:
"Dhruva's heart was pierced by the arrows of his co-mother's words. Because of harboring them in his mind, he did not desire liberation from the Lord of liberation. It is because of this that he became distressed.
30. Dhruva said:
'Even the celibate Sanandana and his brothers[38] did not attain the Lord's abode in one birth through their *samādhi*, whereas I attained the shelter of His feet in six months. But my mind was fixed on some other goal, and so I squandered the opportunity.
31. *Aho!* Just see my materialism. I am so unfortunate: after attaining the lotus feet of the One who can dispel *saṁsāra*, I asked for something that was temporary instead.
[. . .]
33. I perceived reality through the lens of differences,[39] and so, after submitting to the influence of illusion (*daivī-māyā*),[40] I behaved like someone asleep. Even though there are no differences [in reality], I was tormented in my heart by the scourge of enmity toward my brother.
34. I requested Him for something useless—like requesting medicine for someone already dead. The Soul of the Universe is very hard to please, yet, after having managed to please Him with austerities, I then went and requested Him for *saṁsāra*[41]—He who can dispel *saṁsāra*. I am so foolish.
35. Alas! Like a fool who, because of little merit,[42] requests some meager chaffed rice from someone who is a sovereign, I, because of illusion, requested for my pride [to be upheld] from the Lord who was offering me His own personal abode.' "
36. Maitreya said:
"People like yourself, dear Vidūra, who relish the dust of Mukunda's [Kṛṣṇa's] lotus feet, aspire to His servitude with no desire for personal

benefit. They feel satisfied in their minds with whatever comes along providentially.
37. After hearing that his son was returning, as if coming back from the dead, the king could not believe it: 'I am so wretched. How has this good fortune come for me?'
38. But, believing the words of Nārada, the celestial sage, the king was overwhelmed with a surge of joy. In an ecstatic mood, he bestowed a very valuable necklace as a gift to the bearer of the news.
39.–40. Eager to see his son, he mounted his chariot decorated with gold and drawn by trusty steeds, and hastily set out from the city to the sound of conches, drums, flutes, and the chanting of Vedic *mantras*. He was surrounded by *brāhmaṇas*, family elders, ministers, and friends.
41. His two queens, Sunīti and Suruci, adorned with golden ornaments, mounted a palanquin along with Uttama, and also set forth.
42. In the vicinity of the small forest, the king hastily got down from his chariot when he saw his son arriving. He quickly approached Dhruva, immersed in loving feelings.
43. The king, whose mind had long been full of regret and who was breathing heavily, embraced his son with his two arms. Dhruva's bonds of sin had been entirely destroyed by the touch of the lotus feet of the Lord of the Universe.
44. Then, the king, his heart's burning desire fulfilled, smelled his son's head repeatedly,[43] and bathed him with the cold tears from his eyes.
45. Dhruva, the most righteous of people, was lovingly welcomed and honored with blessings. He offered obeisance to his father's feet, and then bowed his head to his two mothers.
46. Suruci picked up the boy who was prostrated at her feet, embraced him, and, with a voice stammering with tears, said: 'May you live long.'
47. Just as water spontaneously [gravitates] to a lower place, all living beings offer respect to one who has pleased the Lord by means of one's qualities, friendly behavior, and such.
48. Uttama and Dhruva, both trembling with love for one another, shed torrents of tears continuously, their hairs ecstatically standing on end from the contact of each other's bodies.

49. Dhruva's mother, Sunīti, embraced her son, who was dearer to her than even her life airs. Full of joy from the touch of his body, she gave up her grief.
50. O hero Vidūra: the breasts of the mother of the hero were moistened by auspicious tears flowing from her eyes, and milk flowed from them continuously.
51. The people praised that queen: 'Your son had been lost for such a long time. But by good fortune he was regained and has removed your anguish. In the future, he will be the protector of the entire earth.' "

Book IV, Chapter 11

Preamble

Dhruva's father eventually retires to the forest at the end of his life to contemplate the ātman, *installing Dhruva on the throne. One day, Dhruva's brother, Uttama, is killed by a celestial* yakṣa *while hunting in the forest. Enraged, Dhruva sets out to the land of the* yakṣas *and challenges them to battle. A furious battle ensues, during which Dhruva slaughters countless* yakṣas. *His grandfather Svāyambhuva Manu, seeing this massacre, and feeling compassion for the* yakṣas *(also known as* guhyakas*), appears before his grandson.*

6. After seeing innocent *guhyakas* (*yakṣas*) being slaughtered by the powerful Dhruva on his amazing chariot, his grandfather Manu approached Dhruva, the son of Uttānapāda, out of compassion, accompanied by sages.
7. Manu said:
"Enough, my child, of this fury. It is sinful and the pathway to *tamas*. Blinded by this, you have abused these innocent, pious people.
8. Such a deed is not befitting our lineage, my dear child, and is forbidden by the righteous. You have undertaken a slaughter of these celestials who have done nothing.
9. Consider, my child: you loved your brother, but, outraged by his murder, many *yakṣas* have been killed by you, simply by dint of their kinship with just one who commited the crime.
10. To butcher living beings like beasts due to thinking the body to be the self is not the way of the saintly (*sādhus*) who are devoted to Kṛṣṇa.

11. You worshipped Hari, the abode of all beings, by means of understanding that He is the *ātman* within all beings; as a result of this you won that supreme abode of Viṣṇu, which is so difficult to attain.
12. You are that same person who did that then. You are beloved by Hari, and you are also highly esteemed by people. How, then, by performing such a censurable act as this now, are you exemplifying the behavior of the saintly?
13. *Bhagavān*, the *ātman* of everything, is pleased by tolerance, compassion, friendship, and equanimity for all creatures.
14. When *Bhagavān* is pleased, a person is freed from the *guṇas* of *prakṛti*, and, liberated, attains *brahma-nirvāṇa*.
15. Men and women are produced from the five great elements, and from the sexual union between them, further men and women are produced in this world.
16. It is from the agitation of the *guṇas* of the *māyā* of the Supreme *Ātman*, O king, that the creation, maintenance, and withdrawal of the universe comes about.
17. The Supreme *Puruṣa*, who is transcendent to these *guṇas*, is merely the efficient cause of this universe of manifest and unmanifest things. It is because of Him that the universe is set in motion, like iron [filings are set in motion by a magnet].
18. That *Bhagavān* projects his power by means of the activities of the *guṇas* through the power of Time. Therefore He creates, but yet is not the doer, and destroys, but is not the destroyer. The deeds of the Supreme Being are difficult to fathom, indeed.
19. Although He Himself is without end in the form of Time, He causes death, and although He is changeless and without beginning, He initiates everything. He causes the birth of progeny through others who were themselves progeny, and causes death to those who inflict death on others.
20. There are no friends or enemies of the Supreme, for He pervades all creatures equally in the form of death. The host of beings are subject to His ways, as He moves things along, just like particles of dust in the wind.
21. It is that Supreme Lord who apportions the growth and decline in life span of all living beings who are suffering [in *saṁsāra*]. But He Himself is self-sufficient and transcendent to both.

22. Some call Him *karma*, O king, others Nature. Some call Him Time, and still others the desire (*kāma*) of men.
23. Who can know the design of He who manifests through his various powers (*śaktis*) but who is inconceivable and immeasurable, my child? He is the source of one's very own being!
24. These *yakṣas*, the followers of Kuvera, the treasurer of the celestials, were not the killers of your brother. Destiny is the cause of the creation and demise of beings, my dear son!
25. It is He who creates, and He who maintains and destroys this universe, yet He Himself is not propelled by the *guṇas* and *karma*, as He is devoid of all ego.
26. He is the *ātman* of all beings, the controller of all beings, and the source of all beings. Employing His power of *māyā*, He creates, maintains, and destroys all beings.
27. My dear Dhruva! Take refuge in Him with your whole being. He is Destiny. He is death and immortality. He is the refuge of the universe. The secondary creators of the world[44] bear offerings to Him, just like bulls who are controlled by a rope through the nose.
28. You, at five years of age, were pierced to the heart by the words of your co-mother, your father's other wife. So you left your own mother, went to the forest, worshipped the transcendent Viṣṇu through austerities, and gained a place at the very top of the universe.
29. O child, seek Him within your heart, freed from anger. He is situated there, beyond the *guṇas*, infallible and unique. He is the Supreme *Ātman*, the seer of the *ātman*. It is within Him that this world appears to be independent and unreal.
30. Therefore, offer your supreme *bhakti* to Him, the Supreme, the inner *ātman*, the infinite *Bhagavān*. He is pure bliss and the possessor of all powers. Then you will gradually pierce through the bonds of ignorance, which have manifested in the form of 'I' and 'mine.'
31. O king, may you be blessed! Anger obstructs your ultimate welfare: restrain your anger by means of immersing yourself completely in the sacred teachings, which act just like medicine in counteracting disease.
32. People are terrified by a person overwhelmed with anger. A wise person desiring to attain a state of fearlessness for himself, does not allow himself to fall under the control of anger.

33. You have committed an offense against Kuvera, the brother of Śiva, because, in a state of fury, you have slaughtered innocent *yakṣas* [his followers] thinking they were the murderers of your brother.
34. Pacify Kuvera immediately, O son, by offering him obeisance, respect, and sweet words, lest the wrath of the great souls consume our family dynasty.
35. After admonishing his grandson Dhruva in this manner, Svāyambhuva Manu received respect from him and then departed to his own city, accompanied by the sages."

Book IV, Chapter 12

1. Maitreya said:
"Upon understanding that Dhruva's anger had subsided and that he had desisted from the slaughter, Kuvera, the lord of wealth, went to that place, praised by the celestial *cāraṇas*, *yakṣas*, and *kinnaras*. He addressed Dhruva, who was standing there with hands folded in respect.
2. '*Bho! Bho!* O faultless warrior prince! You have satisfied me! You have renounced anger on the instruction of your grandfather. It is so hard to relinquish.
3. It is not you who killed the *yakṣas*, nor was it they who killed your brother. It is Time which is actually the controller of the coming and going of all beings.
4. Like a dreaming person, the false notions of "I" and "you" are meaningless; they arise from contemplating the unreal due to a person's ignorance. It is because of this that there is bondage and misfortune.
5.–6. Therefore go on your way, Dhruva. May there be good fortune for you. For liberation from *saṁsāra*, worship *Bhagavān*, Viṣṇu, for He is the destroyer of *saṁsāra*. Do this while contemplating the *ātman* within all beings, as it is He who manifests as the *ātman* within all beings. His feet are worthy of worship. He is connected with his powers—those of *māyā* and of the *ātman*—yet He is separate from them.
7. Dear Dhruva! We have heard that you are inseparable from the feet of Viṣṇu, from whose navel the lotus is born. Choose any wish, O king, anything that enters your mind. Be happy and don't hesitate: you deserve a boon, O son of Uttānapāda.'

8. Urged on by Kuvera, the king of kings, to pick a boon, the high-minded Dhruva, a great *bhāgavata*, chose unwavering remembrance of Hari. It is by this that one easily crosses over *tamas*, which is so difficult to surpass.
9. With a satisfied heart, Kuvera awarded him this boon. Then as Dhruva was watching, he disappeared, and returned to his own city.
10. After this, with sacrificial rites and lavish wealth, Dhruva performed *yajña*, ceremonial rites, for Viṣṇu, who is the bestower of the fruits of ritual. The ritual involved wealth, sacrificial acts, and the celestials.
11. Engaging in intense *bhakti* to the infallible Kṛṣṇa, the *ātman* of everything who is yet separate from everything, Dhruva perceived Him, the Lord, situated in the *ātman* of all beings.[45]
12. The citizens considered Dhruva to be like their father: he was endowed with good character, devoted to the *brāhmaṇas*, compassionate to the less fortunate, and the protector of the codes of *dharma*.
13. He ruled the earth globe for thirty-six thousand years, destroying his pious *karma* through experiencing its fruition, and his impious *karma* through austerity.
14. After ruling the kingdom in this way for many years in a manner conducive to the first three goals of life,[46] the great-souled Dhruva, his senses completely controlled, transferred the royal throne to his son in turn.
15. He considered this universe to be a mental construct produced in dream through ignorance (*avidyā*) caused by *māyā*, like the city of the celestial *gandharvas*.[47]
16. After realizing that his body, wives, offspring, and friends; his power, abundant treasury, harem, and beautiful pleasure groves; and the entire earth bound like a girdle with oceans, were all temporal and subject to Time, Dhruva set out for the holy place Badarikāśrama.[48]
17. He bathed in the pure waters of that place, his senses under control. He set up a sitting place (*āsana*), and with his breath restrained and his senses controlled by the mind, fixed his mind on that image of *Bhagavān* made of the gross elements (the *Virāṭ*[49]). Then, after meditating on this without interruption, he relinquished that form and entered into the state of *samādhi*, beyond thoughts.[50]
18. Carried away by his *bhakti* to *Bhagavān*, Hari, he was continually overwhelmed with tear drops of ecstasy (*ānanda*) flowing ceaselessly.

His body was covered with hairs that stood on end due to bliss, and his heart melted. Freed from the subtle body, he lost awareness of his body.

19. Then Dhruva saw a superb celestial vehicle descending from the heavens, appearing like the full moon illuminating the ten directions.

20. He saw two magnificent celestials standing on that. They had four arms, were blackish in complexion, and their eyes were reddish like the lotus. They were holding clubs, beautifully dressed, and adorned with attractive earrings, armlets, necklaces, and helmets.

21. Upon realizing that they were two servants of Viṣṇu, Dhruva stood up. Out of astonishment, he had forgotten the proper etiquette of welcome; so he offered respects to the two associates of Viṣṇu by reciting the names of Hari, the enemy of Madhu, with hands folded in respect.

22. Sunanda and Nanda, the esteemed servants of the lotus-naveled Viṣṇu, approached Dhruva. His mind was absorbed in Kṛṣṇa, his hands were folded in respect, and his neck was bent in humility. They addressed him.

23. Sunanda and Nanda said:

'*Bho, Bho,* O king, may you be blessed! Listen carefully to what we have to say. When you were five years old, you thoroughly satisfied the Lord with your austerities.

24. We two are the associates of the Lord, who is the wielder of the *śārṅga* bow and the Creator of the entire universe. We have been sent here to bring you to *Bhagavān*'s abode.

25. Come! You have earned that abode of Viṣṇu, which is so hard to attain. The celestials cannot attain it; they can only glimpse at it from afar. The moon, sun, stars, constellations, planets, and all celestial bodies circumambulate it on the right.[51]

26. This realm has never been attained by any of your forefathers, dear Dhruva. Come now to the supreme abode of Viṣṇu, which is glorified by all the universes.

27. You have earned the right to ascend this divine vehicle. It has been sent by the supreme Lord, who is praised in the best of verses.' "

28. Maitreya said:

"After hearing the nectarlike words of those eminent servants from Vaikuṇṭha, Dhruva, beloved of Viṣṇu, took a purifying bath, performed his daily auspicious duties, offered his respects to the two sages, and returned their blessings.

29. After circumambulating that splendid vehicle, Dhruva worshipped it, offered respects to the two Vaikuṇṭha associates again, and assumed a golden form. He then desired to mount up on that carrier.

30. Then Dhruva, the son of Uttānapāda, saw that Death had approached. He put his foot on the head of Death,[52] and climbed onto that marvelous aerial structure.

31. At this, the prominent *gandharvas* resounded their *mṛdaṅga*, *paṇava*, and other such drums, sang, and showered down *kusuma* flowers like rain.

32. As he was about to ascend up beyond the celestial realms, Dhruva remembered his mother, Sunīti, and thought: 'I will give up going to Viṣṇu's realm, even though it is so hard to attain, and go to my poor mother instead.'

33. Having understood his resolve, those two eminent divine beings showed Dhruva that the queen was already proceeding ahead of them in another vehicle.

34. Here and there along the path of ascent, Dhruva saw the planets one by one. As he was proceeding along, he was bestrewed with divine flowers from the celestials in their vehicles as they glorified him.

35. Traversing beyond the three worlds and even the realm of the sages[53] on that celestial vehicle, Dhruva then reached the realm of Viṣṇu beyond all that. He had attained an eternal destination.

36. It was effulgent through its own all-pervading luster—it is on account of that effulgence that these three worlds here shine. Those who are not compassionate to other living entities do not attain that place—only those who constantly perform auspicious deeds attain there.

37. Those dear to Kṛṣṇa, the infallible Lord, are peaceful, equanimous, pure, and affectionate to all beings. Even those who are friends with them easily go to the abode of Viṣṇu.

38. In this way, Dhruva, son of Uttānapāda, who was fully devoted to Kṛṣṇa, became like the crest jewel of the three worlds.

39. The circle of constellations are placed around this realm [the polestar] and revolve around it with great power ceaselessly, like a herd of bulls circle a central post.

40. After seeing the greatness of Dhruva, the eminent sage Nārada sang verses about him at the sacrifice of the Pracetās, while plucking his *vīṇā*.

41. Nārada sang:

'Despite knowing the means to do so, the followers of the Vedas are not capable of approaching the destination attained by Dhruva, the son of the chaste Sunīti, through the power of his austerities—what to speak then of kings attaining this?

42. At the age of five years, he departed to the forest with a heart tormented by the piercing words of his father's co-wife. Following my instructions, he conquered the unconquerable Lord, won over by the qualities of His *bhakta*.

43. When Dhruva was five or six years old, he pleased the Lord of Vaikuṇṭha, and attained His realm. A *kṣatriya* warrior in this world might at best desire to ascend to that realm even after many years, but it was attained by Dhruva in a few days.' "

The Tale of King Pṛthu: The Ideal Monarch

Yoga Blueprint

The teachings in this section continue in the vein of normative Yoga *philosophy. What is noteworthy in this passage is the preeminent regard and respect that is offered to those sages who teach and exemplify such teachings.*

Book IV, Chapter 22

1. Maitreya said:

"While the citizens were extolling King Pṛthu of great fame, the four boy sages (*Kumāras*), who were as effulgent as the sun, approached that place.

2. The king, along with his entourage, saw those perfected masters (*siddhas*) descending from the sky. They were recognizable by their effulgence, and were purifying the worlds of sin.

3. Pṛthu, son of Venu, along with his entourage and followers, jumped up, trying to regain his breath that had been lost from seeing those sages. They appeared just like the *jīva*, lord of the senses, [captivated by] the sense objects made from the *guṇas*.

4. Feeling overwhelmed by their august presence, the king arranged for them to be worshipped once they had accepted seats and other

items used for welcoming guests. With head bowed he was humble and courteous.
5. He sprinkled his hair knot with the water that had washed their feet. By this, he was behaving in the manner of those who are cultured, to demonstrate respect.
6. The king, who was endowed with faith and sense control, was delighted. He addressed the Kumāras, elder brothers of Śiva,[54] who had taken their seats on golden thrones, appearing like the sacred fires in their respective sacrificial hearths.
7. '*Aho!* What auspicious act must I have performed, O you who embody auspiciousness, as a result of which I have obtained your *darśana* (a sight of you). You are difficult to see even by the *yogīs*.
8. What is there that is difficult to attain for anyone when the sages, and Śiva and Viṣṇu, along with their followers, are pleased with that person?
9. The world cannot perceive those sages who wander about, just as the material elements, the causes of this world, cannot perceive the *ātman* that exists in all, and that is the seer of all.
10. Even if they are poor, those saintly householders are blessed whose houses contain water, grass mats, accommodation, servants, and masters that can be offered to saints.
11. But those houses are just like trees which are the abodes of serpents if, despite being replete with all goods, they do not contain water to wash the feet of the Vaiṣṇavas.
12. Welcome, O you best of the twice-born. Desiring liberation, you have been observing vows faithfully. Although you are boys, your minds are fixed and you have attained success.
13. How can there be any auspiciousness in store for us, O masters, who think that the purpose of life is the objects of the senses? Due to our own deeds, we have fallen into this world, which is a reservoir of vice.
14. There is no need to ask after the welfare of your lordships. You enjoy the bliss of the *ātman*, and thoughts of good fortune or misfortune do not arise in you.
15. You are the well-wishers of those in distress, therefore, with faith in you, I ask you: How can salvation be attained in this world of *saṁsāra*?
16. The unborn *Bhagavān* is the revealer of the *ātman*, and, in fact, He is the *ātman* of those who know the *ātman*. It is certain that He

wanders around this world in the form of perfected beings such as yourselves so as to bestow compassion to His devotees.' "

17. Maitreya said:

"After hearing from Pṛthu such praises—gracious, fitting, insightful, and measured—the Kumāras were pleased. Smiling, they replied.

18. Sanat-Kumāra said:

'You have inquired perfectly, O great king, with the welfare of all living beings at heart, even though you know the answers. Such wisdom is befitting the saintly.

19. The association of the saintly is truly beneficial to both parties [speaker and hearer]: the discourses and queries of such association enhance the satisfaction of everyone.

20. O king, it seems that you have an unshakable attraction for reciting the qualities of the lotus feet of Kṛṣṇa, the enemy of Madhu. Such attraction is hard to attain. It clears away the impurities covering the mind in the form of lust.

21. This much is certain, according to the scriptures that have undertaken a thorough inquiry of the matter: the source of welfare for people is detachment from whatever is different from the *ātman*, and firm attraction toward the *ātman* and *brahman,* which is beyond the *guṇas*.

22. [Affection for Hari, who is *Brahman*, transcendent to the *guṇas*, easily develops] by means of faith, by observance of the *Bhagavata dharma*, by inquiry into Truth, by determined application of the *yoga* of transcendence, by unceasing worship of the Lord of *Yoga* (*yogeśvara*), and by pure-hearted discussion about the Lord.

23. By distaste for the company of those who delight in the senses and material possessions and by disinterest in their opinions, by delighting in solitude absorbed in the contentment of the *ātman* except when drinking the nectar of the qualities of Hari.

24. By nonviolence (*ahiṁsā*), by the conduct of the great saints, by remembering the nectar of the great deeds of Mukunda [Kṛṣṇa], by following moral and ethical precepts (*yamas* and *niyamas*), by renouncing lust (*kāma*), by not criticizing, by being free of ambition, and by tolerating the dualites.

25. By continually discussing with devotion the names and qualities dedicated to Hari, which are ornaments for the ears, by disinterest in that which is other than the *ātman*, and in the causes and effects of

the material world, by all these, affection for Hari, who is *Brahman*, transcendent to the *guṇas*, easily develops.

26. When unflinching faith has developed in *brahman*, then a person, under the guidance of a *guru* (*ācārya*), speedily burns up the layers surrounding the *ātman* (*kośas*), making them impotent, like the eruption of fire burns its source. These *kośas*, constituting five aspects,[55] lie in the heart.

27. When the stock of *karma* (*āśaya*) has been burned, and one has been freed from all its qualities, one no longer sees either the internal or external coverings that previously separated the *ātman* from the *Paramātman*, the Supreme—just as, when a dream comes to an end, a person no longer sees the objects within it.

28. It is because the covering in the form of this stock exists, that a person can see nothing other than him or herself, the objects of the senses, and that which is beyond both [the ego]. Otherwise this would not occur.

29. This is like the fact that it is only when a cause is present—such as water or other reflecting things like mirrors—that a person can see the difference between him or herself and the reflection. Otherwise this would not occur.

30. The mind is drawn by objects that attract the senses. When a person is contemplating these objects, the mind diverts the discrimination of the intelligence, just like a dam diverts the water of a pond.

31. When thought (*citta*) is distracted in this way, memory [of the *ātman*] is lost. In the destruction of memory, knowledge is lost. The sages consider this to be the concealment of the *ātman* by the mind.[56]

32. There is no greater loss to a person's self-interest in this world, than the loss of one's own *ātman*; it is for the *ātman* that other things are held dear.[57]

33. Contemplating wealth and the objects of the senses causes the destruction of a person's own self-interest. From the loss of knowledge and realization that occurs because of this, one enters the immovable species of life [plants and the like].

34. One desiring to cross over the depths of *tamas* should not become attached to anything which completely obstructs *dharma*, *artha*, *kāma*, and *mokṣa* (the four goals of life: righteousness, prosperity, sense indulgence, and liberation).

35. Among these, *mokṣa*, liberation, is deemed as the greatest, because the other three goals of life are always subject to the fear of loss.
36. There are higher and lower states of existence for living beings brought about by the agitation of the *guṇas*. But there is no security for any of them, since their hopes are dashed by the Lord [in the form of Time].
37. Therefore you should understand *Bhagavān*, O king. He always shines forth, manifesting everywhere in all hearts and illuminating from within the souls of all moving and non-moving entities,[58] who are covered by mind, intelligence, life airs, senses, and bodies.
38. I surrender to Him. His nature is eternally liberated, transcendent, and pure. *Prakṛti* with all its *karmas* is removed by Him. This universe manifests within Him as *māyā* in the form of cause and effect. This *māyā* illusion is dispelled by discrimination (*viveka*), just as the perception of a snake in what is really a garland is dispelled by discrimination.
39. Worship Vāsudeva; He is your refuge. The saints unravel the knots of accumulated *karma* (*karmāśaya*) through their *bhakti* to His lustrous feet, which are like lotus petals. Those whose minds are separated from Him, in contrast, are not able to control the senses, which flow forth like rivers, even though they struggle to do so.
40. The ocean of *saṁsāra* is filled with the crocodiles of the six senses. Great difficulty awaits those in this world who seek to cross over it by their own struggles without using the boat of *Īśvara*. Therefore, you should make a vessel of the adorable lotus feet of *Bhagavān*, Hari, and cross over this peril in the form of this insurmountable ocean.' "
41. Maitreya said:
"In this manner, the path of the *ātman* was revealed to the king by one of the *Kumāras*, the son of Brahmā, who had insight into the *ātman*. After honoring him, the king replied to him.
42. The king said:
'The compassionate Hari previously granted grace on me, and now, O great *brāhmaṇa*, you have arrived to bestow it upon me.
43. You have accomplished this expertly, O lord; you have been most compassionate. What is there that I can offer you? Everything I own belongs to the great saints, including my very self.

44. My life airs, consorts, offspring, furnished residences, kingdom, power, land, and treasury are hereby all presented to you.
45. One who has realized the Truths of the Vedas and sacred texts deserves control over the army, kingdom, legal jurisdiction, and lordship over all realms.
46. The *brāhmaṇa* eats his own food, wears his own clothing, and gives away his own property. The *kṣatriyas* and other castes consume foodstuffs by the grace of the *brāhmaṇas*.[59]
47. This path of *Bhagavān* pertaining to the knowledge of the *ātman* has been thoroughly presented by them, the knowers of the Veda. They are supremely benevolent and are always content merely with their own deeds. So with what, exactly, can one repay them, other than with a nominal drink of water?' "
48. Maitreya continued:
"Those lords of the *yoga* of the *ātman* were thus honored by the emperor. Then, praising the character of such a king, they disappeared into the sky, before the very eyes of all the people.
49. King Pṛthu, son of Venu, eminent among great souls, became committed to these teachings about the Supreme *Ātman*. Absorbed in the *ātman*, he considered that all his desires had been fulfilled.
50. He performed his duties as an offering to *Brahman*, in accordance with the appropriate time, place, capabilities, protocols, and resources.
51. Fully devoted, he dedicated the fruits of his work to *Brahman* freed from all attachments.[60] He considered himself to be a witness to action, the *ātman* transcendent to *prakṛti*.[61]
52.–53. Just as the sun [is detached from affairs in the world, despite shining upon it], the king did not become attached to the objects of the senses despite living in his home endowed with regality and royal opulence. His mind was free of ego, and he fully performed his duties in this manner while performing the *yoga* of the *ātman*."

Book IV, Chapter 23

1.–3. Maitreya continued:
"Pṛthu, son of Venu, was self-controlled. He was the upholder of the citizens, and by his efforts his kingdom had prospered in all areas. He had provided livelihoods for all moving and non-moving entities and had upheld the law of *dharma* for all creatures. He had fulfilled

the instruction of *Īśvara*, as it was for this reason that he had taken birth. One day, after seeing that his body had succumbed to old age, he transferred the earth to his sons, and set out alone with his wife for the forest to perform austerities (*tapas*). The citizens were disconsolate and the very earth seemed to weep from separation.

4. There, firm in his vow, he immersed himself in severe austerity (*tapas*) recommended by the *Vaikhānasa* texts for the *vānaprastha* phase of life[62]—just as he had previously done when conquering the world.

5. His food consisted of bulbs, roots, and fruits and sometimes dried leaves. Sometimes, for several weeks, he consumed water, and thereafter subsisted only on air.

6. His bed was the bare ground. In the summer, the hero performed the austerity of the 'five fires,'[63] and in the rainy season, the sage tolerated the rains. In the winter he immersed himself up to the neck in water.

7. He was tolerant, with senses restrained and words controlled. He restrained his semen, and controlled his breath. Desiring to propitiate Kṛṣṇa, he performed the highest type of austerity.

8. His accumulation of *karma* and impurities was destroyed by the gradual pursuit of perfection. The six senses were restrained by the practice of *prāṇāyāma*, breath control, and his bonds of *saṁsāra* were cut.

9. Whatever the great Sanat-kumāra had taught him about that highest *yoga* of the supreme self, that bull among men worshipped the Supreme Person accordingly.

10. Undeviating *bhakti* to *Bhagavān*, who is *Brahman*, was performed by that saint. He constantly endeavored with faith in upholding the *bhāgavata-dharma*.

11. In this way, his mind became completely pure by devotional activities for *Bhagavān*. By filling it with remembrance of Kṛṣṇa, knowledge endowed with renunciation arose in his mind. With the penetrating insight from this, he severed the covering (*kośa*) of his *ātman*, which is the abode of doubt.[64]

12. Having realized the nature of his *ātman*, he severed the illusion of being the mind and body and subsequently became freed from all desires. He next even renounced that state, and then severed the realization obtained through this insight in turn.[65] Until an ascetic *yogī*

ceases to be distracted by the processes [and mystic powers] of *yoga*, attraction for the stories of Kṛṣṇa, the younger brother of Balarāma, will not manifest.

13. In this manner, that best of heroes joined his mind with his innermost *ātman*, became absorbed in *Brahman* and, when the due time came, relinquished his own material body.

14. He blocked his anus with his heels, slowly drawing the life airs up through the navel, then the stomach, then fixing it in the heart, then farther up into the throat, then farther up still to between the eyebrows.[66]

15. Raising the air up farther, he settled it in the head, free from all desires. Then he united the air with the totality of air, the body with the earth, and the fire of the body with fire.

16. He merged the cavities of the body with air, and the bodily fluids with water. He returned earth into water, that water into fire, that into air, and that into ether, returning everything to its original source.[67]

17. He merged the mind into the senses, and the senses into the *tanmātra* subtle qualities from which they had originally emerged. He withdrew all these, along with the gross elements, etc., into the great cosmic *mahat* (undifferentiated state of *prakṛti*).[68]

18. He then placed that reservoir of all the *guṇas* into the *jīva* conditioned by *māyā*. Then Pṛthu, a being still covered by *māyā* due to being situated in a body composed of material coverings, finally gave the body up entirely through the force of knowledge and renunciation, and remained situated in his own true nature (*svarūpa*). He was now liberated.

19. The great queen Arci, who was delicate and beautiful and whose feet were not suitable for touching the rough ground, followed her husband to the forest.

20. Although she was severely emaciated by austerities, she did not experience any discomfort because she was true to her vows of *dharma* for her husband, desiring only to serve him. Maintaining her body like a forest sage [with forest fruits and produce], she experienced complete satisfaction in her mind by touching the hand of her beloved husband.

21. When she saw the body of that compassionate lord of both the world and of herself completely deprived of all consciousness and

signs of life, that pious lady wept a little, then placed it on a funeral pyre at the top of a hill.

22. After she had performed the prescribed rites, she bathed in the waters of a river, and offered water oblations to her husband of magnanimous deeds. Then she offered obeisance to the celestials, circumambulated the pyre, and entered the flames, meditating on the feet of her husband.

23. Seeing that chaste lady following her husband, Pṛthu, the best of heroes, the wives of the celestials in their thousands, along with their husbands, showered blessings upon her.

24. Releasing showers of flowers on that hilltop, they extolled her among themselves while celestial drums resounded.

25. The celestial ladies said:

'*Aho!* This spouse is most blessed! She served her husband, the lord of all the kings of the earth, with her whole being, just as Lakṣmī, the Goddess of Fortune, serves her husband, Viṣṇu, the Lord of sacrifice.

26. Just see—following her husband, Pṛthu, son of Venu, she has proceeded beyond us [in the celestial realms] and is going up on high [to Vaikuṇṭha] by dint of her astonishing deeds.

27. What else is there to attain in this world for those mortals who, despite having a flickering life span, have attained the transcendent realm of *Bhagavān*?

28. Anyone in this world who, after obtaining with great difficulty a human form, which can bestow liberation, becomes entangled in sense objects instead, is cheated and has become an enemy of his *ātman*.'

29. While the celestial damsels were praising her in this way, the chaste wife went to the realm her husband had attained. Pṛthu, who had taken shelter of Kṛṣṇa, was the most eminent of the knowers of *ātman*.

30. Such was the glory of that Pṛthu, the best of the *bhāgavata* devotees. His story has now been recounted to you. It is the best of stories.

31. Anyone who reads this extremely auspicious story with great faith, or who recites it or hears it, attains to the realm of Pṛthu (Vaikuṇṭha).

32. By reading it, a *brāhmaṇa* becomes endowed with the potency of *brahman*, a monarch becomes lord of the earth, a *vaiśya* (merchant) becomes master of wealth, and a *śūdra* (laborer) the best of saints.[69]

33. After hearing it three times attentively, one who has no progeny, whether man or woman, becomes endowed with excellent offspring, and a pauper becomes conspicuously wealthy.
34. A person with no claim to fame becomes famous, and a fool becomes a *paṇḍita*. This story becomes the vehicle of bringing good fortune to people and warding off inauspiciousness.
35. It bestows wealth, fame, longevity, access to the celestial realms, and removes the impurities of the age of *Kali*. It provides the perfections of *dharma*, *artha*, *kāma*, and *mokṣa*[70] to those desiring these. One should hear it with faith, as it is the supreme cause of these four goals of human life.
36. A king inclined toward conquest who sets forth on a campaign after hearing this narrative will find other kings presenting tribute to him before he arrives, just as they did to Pṛthu.
37. One should hear, recite, and read the story of Pṛthu, son of Venu, freed from all other attachments, while engaging in pure bhakti to *Bhagavān*.
38. O Vidura! Thus has been narrated this story revealing the glories of the great souls (*mahat*). One who follows it attains the destination of Pṛthu, beyond death.
39. Hearing this story of Pṛthu every day with respect, and reciting it, a person becomes freed from all attachments and attains complete love for the feet of *Bhagavān*, which are the boat for traversing the ocean of *saṁsāra*."

The Allegory of King Purañjana: The Illusion of Sensual Pleasures

Yoga Blueprint

The teachings in this section point to the foolishness and dangers of immersing oneself in romantic reveries and sensual indulgences from the point of view of the ultimate purpose of the human form of life, realizing the ātman. *The allegory illustrates the ephemeral nature of material pleasures, which are inevitably vanquished by old age and death. The final section includes some particularly profound insights into the nature of the mind (IV.29.60–85).*

[*All the items from verse 10 below until chapter 28 have allegorical significance. Their interpretation is given in chapter 28 verse 55ff., so they will make limited sense until then. Nonetheless, the reader is encouraged to peruse chapters 22–25 patiently; while the allegory is somewhat lengthy, it imparts powerful* yogic *teachings.*]

Book IV, Chapter 25

3. Prācīnabarhiṣat's mind was absorbed in ritualistic activities.[71] Once, sage Nārada, who is compassionate and realized in the truth of the *ātman*, went to him to enlighten him:

4. "O king! What real benefit for yourself do you seek from ritual activities? Real benefit is the removal of suffering and the attaining of happiness, but these goals are not achieved from the performance of ritual acts."

5. The king replied:

"O saintly one! My mind has become addicted to ritual activity—I do not know anything else. Please reveal to me the pure knowledge by which I can become free from such ritual activity.

6. The householder life has superficial things as its *dharma*—the mind pursues wealth, wife, and offspring as its goals. A fool who is wandering on the path of *saṁsāra* does not consider anything to be higher."

7. Nārada said:

"*Bho! Bho!* O king! Just look at the hosts of creatures mercilessly slaughtered by you in the thousands as sacrificial animals for the offering—you who are [supposed to be] the protector of creatures!

8. Remembering your butchery, they are all awaiting you [in the next life]: after you have died, they will furiously pierce you with their horns, hard as iron.

9. Now I will relate to you this ancient tale (*itihāsa*). As I narrate, try to gain insight from the story of Purañjana!

10. There was once a king of great renown by name of Purañjana, O king. He had a friend called the Unknown One (Avijñāta), whose activities were unknown.

11. The king wandered over the earth seeking a residence. When he could not find a suitable place, he became somewhat despondent.

12. Desiring pleasure, he did not consider any of the cities that existed on the earth suitable for fulfilling this or that desire of his.

13. Once, on the southern plateaus of the Himālaya mountains, Purañjana saw a city with nine gates, distinctive with good features.

14. It was filled everywhere with ramparts, parks, watchtowers, moats, windows, and with houses whose roofs were made of gold, silver, and iron.
15. The floors of its mansions were inlaid with sapphires, crystals, cat's-eyes, pearls, and rubies; it was like the celestial city of Bhogavatī[72] in beauty.
16. It was endowed with assembly houses, crossroads, highways, playing grounds, resting places, markets, monuments, flags, banners, and coral balconies.
17. In a grove outside the city there were celestial trees and creepers, and a lake with swarms of humming bees, and chirping birds.
18. The city was made beautiful with lotuses, their fresh leaves and stems swaying in a breeze fragrant with the scent of varieties of flowers, and bearing the spray of cool waterfalls.
19. A traveler to that place would think he or she was being called by the cooing of cuckoos. And the place was free of dangers, as the herds of various wild animals had taken the vows of sages [that is, nonviolence].
20. The king happened there by chance, and saw an extremely beautiful maiden approaching. She was accompanied by ten attendants, each of whom was the husband of one hundred wives.
21. She could change her form at will, and was guarded by a five-hooded serpent as bodyguard. Just on the cusp of maturity, the maiden was searching for a male.
22. The maiden had a shapely nose, perfect teeth, comely cheeks, and an exceptionally beautiful face. In her ears, which were symmetrically aligned, she wore attractive earrings.
23. She was dark in complexion, and had wrapped a reddish-colored piece of cloth around her well-formed hips. Walking along with her feet making tingling sounds from their anklets, she seemed like a goddess.
24. Her two breasts, equally rounded and with no space between them, revealed her youthfulness, and she was covering them with the end of her garment out of shyness. She swayed like an elephant in the way she walked.[73]
25. The hero was smitten by the arrows of her tender glances and the dancing of her enticing eyebrows. She looked very beautiful with her bashful smiles. Purañjana gently spoke to her:

26. 'Who are you, with eyes like lotus petals? What is your family lineage? From where have you come, O chaste lady? What do you seek to accomplish here on the outskirts of this city? Please tell me, O shy one!
27. Who are these attendants, with that formidable warrior as their eleventh member? And these beautiful damsels? Who is this serpent that goes before you, O you with beautiful eyebrows?
28. Are you the Goddess Hrī? Or Bhavānī (Parvatī)? Or the Goddess of speech (Sarasvatī)? Or, like a sage in solitude in the forest, are you by chance seeking a husband? If so, he must have fulfilled all his wishes by desiring your lotus feet. [If you are the Goddess of Fortune,] where is the lotus that has fallen from your fingers?[74]
29. You must be someone other than those Goddesses, O you with beautiful thighs, because you touch the ground [with your feet].[75] You should adorn this city together with me—just like the Goddess Śrī with Viṣṇu, the Lord of Sacrifice, in the divine realm [of Vaikuṇṭha]. I am an outstanding hero who has performed many great feats!
30. Therefore, bestow your favor upon me, O beautiful one—my senses have been shattered by your sidelong glances! The mind-born god Cupid, struck by your dancing eyebrows and bashful smiles of love,[76] is harassing me.
31. O you with beautiful eyebrows, your face, encircled by locks of dangling blue curls, has beautiful sparkling eyes and utters sweet words. Please raise it and show it to me, do not turn away out of bashfulness, O you with a bright smile!'
32. 'O hero!' The woman, enchanted by the hero Purañjana—who was begging like one who is not a hero[77]—greeted him smilingly:
33. 'We do not properly know who begot me or these others, O bull among men, nor do we know our family lineage or our name.
34. I do not know by whom this city was constructed, O hero, but it is my refuge. I know only that I am here now and nothing more than that.
35. O respectful sir! These men and women are my male and female friends. This snake remains awake guarding the city when I am sleeping.
36. By chance you have come along and you seek worldly pleasure. May good fortune be yours. I along with my friends will provide these for you, O subduer of enemies.

37. Reside in this city of nine gates for one hundred years, O Lord, enjoying the sensual pleasures that I shall provide.
38. Indeed, whom else should I please other than you? Someone who is not learned? Someone untutored in erotic pleasures? Someone who is not interested in the next life? Or someone like an animal who does not care for the morrow?
39. It is in the here and now that righteous conduct (*dharma*), economic well-being (*artha*), sense indulgence (*kāma*), the joy of children, liberation, and fame are attained as well as the pure celestial realms free of sorrow, which even the knowers of the self (*kevalin*) do not know.
40. The sages say that in this world, the householder stage of life (*gṛhāśrama*), is the only foundation for the well-being of the forefathers, gods, sages, humans, and all beings including oneself.
41. O hero! What woman like me would not accept an available husband who is famous, generous, handsome, and loving like you?
42. O mighty-armed one! Which woman's mind in this world would not cling to your arms, which are like the coils of a serpent? You roam about in order to remove the anguish of the unfortunate with your smiling glances full of compassion.' "
43. Nārada said:
"Thus, the couple entered into a mutual agreement right there and then. Then they entered into the city, O king, and enjoyed for a hundred years.
44. In the hot season, eulogized sweetly by singers while frolicking here and there, the king entered a lake surrounded by women.
45. There were seven upper gates of the city, and two lower, made for the purpose of transporting different objects for whomever was the master of the city.
46. Five of the gates were to the east, or front, one to the south, and another one to the north. I will describe to you the names of the two gates to the west, O king!
47. The two gates to the front, Khadyotā (the left eye) and Āvirmukhī (the right eye), were built in one location. Through these, the king used to go to a country called Vibhrājita (the one made bright), with his friend Dyumān (the shining one).
48. Nalinī and Nālinī (the nostrils) were also built in one location to the front. Through these, the king used to go to the place called Saurabham (fragrance) with his friend Avadhūta (the discarded).

49. The gate called Mukhya (principle) was to the east and the king of the city used to go through that to the two countries Āpaṇa (speech) and Bahūdana (collection of eatables). He was accompanied by Rasajñā (the tongue) and Vipaṇa (the organ of speech).
50. Purañjana went through the southern gate of the city called Pitṛhū (invoking the ancestors), to the country of the southern Pañcālas (the path to the forefathers). He was accompanied by Śrutadhara (the organ of hearing), O king.
51. Purañjana went through the northern gate of the city called Devahū (invoking the gods) accompanied by Śrutadhara, to the country of the northern Pañcālas (the path to the gods).
52. The name of the western gate was Āsurī (penis). Purañjana went through that to the country called Grāmaka (common pleasure), accompanied by Durmadena (drunkard).
53. The name of [the other] western gate was Nirṛti (death). Purañjana went through that to the country called Vaiśasa (destruction), accompanied by Lubdhaka (greedy person).
54. From the citizens, two were blind: Nirvāk (foot) and Peśaskṛit (hand). With these, the lord, the owner of the senses, goes about and performs work.
55. When he went to the inner quarters of the palace accompanied by Viṣūcīna (going in all directions), Purañjana experienced illusion, peace, and joy derived from his wife and offspring.
56. The foolish king, his mind overcome with passion and attached to enjoying the fruits of his actions, was cheated in this way. Whatever the queen wished for, he obliged.
57. When sometimes she drank liquor, he drank, and became intoxicated. When sometimes she ate, he ate; when at other times she took her meal, he took his meal.
58. When sometimes she sang, he sang; when sometimes she cried, he cried; when at other times she laughed, he laughed; when sometimes she gossiped, he gossiped.
59. When sometimes she ran, he ran; when sometimes she stood up, he stood up; when sometimes she lay down, he lay down; and when at other times she sat up, he sat up.
60. When sometimes she listened to something, he listened to it; when sometimes she looked at something, he looked at it; when sometimes she smelled something, he smelled it; and when at other times she touched something, he touched it.

61. When sometimes his wife was grieving for something, he grieved, like a bereaved soul. And when at times she rejoiced, he rejoiced; while when at other times she was delighted, he became delighted.
62. In this way, he was ensnared by the queen and cheated out of all [the qualities] of his own personality and nature. The ignorant fellow, even when unwilling, obliged her out of weakness, like a pet animal."

Book IV, Chapter 26

1. *Śrī* Nārada said:
"The king, who was a great archer, mounted a chariot, drawn by five fleet horses. It had two pole shafts, two wheels, three banners, and five tethers.
2. It had one rein, one charioteer, one chariot seat, two poles, five carriage boxes, seven chariot bumpers, and could perform five types of movements.
3. After mounting the golden vehicle, armed with a quiver of inexhaustible arrows and accompanied by his eleventh general, the king set out for a forest that had five plateaus.
4. Taking up his bow and arrows, the arrogant man roamed about there in the chase. Delighting in the sport of hunting, he left behind his wife, who did not deserve such treatment.
5. Succumbing to a demoniac mentality, his mind became cruel and without compassion, and he slaughtered the wild animals in the forests with his sharpened arrows.
6. It is prescribed in the sacred texts that if a king is greedy, he may hunt animals for sacrifice in sacred places at specified times, O king, but only as many as is necessary for this specific purpose.
7. A learned person who performs actions that have been prescribed by the sacred texts is not tainted by that action, O Lord of kings: on the contrary, knowledge is attained from such actions.
8. But otherwise, an egotistical person who performs actions is bound [by the reactions]. Falling under the control of the flow of the *guṇas*, such a person's wisdom is destroyed and he strays into darkness.
9. Carnage was unleashed on the poor animals in that forest, and their limbs were pierced by arrows with all sorts of feathers. It was an unbearable sight for anyone who was kindhearted.
10. After killing hares, boars, buffalo, gavaya ox, antelopes, porcupines, as well as other animals that were appropriate for sacrifice, the king became exhausted.

11. So, afflicted by hunger and thirst, he desisted and returned to his residence. There, he took bath, ate appropriate foodstuffs, and then lay down to rest until his fatigue passed.
12. Then the king made himself presentable with fragrance, oils, garlands, etc. After this, with all the limbs of his body nicely adorned, he set his mind on his queen.
13. Satisfied, happy, and full of himself, the king's mind was attracted by Cupid. But he could not find his beautiful wife, the lady of the house.
14. Anxious, he inquired from the ladies in the inner quarters, O King Prācīnabarhis: 'Is all well with you, ladies, and with your mistress, too, as before?
15. The opulence of a house does not shine if the mother or the dutiful wife is not present—just like a chariot without its parts. What sensible person would remain in such a place, like a wretch?
16. Where is my charming wife? Illuminating my every step with wisdom, she always lifts me up when I am sunk in an ocean of worries!'
17. The ladies replied:
'O Lord of men! We do know what is going on in your beloved's mind. Look: she is lying over there on the bare floor, O subduer of the enemies.' "
18. Nārada said:
"Purañjana's intelligence was agitated due to attachment to his wife. When he saw his queen lying unkempt on the floor, he fell into a state of great distress.
19. Although he was consoling her with sweet words with a burning heart, the king did not receive any indication from his beloved that she was angry at him out of love.
20. The hero, who was expert in conciliation, gradually consoled her. He touched her two feet, seated her on his lap, and caressed her. Then he spoke to her.
21. Purañjana said:
'Even if they have committed an offense, servants are unfortunate if their masters do not inflict corrective punishment on them on the grounds that the servants are part of the master's entourage, O beautiful one.
22. Punishment meted out on servants by the master is the greatest mercy; only an immature intolerant person does not recognize this to be an act of benevolence toward that person.

23. Please show us your face cast down out of bashfulness and the weight of love, O wise lady. Beaming with smiling glances, and decorated with blue locks of hair like bees, it has beautiful teeth, eyebrows, and nose and utters sweet words. I am yours.
24. I will inflict punishment on whoever has committed an offense against you—unless he be a *brāhmaṇa* or a servant of Viṣṇu.[78] You are the wife of a hero: I will see to it that that person is not joyful or free from fear anywhere in the three worlds or beyond.
25. I have never seen your face without *tilaka* (sacred clay marking), or dirty, joyless, furious out of anger, colorless, or bereft of passion. Nor have I ever seen your two perfectly formed breasts heaving in sorrow, and your red *bimba* fruit–colored lips bereft of their *kuṅkuma* powder color.
26. I am your best friend, but I committed an offense: addicted to the vice of hunting, I went off to the chase on a whim. What woman, eager [for love], would not accept a lover who has come under her control, his manly pride shattered by the force of Cupid's flowery arrows? So please forgive me.' "

Book IV, Chapter 27

1. Nārada said:
"Having brought Purañjana under her complete control by her wiles in this manner, Queen Purañjanī enjoyed her husband, and gave him enjoyment, O great king.
2. The king was delighted when his queen approached him with a bright face, contented, bathed, and auspiciously adorned, O king.
3. Pressed to the bosom of his wife, his neck embraced and his mind stolen away by intimate exchanges, the king was unaware of the speedy passage of insurmountable Time: he was captured by that enchanting woman day and night.
4. Overcome by *tamas* and bound by passion, the noble-minded king lay on a priceless bed with his queen's arms as his pillow. He thought of her as the highest thing in his life, and did not think of his own higher goal.
5. While he was enjoying with his wife in this way, his mind tainted by lust, the king's youth passed by as if it were half an instant, O Lord of kings.

6. Purañjana begot eleven hundred sons in Queen Purañjanī, but half his life was consumed in doing so, O sovereign!
7. He also begot one hundred and ten daughters, O protector of men. Named the Paurañjanīs, and endowed with good qualities, character, and magnanimity, they enhanced the reputation of their mother and father.
8. The king of Pañcāla brokered marriages for his sons, who expanded the family lineage, as well as for his daughters, with suitable young heroes.
9. One hundred sons were begotten to each and every one of his sons, and, through them, the Paurañjana lineage prospered across Pañcāla.
10. Purañjana became attached to sense objects through a growing attachment to his offspring, his inheritors, and his dependents, treasury, and household.
11. Just like you, full of various desires, the king underwent consecration and then offered sacrifices to the gods, forefathers, and lords of beings. These sacrifices were horrific due to the massacre of animals they involved.
12. Then Time, which is not dear to those who hold women dear, approached the king, whose mind was attached to his family, and forgetful of his actual [spiritual] obligations.
13. There was a *gandharva* king called Chaṇḍavega (having impetuous speed). That powerful king had three hundred and sixty *gandharva* warriors.
14. He had a similar number of *gandharva* females, black and white, who were their consorts. They surrounded the city, which had been engineered so as to fulfill all desires, and plundered it.
15. When those followers of Chaṇḍavega began to besiege the city of Purañjana, the serpent Prajāgara (one who stays awake) resisted them.
16. He was the powerful superintendent of Purañjana's fort, and battled single-handedly for one hundred years with the seven hundred and twenty *gandharvas*.
17. But this ally was alone in his fight with many. When he began to weaken, Purañjana and his relatives fell into great anxiety, and so did the citizens of the city.
18. But, imbibing liquor and under the control of women, and seizing tribute from his citizens, the king refused to entertain fear in that Pañcāla stronghold.

19. Meanwhile, O King Prācīnabarhiṣat, there was a certain daughter of Time who desired a husband. She wandered around the three worlds, but no one welcomed her.
20. Because of her personal bad luck, she was known in the world as Durbhagā (the unlucky one). Previously, accepted by the sage-king descendant of Puru, she had bestowed a boon upon him."[79]

Book IV, Chapter 28

1. The king of the *yavanas* was named Bhaya (fear). His soldiers also roamed about the earth along with the daughter of Time, accompanied by the king's brother, Prajvāra (fever).
2. One day, they violently attacked the city of Purañjana, which was replete with material pleasures. It was still guarded by the serpent protector, but he had by now become old.
3. The daughter of Time invaded that city of Purañjana by force. A person overwhelmed by her immediately finds himself bereft of vitality.
4. While it was being ravaged by the daughter of Time, the *yavana* soldiers entered through the gates with great force and poured through all parts of the city from all directions.
5. While she was harassing the city, the proud Purañjana, attached to his family and afflicted with the false sense of "my-ness,"[80] experienced all sorts of intense sufferings.
6. The unfortunate fellow's mind was attached to sense pleasures, and his higher discrimination had been destroyed. Assailed by the daughter of Time, he became bereft of beauty and all his riches were seized by force by the *gandharva* and *yavana* soldiers.
7. Purañjana saw that his city had been destroyed, and that his sons, grandsons, followers, and ministers had lost their respect and had become antagonistic. Moreover, he saw that his wife had lost her affection for him.
8. Purañjana saw the Pañcāla kingdom invaded by enemies. Finding himself in the grasp of the daughter of Time, and overwhelmed by immeasurable anxiety, he could not find a solution to the situation.
9. Caressing his wife and sons, the wretched fellow still craved for sense pleasures, even though these had become useless to him because of the daughter of Time. His interest in the destination of his *ātman* had long been lost.

10. The king began to abandon the city, even though he did not wish to do so. It had been overrun by the *gandharvas* and *yavanas* and devastated by the daughter of Time.
11. Then Prajvāra (fever), the elder brother of Bhaya (fear), arrived there. Desiring to please his brother, he burned down the entire city.
12. As the city was burning, the head of the household with his wife, followers, and goods, along with the citizens, were all tormented.
13. The house of Prajāgara, the city's protector, had been seized by the *yavanas*, and he himself had been consumed by Prajvāra (fever). When the city was overwhelmed by the daughter of Time, he was sorely tormented.
14. Unable to defend the city and under great stress, the serpent Prajāgara trembled intensely, desiring to abandon it, like a snake the hollow of a tree on fire.
15. Seized by the *gandharvas* and assailed by the inimical *yavanas*, the king's limbs became weak, and he cried out.
16.–17. The unfortunate fellow was a householder whose mind was fixed on domestic affairs. He had embraced the notion of "I" and "mine" toward his daughters, sons, grandchildren, daughters-in-law, attendants, and whatever remained of his property in the form of palace, treasury, and possessions. When the time for separation from his wife arrived, he thought:
18. "When I have departed to the other world, how will the mistress of the house survive, deprived of her lord and lamenting for her sons?
19. Unless I had eaten, she would not take her meal; if I had not bathed, she would not bathe before me; if I was displeased, she became very alarmed; and if I was abusive, she remained silent.
20. She enlightened me when I was in ignorance, and she was immersed in sorrow when I had to travel abroad. Even though she has heroes as sons, [without me] she will not wish [to continue] this path of the householder.
21. How will my poor sons and helpless daughters survive when I am gone? It will be like being on an ocean without a boat [for them]."
22. As the king was lamenting with his pitiful intelligence in this way, even though he should have known better, the one known as Bhaya (fear) made up his mind to seize him, and drew near.
23. As he was being dragged away by the *yavanas* like an animal to his fate, the king's followers ran after him, greatly aggrieved and lamenting.

24. At this, the serpent, who had already been seized, abandoned the city and followed him. The city was then destroyed and returned to the elements.
25. As he was being dragged away by the powerful *yavanas*, the king was overcome by *tamas* and could not even remember who had previously been his friends and well-wishers in the past.
26. Those sacrificial beasts that had formerly been slaughtered by him without mercy, now sliced him with their axes in anger, remembering the carnage he had inflicted upon them.
27. Immersed in boundless *tamas*, the king's memory became erased. He then experienced suffering for unlimited years as a result of being corrupted by his attachment to women.
28. Due to his attachment to his wife in his mind [at the moment of death], in his next life Purañjana became a beautiful maiden in the palace of Rājasiṃha of the Vidarbha kingdom.[81]
29. The Pāṇḍya king Malayadhvaja, conqueror of many cities, after defeating other kings in battle, took this maiden [called Vaidarbhī] as wife as a tribute to his heroism.
30. He begot in her a dark-eyed daughter, and seven younger brothers who became kings of the southern lands.
[. . .]
33. The sage-king Malayadhvaja divided the land among his sons, and then, desiring to worship Kṛṣṇa, went to the Kulācala mountains.
34. The ravishing-eyed daughter of the Vidarbha king's name was Vaidarbhī. Renouncing palaces, sons, and pleasures, she followed the Pāṇḍya king, just as moonlight follows the moon.
35.–36. The rivers named *Candravasā*, *Tāmraparṇī*, and *Vaṭodakā* flow in that place. Cleansing himself on both levels (physical and mental) with the sacred waters of those rivers, Malayadhvaja performed austerities (*tapas*). He subsisted on bulbs, fruit kernels, roots, fruits, leaves, grass, and water. This gradually emaciated his body.
37. Seeing everything with equal vision, the king transcended dualities—summer and winter, wind and rain, hunger and thirst, friend and foe, happiness and distress, etc.
38. His passions burned by the cultivation of knowledge and austerity, he controlled his senses, breath and mind by following the *yogic* restraints and observances (*yamas* and *niyamas*). He then united his *ātman* to *Brahman*.

39. He remained stationary in the same spot like a pillar for one hundred celestial years,[82] focusing his attachment on *Bhagavān* Vāsudeva and nothing else.
40. Just like the witness of the emotions of a dream, he perceived that the *ātman* within pervaded but yet was distinct from the body and mind: so he desisted from [identifying with] these.
41.–42. Through the pure lamp of knowledge radiating in all directions, the king could perceive the *ātman* in *Brahman* and *Brahman* in the *ātman*. This knowledge is imparted by Hari as *guru* in the form of instructions spoken directly by *Bhagavān*.[83] Then, after giving up even this ultimate perception, he desisted [from all mental activities].
43. Meanwhile, Vaidarbhī gave up all pleasures and lovingly served her husband, Malayadhvaja, the knower of the ultimate *dharma*.[84] She considered her husband to be her Lord.
44. Her hair became matted, she wore rags and was emaciated from fasting. In the company of her husband, she had become like a flame that becomes extinguished when the fuel is extinguished.
45. Not realizing that her beloved had given up [embodied existence], she attended to him as before. He had been sitting completely motionless on his seat (*āsana*).
46. When she did not feel any warmth in his feet as she was massaging them, Vaidarbhī became terrified, like a deer that has strayed from the herd.
47. Lamenting that she was now forsaken and without any protection, she soaked her breasts with tears of despair and wailed loudly in the forest:
48. "Get up, get up, O sage-king! You are supposed to protect this earth, with its ocean girdle, which is now fearful of robbers and wayward warriors."
49. Lamenting in this way, the young girl, who had followed her husband into the forest, fell at the feet of her husband, crying and shedding tears.
50. Grieving, she assembled a funeral pyre made of wood and burned the body of her husband on it. She had made up her mind to follow him in death by entering it.
51. Then, O master, some friend of hers from before—a *brāhmaṇa* and knower of the *ātman*—[arrived there]. He comforted her with sweet words as she was weeping, and spoke to her.

52. The *brāhmaṇa* said:
"Who are you? Of whose lineage? And who is that lying there for whom you mourn? Don't you know me as your friend with whom you previously used to roam about?
53. O friend! Perhaps you remember your friend called Avijñāta, the unknown one [of IV.25.10]? Attached to worldly pleasure, you abandoned me and left seeking some other destination.
54. We were swans [pure *ātman*], you and I, O noble lady, and our place of refuge was the Mānasa lake. There passed a period of one thousand years when we were without home.
55. You were that swan. You abandoned me, O friend, and set out for the earth, your mind set on worldly pleasures. There you saw a place built by some woman.
56. It had five pleasure groves, nine gates, one protector, three surrounding walls, six families, five marketplaces, five materials, and was governed by a woman.
57. The pleasure groves [in the analogy] are the objects of the senses, and the nine gates are the [orifices of the body for the functioning of the] life airs (*prāṇa*), O master. The surrounding walls are fire, water, and food; and the families are the collection of the six senses.
58. The marketplaces are the connotative organs (*kriyāśakti*),[85] and the five materials are the imperishable elements (the *mahābhūtas* of earth, water, fire, air, and ether). The governor is the intelligence.[86] Once a person enters that place, he is no longer aware [of the real self].
59. Influenced by an attractive woman, you enjoyed in that place, and gave up your memory [as to your real self]. Because of that association, you have attained this miserable state, O master.
60. You are not the daughter of Vidarbha, and this hero is not your real well-wisher. Nor were you the husband of Purañjanī [in your past life] by whom you were trapped in the city of nine gates.
61. It is by *māyā* illusion that you think that man [in your past life, Purañjana] is this chaste woman [that you are now, Vaidarbhī]. You are neither. We are swans [the *ātman*].[87] Please [try to] perceive our real nature.
62. I am you—you are no one else. And see too how you are me. The wise do not see even the slightest difference between us at all.[88]
63. Just as a person beholds the one self as having become two in the reflection of a mirror or an eye, such is the difference between us."[89]

64. In this way, the swan was enlightened by the other swan of the Mānasa lake and regained his memory, which had been lost because of deviating from his original true nature.
65. O Prācīnabarhiṣat! This spiritual teaching has been taught to you in an allegorical manner because *Bhagavān*, the Lord of the Universe, likes to remain beyond the senses.

Book IV, Chapter 29

1. Prācīnabarhiṣat said:
"O Lord! We do not understand your words clearly. The sage-poets understand them, but not us, who are bewildered by ritualism (*karma*)."
2. Nārada said:
"[In the allegory] one should understand Purañjana to be the *puruṣa* (*ātman*). He builds for himself the city (i.e., a body), which has one, or two, or three or four feet, many feet, or no feet at all.[90]
3. The person referred to as Avijñāta, 'the unknown one,' is *Īśvara*, the friend of that *puruṣa*. He cannot be known by people through mundane names, qualities, or actions.
4. Desiring to enjoy the *guṇas* of *prakṛti* in their entirety, the *puruṣa* decided that from all the forms, the one with two hands and feet and nine gates was undoubtedly the best.
5. One should interpret the woman as being the intelligence (*buddhi*), which creates the notion of 'I' and 'my.' Using the intelligence, a person enjoys the *guṇas* in this body through the eye, etc.
6. The male companions are the group of senses that produce knowledge and action (the *jñānendriyas* and *karmendriyas*),[91] and the female companions are their activities. The serpent is *prāṇa*, which has five functions.[92]
7. Know that the greatly powerful one (the eleventh attendant) is the mind. He is the leader of both sets of senses. The *Pañcālas* are the five sense objects, in the midst of which is the city of nine gates.
8. The pairs of gates are the two eyes, the two nostrils, the two ears, the mouth, the genitals, and the anus. [*Prāṇa*] goes out through these to the sense object connected with each respective gate.
9. The two eyes, two nostrils, and mouth are the five gates placed in the front (the east). The right ear is the southern gate, and the left ear is the northern gate.

10. The two lower gates, the penis and anus, have been spoken of as the western gates. The two eyes, Khadyotā and Āvirmukhī, have been built in one location. Through these, the master of the eyes (the *puruṣa*) experiences Vibhrājita, which is form and color.
11. Nalinī and Nālinī are the two nostrils, and smell has been called Saurabha. The sense of smell is Avadhūta; Mukhya is the mouth; Vipaṇa, speech; and Rasavid (Rasajñā), taste.
12. In the allegory, Āpaṇa is [speech associated with] everyday affairs and Bahūdana the varieties of foodstuffs. Pitṛhū is known as the right ear and Devahū the left ear.
13. The lands of the *Pañcālas* are the [two types of] scriptures, one of which teaches the path of material activity and the other the path of renunciation. With the help of Śrutadhara, the ears, one can proceed to the realm of the forefathers, or the realm of the gods [depending on the scriptures one listens to and follows].[93]
14. [In the allegory,] Āsurī is the penis and [Grāmaka] the attachment of common folk to sex. Durmada is said to be the sexual act, and the rectum has been called Nirṛti.
15. Vaiśasa is hell. Lubdhaka is the anus. Now hear from me about the two blind ones: they are the hands and feet. By utilizing them, a person can go about and perform actions.
16. The inner quarters are the heart, and the mind is that which was called Viṣūci (Viṣūcīna). According to the mind's states, one experiences illusion, peace, and joy in the heart.
17. Due to being instigated by the *guṇas*, the mind is transformed [during sleep], or transforms itself [when awake], into various states. The *ātman*, although a witness [and never subject to transformation], identifies with those same states caused by the *guṇas*.
18. The chariot is the body and the horses are the senses. Although motionless, its movement is the passage of the year. The wheels are the two types of *karma* (good and bad), and the banners are the three *guṇas*. The tethers are the five life airs (*prāṇas*).
19. The rein is the mind, and the charioteer is the intelligence.[94] The chariot seat is the heart. The five carriage boxes are the five objects of the senses, and the seven chariot bumpers are the seven bodily constituents (*dhātus*: lymph, blood, flesh, fat, bone, marrow, semen).
20. The five types of external movements are the five organs of actions. With these, one runs after mirages. The army consists of the

eleven senses (the five knowledge acquiring senses, the five organs of action and the mind) and one takes pleasure from five kinds of slaughter. Caṇḍavega is the year, by whom Time is demarcated.
21. His *gandharva* warriors are the days, and the *gandharva* females, the nights. They steal away one's life span by their three hundred and sixty steps.
22. Kālakanyā, whom people do not welcome, is old age in person. The king of the *yavanas* is Death. He adopted Kālakanyā as his sister for the purpose of destruction.
23. His roaming *yavana* soldiers are mental anxieties and illnesses. Prajvāra is fever. It is of two kinds: quick and intense (hot and cold), which are the blight of living beings.
24. In this way, the embodied *puruṣa*, enveloped in *tamas* in the body, is made to suffer for a hundred years through many types of suffering: from the environment, from other living entities, and from one's own mind and body.[95]
25. Although it is without qualities, the *puruṣa* thinks that the qualities of the mind, senses, and life airs are within itself. Therefore it lies [within the body] full of desire, and performs actions thinking, 'I am this' and 'that is mine.'[96]
26. Although it is [capable] of seeing its own true nature, when the *puruṣa* neglects *Bhagavān*, the supreme *guru*, it becomes addicted to the *guṇas* of *prakṛti*.
27. Thinking itself to be a product of the *guṇas*, the *puruṣa* then acts helplessly, and is consequently reborn [in a particular kind of body] according to whether its actions were white (*sattva*), black (*tamas*), or red (*rajas*).[97]
28. Sometimes, as a result of performing white actions, he is born into the celestial realms full of light. At other times, [owing to the performance of red actions], he experiences struggles born of activity, which result in unhappiness; and at other times again [owing to the performance of black action], he experiences immense grief.
29. His intelligence is covered [as to his real nature], in accordance with his mind and the qualities of his actions, and so he sometimes attains the state of a celestial, sometimes of a human, and sometimes of an animal, either as a male, a female or, sometimes, as neither.
30.–31. Just like a wretched dog wanders around tormented by hunger and obtains either [a beating with] a stick or cooked rice [to eat]

in accordance with its destiny, so, in the same, way, the embodied soul (*jīva*), its mind full of desire, traveling on paths that are either high (righteous) or low (nonrighteous), attains either agreeable or disagreeable results in high, middle, or low destinations in accordance with destiny.

32. There is no remedy for the *jīva* being subject to one of the sufferings. These are caused by either its own mind and body, or other living entities, or the environment. And even if there were a remedy, the remedy itself would soon be counteracted [by some other suffering].

33. Any counteraction is of the nature of a person carrying a heavy burden on his head, who then places it on his shoulder [thereby merely shifting the pain from one place to another].

34. O sinless king! Mere action cannot completely counteract another action, just as a dream cannot counteract a dream—both are permeated by ignorance.

35. Even though its reality does not actually exist, *saṁsāra* does not just cease—just as [the unreal experience] of a person roaming about in dream through the medium of the subtle body does not cease [until awakening].

36. *Saṁsāra* is the continued cycle of ignorance of a living being who in reality is *ātman*. The remedy is supreme *bhakti* to the *guru*.

37. When *yoga* is directed exclusively to Vāsudeva, *Bhagavān*, then renunciation and knowledge awaken.

38. Then *bhakti* will manifest for a faithful person absorbed in the narratives (*kathā*) of Acyuta, and always hearing and contemplating them, O sage-king.

39. *Bhakti* is found wherever there are *bhāgavata* devotees, O king. The *bhāgavatas* are saints who eagerly hear and recite the narratives and qualities of *Bhagavān* with pure hearts and minds.

40. In that association, rivers of the nectar of Viṣṇu's narrations recited by the great souls flow everywhere. Those who imbibe these with inundated ears without getting satiated are never affected by illusion, sorrow, fear, or hunger, O king.

41. But the world of embodied beings (*jīvas*), constantly harassed by those sufferings, is not attracted to the ocean of nectar of Hari's narrations.

42.–44. Even up to this very day, Śiva, Lord of the mountain, who is *Bhagavān* himself; Manu; Brahmā; Dakṣa and other progenitors; the lifelong Kumāra celibates headed by Sanaka; Marīci; Atri; Aṅgirā; Pulastya; Kratu; Bhṛgu; Vasiṣṭha; and other such [great sages and divine] beings including I myself cannot see the all-seeing supreme *Īśvara*, even though we see [many otherwise inaccessible things] through our *tapas*, wisdom, and *samādhi* states and we are masters of sacred speech and expounders of the Veda.

45. Those who follow the profound and extensive Vedic sacred texts worship the limited celestial gods in accordance with the prescriptions outlined in the sacred hymns. But such people do not know the Supreme.

46. When *Bhagavān*, who is cherished in the heart of a person, favors that person, then he or she is able to detach the mind, both from the ritualism of the Vedas and from the world.

47. Therefore, O Prācīnabarhiṣat, do not look upon ritualistic actions as being real, even though they have the semblance of reality. They make contact with the ear [as enticing Vedic prescriptions], but do not make contact with the actual Truth.

48. Those whose intelligence is clouded proclaim that the Vedas are all about ritualistic acts.[98] They do not understand the Veda. They do not know that personal realm of Lord Kṛṣṇa (Janārdana).

49. You have covered this entire earth globe with the sacred *darbha* grass facing east [as per the Vedic prescriptions] and have become proud and arrogant, slaughtering many animals. You do not know the higher type of action. That which is for the satisfaction of Hari is [true] action, and the mind fixed on Him is [true] knowledge.

50. Hari is the soul of all embodied beings. He is the *Īśvara* of *prakṛti*. Taking refuge of His feet is the [true] benefit for people in this world.

51. It is He who is the soul, the most beloved One. By taking refuge in Him, one does not experience even the slightest fear. The one who knows this is the learned one. Such a learned one is Hari in the form of the *guru*."

52. Nārada said:

"So, Your question has been dealt with, O best of men. Now please listen to me while I tell you a confidential truth.

53. Consider a deer, its ears enchanted by the sounds of a swarm of bees, excited after mating, and wandering about in a secluded spot full of flowers. But, while grazing on some insignificant [grass], it

remains ignorant of the bloodthirsty wolves ahead of it, and the arrow of the hunter that has been discharged at it from behind.
54. O king, you should see your own self as that deer! The secluded spot is the refuge of women, whose nature is like the flowers. After copulating, your mind is absorbed in them. You seek a tiny bit of happiness—the fruit of ritualistic acts performed out of greed—but this happiness is most insignificant like the [fleeting] fragrance and nectar in flowers. Your ears are completely seduced by the very gratifying words of people—especially women—which are like the sounds reverberated by the swarms of bees. Yet you do not reflect on the small components of time, which bring an end to the days and nights, consuming your life like the pack of wolves. The hunter following you unnoticed from behind as you enjoy in your residences is Death, who finally pierces your heart with an arrow.
55. You are that deer. After considering your own behavior to be like that of the deer, control the [outward] flow of your sense of hearing by your mind, and your mind internally by your heart. Renounce schemes for illicit liaisons that take place in the abodes of women, and please Kṛṣṇa instead. He is the refuge of the swanlike devotees. Gradually desist [from materialistic hankerings]."
56. The king said:
"O *brāhmaṇa*! I have heard and taken to heart all that your honor has spoken. My own preceptors did not know all this, as, otherwise, had they known, why did they not disclose it?
57. You have cleared a major doubt of mine in this matter that was created by them. Even the sages are bewildered when it comes to that which lies beyond the realm of the senses.
58. In this world, a person relinquishes the body with which he or she engages in action, but experiences the consequences of those actions in another body in the next life.
59. This doctrine of the knowers of the Vedas [about *karma*] is accepted everywhere: a prescribed act that is performed is invisible; its [consequence] cannot be seen."
60. Nārada replied:
"The person by whom an act is performed through the subtle body of the mind is the very same one who experiences its [consequence] in the next world. One is not separated from the consequences [because of death].[99]

61. This is just like when a man leaves his living body when sleeping [in dream], and enjoys through a similar or different [dream] body the [seeds of] action that had previously been deposited in the mind [when awake].[100]
62. A person who mentally says, 'I am such and such, and that person is this and that, and these [children] are mine,'[101] receives whatever *karma* is produced [from his actions]. It is as a result of this that there is rebirth.
63. Just as someone's state of mind can be inferred by both the activities and aspirations of that person, so in the same way, the actions performed in a previous life can be inferred from a person's present states of mind (*citta-vṛtti*).
64. Something that has never been anywhere experienced, heard, or seen in one birth might yet appear in the mind if an impression of that thing is imprinted on the mind [from a previous birth].[102]
65. Therefore, O king, you should be aware that an unfamiliar mental image occurring to a person in one body corresponds to [the past-life imprint of that experience recorded] in the subtle body, for the mind is not able to conjure up an object that has never been experienced.
66. The mind reveals the past births of a person, as well as what will come to be and what will not come to be in the future. Blessings upon you!
67. Sometimes, something that has never been seen or heard in this life is experienced in the mind. Whatever this thing might be, it can be inferred that it is based on [something that has been experienced in a different] place, time, and situation.[103]
68. All objects of perception enter the mind sequentially, in groups, and then depart. Everyone is born with a mind [which has been retained with its impressions over countless births].
69. When the mind is exclusively established in *sattva*, absorbed in the presence of *Bhagavān*, then this universe is revealed by that presence. It then shines forth in full manifestation, just like [the sun is revealed] by an eclipse of the moon.
70. This conglomeration of *guṇas*, sense objects, senses, mind, and intelligence [that is, embodied existence] remains in force perpetually, for as long as this notion of 'I' and 'mine' is not given up by a person.

71. This awareness of 'I' is not manifest in deep sleep, swoon, intense pain, in the state of death and fever, nor in the interruption of the movement of breath (*prāṇāyāma*).
72. The subtle body does not manifest as fully in the embryo or in childhood, as it does in youth, because it is then only partially manifest, just as the moon does not manifest as fully when it is a new moon.
73. Although objects do not actually exist, *saṁsāra* does not cease for one contemplating sense objects, just as is the case with objects in dreams [for one still dreaming], even though they are unreal.
74. In fact, the subtle body consists of five parts (the five *prāṇas*),[104] three coverings (the *guṇas*), and sixteen expansions (the ten cognitive and conative organs and the mind). When this subtle body is connected with consciousness, it is called *jīva*.
75. It is through the subtle body that the *puruṣa* receives and relinquishes bodies, and it is through the subtle body that he experiences joy, grief, fear, suffering, and happiness.
76.–77. It is the mind that is the cause of *saṁsāra*, O best of men! Just as a caterpillar does not leave [its footing on one leaf] and proceed on [until it has a secure footing on another leaf],[105] so a person does not relinquish self-identification with the previous body, even while in the actual process of dying, until the *karmas* [associated with the previous body] have completely finished and he or she attains another body.
78. For as long as one remains contemplating [the objects of the senses] and pursuing them through the senses, one accumulates *karma*. And as long as there is *karma*, one remains enmeshed in ignorance and the actions of the non-self (the mind and body).
79. Thus, in order to counteract all this, worship Hari with all your being, realizing this universe to be identical with Him, and that its creation, maintenance, and destruction are all due to Him."
80. Maitreya said:
"The noble Nārada, best of the Bhāgavata devotees, revealed the destination of the swanlike devotees to this king. He then returned to Siddha-loka, the realm of the perfected *yogīs*.
81. The sage-king Prācīnabarhī instructed his sons in the protection of the citizens, and then departed for Kapila *āśrama* to perform austerities (*tapas*).

82. There, freed from all attachments, worshipping the lotus feet of Govinda with concentrated mind and devotion (*bhakti*), the hero attained the state of liberation which bestows the same form as the Lord (*sarūpya*).[106]
83. O Vidura, One who hears or causes others to hear this spiritual allegory of the celestial sage Nārada is freed from the subtle body.
84. It was delivered from the mouth of the celestial sage, and cleanses the mind, purifying the worlds with the glories of Mukunda. Anyone who hears it narrated attains the supreme destination. Freed from all bondage, that person no longer wanders about in *saṁsāra*.
85. I studied this wonderful spiritual allegory. Through it the question about a person's householder life has clearly been dealt with."

Book V

The Teachings of the Ṛṣabha Incarnation: The Ascetic as Madman

Yoga Blueprint

This narrative, like others, emphasizes again the illusory nature of sensual pleasures and family happiness. The passage stresses the importance of devoting at least the last years of life to renunciation and the pursuit of higher truths. Of interest here is the preeminence given to the brāhmaṇa *caste, but what is especially noteworthy in this regard is the* Bhāgavata's *expectations pertaining to the qualifications of the true* brāhmaṇas *that make them respectworthy in the first place in 5.24–25.*

The setting of the passage is Ṛṣabha about to renounce his kingdom and leave for the forest. He enthrones his eldest son, Bhārata, and requests his other sons to cooperate with their elder brother. Here we find him delivering parting spiritual teachings to them all.

Book V, Chapter 5

1. Ṛṣabha said:
"My dear sons! This body possessed by embodied beings in the world of men is not meant to be used for pleasures, which create so much trouble, and which are available to stool-eaters [such as hogs]. It is meant for divine austerities. By performing these, one purifies the mind, and one attains the eternal bliss of *Brahman*.
2. The sages say that service to the great souls is the door to liberation. Keeping company with those who are attached to women in

contrast is the door to *tamas*. The great-souled ones are those who are equanimous, peaceful, devoid of anger, a good friend [to all], and righteous.

3. Their goal in life is to establish love for Me, the Lord, not [to seek the company of] people who are attached to children, wife, and home, and are only occupied with maintaining the body. Such people take no pleasure in anything beyond whatever is necessary to maintain the body.

4. Indeed, that person who seeks fulfillment in the satisfaction of the senses is constantly bewildered, and engages in bad *karma*. I do not consider this mind-set wise, as this body, even though temporary, is the very thing which bestows suffering on the *ātman*.

5. Ignorance remains present for as long as there is no understanding of the Supreme; consequently, one does not inquire into the nature of the *ātman*. And as long as there is action [in pursuit of fulfilling desire], the mind remains absorbed in *karma*, and, consequently, is bound to a body.

6. Due to the soul being enveloped by ignorance in this manner, the mind functions, bound by *karma*. But one is not freed from being bound by the body for as long as love for Me, Vāsudeva, does not develop.

7. Even if one is learned, for as long as one is deluded about one's real self-interest and cannot see that endeavors performed under the influence of the *guṇas* never end up as had been anticipated, one's [higher] memory is lost. Consequently, a fool pursues a home and sex life, but finds only suffering instead.

8. This attraction to sex indulgence between a man and a woman, the wise say, is the knot in the heart that binds them. From this, comes this illusion of 'I' and 'mine,' which takes the form of a person's home, property, offspring, and the acquisition of ample resources.

9. When a sober person loosens the bondage of *karma* stemming from this knot in the heart in the form of the mind, and when he has turned his back on this [desire for sex and the like], then he has transcended its cause. At this point one is liberated and attains the Supreme.

10.–13. An intelligent person, endowed with resolution, perseverance, and *sattva*, should remove the characteristic known as the ego. This can be accomplished through the following ways: obeying Me, the supreme swanlike *guru*, with love; becoming free of desire; tolerating the dualities [of the world]; understanding the suffering of beings everywhere; inquiring into Truth; austerity; renouncing ambition; performing activities for Me; constant narrations about Me; associating with those who have Me as their Lord; glorifying My qualities; being free of enmity; equanimity; peacefulness; desiring to remove the understanding of the self as body and homestead; study of the sacred texts whose subject matter is the *ātman*; living in solitude; control of the mind, senses, and life breath; faith in Truth; undeviating celibacy; attentiveness; control of speech; perceiving my presence everywhere; knowledge illuminated with wisdom; and the practice of *yoga*.

14. With diligence, by means of this *yoga* practiced as indicated above, one should completely sever the bonds of the knot in the heart produced by ignorance. This knot is the reservoir of all *karma*. Once this is accomplished, one can desist from *yoga*.

15. The king and the teacher who are desirous of attaining My abode, and whose goal of life is My grace, should teach all this to their sons and disciples who do not know it, without getting impatient. They should not engage those who are bewildered by *karma* to perform more acts of *karma*. What benefit does a human being gain by causing one whose vision is lost to be engaged in *karma*, and thereby causing that person to fall farther into the abyss (of *saṁsāra*)?

16. One intent on fulfilling desires, who strives after material objects, is a person whose vision is lost as to his own personal true benefit. Creating enmity with others for the sake of a little happiness, a fool does not see the endless suffering [this engenders].

17. What learned person, who is compassionate and personally knows the Truth, upon seeing a person of limited understanding immersed in ignorance, would again direct that person, who is like a blind man, back on the wrong path?

18. One should not be a *guru*, one should not be a relative, one should not be a father, one should not be a mother, one should not be a celestial being, and one should not be a husband, if one cannot liberate [one's dependents] from involvement with the process of death (*saṁsāra*).

19. This body of Mine is hard to comprehend;[1] indeed, *sattva* is My heart and it is there that *dharma* resides. *Adharma* has been relegated

to a long distance behind me. Therefore, the Āryas call me Ṛṣabha (best of beings).

20. You have all been born from My heart. Therefore, serve the noble Bharata, who has been born from the same womb as you, with uncontaminated (*akliṣṭa*) mind. Doing this will constitute service and support for the population.[2]

21. Among created beings, creeping creatures (like snakes) are higher than plants; higher than these are those who are endowed with intelligence; higher than those are human beings; higher than them are the *pramatha* demons; higher than these, the *gandharva* celestials; next in the hierarchy are the *siddha*, perfected beings; and then come the attendants of the gods [such as the *kinnaras*].

22. The celestials, whose chief is Indra, are higher than the *asura* demons, and greater than these is Dakṣa and the sons of Brahmā. Śiva, the son of Brahmā is greater still. Śiva holds Me to be the supreme and, although I am the supreme Lord, I Myself hold the *brāhmaṇas* to be My lords.

23. I do not find any other being comparable to the *brāhmaṇas*, so what else could I consider superior? Whatever is offered to a *brāhmaṇa* by people with faith, I eat with relish—but this is not the case with [the oblations offered] in the Vedic *agni-hotra* fire ritual.[3]

24. It is the *brāhmaṇas* who have transmitted My ancient glorious body in the form of the Vedas. They are manifest *sattva*, the highest pure quality, along with peacefulness, discipline, truthfulness, compassion, austerity, tolerance, and realization of Truth.[4]

25. The *brāhmaṇas* engage in My devotion and, although they are destitute, [they do not seek anything from Me], even though I am unlimited, completely supreme, and the bestower of the celestial realms as well as of liberation. So what would they possibly seek from anywhere else?

26. O sons! With a pure mind, you should consider all creatures, whether moving or non-moving, to be worthy of respect due to being the abodes of Me in person. This, in truth, is the offering that is to be made to Me.

27. My worship consists of directly offering the activities of sight, words, and mind to Me. Without doing this, a person is not able to free him or herself from the great illusion, in the form of the bonds of death.

28. For the benefit of instructing society at large, the completely realized and magnanimous *paramahaṁsa* Bhagavān Ṛṣabha instructed His sons in this way, even though they themselves were highly educated. Then, for the great sages whose nature is peaceful, and who have desisted from all ego-based activity, He taught the *dharma* of the *paramahaṁsa* (topmost swanlike devotees). This *dharma* is characterized by detachment and by knowledge in *bhakti*. After this, He consecrated the eldest of His hundred sons, Bharata, for the governance of the world. Bharata was dedicated to the devotees of *Bhagavān* and he, too, was a topmost *Bhāgavata* devotee. Ṛṣabha Himself then renounced his home, retaining possession of only His body. He then internalized the sacred *āhavanīya* sacrificial fire within Himself,[5] and wandered forth from *Brahmāvarta*, the land of *Brahman*, like a madman, His hair disheveled, and with only the air as His clothing.
29. In the garb of an *avadhūta* (extreme ascetic), Ṛṣabha acted like a blind, dumb, deaf, stupid, and insane person. Since He had taken a vow of silence, He remained silent even when addressed by people.
30. He wandered about the earth traveling alone. Wherever He went—towns, villages, mines, fields, parks, mountain villages, army encampments, cowpens, herdsmen stations, merchant caravan sites, mountains, forests, and hermitages, etc.—He was surrounded along the way by the lowest of men, like a forest elephant surrounded by flies. He ignored their insults; farts; hurling of dust, stones, and feces; spitting, urinating, beatings, and derision. His mind was never disturbed by displaying any pride of 'I' and 'my,' since He was situated in His own glory, His own true nature. Realizing both the real and the non-real, He perceived this body, which is referred to as real, to actually be an unreal form.
31. He was an extremely handsome young man: His hands, feet, chest, long arms, shoulders, throat, face, limbs, and other bodily parts were [beautifully] composed. His face had a spontaneous smile, and was naturally attractive. His charming wide eyes were reddish and cooling, like fresh full-blown lotuses, and His nose, throat, ears, and forehead were perfect and delicate. His cheerful face and discreet smile cast Cupid, the holder of the flower bow, into the minds of the ladies in town. With His mass of brown, matted and curly hair hanging down, and His body dirty like that of an *avadhūta* ascetic, He appeared as if possessed by a demon.

32. Whenever *Bhagavān* Ṛṣabha saw that this world was antagonistic toward his type of *yoga*, He nonetheless considered compromising it to be unacceptable. He took the python vow: lying down, He ate, drank, chewed, urinated, and evacuated [in the same place], rolling His limbs around until His body was smeared in feces.
33. Yet the fragrant aroma of His sweet-smelling feces percolated that region for a distance of ten *yojanas* in all directions with a pleasant smell.[6]
34. In this way, adopting the behavior of a crow, deer, or cow while wandering about, standing, sitting or lying, He drank, ate, and urinated in the manner of crows, deer, and cows.
35. *Bhagavān* Ṛṣabha, the Lord of liberation, exemplified in this way the various behaviors of *yoga*. He experienced supreme absolute uninterrupted bliss in *Bhagavān*, Vāsudeva, who exists in the hearts of all creatures as the *ātman*. Because in His mind there was oneness and no separation or difference between Himself and that *ātman*, He was fully endowed with the attainment of all the *siddhi* mystic powers. These are the mystic powers of *yoga* attained spontaneously, such as flying through the air, [moving] at the speed of mind, disappearing, entering into the bodies of others, grasping things from afar, etc.[7] But, O king, He did not actually welcome these in His heart."

Book V, Chapter 6

1. King Parīkṣit said:
"But the mystic powers are attained spontaneously when the seeds of *karma* are burned up by the knowledge manifesting from the practice of *yoga*, O Lord. Surely they ought not to again become disturbances [to the path: so why did Ṛṣabha renounce them?]!"[8]
2. Sage Śuka replied:
"What you have said is true. Nevertheless, some [sages] never place faith in the fickle mind here in this world—just as a wicked *kirāta* hunter [does not place faith in a captured deer not escaping]!
3. Therefore it is said:
'One should never make friends with the fickle mind. From trusting it, the *tapas,* austerity, practiced for a long time by great Lords [such as Śiva and Saubhari[9]], was lost.

4. For the *yogī* who has made friends with it, the mind always creates a space for lust and the other enemies that follow it [anger and so on], just like a husband's wife who goes with other men.
5. Lust, anger, pride, greed, sorrow, illusion, and fear are the bonds of *karma*, and they have the mind as their root. So what sensible person would accept the mind [as trustworthy]?
6. Thus, although He was the topmost of all the lords of the universe, the majesty of *Bhagavān* Ṛṣabha went unnoticed due to His behavior, speech, and garb of an *avadhūta* ascetic, which appeared like those of a simpleton. Perceiving with perfect internal vision that the *ātman* was non-different from the [Supreme] *Ātman*, and desiring to abandon His own body and so teach to *yogīs* the method of leaving the body, He gave up identification with His body.
7. *Bhagavān* Ṛṣabha was freed from identification with His subtle body, but His body continued to wander about this earth with a semblance of ego, due to *vāsanas*, memory imprints, caused by *yogamāyā*.[10] He haphazardly traversed the regions of Koṅka, Veṅka, and Kuṭaka, and the regions of South Karṇāṭaka and arrived at a forest on the Kuṭaka mountain. He placed a stone in his mouth like a madman, and, naked and with scattered hair, roamed about there.
8. Then, a fierce forest fire broke out from the friction of the bamboos, which spread by the force of the wind. Engulfing that forest, it burned it up along with Ṛṣabha.
[. . .]
15. Which other *yogī* even in his imagination could follow the example set by the birthless Ṛṣabha? The *yogī* desires the powers of *yoga*, which were discarded by Ṛṣabha because they pertain to the realm of the unreal,[11] even though they endeavored [to present themselves to Him].
16. Thus has been narrated the spotless story of *Bhagavān* by name of Ṛṣabha, the supreme *guru* of all cows, *brāhmaṇas*, celestials, worlds, and Vedas. This account contains the highest and ultimate auspiciousness and purifies all the bad actions performed by people. Exclusive *bhakti* for *Bhagavān*, Vāsudeva, develops in both the one who hears and the one who recites this story attentively with growing faith.
17. It is in *bhakti* that sages continually immerse their minds, which are otherwise constantly tormented by the sufferings of *saṁsāra* with its various vices. Because of the insurmountable bliss of *bhakti*, they

have no interest even in final liberation, which is the supreme goal of life.[12] Liberation anyway manifests itself [as a by-product of *bhakti*], so all goals are fulfilled by dint of devotion to *Bhagavān*.

18. O king! *Bhagavān* Mukunda is the Lord, *guru*, beloved deity, lineage master, and sometimes servant of you and the Yadu dynasty. Howsoever that may be, my dear one, He sometimes awards *mukti*, liberation, to those who worship Him, but not *bhakti yoga*.

19. Ṛṣabha's desires were extinguished, since He had attained experience of His own eternal self. Out of kindness, He explained about the realm of the *ātman*, which is free from fear, to people of the world whose intelligence has been asleep for so long, due to [indulging in] fantasies of unreality [that is, taking the body to be the self]. Reverence to him, *Bhagavān* Ṛṣabha."

The Tale of King Bharata: The Mind at the Moment of Death

Yoga Blueprint

There are a number of yogic *elements in the story of King Bharata. The first, underpinning the cultural context of the* Bhāgavata, *reflects the Vedic notion that individuals are ideally expected to go through four stages of life (*āśramas*), each lasting twenty-five years. The first of these is* brahmacarya, *celibate studentship;*[13] *the second* gṛhastha, *householder;*[14] *the third,* vānaprastha, *forest dweller;*[15] *the fourth and final stage,* sannyāsa, *full ascetic renunciant. As we will find in the story of King Bharata, in the last stages, a person severs all attachment to home, hearth, and family and devotes the remaining years of life to cultivating* yoga *practices, performing austerities, and meditating in solitude. Additionally, the sacred texts advise one to undertake such practices in a holy place, where, in addition to worldly distractions being minimized, the atmosphere is pervaded by associations with divinity, as we will encounter in our story.*

The main yoga *lesson of the story, expressed in chapter 8, is the principle that the state of one's mind at the moment of death determines one's next life. In the* Bhagavad Gītā *(VIII.6), Kṛṣṇa states: "Whatever state of being one remembers when one leaves the body at the end of life, is the very state one will attain in the next life." Since he allowed himself to become excessively attached to a young fawn to the point where he became consumed with thinking about it constantly, Bharata's mind was absorbed in thought of the fawn when Death came to claim him, and thus his mind and consciousness were transferred into the body of a deer in his next life.*

There are, of course, other variables that feed into determining one's next birth, as outlined in the Yoga Sūtras *II.12–14, such as the pious and impious deeds performed in life, which, in Bharata's story, qualified his next births, granting him the boon of remembering the cause of his condition. Consequently, in his last birth, he exhibited the full symptoms of complete detachment from all things material, as expressed in* Yoga Sūtras *I.15–16. A further feature in this final life illustrates a foundational principle of* bhakti*: divinity can personally transubstantiate and manifest through material elements, such as the deity, as will be found in this story.*

Book V, Chapter 7

1. *Śri* Śuka said:
"Bharata, the great devotee of Lord Viṣṇu, was dedicated to ruling the earth. When he was deliberating on how to govern it [on the orders of his father] *Bhagavān* Ṛṣabhadeva, he took as his wife, Pañcajanī, the daughter of Viśvarūpa.
[. . .]
3. This continent was [previously] named Ajanābham, but since the time of Bharata, they designated it 'Bhārata.'[16]
4. Bharata, the Lord of the earth, had vast knowledge. Following his own *dharma* (duty), he governed the citizens with great affection, just as his father and grandfather had done. They, in turn, were following their own respective duties.
[. . .]
8. He enjoyed in this way for ten million years, at which time he perceived that the appropriate moment for extinguishing his *karma* [had arrived]. At this point, he divided among his sons his personal wealth, bestowed by his father and grandfather, according to the norms of inheritance. He then set out from his home, the abode of all kinds of opulence, to the holy place Pulaha.
9. Actually, even today, out of affection, Lord Hari appears to His devotees who reside there in that place, in whatever form they desire.

[. . .]
11. Bharata lived alone in the grove around that place known as Pulaha-*āśrama*. He dedicated himself to the worship of Lord Viṣṇu with varieties of flowers, shoots, *tulsi* leaves, and water, and with offerings of bulbs, roots, and fruits.[17] Detached from desires for sense objects, he cultivated peacefulness of mind and attained ultimate bliss.
12. By such uninterrupted worship of the Supreme Being, Bharata became calm and his heart melted from the surge of his growing love for God. All the hair on his body was seen to stand on end due to the force of his ecstasy, and his vision became obstructed by tears of affection caused by his contemplation.[18] His intelligence was absorbed in his heart,[19] which was like a deep lake overflowing with supreme bliss from his devotional practices of ever increasing meditation on the red lotuslike feet of his beloved Lord. In this state, he even sometimes forgot the very service to the Lord that he was supposed to be performing."

Book V, Chapter 8

1. *Śrī* Śuka said:
"Once, after finishing his customary duties and taking his bath in the great river, Bharata sat down on the water bank, reciting the sacred syllable *oṁ* for a period of three *muhūrtas* (two and a half hours).[20] *Oṁ* is the Absolute Truth *Brahman* manifest as sound.[21]
2. Just then, O king, a deer arrived at that body of water at that spot, desiring to drink.
3. Just at the very moment that she was drinking the water, the fierce sound of a lion's roar burst forth nearby, striking terror in all creatures.
4. The doe was by nature timid. When she heard that sound, her heart immediately became alarmed, her thirst was pushed aside, and her eyes became restless with trembling glances. Overwhelmed by fear of the lion, she suddenly leaped up in terror.
5. The deer happened to be pregnant. The embryo, dislodged due to her great fear, emerged from her womb and fell into the waters.
6. Separated from her herd, and traumatized by exhaustion and fear, as well as by the leap and the birth, the black doe then dropped down dead in some cave.

7. The kingly sage Bharat saw that the deer's offspring had been discharged by its parent and was being helplessly carried away by the current. So, with the compassion of a well-wishing soul, he lifted it out and took it to his *āśrama* hermitage, understanding that it was motherless.

8. Indeed, Bharata became personally extremely attached to the deer's offspring. Because of his contemplating, petting, fondling, protecting, and nurturing it day by day, his spiritual practices—adherence to the moral *yama* vows[22] and worship of the Supreme Being, etc.—were discarded, one by one. Finally, after the passing of some days, all of them were abandoned.

9. The king thought: 'Alas, this helpless offspring of a deer has been separated from its friends and herd by the Lord's power of Time, which is like an ever-moving chariot wheel. It has approached me for protection, and sees me as parent, brother, kinsman, and herd companion. It knows no one else and has full faith in me alone. Therefore, since it has taken refuge of me, it is fitting that I attend to its petting, fondling, protection, and nurture. I am not callous, and I know the sin of neglecting one's dependents.[23]

10. Surely those who are noble saintly Āryas,[24] peaceful in nature and benevolent to the helpless, sacrifice their own needs, even if they are very important, for a need such as this.'

11. In this way, Bharata became attached to the young deer while eating, bathing, wandering about, sleeping, and sitting, and his heart became bound by affection.

12. When he was about to go and collect *kuśa* grass, flowers, leaves, fruits, roots, or water, he became apprehensive about the threat of wolves and dogs [in his absence] and so he went into the forest accompanied by the young deer.

13. When, due to its simple nature, the deer became stuck here or there on the trails, Bharata would carry it on his shoulder out of kindness, his heart burdened with excessive love. Similarly, he would place it on his lap or chest and experienced great joy in petting it.

14. Even while he was in the middle of performing his religious rites, the emperor would get up midway and cast a glance at her. At such times, his mind reassured, he prayed for blessings for the fawn, saying: 'May there always be good fortune for you.'

15. At other times [when he could not see the fawn], he became like a miser who had lost his wealth. Pining over the fawn because of his affection and compassion, his heart would become afflicted with distress from being separated from her. Overwhelmed with intense anxiety, he then spoke as follows:
16. 'Oh alas! The helpless fawn, offspring of a dead doe, placed her faith in me. I have done nothing to merit this: on the contrary, I have the mentality of a deceitful *kirāta* hunter.[25] Will it return and, like a noble person, disregard all this by trusting me again?
17. Will I see it again wandering tranquilly on the fresh grasses of the gardens of this hermitage, under divine protection?
18. I hope that no wolf or wild dog or other such creature, wandering about alone, devours it.
19. The sun, lord [of the heavens], which is the soul of the three [Vedas][26] and which arises for the welfare of the entire world, is now setting, but the fawn has not returned. She was entrusted to me by the doe.
20. Or perhaps the fawn princess will yet return, and bring me delight—driving away the pining of its well-wisher with its various pleasing and attractive fawnlike frolics—even though I have done nothing to deserve this?
21. While it was playing, it would approach me in great alarm whenever I would close my eyes in a feigned state of *samādhi* meditation. On those occasions, agitated with affection, it would strike me with the tips of its horns, soft as water drops.
22. When the oblations for the fire sacrifice that had been placed on the sacred *kuśa* grass had been polluted [by it][27] and it was reproached by me, it became very frightened. It immediately stopped its frolics, and remained with all of its senses restrained, like the son of a sage.'
[. . .]
26. With his heart bewildered by such unsustainable delusions manifesting in the form of the fawn due to the force of his previous *karma*,[28] Bharata abandoned his *yogic* practices, his performance of *yogic* austerities, and the specifics of his worship of *Bhagavān*. How could this unnatural attachment to the fawn—a member of a different species—become an obstacle like this for the sage-king Bharata, who had taken up the practices of *yoga*? Bharata had already renounced even his own sons, as obstacles to his realization of the Ultimate

Truth, and they are so difficult to give up. But yet, he ended up neglecting his soul, *ātman*, due to his attachment to petting, pleasing, rearing, and nurturing that fawn. Finally, unsurpassable Death in the form of Time, voracious and consuming, appeared before him, like a snake before a mouse hole.

27. At that time, gazing at the deer who was lamenting at his side like a son, his mind completely absorbed in the deer, Bharata left this world, and with it the deer. He subsequently himself obtained the body of a deer.[29] However, along with losing the dead body, he did not lose the memory of this past life, as others do.

28. In that next birth, as a consequence of his previous efforts to worship God, Bharata was able to remember that he himself was the cause of attaining that state as a deer.[30] He lamented profusely:

29. 'Alas, what misfortune! I have fallen from the path of those who have attained self-realization. I had taken refuge in a sacred forest in solitude, had freed myself from all attachments, and had realized my own *ātman*. For a long time my mind was completely and utterly absorbed in Kṛṣṇa, the inner Soul of all souls by means of the *yogic* practices of hearing about him, reflecting upon him, chanting his glories, worshipping Him, and remembering Him all the time in all possible ways. But I let that same mind again flow away after a fawn from some distant place. What a fool I am!'

30. In this way, his detachment from worldly objects concealed [by his birth as a deer], Bharata left his mother deer and returned again from Kālañjara to the *āśrama* of the sages Pulastya and Pulaha. It was a sacred place, where the sacred *śālagrāma* stone is found,[31] a place favored by groups of tranquil-minded sages.

31. Subsisting on dry leaves, grass, and plants, and with only his own *ātman* as companion, Bharata awaited Death in that place, very fearful of [developing] any attachments. Counting [the days until] his deliverance from the *karma* that had caused this state of being a deer, when the time came, he gave up his deer body, which was wet from bathing in the waters of that holy place."[32]

Book V, Chapter 9

1. There was a certain *brāhmaṇa* in the lineage of sage Aṅgirā.[33] He was endowed with the qualities of peacefulness, self-control, austerity, the study and recitation of the Vedic texts, renunciation, contentment,

tolerance, humility, wisdom, non-enviousness, knowledge of the self, and joyfulness.[34] He begot nine sons from his elder wife, all with his same qualities of learning, character, behavior, handsomeness, and magnanimity. And in his younger wife, twins were born.

2. One of these was a male. They say that he was Bharata, best of the sage-kings, an exalted devotee of the Lord, who had given up the body of a deer and taken birth in a *brāhmaṇa* family as his final birth.

3. In that birth, too, he was very fearful of attachments to his kinsmen. So he fixed his mind on the lotus feet of the Lord, who destroys the bonds of *karma*, engaging in hearing, remembering, and reciting His qualities. By the grace of the Lord, he remembered the series of his previous births, and so, always concerned about obstacles to [the realization of] the *ātman*, he presented himself to the world as mad, stupid, blind, and deaf.

4. After his son had received the sacred thread of the twice-born,[35] the *brāhmaṇa*, his mind bound by love for his son, performed the sacred rites of passage for him culminating in the rite celebrating the completion of Vedic studies. This was in accordance with custom;[36] after all, the training of the son is to be undertaken by the father. He also arranged for his son to be taught the rules pertaining to cleanliness and mouth-washing, etc., and the rules of correct behavior, even though the son did not accept them.

5. Bharata, even in the very presence of his father, did not learn all this correctly. The father wanted to teach him the *gāyatrī mantra*, beginning with *oṁ* (*praṇāva*) and containing the words *bhūr, bhuvaḥ, svaḥ*,[37] but even over a period spanning the spring and summer months, he could only make Bharata grasp it incorrectly.

6. In this way, the father's mind was absorbed in affection for his son, whom he considered to be his very self, and he clung to the illusory notion that Bharata had to be educated. So he taught his son all the duties of the graduating Vedic student (*brahmacārya*)—cleanliness, study, the taking of vows, regulatory principles, and service to the *guru* and sacred fire, etc. But his hopes remained unrealized in all that time, as Bharata did not apply himself to them. Then the *brāhmaṇa* himself, forgetful [of his own *ātman* self] due to his attachment to his household, was taken away from his home by Time, which is never forgetful.

7. Thereupon, the chaste younger wife, entrusting the twins to her co-wife, herself went to the realm of her husband by following him.[38]
8. After the father had passed away, the other brothers desisted from the obligations of instructing their brother Bharata, thinking him to be dull-witted. Their sphere of understanding was limited to the ritualistic knowledge of the three Vedas,[39] not the higher knowledge of the Self, and so they were ignorant of Bharata's greatness.
9. When vulgar, beastly people called him names such as "mad," "dull-wit," "deaf," or "dumb," Bharata responded with behavior in accordance with their expectations. When he was made to work by the will of others, he worked. He ate whatever food came his way—whether from forced labor, or as wages, or by begging, or by Fate, and irrespective of whether it was a large or small amount, tasty or spoiled—but he never did so motivated by the gratification of the senses. He had gained mastery over his own *ātman*, which is blissfully experienced, pure, perfect in its own right, and untouched by cause and effect (the law of *karma*). He never identified himself as being the body in its experiences of happiness and distress, which are caused by the dualities.[40]
10. Bharata wandered about with only his buttocks covered with a loincloth, without covering his body in heat or cold, wind or rain. He was built like a bull, solid in limb and muscular. His *Brahman* effulgence, like a precious gem, was covered over by dirt from lying down on the ground and from not washing or massaging. With his sacred *Brahman* thread black from grime, he was considered "fallen, a *brāhmaṇa* in name only" by those who did not know who he really was.
11. When he was put to work even by his own brothers in field labor, he did it, but he was not aware of whether [the ground he was given to clear] was even or uneven, excessive or inadequate. When he sought food from others as wages for such work, he would eat a single grain, or an oil cake, or husk or rotten grain, or even the sediment left in the pot after cooking, and other such things, as if they were nectar.
12. As it happened, one day, the leader of a band of thugs, desiring a son, was about to offer a man as sacrificial beast to the Goddess Bhadrakālī.[41]
13. After this sacrificial "beast" by chance escaped, the chief's followers, who were pursuing him but unable to find their quarry—it

being midnight and covered in darkness—espied Bharata, by the unexpected hand of Fate. That descendant of the distinguished Aṅgirā lineage was standing guard, protecting the fields from deer and boars.
14. After evaluating Bharata's perfect [physical] qualities, the thugs bound him with ropes, thinking he would accomplish their master's task, and joyfully brought him back to Kālī's (Caṇḍikā's) temple, their faces beaming with joy.
15. The thugs then fed him, anointed him in accordance with their rites, dressed him in fresh cloth, and made him ready with ornaments, ointments, garlands, sacred clay, and so forth. Then they brought the human sacrificial animal before Goddess Bhadrakālī, to the accompaniment of the sounds of cymbals, drums, hymns, and songs, along with offerings of incense, lights, garlands, parched grains, shoots, sprouts, and fruit, in accordance with the prescriptions for a great sacrificial slaughter.
16. Then, the leader of the thugs, about to propitiate Goddess Bhadrakālī with the sacrifice of blood wine from the human beast, took up a terrible sword, which had been sharpened and consecrated for the occasion.
17. As is evident, the nature of these thugs was *rājasic* and *tāmasic*[42]—their minds had become proud from the passion of possessing wealth. They delighted in violence, and had willfully taken the unrighteous path, contemptuous toward the foremost (*brāhmaṇa*) caste, who are rays of God. The Goddess Bhadrakālī saw this extremely cruel act against Bharata, who was self-realized, without enemies, a well-wisher to all beings, and the direct descendant of a *brāhmaṇa* sage (Aṅgiras). Such an act had no sanction or support [in sacred scripture]. Just at the last moment, She suddenly burst forth [from the deity] in a scorching form, intolerable to bear due to its *Brahman* potency.
18. She burst forth, as if desiring to destroy the world. Her terrifying face had swollen red eyes and eyebrows like curved arches quivering with the force of the intense rage and intolerance that possessed Her. Then, with that very same sacrificial sword, She severed the heads of those sinful evildoers. Furiously emitting a resounding laugh, She drank the hot blood wine pouring out of the thugs' necks with her companions.[43] Staggering with the intoxication of excessive drinking, She sang raucously with Her associates, danced, and sported playfully with their heads as balls.

19. In this way, the offense of directing black rites against great souls completely rebounds back on the performer.
20. O King Parīkṣit, devotee of Viṣṇu, it is not, in actual fact, so amazing that Bharata remained unperturbed, even when his head was about to be severed. How can any fear exist for the supreme devotees of Hari (*paramahaṁsas*),[44] who are freed from the extremely tight knot in the heart caused by misidentifying the true *ātman* self with the body? They are the well-wishers of all living beings, without enmity, and have taken refuge at the Lord's lotus feet. So they are protected in all such situations by *Bhagavān* Himself in the form of His ever vigilant weapon of Time.

The Teachings to King Rahūgaṇa: The Illusion of Social Status

Yoga Blueprint

The main yogic *teachings imparted in this section focus on the illusory nature of social status and, of course, bodily identification in general. Of interest in the story is the great care Bharata took not to step on insects, reflecting the extreme sensitivity of enlightened saints to not inflicting violence on other creatures, even ants on the road. This principle of* ahiṁsā *is the very first of the yamas, which are the first of the limbs of yoga. It is thus the first step on the* yogic *journey and considered nonnegotiable by the* yoga *tradition (*Yoga Sūtras *II.31). Finally, the passage sends out a warning of not offending saints, even if they are wandering among us unbeknownst!*

Book V, Chapter 10

1. *Śri* Śuka said:
"One day, as Rahūgaṇa, the ruler of the Sindhu and Sauvīra kingdoms, was traveling along the banks of the *Ikṣumatī* river [to the *āśrama* of Kapila], Bharata, best of the *brāhmaṇas*, was spotted by chance by the chief of the king's palanquin bearers, who happened to be seeking a bearer at that time. Considering Bharata to be stout, young, of solid limbs, and capable of carrying a burden like a cow or an ass, he brought him back. So Bharata was seized, like the other bearers who had been pressed into forced labor before him, even

though he did not deserve such treatment. But that great soul just carried the palanquin.

2. Bharata was looking carefully ahead for the distance of an arrow [so as to avoid stepping on any insects]. When his stride was no longer in step with that of the other men, Rahūgaṇa noticed that the palanquin's motion was uneven and yelled to the men carrying the palanquin: 'Hey bearers! What is this? Walk properly! Carry the vehicle evenly.'

3. At this, hearing the chastising words of their master, the bearers' minds became fearful of punishment. So they informed the king as follows:

4. 'It is not us who are being careless, O lord of men. We are carrying the palanquin properly in accordance with your instruction. It is this person here who is not walking quickly, although he was just employed fresh today. We are not able to carry the palanquin evenly with him.'

5. After hearing the words of the poor fellows, Rahūgaṇa realized that the irregular [motion] of one person linked with others obviously creates irregularity with all those who are connected with him. Although he had served his elders [and so should have known better], his anger was somewhat aroused by the force of his kingly nature. His mind overcome by *rajas*, he [sarcastically] addressed Bharata, whose *Brahman* potency was concealed, like a fire [covered by ashes]:

6. 'Hey, brother! This is obviously a major inconvenience [for you]. The path is long and you have been carrying the load all alone for a long time as these other co-workers are not behaving as friends. You are not very stout, nor are your limbs solid, and you are assailed by old age.' Although he was sarcastically insulted in this way, Bharata continued carrying the palanquin silently as before. He had never projected the false notion of 'I' and 'mine' on this worthless body—which was to be his last. The body is, after all, just a residence created because of ignorance [of the true *ātman* self]. It is made specific [to each embodied being] by the *guṇas* out of material substances in accordance with *saṁskāras* and *karma*.[45]

7. Then, after some time, when the movement of the palanquin again became disrupted, Rahūgaṇa, furious, exclaimed: 'Hey! What is going on? You have disobeyed my order. By disregarding me, you are as

good as dead. I will teach you a lesson so that you will regain your senses, you deranged fool, just as Yama, the god of death with rod in hand, inflicts on the people in general.'

8. Although the king spoke in this uncontrolled way, he considered himself to be learned. Thinking himself lord of men, due to arrogance born of *rajas* and *tamas*, he had in the past rebuked all those who were devotees of *Bhagavān*. Bharata was a supremely powerful *brāhmaṇa*. He had realized his *Brahman* nature as *ātman* and was the dear friend of all beings. Half smiling, he spoke to the king, who was not very familiar with the behavior of perfected *yogis*.

9. The *brāhmaṇa* replied:

'What you have said is not sarcastic but in fact would be true, O hero, if, in fact, there were in reality a burden borne by me a bearer, and if there were indeed a path to be walked by me a walker [but, in reality, I am an *ātman* and thus have nothing to do with such things]. However, the wise do not talk about such qualities as "stout," pertaining to the body.

[*The* brāhmaṇa *here and in the following verses deconstructs from the perspective of* yogic *wisdom each of the phrases the king had just uttered, in order to enlighten him*.]

10. Stoutness, thinness, disease, anxiety, hunger, thirst, fear, quarrel, desire, old age, sleep, attachment, anger, ego, illusion, grief—these all apply to one who is born with a body; they do not apply to me [the *ātman*].

11. [With regard to your comment about being "as good as dead"], you are correct, it is in fact seen that all created things have a beginning and an end. And if the relationship between master and servant were forever fixed, O honorable king, then it would indeed be appropriate to speak of "obeying an order."

12. We do not find the slightest grounds for the notion of any real difference [between king and servant], other than what is assigned by social convention. Therefore, who is really a "ruler"? And what is really "servitude"? Nevertheless, despite all this, O king, tell us: What can we do for you?

13. What would be the benefit of your "remedy" for me, O hero, if, in fact, I have attained my true *ātman* self but am only acting like a

mad, deranged fool? And if, on the other hand, I actually really am a mad dullard, then your "remedy" will be like grinding the already ground [a waste of time].'

14. In this manner, Bharata, the best of the sages, responded by redirecting the king's statements back to him. His demeanor was calm, as ignorance—the root cause of forgetfulness of the *ātman*—had ceased to affect him. Thereafter, he continued carrying the king's vehicle as before, wishing to finish up his stock of activated *karma* by accepting this task as its fruits.[46]

15. The Pāṇḍu king, lord of the Sindhu and Sauvīra kingdoms, heard these words of the *brāhmaṇa*. They were in accordance with all the sacred texts on *yoga* and had the potency to cut through the knot [of ignorance] in the heart. Despite what had just transpired, because of his genuine faith, he hastily got down and touched his head at Bharata's feet, begging forgiveness, his kingly pride evaporated. The king at this point became fully qualified to inquire into Truth. He said:

16. 'You bear the sacred thread of the twice-born *brāhmaṇas*—so who are you, who wander about in disguise? Are you some ascetic renunciant? Whose son are you? From where have you come here, and for what purpose? If it is to uplift us, then are you perhaps the sage Kapila Himself?

17. I do not fear the thunderbolt of the king of the gods, Indra; nor the trident of the three-eyed God, Lord Śiva; nor the rod of Yama, god of death; nor the weapons of the gods of fire (Agni), sun (Sūrya), moon (Chandra), nor wind (Vāyu); nor the treasurer of the Gods (Kuvera). But I greatly fear offending the *brāhmaṇa* caste.

18. You have no attachments and roam about like a dullard with the extraordinary potency of your wisdom remaining concealed. Please explain your words, which deal with *yogic* concepts—they are incomprehensible to my mind.

19. I am traveling [on pilgrimage] to ask Kapila this question: "What is the refuge [for those suffering] in his world?" Kapila is the ultimate *guru* of the sages who know the truth about the *ātman*. He is the Lord of *yogīs*. He is Lord Hari [Viṣṇu] Himself, incarnating His quality of knowledge in the form of Kapila.[47]

20. Is it possible, good sir, that you are none other than He, Kapila? He wanders around, His true characteristics concealed, observing the condition of the world. How can someone whose spiritual intelligence

is blind and who is bound up with attachments to hearth and home, understand the ways of the Lords of *yoga*?

21. [Responding to Bharata's comments in verse 9:] It is well-known that fatigue is experienced by someone engaged in work, and so I infer that fatigue must be experienced by you, good sir, walking along carrying a burden. The ways of conventional reality must at least be acknowledged as really existing on some level, since it is not possible to fetch nonexistent water in a nonexistent pot.[48]

22. From heat applied to the cooking pot, the water inside is heated. From the heat applied to that water in turn, the grains of rice within become cooked. In the same way, *saṁsāra* ultimately does affect the *ātman*, since the *ātman* is after all bound by *saṁsāra* through its connection with the mind, life airs, senses, and body.

23. A king, who is a protector and ruler of the citizens, if he be a servant of God, does not "grind the ground" [as you claimed]. By striving to perform his duties as worship of Kṛṣṇa, he is released from masses of sinful *karma*.

24. Good sir, I have humiliated an exceptional saint due to my arrogance in thinking I am a lord of men. Please bless me with a favorable glance of compassion so that I might be absolved of the sin of offending a saint. You are the well-wisher of the lowly.

25. You may be undisturbed [by all this], since you are completely free from pride, and are the dearmost friend of the world. But someone like me, even if I be Lord Śiva, the bearer of the trident, will perish very quickly because of the offense I have performed against a great soul.' "

Book V, Chapter 11

1. The *brāhmaṇa* (Bharata) said:

"You would not be considered noteworthy in the company of those who are really learned because you are not wise, even though you are trying to speak the type of words spoken by the wise. Those who are sages, in their reflections on Truth, do not speak in the way you have about mundane relationships [as between king and subject].

2. Along the same lines, O king, a pure saint free from desire, who is a knower of Truth, usually does not take any satisfaction in the rhetoric of the ritualistic portions of the Veda, even though these give the

appearance of great knowledge by presenting abundant information on elaborate householder rituals.[49]

3. But, for one who does not come to the conclusion that the [ephemeral] happiness of the householder should be renounced voluntarily, just like a dream, not even the wisest Vedic words [the Upaniṣads][50] are sufficient for realizing the direct experience of the Truth of the self.

4. As long as a person's mind is untamed and overwhelmed by *sattva*, *rajas*, and *tamas*, it produces merit and demerit—good and bad *karma*—because of the desires of the mind.

5. The mind is filled with past-life memory impressions (*vāsanās*[51]). It is pervaded by desires for sense objects. It is subject to the flow of the *guṇas*, and it is always undergoing change [because of desires and the like]. It is chief among the sixteen categories of Sāṅkhya (the five working senses, five knowledge-acquiring senses, and the five gross elements that constitute the makeup of material bodies).[52] Taking on different forms [in *saṁsāra*] with different names [man, beast, bird, and so on], some high, some low, the mind manifests in different bodies.

6. This mind, which is a creation of *māyā* (illusion), envelops the *ātman* with which it is associated. In due course of time, it causes the experience of the fruits of action in the form of intense happiness and distress and all the shades that lie between them. It is the cause of the illusion of the cycle of birth and death.

7. For as long as this mind exists, conventional reality (*saṁsāra*) remains manifest and ongoing, and the *ātman* (*kṣetra-jña*) is subject to the experience of gross and subtle bodily forms. It is because of this that the wise say that this mind is the cause both of lower experience under the influence of the *guṇas*, as well as of higher existence, liberation, the state beyond the influence of the *guṇas*.[53]

8. If the mind is influenced by the *guṇas*, it leads the living beings to calamity. If it transcends the *guṇas*, it leads to liberation. It is just like a lamp, which emits a smoky flame when it is consuming its ghee wick, but otherwise [once it has burned up all the ghee] enjoys its own nature [burning purely]. In the same manner, when the mind takes recourse to its various states, *vṛttis*, it is bound by *karma* and the *guṇas*, but when it does not, it resorts to its own true nature.

9. The mind has eleven *vṛttis*: five related to the knowledge-acquiring senses, five related to the working senses, and one related to the ego.

They say that these *vṛttis* have eleven fields of activity: the five organs of action, the five sense objects, and the ego.[54]

10. Smell, form, touch, taste, and sound—the objects of the knowledge-acquiring senses—and evacuation, sexual intercourse, locomotion, speech, and grasping—the functions of the working senses—along with accepting the body as 'mine' (the ego) are the eleven. But some say this sense of 'I' is the twelfth.

11. These eleven functions of the mind multiply into hundreds and thousands and millions [of derivative states] in accordance with Time, *karma*, latent *saṁskāras*, nature, and specific material objects. But they do not exist for themselves, or for each other: they exist for the sake of the *ātman*.[55]

12. The *kṣetra-jña*, although pure, witnesses these never ending states of the mind, which are sometimes manifest, and sometimes unmanifest [as in deep sleep]. The mind is created by *māyā* as a covering of the *jīva* soul, and is an impure agent [subject to ignorance and the like].[56]

13. There is a [supreme] *kṣetra-jña*, who is an *ātman* and a *puruṣa*. He is primordial, unborn, self-luminous, directly experienced, and Lord of all. He is known as Nārāyāṇa, *Bhagavān*, Vāsudeva. He controls through his *māyā* power, from within the *ātman*.[57]

14. Just as air, after entering within all moving and non-moving entities, controls them from within in the form of breath, so does the Supreme, *Bhagavān*, Vāsudeva, the Supreme *Ātman*, and *Kṣetra-jña* (knower of the field of *prakṛti*), enter into this world.

15. O Lord of men, as long as an embodied being has not shaken off this *māyā* by means of awakening knowledge, has not conquered the six enemies [noted in the next verse] and become free of all attachment, and has not realized the true nature of the *ātman*, he or she must wander in this world of *saṁsāra*.

16. Such a person continues wandering in *saṁsāra* until he or she realizes that the mind, which masquerades as the self, plants the seeds of suffering in *saṁsāra*. It causes enmity, greed, desire, disease, illusion, and sorrow. It is the creator of the sense of ownership, the ego.

17. With diligence, defeat this enemy of the mind with the weapon of the worship of the lotus feet of Hari, the supreme *guru*. This mind is extremely powerful, and has become stronger by neglect. It is an impostor, and presents itself as if it were the true self."

Book V, Chapter 12

1. Rahūgaṇa said:

"Homage, homage to You. Your [ultimate] form is the cause of the universe and yet Your [present] form minimizes Your real nature.[58] Homage to You, O renunciant. Your eternal realization is concealed under the guise of a fallen *brāhmaṇa*.

2. My vision has been poisoned by the serpent of pride in this foul body, O *brāhmaṇa*. Your words are a nectarlike remedy for me. They are just like powerful medicine for someone who is afflicted by the fever of a disease, or ice water for one scorched by the heat of the summer.

3. Later, I shall raise a question pertaining to a doubt that I have, good sir. For now, please explain to me, in a manner that is easy to understand, that which You previously spoke about on the subject of the *yoga* of the highest self. My mind is eager to hear.

4. O Lord of *yoga*, You said that the relationship between apparent cause [bearing the palanquin] and effect [fatigue] is only based on conventional reality, but that this relationship is not easily defensible when an inquiry into [higher] reality is conducted. My mind is bewildered in this matter, sir."

5. The *brāhmaṇa* replied:

"This thing known as a 'person' is nothing other than something made out of earth walking upon the earth—a thing made of earth due to whatever cause. On top of the two feet of this thing are ankles, calves, knees, thighs, waist, neck, and shoulders.

6. On top of these shoulders sits a wooden palanquin, and inside that, one who is known as 'the king of the Sauvīra.' He, sir, is pervaded by arrogance; blinded by pride, he thinks: 'I am the king of the Sindhus.'

7. Forcing these pitiful people, who are already afflicted by extreme hardships, into compulsory labor while boasting that 'I am the protector of the people,' you are in fact without pity. You would not make a favorable impression in an assembly of the wise.

8. We know that the beginning and end of all moving and nonmoving entities is always just the earth—anything else is simply a label that is assigned based on convention. Let it be demonstrated if [any other cause] can be inferred from [observing] the true nature of reality.

9. In the same manner, the existence of that which is denoted by the word 'earth,' in turn, can be understood as unreal, because from the dissolution of earth, what remains are subatomic particles.[59] It is only when these atoms combine that specific things [such as earth] are formed. But atoms, too, are conjectured by the mind out of ignorance [of ultimate reality].

10. You should understand anything else—thin and fat, small and big, real and unreal, animate and inanimate—in the same manner. Anything in the realm of dualities is [in its essence] made of *prakṛti* under the labels: of substance, nature, the subconscious mind, Time, and *karma*.[60]

11. Knowledge is *Brahman*: it is pure, the supreme goal of life, one, undivided, without any inside or outside, Truth, complete, the innermost, and peaceful. It is known by the name *Bhagavān* and the sages know it as Vāsudeva.[61]

12. O Rahūgaṇa, this knowledge is not attained by penances, the performance of ritual sacrifices, the offering of libations, the fulfilling of household duties, the chanting of Vedic *mantras*, or by extreme austerities involving water, fire, and sun.[62] It is only attainable from the dust of the feet of the great devotees.[63]

13. Among such souls, discussion of the qualities of Viṣṇu, whose glories are praiseworthy, are relished, and mundane topics are avoided. By cultivating these discussions daily, the pure mind of the seeker of liberation becomes inclined toward Vāsudeva.

14. I too was previously a king by name of Bharata. I had attained liberation from the bondage of attachments to all material things, whether experienced or heard about.[64] Although engaging in the worship of *Bhagavān*, due to attachment to a deer I became a deer, and my goal was ruined.

15. Because of the potency ensuing from my worship of Kṛṣṇa, the memory of my previous life was not lost even in the deer's body, O hero. Therefore, now, being fearful [of attachments] I avoid the company of people, and wander about in disguise.

16. Therefore a person should destroy illusion here in this world with the sword of knowledge produced from the association of those who are detached from all attachments. Having regained one's memory of God, by hearing and speaking about the glories of His activities, one attains the supreme destination."

[Bharata's teachings are continued in the next chapter in the Allegory of the Forest.]

The Allegory of the Forest: The Illusion of Family Life

Yoga Blueprint

Bharata continues to instruct the king, using the story of a caravan lost in a forest to portray the ultimate impossibility of attaining satisfaction and fulfillment in family affairs and the pursuit of happiness through material ambitions, a consistent theme in the Bhāgavata. *As with the story of Purañjana, this is an allegory. The interpretation of the various elements presented in this chapter are explained in the next chapter.*

Book V, Chapter 13

1. The *brāhmaṇa* [Bharata] said:

"Seeking activities that vary according to the qualities of *sattva, rajas*, and *tamas*, a caravan of merchants is made by *māyā* to follow a trail that is very difficult to traverse. Wandering about pursuing the goal of wealth, it enters a forest; but it finds no happiness there.

2. In that forest, there are six robbers, O lord of men. They forcefully plunder the merchant caravan, which is led by an evil leader. Jackals there steal away the foolish merchants, like wolves a sheep.

3. In that forest, dense with abundant thickets, grasses, and creepers, the merchant caravan is harassed by intense mosquito bites. Sometimes it sees a city of the celestial *gandharvas* [an illusory castle in the sky] and other times demons that appear like fast-motion firebrands.

4. With the intention of [appropriating] wealth, water, and residences for themselves, the members of the caravan run here and there in the forest. Sometimes, the caravan's vision is covered by dust and obscured by grit stirred up by storms, and it cannot determine its direction.

5. Its members' ears are pained by the sound of invisible crickets, and their minds are deeply distressed by the hoots of owls. Afflicted by hunger, the caravan resorts to inauspicious trees[65] [that provide no fruit], and sometimes, it chases after water that is a mirage.

6. Sometimes it approaches riverbeds, but they are depleted of water, or else, when bereft of food, begs from others. At other times, it en-

counters a forest fire and is tormented by the flames, or it becomes desperate and is deprived of life by the *yakṣas*.[66]

7. Sometimes, the caravan's possessions are seized by other powerful men, and the minds of its members are plunged into despair. At such times, lamenting and falling into delusion, they faint. At other times, the caravan enters into the city of the celestial *gandharvas* [a castle in the sky] and enjoys for a moment like someone who is happy.

8. The merchants' minds become distraught when they wish to climb a mountain but their feet [are pained] by gravel and thorns as they are walking along. Tormented at every step by the inner fire of hunger, the householder erupts into anger against his own family.

9. Sometimes a person is swallowed by a boa constrictor, and in complete confusion is left discarded in the forest. He lies down, and is bitten by snakes. Then, bereft of sight, he falls into a blind well of dense darkness.

10. Sometimes, seeking some meager enjoyment such as honey, the caravan is assailed by bees and becomes completely frustrated. And if its goal in that endeavor is attained with great difficulties, others then forcefully plunder that honey from it.

11. Sometimes the merchant caravan remains incapable of counteracting cold, intense heat, wind, and rain. At other times, while trading something with others, its members end up developing enmity because of cheating one another for money.

12. Sometimes, when money becomes scarce in that forest, and when beds, seats, houses, and transportation become hard to come by, the merchant caravan begs from others. But, eyeing the possessions of these others, it is left with its desires unfulfilled, and receives humiliation instead.

13. As it wanders on this path distressed by money woes and great difficulties, relations of enmity develop because of reciprocal monetary dealings with others, even as they intermarry.

14. The merchant caravan discards here and there those who are dead, and clutches tight those who are born. Even up to this day, O hero, no one has returned from that forest, nor has anyone taken up the practice of *yoga*, which leads to the highest goal.

15. Ambitious men, who have forged enmity with others, and conquered the ends of the earth, thinking, 'Everything in the world is mine,' do not attain to that place [the abode of Viṣṇu] once they end

up lying dead on the battlefield. Only one who has laid down his rod of kingship and renounced enmity attains that place.
16. Sometimes the caravan clings for shelter to the arms of creepers, desiring to hear the muffled sounds of birds who nestle there. Sometimes, being afraid of a pride of lions in some place, it establishes friendship with cranes, herons, and vultures.
17. Cheated by them, it enters into the company of swans, but then, not finding their behavior pleasing, it approaches the monkeys. The members of the monkey troupe gaze into each other's faces, oblivious of the end of life [that looms], their senses gratified by the indulgences of that species.
18. As one member is about to enjoy in the trees, affectionate to wives and sons, and emasculated by his attachment to them, he falls into some mountain pit out of carelessness, depleted by sexual indulgence. Grabbing hold of a creeper, he remains [suspended], terrified of an elephant.
19. Subsequently, if somehow he becomes freed from this calamity, he once again enters into the company of the merchant caravan. No person who has entered this path created by *māyā* and is wandering about on it knows [the ultimate Truth] even until this very day, O conqueror of foes!
20. O Rahūgaṇa! You also are on this path! By renouncing your rod of kingship, and making friends with all living entities, and with a mind that has conquered illusion, take up the sword of knowledge sharpened by service to Hari. Then you will cross over to the Ultimate Truth."
21. The king said:
"*Aho!* The human birth is the most excellent of all births. What good is there in other births—even in that other world, the celestial realm—if there is not the plentiful association of great souls, whose minds are purified by the glories of Hṛṣīkeśa [Viṣṇu]?
22. There is nothing to be amazed at in the fact that sins are destroyed and pure *bhakti* to Adhokṣaja [Viṣṇu] manifests from the dust of your lotus feet. My ignorance, which was rooted in false reasoning, has been dispelled by just a moment of your association.
23. May those *brāhmaṇas* who wander the kingdom in the garb of *avadhūta* ascetics be blessed. Reverence to [such *brāhmaṇas*] who are elderly, reverence to those who are children, reverence to those who are youths, and reverence to those who are boys."

24. *Śrī* Śuka said:
"The son of the *brāhmaṇa* sage was in the highest state of enlightenment. After he had instructed knowledge of the self to the Sindhu king with great compassion, even though he had been belittled by him, his feet were worshipped by Rahūgaṇa with humility. He then wandered off about the earth, his mind free from the waves of sensual attraction, like an ocean full to abundance.
25. The king of the Sindhus cast off the notion of the body as being the self—a notion that is superimposed on the self by ignorance (*avidyā*). He had received the knowledge of the supreme self from a perfected being. This is the process of enlightenment for people who have taken guidance from those who, in turn, have taken shelter of *Bhagavān*."
26. The king said:
"O great devotee! This path of *saṁsāra* in the world of the *jīvas* that you have explained with great erudition is esoteric. The subject matter is allegorical and appropriate for learned Āryans—its meaning cannot be understood easily by laymen. Since it is difficult to interpret, kindly explain the symbolic meaning embedded in it."

Book V, Chapter 14

[*Interpretation of the elements of the allegory.*]
1. Śuka said:
"This world of *jīvas* is like the caravan of merchants [in the allegory] intent on wealth who have entered the forest of *saṁsāra*—a most inauspicious place, like a burial ground. It is due to *māyā*, which functions under the control of *Bhagavān*, *Īśvara*, Viṣṇu, that the caravan has stumbled onto this path of *saṁsāra*, which is difficult to traverse, like an unpassable forest trail. The merchants subsequently experience the *karma* produced by their bodies. For those who think the body to be the self, the group of six senses are like gates through which *saṁsāra* is experienced. This *saṁsāra* is beginningless and consists of attaining and relinquishing a series of differing bodies, which are produced by the performance of auspicious and inauspicious deeds, themselves the products of the particular qualities of the *guṇas* of *sattva*, *rajas*, and *tamas*. Although the efforts of the merchants are fruitless and full of hardships, still, even up until now, they do not attain the path that is followed by the bees at the feet of Hari

and the *guru* [the *bhāgavatas*]. It is this that brings peacefulness to the hardships of *saṁsāra*.

2. In that forest, those who go by the name of the six senses, are in reality robbers. For whatever wealth is attained after much difficulty is really meant for the pursuit of *dharma*. And the wise declare that *dharma* is that which is conducive to the other world and characterized by the direct worship of the Supreme Person. But, just like robbers plunder a caravan of merchants, [the senses] of a misguided person of uncontrolled mind plunder that rightly earned wealth for mundane sense enjoyment in the household, and through plans and the pursuits of activities involving seeing, touching, hearing, tasting, and smelling.

3. In that forest, the household members, who are wives and children by name, but wolves and jackals by deed, seize the wealth of the miserly householder, even as he is watching and resisting, [like wolves and jackals seize] the sheep in the allegory even though it is being well protected.

4. Just as a field, although it is plowed every year, becomes once again like a thicket of plants, grass, and creepers by the time of sowing unless the seeds [of weeds and such] have been burned with fire, so, in the same way, the householder *āśrama* is a *karma* field in which seeds of *karma* never disappear. The householder situation is a storehouse of *karma*.

5. Placed in that situation, the householder's wealth, which is like his very life breath, is harassed by the mosquito stings of ill-bred men, and by the thieves of rats, birds, and locusts. Sometimes, with mind influenced by actions, desires, and ignorance, the householder wanders about on that forest path without attaining his goals, and, in a state of illusion, looks upon the world of men as if he had attained the celestial city of the *gandharvas*.

6. There, lusty after pleasures such as drink, food, and sex, he chases after sense objects, which are mirages.

7. Sometimes, just as one in distress desires fire, a person whose mind is predominated by the *guṇa* of the same color (the red of *rajas*) wishes to gain gold. But gold is a kind of stool [that is, a by-product of fire], and is the abode of unlimited evils.[67]

8. In this way, a person devoted to the various means of subsistence such as home, beverages, wealth, and so on, sometimes runs around here and there in this forest of *saṁsāra*.

9. At times, mounted upon the hips of a lusty woman, his eyes enveloped in *rajas*, he becomes obscured by the passion (*rajas*) of the moment, which is comparable to a whirlwind, and transgresses moral behavior. His mind completely enveloped in *rajas*, he is not aware of the *dig-devatā*, the celestial beings who oversee all corners of the universe.
10. At other times, he suddenly gains realization of the falseness of sense objects. But he then again loses his memory [of this realization] due to considering himself to be something he is not [that is, the body], and then once more chases after those same sense objects, which are like the water in a mirage.
11. Sometimes his heart and ears are tormented by the rebukes of government officers and enemies, directly or through second parties. These are [delivered with] arrogance, harshness, and aggression, like the sounds of the owls and crickets [of the allegory].
12. Even though he himself is dying while living, when his pious *karma* from the past becomes diminished, he seeks recourse in the form of wealth from those who are also dead, though alive. But such wealth is devoid of value in both worlds[68] and so is like a poisonous well, or like impious [poisonous] trees and creepers such as the *kāraskara* and *kākatuṇḍa* [in the allegory].
13. Once in a while, his mind becomes corrupted by association with bad company, and he takes recourse of heretics. But this simply produces grief in both worlds [here and the hereafter], and is comparable to stumbling into a river that has no water.
14. When he cannot procure food for himself by means of causing distress for others, he then devours those who possess even a blade of grass belonging to his son or father—or he may devour even his son or father themselves.
15. And sometimes, approaching the home, which is devoid of desirable things and causes misery, like a forest fire, he falls into a state of despair, and is scorched by the fire of anguish.
16. At other times, when his wealth, which is his very life air, is seized by fiendish government officials, who have become hostile due to the workings of Time, he becomes like a corpse, deprived of all signs of life.
17. Sometimes he experiences the type of happiness found in dreams, and due to hallucinating, imagines his deceased father or grandfather to be present.

18. At other times, desiring to climb the enormous mountain of regulations dealing with the duties of the householder, his mind becomes attracted to mundane addictions. At such times, he laments, as if entering a field of thorns and gravel.
19. Sometimes, depleted of strength by the [gastric] fire within his body, he erupts into anger against his own family.
20. Seized by the boa constrictor of sleep, he becomes immersed in the darkness of *tamas*, and lies like a corpse that has been discarded in a desolate forest [of the allegory], unaware of anything.
21. At other times, the teeth of his pride are broken by malignant people, and he cannot attain a moment's sleep. His lucidity is obscured by a disturbed heart, and he becomes like a blind person who has fallen into a dark well.
22. At any opportunity he searches for drops of honey in the form of lust, taking someone else's wife or wealth. For this he is beaten by the king or husband, and falls into a bottomless hell.
23. Actually, they say that the sowing of the seeds of *saṁsāra* for a person on this path, is *karma* of both types [pious and impious].[69]
24. If he is freed from bondage, Devadatta[70] snatches away [the wife or wealth] from someone, and Viṣṇumitra does the same from him in turn, and in this way these possessions remain transient.
25. Sometimes, incapable of warding off one's conditions of cold, wind, and other various *adhidaivika* and *adhibhautika* problems (caused by other living entities, or the environment), one sinks into a depressed state of unlimited anxiety.
26. At times, in dealings among themselves, or if one takes away any money from another—even just a *kākiṇi* coin (farthing), or anything at all—one creates enmity, because of fraudulent business dealings.
27. On this path there are obstacles such as happiness, distress, desire, aversion, fear, pride, delusion, madness, sorrow, illusion, greed, envy, jealousy, insult, hunger, thirst, anxieties, disease, birth, old age, death, and more.
28. At times, embraced by the creeperlike arms of a woman, who is the divine *māyā*, a person's wisdom and discrimination spill away, and his heart becomes bewildered in efforts to create a pleasure house for her. Then his mind becomes captured by the behavior, glances, and words of his wife, daughters, and sons, who are attached to him

for sustenance. Because his mind is uncontrolled, he casts himself into a bottomless dark hell.

29. On occasion, his mind is terrified by the discus of *Īśvara*, Viṣṇu, *Bhagavān*, known as the Time factor through its churnings. The units of Time begin with the smallest atom, etc., and end with the two halves of Brahmā's life (*dvi-parārdha*).[71] With great force, and without even blinking, Time snatches away the ages of all beings from Brahmā to the straw or clump of grass from under their very eyes. Contemptuous of *Bhagavān* himself, *Īśvara*, whose personal weapon is the wheel of Time, and who is the Supreme presiding Being of sacrifice, a person resorts to the gods of the heretics, who are rejected by the unanimous opinion of the Āryans. These are analogous to the herons, vultures, cranes, and *vaṭa* birds [in the allegory].

30. If the person is cheated by those heretics, who have cheated their own selves, he resides with the *brāhmaṇa* caste. They engage in activities such as worshipping *Bhagavān* the Supreme enjoyer of sacrifice, following the activities prescribed in the *Śruti* and *Smṛti* sacred texts,[72] and undergoing the sacred thread ceremony for the twice-born. Not finding their character pleasing, he joins company with the *śūdra* caste. His absorption in thoughts of sex and the means of supporting the family is considered impure according to the codes of conduct of the sacred texts, like that of the monkey race [in the allegory].

31. There, too, the unfortunate minded person enjoys himself freely and without restrictions, gazing into the faces of others and indulging in vulgar activities, forgetful of his impending end wrought by Time.

32. Sometimes, frolicking in the household, which, like the trees [in the allegory], only contains objects of this world, he is enamored by his sons and wife, and spends his time in sexual pursuits, like the monkeys.

33. Bound to his path, he is trapped in darkness, analogous to the cave in the mountain [of the allegory], by the fear of the elephant of death.

34. At times, unable to counter the sufferings of cold and wind and the *adhidaivika* and *adhyātmika* miseries (caused by one's own body and mind, or by the environment) inflicted on him, he broods over endless sense objects.

35. Sometimes, whatever wealth he obtains in dealings among others is through fraudulent business transactions.

36. At other times, when his wealth is depleted and he becomes deprived of objects of enjoyment such as beds, seats, foodstuffs, etc., he resolves to seize by force the objects of his mind's desire that are lacking.
37. In this way, due to the influence of past life impressions (*vāsanās*), he again enters into fresh relationships of marriage with and separations from others, even though relations of enmity had previously been created with them on account of business transactions.
38. On this path of *saṁsāra*, a person is bound by various troubles and obstacles. Wherever he meets his death, the others abandon him in that place. Holding tight to each newborn, one grieves, is deluded, is afraid, quarrels, weeps, rejoices, sings, and is bound up by life. No one has yet up to today returned to the place where the caravan of worldly men initially began, a place avoided by the saintly in the first place. It is also the place where the path ends, say the wise.[73]
39. He does not take to the path of *yoga*, or attain that place which the sages, who have renounced violence, whose natures are peaceful, and whose minds are controlled, attain.
40. Although sage-kings sponsored great sacrifices and conquered all the corners of the earth, they leave it behind when they themselves are killed and lying [lifeless] in battle with others on that very same earth. They had thought they owned this earth, and had created relationships of enmity for possessing it.
41. Grabbing the creepers of *karma*, if one is somehow freed from hell after this calamity, one once again joins the caravan of men in the world and finds oneself on this path of *saṁsāra* all over again. The same also goes for one who has gone to the celestial realm beyond.
42. They sing thus, about Bharata:
'No one is able to follow the path of the great-souled sage-king, son of Ṛṣabha, not even in one's mind, O king, any more than a fly can imitate Garuḍa (the eagle carrier of Lord Viṣṇu).
43. Even though he was in the prime of life, in his total devotion to Lord Viṣṇu, whose glories are supreme, Bharata renounced the things dear to his heart—kingdom, friends, sons, and wife, which are so difficult to give up—as if they were excreta.
44. He did not desire the things that are normally so difficult to renounce—earth, sons, kinsmen, possessions, wife, and even the

Goddess of Fortune, who is sought by the best of the celestials, even though Her glance was merciful [upon him], O king. This is befitting those whose minds are absorbed in devotion to Lord Viṣṇu, the enemy of Madhu;[74] for them even liberation is a trifle.

45. Even at the moment that he was giving up his birth as a deer, he uttered, smiling: "Reverence to Nārāyaṇa, Hari, the enjoyer of sacrifice, the Lord of *dharma*, the authority on codes of conduct, the [goal of] *yoga*, the conclusion of Sāṅkhya, and the Lord (*Īśvara*) of *prakṛti*." '

46. The sage-king Bharata's deeds and pure qualities are honored by the *Bhāgavata* devotees. Whoever hears, recites, and glorifies this story attains all blessings for himself: he does not need to seek anything from anywhere else. This story brings good fortune, long life, wealth, fame, the celestial realms, and liberation."

Book VI

The Tale of Ajāmila: The Power of *Mantra*

Yoga Blueprint

The primary teaching imparted in this narrative pertains to the inherent power of mantra, Īśvara's *names. Chanting* mantra *is the principal form of meditation not only in* bhakti, *but also in generic Patañjali-type meditational* yoga.[1] *It is the primary, simplest, and most immediate method of directly contacting* Īśvara *as manifest in sonic presence. That Ajāmila attained liberation merely by inadvertently calling out the name of Nārāyaṇa transmits a powerful message about the superexcellency of reciting such names. The passage informs the reader that there is no other* yogic *method that purifies the mind in a comparable way: whereas other processes and acts of atonement may cancel the negative effects of* karma*—the negative effects accrued from* adharma*—they do not remove the underlying desires that cause the mind to engage in compromised* karma *in the first place.* Īśvara *in the form of sound does, however (see* "Kīrtana *[Chanting]" for further discussion on* mantra*).*

This section also contains an excellent analysis of the general process of karma *and reincarnation. A further noteworthy element in this tale is the clear distinction that* Yama, *the god of death, makes between gods such as himself—namely, powerful celestial beings—and God as* Īśvara, *the ultimate Supreme Being. Yama is the Indic equivalent of Pluto. Unlike the Greco-Roman and other Indo-European gods that were swept aside by the spread of monotheistic Christianity, the* *monotheistic traditions of India retained the gods but relegated them to temporal spheres that, while supernormal, were nonetheless clearly inferior and subservient to Viṣṇu and the realm of Vaikuṇṭha. Of interest, too, in this passage, is that Ajāmila attained a form (*svarūpa*) as an associate of* Bhagavān. *As discussed in "The Divine* Brahman *Realms of Vaikuṇṭha and Goloka," the liberated state in* Bhāgavata *theology involves receiving a* Brahman *form such that the relationship with* Bhagavān *can continue for eternity* in *Vaikuṇṭha.*

Book VI, Chapter 1

6. *Śrī* Parīkṣit said:
"Now, O blessed one, please kindly explain how a person here in this world might avoid going to the hellish realms, where there are intense and varied forms of punishments."[2]
7. *Śrī* Śuka said:
"If someone who has committed sin in thought, word, or deed does not perform an act of atonement while still here in this world that is appropriate to the sin, then that person will undoubtedly go to the hellish regions, where there are severe punishments, as described to you previously.[3]
8. Therefore, before the body succumbs to the ravishment of death, one must ascertain the severity or lightness of one's errors and quickly endeavor to atone for one's sins in this world appropriately—just as a doctor who knows the cause of sickness should prescribe appropriate medicine for a disease."
9. The king said:
"Yet a person keeps committing sin again and again, as if powerless, even though knowing from direct experience or from hearing from others[4] that this is detrimental to him or herself. So what, ultimately, is the use of atonement?
10. At times one ceases from inauspicious activities, but then at other times one engages in them again. Therefore it seems to me that atonement is useless, just like an elephant taking a bath is useless."[5]
11. *Śrī* Śuka, son of Bādarāyaṇa (Vyāsa), replied:
"It has never been stated that [sinful] action can be completely annulled by [other] action. In fact, this [type of process] is appropriate only for those who lack knowledge of the self. [Real] atonement is in fact knowledge of the self.[6]

12. Just as diseases do not overcome a person who is eating healthy foods, so one who follows the sacred prescriptions, O king, slowly becomes eligible for liberation.
13.–14. By means of austerity (*tapas*), celibacy (*brahmacarya*), meditation, sense control, renunciation, truthfulness (*satya*), cleanliness (*śauca*), the moral and ethical restraints (*yamas* and *niyamas*), the wise, who are knowers of *dharma* and endowed with faith, eliminate sin caused by body, word, or thought—even great sin—just like fire destroys a cluster of bamboos.
15. Some people—those dedicated to Vāsudeva [Kṛṣṇa] with unswerving devotion—dispel sin completely, just as the sun dispels fog.
16. Actually, a sinful person does not purify himself as much through such things as austerity, O king, as does one whose life is devoted to Kṛṣṇa by service to Kṛṣṇa's devotees.
17. This is certainly the best path in this world: it is safe and free of fear. Benevolent saints who are devoted to Nārāyaṇa are found on this path.
18. O Lord of kings, the performance of acts of atonement does not purify one who is averse to Nārāyaṇa, any more than river water purifies a vessel that has contained liquor.[7]
19. Those who have even once devoted their minds to the lotus feet of Kṛṣṇa, attracted to His qualities, have performed [complete] atonement. Not even in dreams do they see Yama, the Lord of death, and his minions, who carry nooses.
20. [The sages] give as an example in this regard, this ancient legend (*itīhāsa*); it is an exchange between the messengers of Viṣṇu and those of Yama. Listen as I recount it.
21. In the town of Kānyakubja lived a twice-born *brāhmaṇa* by name of Ajāmila. He became the husband of a prostitute servant girl, and so his high character became destroyed, polluted by that relationship.
22. Adopting a despicable livelihood, the corrupt fellow maintained his family by kidnapping, fraud, theft, and causing distress to other beings.
23. A long period of eighty-eight years passed by as Ajāmila was maintaining himself in this manner and indulging his sons from that woman, O king.
24. That old man had ten sons. From these, the youngest, a lad whose name happened to be Nārāyaṇa, was the great favorite of his parents.

25. The old man's heart was attached to that toddler, with his broken sentences, and he took great pleasure in gazing on his childish play.
26. Whenever he was eating and drinking, he used to feed the boy by offering him food and drink, his heart bound by affection. The foolish man did not see death was approaching.
27. Passing his life in this way, when the time of death presented itself, the ignorant man fixed his mind on his son—the boy whose name was Nārāyaṇa.
28. At that time, he saw three very dreadful beings [the servants of Yama, Lord of death] bearing nooses in their hands. They had twisted snouts, erect hair, and had come to take him away.
29. With his senses thrown into confusion, Ajāmila called out loudly in a labored voice to his son, who was absorbed in play some distance away—the one called Nārāyaṇa.
30. Upon hearing the repetition of Hari *kīrtana*—the name of their Lord—from the mouth of the dying man, O great king, the servants of Viṣṇu immediately appeared there.
31. The messengers of Viṣṇu forcefully obstructed those who had been dispatched by Yama as they were dragging Ajāmila, husband of a prostitute, from the interior of the heart region.[8]
32. Thwarted in their task, the attendants of Yama said to them: 'Who are you to be obstructing the order of Yama, Lord of *dharma*?
33. Whose men are you? From where have you come? Are you celestial gods, demigods, or are you perfected beings (*siddhas*)? Why are you preventing us from taking this man?
34. You both have eyes like lotus petals, and are dressed in yellowsilken garments. You wear helmets, earrings, and bright lotus garlands.[9]
35. You are both youthful, and you have four beautiful arms. You bear bow, quiver, sword, club, conch, and lotus. Your appearance is majestic.
36. You are illuminating the darkness in all directions with your personal effulgence. For what reason do you impede us, the servants of Yama? Yama is the guardian of *dharma*.' "
37. *Śrī* Śuka said:
"Upon being addressed in this way by the messengers of Yama, those attendants of Vāsudeva smiled. Then they replied as follows, in voices that resounded like thundering clouds.

38. The messengers of Viṣṇu said:
'If you are indeed the order carriers of Yama, king of *dharma*, then explain to us the facts about *dharma*, righteousness, and also the characteristics of *adharma*, unrighteousness.
39. How do you think punishment should be enforced? And what is the appropriate circumstance for it? Moreover, among those who perform deeds, who is subject to punishment: only certain men or everyone?'
40. The messengers of Yama replied:
'*Dharma* is that which is enjoined in the Vedas, and *adharma* is its opposite. The Vedas are self-manifest, and are Nārāyaṇa Himself. This is what we have heard.
41. It is by Him in His supreme abode that all these entities made of *rajas*, *sattva*, and *tamas* are manifest in their various forms, activities, names, and qualities in the ways that they are.
42. The gods of the sun, fire, sky, wind, moon, twilight, day, and night, cardinal directions, water, and earth, as well as Yama, god of *dharma* himself, all of these are the witnesses of embodied beings.
43. It is by them that whatever constitutes *adharma* is determined, and the basis established for whatever is appropriate for punishment. And everyone who performs actions is eligible for punishment in accordance with the nature of their actions.
44. Those who act perform both benevolent actions and nonbenevolent sinful ones. No embodied being can refrain from performing action: this is the consequence of the influence of the *guṇas*.
45. Whatever be the nature and degree of *dharma* and *adharma* performed by a person in this life, that same person experiences the fruit of the very same nature and degree in the next life.[10]
46. O best of celestial beings! Just as there are three types [*sattva*, *rajas*, and *tamas*] perceived among beings in this world on account of the differences in the *guṇas*, so it can be inferred is the case in other worlds.
47. Just as the present state of Time gives an indication of the nature of past Time [that preceded] and future Time [that will succeed it], so the present life [of a person] indicates the *dharma* and *adharma* of past and future births.[11]
48. Our Lord [Yama], abiding in his city, clearly discerns a person's previous life through [the power of] his mind, and evaluates what will

be that person's next life through the power of his mind. He himself is supreme and not subject to rebirth.

49. Just as in a dream [a person identifies with the dream body and loses awareness of the waking body], so, an ignorant person immersed in *tamas* considers himself to be the physical body and is not aware of previous and future bodies, since the memory of past lives is lost.

50. The *jīva* accomplishes its purposes with the five [organs of actions], and knows the five [sense objects] with the five [knowledge-acquiring organs].[12] Accompanied by the sixteenth [the mind], the *jīva* alone is the seventeenth, and it is he who experiences these three—the five instruments of action, five instruments of knowledge, and the five sense objects.[13]

51. This subtle body made of these sixteen parts,[14] which are constituted by the three *śaktis* (*sattva*, *rajas*, and *tamas*), is insurmountable. It is the cause of *saṁsāra* for a person—in other words, of the experiences of joy, sorrow, fear, and affliction.

52. The embodied *ātman*, whose six instruments of mind and senses have not been controlled, ignorant of its true nature, engages in action even if not wishing to do so. Like a silkworm in its cocoon, a person is covered by his or her activities, and is bewildered.[15]

53. Not a single being can ever exist for even one moment without performing action. One performs action even against one's will, due to the impulses of one's nature and the force of the *guṇas*.[16]

54. As a result of these impulses of one's nature, and with unseen *karma* as the underlying cause,[17] a gross and subtle body is attained in conformity with the [mother's] womb and [father's] seed.

55. This compromised state of the *puruṣa* comes about from association with *prakṛti*. But it is dissolved very quickly from association with the Lord.

56. This Ajāmila was once endowed with Vedic learning, and was a repository of good character, conduct, and qualities. He honored his vows, was gentle and self-controlled, clean, truthful in speech, and well versed in the sacred utterances of the Vedas.

57. He was humble and diligent in serving the elderly, guests, sacred fire, and teachers. He was a friend to all beings, saintly, of measured speech, and free of envy.

58. One day, this twice-born *brāhmaṇa*, obeying his father's request, went to the forest and returned carrying fruit, flowers, kindling sticks, and *kuśa* grass [for the performance of Vedic ritual].
59. He saw some shameless *śūdra* with a servant girl, whose eyes were fluttering about in intoxication, due to having drunk *maireya* liquor.
60. Fallen [from civilized behavior] and shameless, he was flirting, singing, and laughing in the company of that woman. Her cloth had become loosened.
61. After seeing that woman embraced by the arm of the *śūdra*, which was smeared with erotic [turmeric powder], Ajāmila immediately fell under the control of [dormant desires] lying in his heart, and became infatuated.
62. Struggling to the best of his abilities to restrain his mind with his mind in accordance with the instructions of the sacred texts, he was yet not able to bring it under control. His mind had become agitated by Cupid.
63. Possessed as if by a malevolent spell in the form of infatuation provoked by that woman, Ajāmila lost control of his senses. Fixated only on her in his mind, he abandoned the performance of his prescribed *dharma*.
64. With the entirety of the wealth inherited from his family, Ajāmila indulged her with vulgar sensual pleasures stimulating to her fancy, in whatever way might be pleasing to her.
65. His rightful wife was a young *brāhmaṇa* lady from an excellent family. But this sinful fellow soon abandoned her, his better judgment shattered by the coquettish glances of that wanton woman.
66. In whatever way he could, [after squandering his inheritance,] this foolish man obtained money through fair or foul means, and supported the family of that woman, as she had other children [from different men].
67. This person became corrupt because of impure association. He has led a sinful life and has transgressed the rules of the sacred texts. He has kept going on like this for a long time with unrestrained and utterly vile behavior.
68. This person has committed many sins and has not performed atonement, therefore, we are bringing him before Yama, the bearer of the rod, where he will be purified by punishment.' "

Book VI, Chapter 2

1. *Śrī* Śuka, son of Vyāsa, said:
"Those messengers of *Bhagavān* Viṣṇu were skilled in the codes of human affairs. After considering everything that had been spoken by the messengers of Yama, they responded as follows:
2. The messengers of Viṣṇu said:
'*Aho!* What a shame it is that unrighteousness, *adharma*, taints the assembly of those who are knowers of *dharma*, for punishment is being wantonly inflicted by them upon a sinless person who does not merit punishment.
3. Those who are authorities are the guardians of living beings, and [are supposed to be] saintly and impartial. If injustice exists among them, to whom will the citizens go for protection?
4. However a superior person behaves, others will strive to emulate. Whatever he or she establishes as standard, common people will follow.[18]
5. A common person places his head on the lap [of his protector] and so sleeps securely, like an animal does. He himself does not know what is *dharma* and what is *adharma*.
6. How can such a superior person, if he or she is worthy of being trusted by all beings, act contemptuously and inflict suffering on a simple-natured person who has formed friendship with and placed trust in him or her?
7. This person Ajāmila has performed atonement for sins performed even in countless past lives because, in a helpless condition, he uttered the name of Hari, which bestows liberation.
8. When he chanted the four syllables "Nā-rā-ya-ṇa," the annulment of sins was accomplished by this act—even for this sinful man.
9.–10. A thief; a drunkard; a murderer of friends; a killer of *brāhmaṇas*; one who defiles his *guru's* bed; a murderer of a woman, king, parent, or cow; all these and other types of sinners—indeed for every kind of evil person—the chanting of the name is the best atonement; the mind of Viṣṇu [is attracted] by that sound.
11. A sinful person is not purified by the acts of atonement and vows prescribed by the experts in Vedic knowledge, as much as by the reciting of the syllables of the name of Hari. The name reminds one of the qualities of Viṣṇu, whose glories are supreme.

12. Under normal circumstances, even when atonement is performed, it is not fully effective if the mind again runs along the path of unrighteousness. For one who desires to eliminate all *karma*, it is in fact the repetition of the names and qualities of Hari that makes the mind pure (*sāttvika*) [and hence one loses the desire to perform unrighteous acts in the first place].
13. Therefore, do not take him away. Because this man mentioned the name of *Bhagavān* as he was dying, he has accomplished atonement for all of his sins.
14. The sages know that reciting the name of Viṣṇu, the Lord of Vaikuṇṭha, removes all sin, even if uttered as a designation for someone else, jokingly, inserted in a song, or disrespectfully.
15. If a person utters "Hari," even unconsciously, when falling, tripping, injured, bitten, burned, or struck, that person is not eligible for suffering in hell.
16. Atonements for sins have been prescribed by the sages: severe atonements for severe sins, and minor atonements for minor sins.
17. However, although such sins are purified by acts such as austerity (*tapas*), charity, and the performance of vows, their causes [desires], born of unrighteousness, are not cleansed from the heart. But they are cleansed by service to the lotus feet of *Īśvara*.
18. Viṣṇu's glories are supreme. Chanting His name, whether knowingly or unknowingly, burns the sins of a person, just like fire burns kindling wood.
19. Just as the most potent medicine manifests its inherent effects, even if consumed by an ignorant person, so is the case with *mantra* when uttered.' "
20. *Śrī* Śuka said:
"After establishing very clearly the nature of *Bhāgavata dharma* in this way, O king, the servants of Viṣṇu freed that *brāhmaṇa* from Yama's bonds, and released him from death.
21. After receiving this response, the servants of Yama went back for an audience with Yama. They informed King Yama about everything that had happened, O subduer of enemies.
22. The *brāhmaṇa*, freed from the bonds, regained his senses and his fear was dispelled. He bowed his head to the servants of Viṣṇu, overwhelmed in ecstasy by the vision of them.

23. The servants of the great Lord Viṣṇu, perceiving that Ajāmila was desiring to speak, suddenly disappeared from there right in front of his eyes, O sinless Parīkṣit!
24. In this way, from the conversation between the messengers of Viṣṇu and those of Yama, Ajāmila heard both about the pure *dharma* associated with *Bhagavān* free from all self-interest, and also at the same time about the *dharma* associated with the three Vedas, which is based on the *guṇas*.[19]
25. Since he had heard about the wonderful greatness of *Bhagavān*, Ajāmila immediately became infused with *bhakti*, devotion, and became greatly repentant about his sinful self:
26. '*Aho!* After losing control of my senses what great wrong I did! As a result, I ruined my *brāhmaṇa* status and begot sons in a woman of low morals.
27. Curses upon me! I am a stain on the reputation of my lineage and condemned as a scoundrel by the righteous. I abandoned my son and chaste wife, and went with an unchaste woman given to drinking.
28. *Aho!* I have also deserted my old parents by neglecting their order. They are without protectors or other relatives and have suffered great hardship. I am a worthless rascal.
29. It is clear that a person such as I will fall into the hell called *Aruṇa*, where lusty people who break the codes of *dharma* undergo the punishments of Yama.[20]
30. *Aho!* Was this a dream, or did I actually perceive this wonderful occurrence here? Where have they now gone, those who were dragging me away holding bonds?
31. And where have those four beautiful perfected beings (*siddhas*) gone, who freed me as I was being led away to the lower regions, bound by fetters?
32. Although I am a wretched fellow, I must have performed some auspicious deed causing me to have that vision of those most learned beings. My mind has become filled with joy because of them.
33. Otherwise, it would not be possible for the tongue of someone like me to utter the name of Viṣṇu, Lord of Vaikuṇṭha, as I was dying. I am a degraded keeper of a harlot.
34. I am a shameless sinful rascal who has destroyed his *brāhmaṇa* heritage. What am I in comparison to that name of *Bhagavān*, "Nārāyaṇa," which is auspicious?

35. Such is the person that I am. Therefore, keeping my breath, senses, and mind controlled, I will conduct myself in such a way that my life will never again sink into deep *tamas*.
36. Having freed myself from this bondage born of *karma*, lust, and ignorance, I shall regain control of myself and become peaceful, a true friend to all beings, amiable, and compassionate.
37. I am a wretch. My soul has been seized by *māyā* in the form of a woman, by whom I have been made into a plaything, like a pet deer. I am going to commit to freeing myself.
38. I will give up the illusion of "I" and "mine" in the form of the body and its possessions, and dedicate my mind to *Bhagavān*, purified by chanting his glories (*kīrtana*). I will become determined to keep my intelligence fixed only on things that are not false.'
39. From just a moment's association with saintly beings (*sādhus*), complete detachment arose in Ajāmila in this way. Freed from all bondage, he set out for Hardvāra, the door of the *Gaṅgā* river [in the Himālayas].
40. In that divine abode, Ajāmila took his seat and situated himself in *yoga*. He withdrew the five senses [from their objects], and fixed his mind on the *ātman*.
41. Then he detached his mind from the *guṇas* through complete absorption on the self (*samādhi*), and attached it to the form of *Bhagavān*, who is *Brahman*, the Soul of experience.
42. When his mind was fully fixed, he then again saw those beings from before. Realizing that he had seen them previously, the *brāhmaṇa* offered them homage by bowing his head.
43. After that vision, Ajāmila gave up his body at a sacred place on the banks of the *Gaṅgā*. Immediately he received a spiritual body of the type attained by the associates of *Bhagavān* [in Vaikuṇṭha].[21]
44. The *brāhmaṇa* climbed onto a golden vehicle, and departed through the celestial realms along with those servants of Viṣṇu, the Great Being. He went to where Viṣṇu, the Lord of Śrī, the Goddess of Fortune (Lakṣmī) resides [Vaikuṇṭha].
45. Ajāmila had abandoned his vows and strayed away from all *dharma*. As the fallen husband of a harlot engaging in forbidden activities, he was falling into hell. But he was immediately liberated by uttering the name of *Bhagavān*.

46. For those desiring liberation, there is nothing superior for severing the bonds of *karma* than this reciting (*anukīrtana*) of [the names] of Viṣṇu, the Lord of all holy places.
47.–48. This supremely intimate narrative destroys all sins. Any *yogī* who hears and recites it with faith will not go to hell or see the servants of Yama. Howsoever an ill-fated human one might have been, he or she will be considered great in Vaikuṇṭha, the abode of Viṣṇu.
49. Ajāmila, even though referring to his son, uttered the name of Hari while dying. What, then, to speak of uttering it with faith?!"

Book VI, Chapter 3

1. The king said:
"When Lord Yama, king of *dharma*, heard this account from his servants, how did he respond to them? Everyone in this world is under his control, yet his servants were obstructed and his order disobeyed by the order carriers of Viṣṇu.
2. Such flouting of the order of Lord Yama has never been heard of ever before by anyone, O sage! I am certain that other than you, noble sir, no one can resolve this anomaly in the minds of common people."
3. *Śrī* Śuka replied:
"The servants of Yama, O king, whose mission had been thwarted, related everything to their master Yama, the Lord of the city of Saṁyamanī.
4. The messengers of Yama said:
'O master: how many rulers in this world actually are there responsible for awarding the fruits of action for living beings engaged in the three kinds of activities?[22]
5. If there are many rulers who uphold justice in the world, who would get to bestow death [hell] and who the celestial realm [in the event there were a disagreement among them]?
6. And if there be a plurality of rulers for the multitude of beings who act, then rulership would become a minor position in name only, like that of the governor of a province.
7. Therefore [as far as we are concerned] you are the one supreme Lord among all beings, including the celestial demigods. You are the ruler, awarder of justice, and arbitrator of what is auspicious and inauspicious for humankind.

8. The authority of that ruler—that is, of you—has been transgressed and as of today is no longer upheld in the world: your order has been transgressed by those four messengers—those perfected beings.
9. They forcefully cut the bonds from that sinful wretch as he was being taken by us to the torture chambers under your order, and then they freed him.
10. Upon him calling the name "Nārāyaṇa," they swiftly arrived, telling him: "Do not fear." We wish to know who they are, if you feel we are competent to know.' "
11. *Śrī* Śuka, son of Bādarāyaṇa, said:
"Questioned in this way, Lord Yama, who is the judicator of created beings, became pleased with his messengers. He replied smilingly, remembering the lotus feet of Hari.
12. Yama said:
'Higher than I is the Supreme Being of all moving and non-moving things. In Him the universe is sewn, lengthwise and crosswise like a cloth.[23] Viṣṇu, Brahmā, and Śiva, the Maintainer, Creator, and Destroyer of this world, are His partial expansions.[24] This world is under His control, like a bull with a rope through its nose.
13. By means of the respective caste designations which are found in His words [the Vedic injunctions] consisting of regulations,[25] He binds people just like cows are bound by means of ropes. Bound by the restraints of their duties and actions, people bear offerings to Him fearfully.
14.–15. I, the great Indra, Nirṛti, the Pracetas, Soma, Agni, Śiva, Pavana, Viriñci [Brahmā], the [twelve] Ādityas, the Viśvas, the [eight] Vasus, the Sādhyas, the host of Maruts, the host of Rudras, the *siddhas*, perfected beings, along with others such as the creators of the universe [like Marīci], and the lords of the celestials, as well as Bhṛgu and others,[26] none of us understand His intention, since we are affected by *māyā*, even though we are predominantly in *sattva* and untouched by *rajas* and *tamas*. What then to speak of others?
16. He is transcendent. Even though He exists in the heart within the self of all beings, a living being cannot perceive Him through the senses, mind, life airs, intellect, or [Vedic] words—just as physical forms cannot perceive the eyes.
17. Hari is self-dependent, the Supreme Lord, transcendent, the ultimate controller of *māyā*, the Supreme Soul. His messengers often

wander about here in this world. They have the same nature, qualities, and form as He,[27] and so are very attractive to the mind.

18. Viṣṇu's associates are worshipped by the celestials. Their forms are wondrous, and it is very hard to attain a vision of them. They protect the mortal devotees of Viṣṇu from enemies and from everything—including even from I myself.

19. The codes of *dharma* are decreed by *Bhagavān* Himself. Neither the *ṛṣi* sages, nor the celestial demigods, nor the best of the perfected *siddhas*, nor the demons or humans understand them, what then to speak of the angelic *vidhyādharas*, *cāraṇas*, and other celestials?

20.–21. The self-manifest Brahmā, Nārada, Śiva, Sanat-Kumāra, Kapila, Manu, Prahlāda, King Janaka, Bhīṣma, Bali, Śuka, and I myself, only we twelve know the *Bhāgavata dharma*,[28] my men. It is intimate, completely pure, and difficult to understand; but, having known it, one achieves the nectar of immortality.

22. It is this alone that has been handed down as the ultimate *dharma* for humankind in this world: *bhakti yoga* for *Bhagavān* by reciting His name and other such devotional activities.

23. Just see the greatness of chanting the name of Hari, my sons! By this, even Ajāmila was freed from the bonds of death!

24. Just this much alone is sufficient to remove the sins of human beings—the reciting of the names, deeds, and qualities of *Bhagavān*. Even though he was actually calling out to his son, the sinful Ajāmila said "Nārāyaṇa" and so attained liberation.

25. That other great being [Manu, the compiler of the conventional *dharma* texts] often did not know this truth. Alas, his intelligence was bewildered by the divine *māyā*! Performing rituals in the form of great sacrifices involving the three sacred fires[29] in accordance with the sweet flowery words of the three Vedas, his mind became dull.[30]

26. After considering all this, those who are intelligent engage in loving devotion to the unlimited *Bhagavān* (*bhāva-yoga*) with all their heart. Even if there is some sin among them, nevertheless, such people do not deserve any punishment from me: the chanting of the name of Viṣṇu will destroy it.

27. Those saintly devotees of *Bhagavān* see all beings equally. Praises of their purity are sung by the *siddhas*, perfected beings, as well as by the celestials. You should never approach them—they are protected by the club of Hari: neither we nor Time have jurisdiction over them.

28. The nectar of the lotus feet of Mukunda [Kṛṣṇa] is forever pleasing to the community of the highest renunciants, who are devoid of all material possessions. Bring to me the unrighteous who are averse to relishing these stories, but who instead relish the bonds of the household, which is the pathway to hell.
29. Bring to me those unrighteous souls whose tongues have never spoken of the name and qualities of *Bhagavān*, whose minds have never remembered His lotus feet, whose heads have never bowed down to Kṛṣṇa even once, and who have never done any service for Viṣṇu.
30. May that *Bhagavān*, *Nārāyaṇa*, the primeval Person, forgive the offenses performed by us through our servants. Forgiveness is fitting for Him. He is magnanimous on His foolish servants, and we hold out our hands in supplication. Reverence to the Supreme Person.' "
31. [*Śrī* Śuka said:]
"Therefore, O descendant of the Kuru dynasty, you should know that the only atonement for all sins, even great ones, is the reciting of the names of Viṣṇu (*saṅkīrtana*). This brings auspiciousness to the world.
32. The mind is not purified as much by vows and other such things as it is by the exemplary devotion of those who always hear and chant about the great deeds of Hari.
33. One who has tasted the nectar of the lotus feet of Kṛṣṇa never again enjoys the *guṇas* of *māyā*. These lead to vice and have been renounced by them. Others, on the other hand, afflicted by lust, strive to clean the *rajas* from the mind by [material] action. But from doing this, only more *rajas* is produced anew.
34. The servants of Yama, their minds struck with awe, from then on remembered the glories of *Bhagavān* as described by their master. Being afraid of those who have devoted themselves to Acyuta [Kṛṣṇa], they do not dare to look at them from that time henceforth, O king.
35. The great sage Agastya recited this intimate story when seated in the Malaya hills worshipping Hari."

The Tale of King Citraketu: The Dead Son Returns

Yoga Blueprint

This passages continues in the vein of a number of the previous teachings in terms of illustrating the illusory and ephemeral nature of family relationships and attachments. The stark and blunt message it adds to this is that once even the most intimate relationships are severed by death, the departed ātman *pursues its trajectory into the next life and does not even remember its previous relationships, even if reencountering those same people.*

The opening verses below point to the rarity of those who seriously commit their lives to seeking truth.

Book VI, Chapter 14

1. *Śrī* Parīkṣit said:

"Vṛtra was sinful and his nature was *rājasic* and *tāmasic*. How did unwavering devotion to Nārāyaṇa, *Bhagavān*, arise in him, O *brāhmaṇa*?

2. Devotion to the lotus feet of Mukunda rarely manifests even among the celestials who are in pure *sattva*, or among the sages whose hearts are untainted.

3. Living entities are as innumerable as the particles of dust on the earth. From those among them who are human, only a few strive for higher goals.

4. From these, for the most part, there are only a few who seek liberation, O best of the *brāhmaṇas*. And from thousands who seek liberation, only one becomes perfected and attains liberation.[31]

5. And even among thousands who are liberated and perfected, a peaceful soul who is devoted to Nārāyaṇa is very rare, O best of the sages.

6. So, given all this, how did the sinful Vṛtra, the tormentor of all the worlds, become someone with such unwavering devotion to Kṛṣṇa in that terrible conflict [with Indra]?[32]

7. I am greatly puzzled by this, O master, and eager to hear. Vṛtra impressed Indra of the thousand eyes,[33] by his valor in the battle."

8. *Śrī* Sūta replied:

"The great Śuka, son of Vyāsa, was pleased by the question of the faithful Parīkṣit. He honored him and spoke these words.

9. *Śrī* Śuka said:

'Listen attentively to this narrative, O king, which I heard from the mouths of Vyāsa, Nārada, and also of sage Devala.

10. There once was an emperor among the *Śūrasena* people known as Citraketu who ruled over the earth, O king. During his reign, the earth provided all needs.

11. He had many wives.[34] However, although he wanted progeny, he could not obtain any offspring from them.
12. Consequently anxiety afflicted this king, even though he was endowed with all desirable qualities such as good looks, youthfulness, generosity, nobility, learning, opulence, and wealth.
13. Neither his opulence, nor all his queens with their lovely eyes, nor this earth of which he was sovereign could give the emperor any satisfaction.
14. Once, the great sage Aṅgirā, who happened to be wandering around those realms, arrived unexpectedly at his palace.
15. The king honored Aṅgirā according to custom by rising to greet him and making offerings and other such things. Then, after the sage had received hospitality and was comfortably seated, the king sat nearby with attentive mind.
16. When the king had respectfully bowed down on the ground and had taken his seat, Aṅgirā returned respect to the king. He then addressed the king by speaking as follows, O king.
17. *Śrī* Aṅgirā said:
"Are you and your citizens well and in good spirits? Just as a person is protected by the seven evolutes of *prakṛti* (*buddhi*, *ahaṅkāra*, and the five *tanmātras*),[35] so is the king protected by seven *prakṛtis* (constituents of statehood: kingship, ministers, allies, treasury, fortress, army, territory).[36]
18. Truly, when a king entrusts himself to these *prakṛtis*, he secures the highest well-being. Reciprocally, the *prakṛtis*—ministers, etc.—are delivered of their cares by the king, O Lord of men.
19. Are your wives, ministers of state, servants, merchant guilds, counselors, citizens, communities, regional kings, and sons under your control?
20. If one is in control of oneself, then all these other things come under one's control; the worlds, along with their rulers, all enthusiastically offer such a person tribute.
21. But I can see that your mind is not at peace. Whether on account of yourself or of others, your face is disturbed by worry. You have some desire that has not been fulfilled."
22. Upon being confronted in this way by the sage, who actually already knew the cause, O king, Citraketu, desiring offspring, responded to him bowed down in humility.

23. Citraketu said:
"Your holiness! The sins of *yogīs* have been destroyed by dint of their austerities, knowledge, and *samādhi* insight. What is there that is not known by them about embodied beings, whether internal or external?
24. Nevertheless, since you have requested, O *brāhmaṇa*, I will disclose what is disturbing my mind, obliged by the order of your holiness, even though you already know.
25. Because I am without progeny, my possessions, majesty, and kingdom, which are so sought after by rulers of the world, do not bring any solace to me, just as things unrelated to nourishment do not bring solace to those who are hungry and thirsty.
26. Therefore please protect me, O blessed one, as I am falling into a dark [hell] along with my ancestors.[37] Instruct me as to how to overcome such a destiny by means of progeny, as otherwise such a fate is very difficult to avoid." '
27. *Śrī* Śuka said:
'Beseeched in this manner, Aṅgirā, the saintly and venerable son of Brahmā, being compassionate, offered rituals to Tvaṣṭā,[38] including a sweet dish he had cooked for him.
28. The principal and eldest of the king's queens was called Kṛtaduti, O descendant of Bharata. The twice-born sage gave the remnants of the sacrifice to her.
29. Then he said to the monarch: "A son will be born to you, O king. He will be a source of joy and also of sorrow to you." At that, Angirā, the son of Brahmā, departed.
30. And so it came to be: just from eating that sweet dish, Queen Kṛtadyuti became pregnant from Citraketu, just as Kṛttikā did for Agni.[39]
31. Because of the potency of the king of the *Śūrasenas*, her pregnancy grew gradually every day just like the waxing moon, O king.
32. In due course, the time arrived, and a son was born, causing great joy among the *Śūrasena* citizens who heard the news.
33. The king was overjoyed. When his son had been bathed, cleansed, and decorated, the king had benedictions chanted by the *brāhmaṇas*, and then arranged for the birth ceremony to be performed.
34. He bestowed upon the *brāhmaṇas* gold, silver, garments, ornaments, villages, horses, elephants, and six crores of cows.

35. The magnanimous regent also showered desirable things on the other citizens for the prosperity, fame, and longevity of his son, just like rain clouds shower on living beings.
36. Since the son had been obtained with difficulty, the affection of the saintly king for him grew every day, just as does the affection of a poor man for wealth when it is attained with difficulty.
37. And excessive affection born out of ignorance also grew in the mother, Kṛtadyuti, for her son. Meanwhile, a fever of desire for bearing children burned in her co-wives.
38. As he fondled his son every day, special affection for the wife who had given him birth grew in the king. This was not matched toward the other wives.
39. Overwhelmed by envy, by the distress of being childless, and by the indifference of the king, the other wives lamented their situation:
40. "Woe betide an unfortunate woman who is childless and not respected in her home. She is neglected as if she were a servant by the co-wives who have beautiful sons.
41. In fact, what distress is there for servant girls who are respected for their steady service of the master? But an unfortunate woman is like a maidservant of a maidservant."
42. In this way, intense hatred arose in the queens. They were tormented both by their co-wife's blessing of a son and by being neglected by the king.
43. Being unable to tolerate the king anymore, the cruel-hearted women administered poison to the infant. Their good sense had become destroyed by hatred.
44. Unaware of the great sin performed by her co-wives, Kṛtadyuti looked at her son and, thinking he was just sleeping, wandered about the house.
45. Eventually, thinking that the boy had been sleeping rather a long time, the intelligent woman requested the nurse: "My dear, please bring me my son!"
46. After approaching the supine child, the nurse saw that his eyes were turned upward and that his life airs, powers of senses, and mind had passed away. "I am doomed," she said, and fell on the ground.
47. Upon hearing the highly distressed cry of her maid, who was also wildly beating her breast with her two hands, the queen hastily entered the room and approached her son. She saw that he had suddenly died.

48. Overwhelmed by shock, she fell to the ground and lost consciousness, her hair and clothes in disarray.
49. Thereupon, after hearing the commotion, all the people living in the king's palace, men as well as women, came to the scene. They too became overwhelmed with grief, sharing in the calamity. Those who had committed the evil deed also wailed falsely.
50. When he heard that his son had died of unknown causes, the king became blind with grief. He rushed there, stumbling on the way due to intense grief inflamed by the bonds of affection.
51. Surrounded by his ministers and *brāhmaṇas*, the king fell unconscious at the feet of his dead son. Taking long-drawn-out breaths, he was not able to speak. His voice became choked up and muffled with tears, and his clothes and hair were thrown into disarray.
52. At this, when the pure-hearted queen saw her husband overwhelmed with this great grief over the dead boy, his only son, she lamented in various ways. This increased the heartfelt pain of the ministers and citizens.
53. She bathed her two breasts, beautified with ointment and *kuṅkuma* powder, with mascara-laden teardrops. Tearing at her hair, her garland in disarray, she lamented in various ways for her son in her lovely voice, like a *kurarī* bird:
54. "*Aho*, O Creator! You must be really foolish: since this death comes to the subsequent [generation] while the previous one still lives, you are acting against [the rules] of your own creation! And if this is not the case, then you must surely be an enemy!
55. Perhaps the fact is that there is no chronological order in this world in the birth and death of embodied beings, and that things happen in accordance with personal *karma*. Even then, you have severed the bond of affection for this child—and this bond was made by you yourself for the growth of your creation [in which case you must be really foolish!].
56. My darling son—after seeing your father overwhelmed with grief, you should not abandon me. I am inconsolable and helpless. Through you, we will easily cross over this darkness of [*saṁsāra*]—it is difficult to cross over without offspring.[40]
57. Get up, darling. These friends of yours of your age are calling you to play. You have surely slept for long enough and are ravished

by hunger. Eat. Drink from my breast. Remove our sorrow, and that of our friends and family, O joy of your father.
58. My good fortune is gone, O son, for I cannot see your innocent smile, happy eyes, and lotus face. I do not hear your charming voice. Or have you been taken by that cruel one [Yama, Lord of death]? Have you gone to the next world, from where there is no return?" '
59. *Śrī* Śuka said:
'As his wife was mourning the dead son with various laments of this sort, Citraketu, greatly aggrieved, wailed at the top of his voice along with her.
60. As that husband and wife were lamenting, all their attendants, men and women, wept. Everything became deprived of life.
61. The sage known as Aṅgirā knew that the king had fallen into this state of despair, that his peace of mind was destroyed, and that he was without a guide. So he arrived there with Nārada.' "

Book VI, Chapter 15

1. *Śrī* Śuka said:
"The king, overwhelmed with grief and lying next to the dead body, seemed equally dead himself. The two sages spoke to him, and enlightened him with words of wisdom:
2. 'This person for whom you grieve, O king, whom do you suppose he was to you in a previous life, or is at present, or will be in a future life? And who are you to him?
3. Just as grains of sand are brought together and then thrust apart by the force of the current, so, in the same way, embodied beings are joined and separated by Time.
4. Just as among seeds of grain, [some] seeds are productive and [some] are not productive, similarly among living beings, impelled by the *māyā* of the Lord, [some] living beings survive and [some] do not.
5. You, we, and all these moving and non-moving entities who appear contemporaneous do not [factually] exist even in the present, O king, just as we did not exist before our births and deaths, nor will we exist after them.
6. Although He is impartial like a boy [at play], the Lord of beings creates, preserves, and destroys beings by means of other beings. These beings are not independent but created from Himself.

7. The body of the embodied one is born from a body [the mother] by means of another body [the father], just as a seed is generated from another seed. But the embodied one is eternal, just as objects [like the atoms of the earth] are eternal.[41]

8. This distinction between the embodied one and the body is construed by lack of discrimination (*viveka*) and is primordial. It is imagined, just as is the distinction in an object between its universal and its individuator.' "[42]

9. *Śrī* Śuka said:

"Consoled in this way by these words spoken by the *brāhmaṇa*, King Citraketu wiped his distraught face with his hands and responded.

10. The king said:

'Who are you two who have arrived disguised in the garb of ascetic mendicants? Full of wisdom, you are the most distinguished of the distinguished.

11. There are certainly *brāhmaṇas* who are dear to *Bhagavān* roaming the earth at will disguised as madmen, enlightening those such as I who have dull understanding.

12.–15. [Such sages are] Kumāra, Nārada, Ṛbhu, Aṅgirā, Devala, Asita, Apāntaratamā, Vyāsa, Mārkaṇḍeya, Gautama, Vasiṣṭha, *Bhagavān* Rāma,[43] Kapila, Bādarāyaṇi [Śuka], Durvāsā, Yājñavalkya, Jātukarṇa, Āruṇi, Romaśa, Cyavana, Datta, Āsuri, Patañjali, sage Vedaśirā, the sage Bodhya, along with Pañcaśirā, Hiraṇyanābha, Kauśalya, Śrutadeva, and Ṛtadhvaja. These perfected masters wander about for the sake of [imparting] knowledge.

16. Therefore, O masters, please bestow the light of knowledge upon me; I am a vulgar beast, my intelligence is dull, and I am immersed in obscuring *tamas*.'

17. *Śrī* Aṅgirā said:

'I am Aṅgirā, O king, the one who bestowed a son upon you in the first place, when you desired one! And this is his lordship sage Nārada himself, the son of Brahmā.

18.–19. You are now immersed in *tamas* because of grief over your son. It is difficult to overcome. But we did not forget you, and have come here, O master, to show kindness to you. You are a servant of the Supreme Being and do not deserve to be in this situation. Do not lament: you are a *bhakta* of *Bhagavān*, devoted to the *brāhmaṇas*, O master.

20. When I first came to your house, I could have given you supreme knowledge at that time. But when I understood that you were intent on something else, then I just gave you a son.
21.–22. So now you are experiencing the suffering of those who have sons. The same holds true for those who have wives, homes, riches, prosperity, and powers of various sorts, the temporary objects of the senses such as sound—the opulences of kingship, a mighty kingdom, strength, treasury, servants, ministers, and friends.
23. These all bestow trouble, fear, illusion, and grief, O Lord of the Śūrasenas; they are dreams, *māyā*, concoctions of the mind. Their appearance is like the city of the *gandharvas* [a castle in the sky].
24. They are creations of the mind. Although they are perceived, they are not real, since they are without enduring substance. A person contemplates them with the mind, due to the force of past *karma*, and then produces further varieties of *karma*.[44]
25. In fact, this body of the embodied one is made of the gross elements of matter, the knowledge-acquiring senses and action-performing senses. It is said that it brings suffering and various afflictions to the embodied one.
26. Therefore, reflect on the true situation of the *ātman* with a sound mind. Give up the conviction that objects in the world of duality are stable. Then you will attain a state of peacefulness.'
27. *Śrī* Nārada said:
'Please accept the teaching (*upaniṣad*) of this *mantra* that I bestow on you. Meditating upon it, you will have a vision of the Supreme Lord Saṅkarṣaṇa [Viṣṇu].[45]
28. Draw near to the soles of His feet, O lord of men. In the past, Lord Śiva and other gods, after freeing themselves from this illusory world of duality, immediately attained to His glory, which is incomparable and supreme. You too will also attain the Supreme without delay.' "

Book VI, Chapter 16

1. *Śrī* Śuka, son of Badarāyaṇa said:
"O king, after this, the celestial sage granted a vision of the king's dead son to all the grieving kinsmen. Then he spoke.
2. *Śrī* Nārada said:
'O *jīvātman* (embodied soul),[46] blessings upon you! Just look at your mother and father, and your friends and relatives burning with intense grief because of what you have done.

3. Take back possession of your body for the remainder of your life. Surrounded by your kinsmen, indulge in the enjoyments bestowed by your father, and eventually ascend on to the throne of the king yourself!'

4. The *jīva* (soul) said:

'In accordance with *karma*, I have been transmigrating through numerous births—as a celestial being, animal, and human. In which birth were these two my father and mother?

5. Kinsmen, relatives, enemies, those who are neutral, friends, the indifferent, and adversaries—everyone becomes each of these in turn, in mutually reciprocating roles with everyone else.

6. Just like objects such as articles of trade or gold move about from here to there among people, so does the *jīva* move about in [various] wombs and procreators.

7. The relationships with objects and living beings among people is clearly seen to be impermanent. Yet for as long as there is a relationship with these things, there is a sense of "mine-ness" over them (that is, ownership).

8. The *jīva* is eternal and without any sense of I-ness (ego), yet when it attains a particular birth, a sense of "this belongs to me" develops in it for as long as it finds itself in that particular birth.

9. This soul is eternal, imperishable, subtle, the support of everything, and self-aware. Being a master, it creates its own universe for itself, through its own *guṇas* of *māyā*.

10. No one is dear to it, no one its enemy, no one its kin, no one foreign to it; it is the one seer (*draṣṭṛ*) of all the minds of the performers of virtuous and faulty acts.

11. The soul does not in fact accept the fruits of activity, virtuous, or faulty. It is the lord who is seated neutrally as the witness of cause and effect.' "

12. Śuka, son of Badarāyaṇa, said:

"After uttering these words, the *jīva* then departed, and its relatives were struck with amazement. They severed the bonds of personal affection, and were freed from their sorrow.

13. After removing the dead body of their relative and performing all the appropriate rites, the kinsmen gave up their affection. It is the giver of grief, illusion, fear, and distress, yet it is so difficult to give up.

14. Remembering the words of the sage, the killers of the child, who had lost their luster because of the child's murder, became ashamed.

Under the direction of *brāhmaṇas* they undertook the penance for infanticide there on the banks of the *Yamunā* river.

15. When Citraketu's mind was enlightened in this way by the words of the *brāhmaṇa*, he stepped out from the dark well of household life, like an elephant from the mud of a lake.

16. After bathing in the *Kālindī* river in the prescribed manner and performing pious rites with water, Citraketu worshipped the two sons of Brahmā silently with controlled breath (*prāṇa*).

17. The venerable Nārada, pleased that the *bhakta* king had controlled his mind and submitted to their instructions, gave him the following [prayer] to recite:

18. 'Reverence to You, *Bhagavān* Vāsudeva; let me contemplate You. Reverence to Pradyumna, Aniruddha, and Saṅkarṣaṇa.

19. Reverence to You who are absolute wisdom. You have a form of supreme bliss, and You delight in your own nature. You are peaceful and Your knowledge transcends duality.

20. Reverence to You who are situated beyond the waves of *śakti* (*māyā*) in the experience of Your own bliss. Reverence to You, Lord Hṛṣīkeśa, the Supreme. Your form is unlimited.

21. He is the One who is still not understood when words have exhausted themselves, along with the mind.[47] He has no material name and form (*nāma-rūpa*), is pure consciousness (*cit*), and transcends cause and effect. May He be favorably disposed toward us.

22. From Him this world is born, and in Him it rests and is dissolved, just like the earth with regards to the things made of earth. Reverence to that *Brahman* which is You Yourself.

23. The life air, senses, intelligence, and mind cannot know Him or touch Him. He pervades within and without, like the sky. I offer reverence to Him.

24. The body, senses, life airs, mind, and intellect, these perform activities when pervaded by His rays. Otherwise they cannot do so, just like iron cannot perform functions when it is not heated. That which is known as "the seer" (*draṣṭṛ*) in the states of consciousness [waking, sleeping, deep sleep, pure consciousness] is Him.

25. *Oṁ*. Reverence to *Bhagavān*, the Supreme Person, the almighty and omnipotent Lord. Your two lotus feet are tenderly massaged by the lotus budlike hands of the multitudes of devotees surrounding You. You are the Ultimate Supreme Being.' "

26. *Śri* Śuka said:
"After Nārada had taught this practice to the submissive *bhakta* king, he departed with Aṅgirāsa to the abode of the self-manifest Brahmā.
27. So for seven days, imbibing only water, Citraketu meditated with focused attention on that practice in the manner instructed and imparted by Nārada.
28. Then, O king, at the end of seven days, by concentrating on that practice without interruption, he attained the position of lordship over the celestial *vidyādharas*.[48]
29. Thereafter, a few more days later still, the flow of his mind became enlightened, and he attained the presence of the feet of the God of gods, Śeṣa.[49]
30. He saw the Lord, who was as white as a lotus fiber, wearing blue garments, and adorned with a radiant headdress, armlets, belt, and bracelets. He had a smiling face, and reddish eyes, and was surrounded by an entourage of perfected *yogī* masters.
31. All the king's sins were destroyed from seeing the Lord, and his subtle body became pure and cleansed. His eyes filled with tears of love from intensified devotion, and his hairs stood on end. He approached silently, and offered homage to that primordial Being.
32. With teardrops of love, he continually dampened the footstool of the lotus feet of the most praiseworthy Lord Viṣṇu. He was so choked up with love, he was incapable of offering homage for a long time as no words issued forth.
33. Then, recovering his speech, the king controlled his mind with his higher reason, and restrained his senses from external engagement. Then he spoke the following words to that personal Being, the *guru* of the universe, who is described in the scriptures of the Vaiṣṇavas.[50]
34. Citraketu said:
'O unconquerable One! Although You are unconquerable, Your Lordship is conquered by the saints (*sādhus*) whose minds are controlled. Their hearts, in turn, have been conquered by You. You are so merciful that You give Yourself to those who always engage in Your *bhakti* without any personal desire.
35. O *Bhagavān*! The emergence, preservation, and dissolution of the universe is nothing other than an expression of Your power. The [secondary] creators are partial manifestations of partial manifestations

of You.[51] Because of thinking themselves independent, they vie among each other in vain.
36. It is You who exist at the beginning, middle, and end of [everything from] the smallest atom to the entire cosmic manifestation, even though You are immune from these three [states of change]. That which remains permanent throughout the beginning, termination as well as intervening period of all beings, is none other than You alone.
37. This egglike universe is covered by seven layers of earth atoms, etc., each one ten times thicker than the previous one.[52] That place where it, along with billions and billions of other universes exist like miniscule atoms, is Ananta, the unlimited One [You].
38. There are those, thirsty for sense gratification, who [have the appetites] of animals even though they are in human forms. They worship the lower celestial beings, rather than You, the Supreme. But those blessings received from the celestials, O Lord, come to an end when the celestials themselves come to an end—just like the boons received from a royal family [when the dynasty is destroyed].
39. [Even if] desires for sensual pleasure are offered to You, O Supreme Being, they do not generate *karma*, just as cooked grains do not germinate. [This is because] You are not made of the *guṇas* but are pure awareness, while the snares [of *karma*] of the world of duality (*saṁsāra*) are attributes of the *guṇas*.[53]
40. O unconquerable One! [*Saṁsāra*] was conquered by You when You delivered the flawless teachings of *Bhāgavata-dharma*. Those sages who are free of all desires and delight in their own *ātman*, worship You for liberation.
41. The attitude of discrimination—making distinctions of I, you, mine, yours—which is found elsewhere, does not exist here among the people [following the *Bhāgavata-dharma*]. Actions performed with an attitude of discrimination are impure, temporary, and characterized by non-*dharma*.
42. What benefit is there in notions of "mine" and "other"? How much value is there in *dharma* [systems] that are harmful to oneself and others? [Such systems] are actually non-*dharma* because they are harmful to oneself, inflict suffering on others, and cause Your displeasure.
43. Your principles, which you established by means of the *Bhāgavata dharma*, do not change. The Āryans, who see no differences

between the multitude of moving and non-moving entities, worship You.
44. After seeing You, all the sins of men are destroyed, O *Bhagavān*. This has always been the case. Even a *pukkaśa* tribesman, after hearing Your name once, is freed from *saṁsāra*.
45. Therefore, O *Bhagavān*, today we have had all the impurities in our minds wiped away by seeing You. How could that which was spoken by Your devotee the celestial sage Nārada turn out to be otherwise?
46. O Unlimited One, Soul of the Universe, everything performed by people in this world is known to You. What is there that can possibly be revealed to the Supreme *Guru*, just as what can be revealed to the sun by fireflies?
47. Reverence to You, *Bhagavān*, the Lord of creation, maintenance, and dissolution of the universe. The true nature of Your Being cannot be understood by imperfect *yogīs* because of their seeing things as different [from You].
48. The creators of the worlds are animated when You breathe, and when You perceive, their organs of perception awake to perception. The sphere of the universe appears like a mustard seed upon the head of Śeṣa. To Him, the Being with a thousand heads, I offer reverence.' "
49. *Śrī* Śuka said:
"*Bhagavān* Ananta was pleased when He was glorified in this way, and spoke to Citraketu, the Lord of the *vidyādharas*, O upholder of the Kuru dynasty.
50. *Śrī Bhagavān* said:
'You have attained perfection by accepting the teachings about Me delivered to you by Nārada and Aṅgirā, as well as by following that technique, and also by seeing Me.
51. I am the soul of all beings, and I cause the welfare of all beings. I am *śabda-Brahman* [the Veda] and the Supreme *para-Brahman*. These are both My eternal forms.
52. The *ātman* infuses the world, and the world envelops the *ātman*. Both of them are pervaded by Me, and both are created in Me.
53. This is just like a person deeply sleeping who sees the whole universe in himself, but, upon waking, realizes that his self is only situated in one place.
54. Such is the case with the *ātman*: when one realizes that the *jīva*'s states of consciousness, such as wakefulness, etc., are expressions of

māyā (illusion), then one should remain fixed in the knowledge that the seer is transcendent to these states.

55. Know me to be that *ātman*, by dint of whom the *puruṣa* understands the dream to be his when in the state of dreaming.[54] I am *Brahman*, bliss, beyond the *guṇas*.

56. That awareness of both the states of dream and of awakening for a person remembering them, which pervades and goes beyond them, is *Brahman*, the Supreme.

57. It is due to the forgetfulness of this My nature that *saṁsāra* exists for a person who thinks of himself as separate. It is because of this forgetfulness that a person undergoes body after body, and death after death.

58. After having attained a human birth where there is the possibility of knowledge and wisdom, if one does not awaken to the *ātman*, one does not obtain any [ultimate] benefit [from this birth].

59. Keeping in mind the hardships [accruing from chasing] desires in this world, of the contrary results that arise from them, and of the freedom from fear that comes from not pursuing them, a sage should desist from desires.

60. A husband and wife perform actions for the sake of happiness and to avoid unhappiness. But there is neither the cessation of unhappiness nor the attainment of happiness from this.

61.–62. Realizing in this way the opposite results attained by those people who think themselves clever, and realizing the subtle nature of the *ātman*, which transcends the three states [of waking, sleep, and deep sleep], and freed by one's own willpower from sense objects whether seen or heard about, a person should become My devotee and take satisfaction in knowledge and wisdom.

63. This is what is to be known as the true self-interest of those who have taken a human birth: perceiving with all one's being the oneness of the *ātman* with that Supreme. This perception is attained by means of skillful intelligence and the practice of *yoga*.

64. By contemplating these words of mine, O King, with faith and without confusion, you will quickly become perfected with knowledge and realization.' "

65. *Śrī* Śuka said:

"As king Citraketu, who had been inspired in this way, was watching, Hari, *Bhagavān*, who is the *Guru* of the universe and soul of everything, disappeared from there."

Book VII

The Teachings of Yamarāja: Lament of the Widowed Queens

Yoga Blueprint

This pithy story, which contains a fable within it, illustrates the futility of grieving for a deceased loved one, given that the body is still present, while the soul had never been perceived in the first place. The teachings also stress the importance of accepting one's karma.

Book VII, Chapter 2

27. People recite this ancient legend (*itihāsa*); it involves a conversation between Yama and the relatives of a dead person. Please listen to it.
28. There was a renowned king called Suyajña in a kingdom called Uśīnara, who was killed by his enemies in battle. His relatives gathered round his body.
29. His jewel-laden armor was shattered, and his garland and ornaments were in disarray. He was lying covered in blood, his heart pierced by arrows.
30. His hair was scattered, his eyes glazed, and his lip bitten in fury. His lotus face was darkened with dust and his arms and weapons had been severed in the battle.
31. The lord of the Uśīnara kingdom had been reduced to this state by Fate. His queens were distraught upon seeing him. "Our lord has been killed," they said. Beating their chests forcefully with their fists again and again, they fell at the feet of the king.

32. Crying loudly, the poor queens bathed his lotus feet with their tears, reddened with the *kuṅkuma* powder from their breasts, their ornaments and hair in disarray. They wailed, invoking people's pity by their laments.
33. "*Aho!* O lord, you have been taken away from our sight by cruel Fate. You, who were previously the maintainer of the citizens of Uśīnara, have now been reduced to the source of their lamentation.
34. How will we exist without you, our dear friend and guide, O great king? Tell us the means of following your steps, O hero, to wherever you will go. We are your faithful servants."
35. The queens, embracing their husband and lamenting in this way, were resisting carrying away the dead body; then the sun finished setting.
36. After hearing such lamentation by the relatives of the dead man, Yama, the god of death, assumed the form of a young [orphan] boy and personally came there. He addressed the queens.
37. *Śrī* Yama said:
"*Aho!* Just see the bewilderment of these queens who are mature in age, even though they know the laws of nature. These queens lament uselessly, even though they themselves are bound by the same rules. This dead man has gone back to wherever he came.
38. *Aho!* We ourselves are most fortunate, because even though we were abandoned by our parents, we are not in anxiety. Even though we are weak, we have not been devoured by wolves and wild animals. That Being who protects us in the womb, will protect us now.
39. Out of His desire, that imperishable Lord creates this universe, and He protects and dissolves it. They say that this is the play of that Lord, O women! He is the Controller in the coming together and dissolution of moving and non-moving beings.
40. In some cases, even if fallen by the roadside, one lives when protected by Fate, in others, even if safely situated at home, one meets destruction when neglected by Fate. An orphan in the jungle survives when protected by Fate, while one secure at home does not live when struck by Fate.
41. Without exception, living bodies appear and then disappear in time in accordance with their respective *karma* and particular births. Although embedded in *prakṛti*, the *ātman* is completely different, and is not actually bound by its *guṇas*.

42. This body made of material elements is produced by illusion and is different from the *puruṣa*, just as a person is different from a house made of earth, water, and fire. A person is born, undergoes some changes, and then dies in due course of time.
43. Just as fire manifests in pieces of wood but is different from them; and just as air enters the body but exists distinct from it; and just as the sky, which is omnipresent, is not tainted by anything; so a being, who is the support of all the *guṇas* is yet transcendent to them.
44. O foolish people! That Suyajña for whom you lament still lies here. But [the consciousness of] the one who was the hearer and the responder was never perceived in the first place.[1]
45. The primary life air in the body, even though essential, is also not the hearer or responder. It is the *ātman* who is the possessor of the senses, and it is different from the body and life airs.
46. By its own potency, the omnipresent *ātman* possesses bodies in higher and lower births characterized by mind, senses, and material elements but yet is different from them.
47. For as long as the *ātman* is connected with the subtle body, it is bound by *karma*. As a result, it is subject to error, defects (*kleśas*), and the influence of *māyā*.
48. This ego, which perceives and speaks of objects in the *guṇas*, is illusory. It is like a dream, which is a mental concoction. All things made of the material elements are false.
49. Those who understand the truth do not lament for anything in this world, whether permanent or impermanent. But the nature of those who lament is to say, 'It is not possible to do anything other than lament.'
50. Once upon a time, some hunter—the harbinger of death to birds—spread out his nets and placed them about in the forest, setting bait here and there.
51. He saw a pair of *kuliṅga* birds wandering about there. The female one of them was suddenly allured by the hunter.
52. She became trapped, O queens, bound by Fate in the cords of the net. The male *kuliṅga* bird, seeing her fallen into this calamity, was greatly aggrieved out of affection. Unable to do anything, the poor thing lamented for his poor mate:
53. '*Aho!* Fate is cruel. What will the Supreme Lord do with me, an unfortunate soul, and with my poor wife who is so kind she is lamenting for me?

54. Let Fate take me as it pleases. What is the use of living miserably with only half of myself? There will only be suffering from such a bereaved life.
55. My poor offspring are awaiting me in the nest. How will I maintain the chicks, whose wings have not yet grown, now they have been bereft of their mother?'
56. Propelled by the Time factor, the hunter had hidden nearby. While the *kuliṅga* bird was lamenting in this way, its throat choked up with tears due to being afflicted by this separation from its beloved, the fowler pierced it with an arrow.
57. In the same way, you queens will not get your husband back even if you lament for hundreds of years; meanwhile you are foolishly not perceiving your own imminent death."
58. While the young boy was discoursing in this way, all the relatives' minds were struck with astonishment. They realized that everything is temporary and situated in unreality.
59. After Yama had imparted these instructions, he disappeared from there. Then the relatives of King Suyajña performed the funerary ceremonials.
60. Therefore, free from bodily ignorance in the form of clinging (*abhiniveśa*[2]) to notions of self and other—such as "Who am I and who is other?" or "What is mine, here, and what belongs to others?"—you should not lament for your own body or anyone else's.

The Tale of Child Prahlāda: Viṣṇu Protects His *Bhaktas*

Yoga Blueprint

The story of Prahlāda is one of the best-known bhakta *stories in Hinduism. As with Dhruva, Prahlāda was a child* bhakta, *in addition to which he was born into a family of* asuras *(demons). This once again underscores the principle that neither age nor birth nor any other factor disqualifies one from the path of* bhakti. *In fact, the text selects Prahlāda to formally articulate the nine practices that form the core of* vaidhī bhakti *discussed in part 1. Significant here is Prahlāda advising his fellow boy students not to fritter away even a moment of human life, but to start thinking about the purpose of life even as children.*

We find here another example of the Bhāgavata's *disinterest in the standard goal of* yoga*—realization of the* ātman *(VII.6.25), not* *to mention any sort of more mundane blessings, even if offered by Viṣṇu himself (VII.9.55). But we find in this passage, too, a second reason Prahlāda is disinterested in liberation. We know that one of the* Bhāgavata*'s repeated subthemes is the promotion of immersing the mind in* Īśvara *as being far more blissful than awareness being absorbed in its own nature, which is why* bhaktas *reject the standard goals of* yoga. *But Prahlāda expresses disinterest in liberation not just because of the greater experience of bliss for oneself, but because it entails abandoning other living entities to suffer in* saṁsāra *(VII.9.44). In this, he exemplifies an attitude often associated with the* Boddhisattva *in Buddhism. Of significance, too, is that the passage makes a dismissive comment about those who teach and perform the various activities associated with* yoga *and the like simply to make a living.*

[*This narrative is recounted to King Yuddhiṣṭhira by sage Nārada.*]

Book VII, Chapter 4

30. Hiraṇyakaśipu had four very wonderful sons. On account of his qualities, Prahlāda was the greatest of these. He was a worshipper of the Supreme.

31. He was devoted to the *brāhmaṇas*, endowed with good character, committed to Truth, had controlled senses, and acted as the well-wisher and best friend to all beings, as if they were his own self.

32. Toward Āryans (cultured people) he was dutiful, like a servant; toward the needy, he was kind, like a father; toward equals, he was affectionate, like a brother; and toward teachers, he had a respectful attitude. Although he was blessed with learning, wealth, beauty, and good birth, he was without any sense of pride or arrogance.

33. His mind was not disturbed in calamities, and he was free of cravings—both of things he had experienced and of those he had heard about—as he perceived the ephemeral nature of the *guṇas* that produce them. His senses, life air, body, and intelligence were always controlled and his desires appeased. Although an *asura*, demon [by birth], he did not possess [the qualities] of the *asuras*.

34. The great qualities found in Prahlāda are constantly being glorified by poets—they have not been forgotten [by Time] even up to today—just as is the case with the qualities of *Bhagavān*, *Īśvara*.

35. Even the *sūras*, celestials, who are enemies [of Prahlāda's lineage of *asuras*], pay homage to him, O king—not to mention others such as your good self.
36. He had innate devotion for *Bhagavān* Vāsudeva. From his innumerable qualities, this much alone is enough to indicate his greatness.
37. As a child, he was not interested in toys, and acted like a simpleton, on account of his mind being absorbed in God. His mind appeared possessed [as if] by the planet Kṛṣṇa,[3] and so he did not perceive the world as it is conventionally perceived.
38. While sitting, wandering about, eating, lying down, drinking, and eating, he was not consciously planning these [activities], as he was in the embrace of Govinda [Kṛṣṇa].
39. Sometimes his mind would become pervaded by anxiety for Kṛṣṇa, the Lord of Vaikuṇṭha, and he would cry. Sometimes he would laugh from joy at thoughts of Him, and sometimes he would burst into song.
40. Sometimes he would yell at the top of his voice, sometimes he would dance without shame. At other times, his mind fixed on Kṛṣṇa, he identified with Him so much that he imitated His activities.
41. Sometimes he remained silent, his hair standing on end in ecstasy. At such times, experiencing bliss from contact with the Lord, his eyes filled with tears of joy and love and remained fixed and unblinking.
42. Continuously radiating with internal ecstasy attained through service to the lotus feet of Viṣṇu and through the association of devotees who desire nothing for themselves, Prahlāda bestowed peace of mind on those who were miserable due to keeping bad company.
43. Hiraṇyakaśipū inflicted violence on Prahlāda, his own son, who was a great illustrious soul and *bhāgavata* devotee.
44. *Śrī* Yuddhiṣṭhīra said:
"O celestial sage! We wish to understand from you, who are true to your vows, how the father inflicted harm on his own son, a pure *saddhu* (saint).
45. Fathers are affectionate to their own sons, and only reproach them if they are disobedient with the goal of imparting a lesson—never to harm them as if they were an enemy!
46. This should be all the more so for obedient saintly sons like Prahlāda, who respect their teachers as gods, O master. Please dispel this curiosity of mine, O *brāhmaṇa*: What animosity impelled a father to take the life of a son?"

Book VII, Chapter 5

1. *Śrī* Nārada replied:

"The great Kāvya (Śukrācārya) was selected by the *asuras* (demons) as the chief priest (*purohita*). His two sons, Ṣaṇḍa and Amarka, lived near the palace of the *daitya* (demon)[4] king.

2. They instructed various courses of learning to the boy Prahlāda, who was already well behaved. Along with other young *asura* boys, Prahlāda had been entrusted to them by the king.

3. Whatever was taught by the teacher there, Prahlāda heard and repeated, but in reality he did not accept the teachings in his mind, as they were grounded in the illusion of 'mine' and 'other.'[5]

4. One day, O son of Pāṇḍu, the king of the *asuras* seated his son on his lap, and asked: 'Tell me what you think is good, my son.'

5. *Śrī* Prahlāda said:

'The minds of embodied beings are beset with anxieties because of being captured by illusion, O best of the *asuras*. What I think is good is that they renounce the blind well of the household,[6] which causes the downfall of the soul, and go to the forest, where they can take shelter of Hari.' "

6. *Śrī* Nārada said:

"When he heard the words of his son, which resonated with those of the enemy [the *sūras*, celestials, who are favorable to Viṣṇu] the *daitya* laughed: 'The minds of the boys have been influenced by the views of the enemy.

7. The boy should be kept apart in the house of the *guru*, so that his intelligence does not become influenced by *brāhmaṇas* favorable to Viṣṇu from the other side in disguise.'

8. When Prahlāda had been brought back to their home, the *daitya*'s priests summoned him and flattered him with slippery words. Then they asked in reassuring tones:

9. 'Prahlāda, dear boy! May you be blessed! Now, speak truthfully, do not tell lies: From where did this misguided idea come to you? It is beyond the normal comprehension of young boys.

10. O joy of your lineage, has this disturbance in your understanding been caused by someone else, or was it just spontaneous? Tell us—we your teachers are eager to hear.'

11. *Śrī* Prahlāda said:

'Reverence to that *Bhāgavan*, by whose *māyā* the false conception

of "mine" and "other" manifests in people. It is seen in those who have deluded intelligence.
12. This beastlike understanding of "that person is different from me, and I am different from him" is destroyed when He is favorably disposed to people. It is a false understanding, a petty attitude that makes distinctions.
13. It is *Bhāgavan* who has "disturbed my understanding." He is actually the *ātman*, which is misperceived because of false understanding of "mine" and "other." His ways are unfathomable—the reciters of the Vedas and all beings from Brahmā down are bewildered about his ways.
14. Just as iron moves itself when in the vicinity of a magnet, O *brāhmaṇa*, so in the same way my consciousness is disturbed according to the will of Viṣṇu, the wielder of the *cakra* discus.' "
15. *Śrī* Nārada said:
"After speaking these words to the *brāhmaṇa*, the high-minded Prahlāda fell silent. Then that wretched servant of the king, furious, threatened him:
16. 'You are bringing disrepute to us. The fourth method, punishment,[7] has been prescribed in the sacred texts for a fool who acts like a firebrand in the family lineage. Bring us the rod!
17. This boy is like a thorn tree born in the forest of sandalwood of the *daityas*. He is the handle of the axe of Viṣṇu who [wishes] to fell us at the roots.'
18. In this way the demon *brāhmaṇa* intimidated Prahlāda through threats and various other such means. Then he made him learn the philosophy behind the first three goals of life (righteousness, material well-being, and sense gratification).[8]
19. After this, the teacher ensured that the boy learned the fourfold things to be known [by kings—namely, pacification, bribery, divide and rule, and punishment]. He then brought him forward, washed and decorated by his mother, to the *daitya* king once again.
20. Prahlāda bent low at his feet, and the *asura* welcomed the boy with blessings. Embracing him for a long time with his arms, the king felt intense pleasure.
21. Seating upon his lap his son whose face was beaming, he kissed his head, wetting it with his tear drops. Then he spoke as follows to his son.

22. Hiraṇyakaśipu said:
'O Prahlāda, my son, may you live long. Tell me something about the highest learning from whatever you have studied from your teacher over the course of time up to now.'
23.–24. Prahlāda replied:
'The nine characteristics of *bhakti* that people can offer to Viṣṇu are: hearing about Him, singing about Him, remembering Him, serving His feet, worshipping Him, glorifying Him, considering oneself His servant, considering oneself His friend, and surrendering completely to Him. When these are offered to *Bhagavān*, then I think this to be the highest learning.'
25. Upon hearing these words of his son, Hiraṇyakaśipu's lip trembled, and he said as follows to the son of his *guru*:
26. 'You excuse for a *brāhmaṇa*. What is this that you have done by deceitfully siding with the enemy? You have disrespected me, and caused this boy to learn nonsense, you fool!
27. There are dishonest persons in the world—untrue friends wearing false garb. Their deception reveals itself in the course of time, just like a disease does in sinful people.'
28. The son of the *guru* replied:
'He was not taught this by me, nor was he taught by anyone else. This son of yours, O enemy of Indra, says that this understanding of his is innate. Control your anger, O king, do not lay the blame on us.' "
29. *Śrī* Nārada said:
"After receiving this reply from the teacher, the *asura* again spoke to his son: 'If these ideas did not come from the mouth of your teacher, then whose perverse opinion is it, you wretched boy?'
30. *Śrī* Prahlāda said:
'For those who have taken vows of commitment to householder life, an understanding of Kṛṣṇa is not attained either from someone else, nor spontaneously, nor from reciprocal dealings among each other. Such people are chewing again and again that which has already been chewed, and end up entering a hellish condition because of their uncontrolled senses.
31. Those who seek the goal of life externally, their hearts tainted [by desire], do not understand Viṣṇu to be the goal of their real self-interest. They are like blind people being led by the blind; but they

are nonetheless still constrained by the formidable ropes of the Lord's laws.

32. Until such people make the decision to bathe their minds in the dust of the feet of the great selfless devotees, their understanding will never be able to touch the lotus feet of Viṣṇu. These have the quality of eliminating all contamination [from the heart].'

33. No sooner had Prahlāda finished speaking than Hiraṇyakaśipu hurled his son from his lap onto the ground, his mind blinded with fury.

34. Consumed with indignation and fury, his eyes turning red, he cried: 'Demons! Let this doomed person be executed. Take him away!

35. This offensive boy is [to all intents and purposes] the killer of my brother as he worships Viṣṇu, the killer of his uncle,[9] like a servant. He has abandoned his own well-wishers.

36. If, at five years of age, he has rejected the affection of his father, which is so hard to renounce, then what good will this useless fellow be able to do for Viṣṇu?

37. The [offspring of] another person, if he or she acts in one's interest, can be considered one's own child—just like medicine. But even one's own child, if not acting in one's interest, is like a disease. One should cut off that [diseased] limb for one's own interest so that the rest [of the body] can live happily after it has been severed.

38. An enemy masquerading as a friend is like an uncontrolled sense for a sage. He should be killed by any means—whether he is eating, lying down, or sitting.'

39.–40. Those demons had fierce teeth, cruel faces, copper beards and hair, and bore tridents in their hands. Commanded by their lord, they attacked Prahlāda in all his vital places with their tridents uttering terrifying roars and yelling: 'Cut him! Pierce him!'

41. But these were ineffective on Prahlāda, who had his mind fixed on *Bhagavān*, the Soul of everything, the Supreme imperceptible *Brahman*.

42. When all the attempts proved futile, the king of the *daityas* became greatly alarmed, and made further murderous attempts with determination, O Yudhiṣṭhira.

43.–44. When the *asura* could not kill his innocent son by means of elephants, serpents, sorcery, hurling him [from high places], magic, confinement, administering poison, food deprivation, ice, wind, fire,

water, or hurling boulders at him, he became completely distraught. He could not find a means to accomplish this goal.
45. 'This boy has been verbally abused by me, and I devised various means to murder him; but he freed himself from all those lethal attempts by his own power.
46. Although he is only a boy, this one is very intelligent and will not forget my non-Āryan (uncivilized) behavior, just like Śunaḥśepa.[10] He is powerful, and he is living with me, not in some distant place.
47. This boy is invulnerable, and fears nothing. His power is immeasurable. He will certainly be the bearer of my death for being his enemy—or perhaps he will not.'
48. Hiraṇyakaśipu's downcast face became haggard on account of anxiety. Ṣaṇḍa and Amarka, the two sons of Śukra, the *guru* of the demons, spoke to him in private:
49. 'The three worlds were conquered by you single-handedly. All the regions of the celestials were thrown into turmoil just by your frown. We do not see anything to worry about from Prahlāda, O master. There are no grounds [to fear] the good or bad qualities of children.
50. Bind this boy with the bonds of Varuṇa,[11] and keep him so that he does not flee away in fear until Śukra, the *guru* of the Bhārgava clan arrives. The intelligence of people matures with age, and through rendering service to Āryans.'
51. 'Do just that,' Hiraṇyakaśipu said, accepting the words of his *guru*'s sons. 'And make sure that the *dharma* of kings who are householders is taught to him.'
52. So they taught everything about appropriate behavior, material gain, and sense indulgence (*dharma*, *artha*, and *kāma*) in proper order to Prahlāda, O king. Prahlāda remained humble and obedient.
53. During the instruction of these three topics to him by his teachers, Prahlāda never considered them to be the real truth, as they are prescribed for those who delight in dualities.
54. When the teacher went back to his home to attend to his household duties, Prahlāda was called by the young boys at the school of his same age. They had been waiting for the moment.
55. The wise Prahlāda replied to them with sweet words. Smiling, he spoke to them kindly, knowing their devotion to him.
56. Out of their respect for him, all the boys put aside their toys and play paraphernalia. Their intelligence had not been polluted

by the words and actions of those [in ignorance] who delight in dualities.

57. They surrounded Prahlāda, O king, fixing him in their eyes and hearts. That great *bhāgavata* devotee, although an *asura*, was a friend to all. He spoke to them kindly."

Book VII, Chapter 6

1. *Śrī* Prahlāda said:

"A wise person should practice the *dharma* of *Bhagavān* from childhood. A human birth is rare, and even though it is temporary, it can bestow the true goal of life.

2. Therefore, a person born into this world should approach the feet of Viṣṇu: He is one's *Īśvara*, the dearest friend, and beloved of all beings.

3. O sons of demons! The sensual pleasures of embodied beings are available everywhere without endeavor. They arise naturally from the connection with the body; and the same is the case with suffering.

4. Any endeavor, which, in the final score, leads to the complete waste of one's life, should not be pursued. This is not the way to attain one's [real] well-being—the lotus feet of Mukunda [Kṛṣṇa].

5. Therefore, a wise person who has ended up in *saṁsāra* should strive for this well-being while the body is still vigorous and strong and has not deteriorated.

6. The life of a person is one hundred years. For a person whose senses are not controlled, half of this is useless, subjected to the darkness of *tamas* when sleeping at night.

7. For a foolish person, a further twenty years are frittered away in childhood and boyhood engaging in play, and twenty more years are lost when the body is seized by old age and becomes incapable.

8. For one who is deluded [about the true self] and attached to household life, the remaining balance of life is wasted in deep ignorance [of the goal of life] by chasing desires, which are difficult to fulfill.

9. What person is able to free the self when it is attached to the household with uncontrolled senses, bound by the strong bonds of affection?

10. Who, in truth, will renounce his thirst for wealth, which is dearer than life itself? Merchants, servants, and thieves barter their dear life for wealth.

11. How can a man renounce intimate association with his sympathetic, considerate wife and her charming words of council? And his bonds of affection with his friends? And what of his attachment to his toddlers with their broken baby babble?
12. And how can one renounce thinking in one's mind of sons? And those cherished daughters? And how about brothers, sisters, or helpless parents? And what of homes and all one's meaningful possessions, family occupations, herds of cattle, and servants?
13. Like a silkworm [bound in its own cocoon], one struggles to perform actions—placing great importance on the pleasures of the tongue and genitals—but one's desires always remain unsatisfied due to insatiable greed.
14. In delusion, one does not discern that one's own life span is flying past in the maintenance of one's family, and in the end one's goals are brought to ruin. Delighting in one's family, one does not realize that one is beset on all sides by the threefold sufferings.[12]
15. One's mind is always absorbed in matters of wealth. And although knowing the negative repercussions both here and in the next world of stealing the wealth of others, the householder whose senses are uncontrolled and whose lust is never quenched, nonetheless steals.
16. Even a learned person who maintains his own family does not attain his [highest] destination, O *dānavas* (demons). Due to the mind-set of making distinctions between what is one's own and what is another's, he too is subject to *tamas* just like any deluded person is.
17. No one, anywhere, who is bound to offspring and kept like a pet for the enjoyment of sensual women is ever capable of completely freeing his own self. Such a person is helpless.
18. Therefore, O *daityas* (demons), one should approach Nārāyaṇa, the Supreme God, keeping at a distance the *daityas* whose minds are absorbed in sense gratifications. It is He who is the liberation sought for by those who are freed from all attachments.
19. O sons of the *asuras* (demons), it does not take a great effort to please Acyuta [Kṛṣṇa]. It can be accomplished in so many ways. He is the innermost soul of all beings.
20.–21. There is one Supreme *Ātman*, *Bhagavān*, the imperishable *Īśvara,* who exists in all higher and lower beings from Brahmā to the immovable entities [like plants]. He is in the material elements and

in the transformations of the material elements starting with the *mahat* [the first transformation of *prakṛti*]. He is the *guṇas* themselves, He is the *guṇas* when they are in equilibrium, and He is the *guṇas* when they are mixed into activity.
22. Through Himself in the form of the inner self as the seer, and also through taking the form of the seen,[13] He is both the One who pervades and that which is pervaded. He is describable and nondescribable. He is manifold.
23. *Īśvara*, the Supreme Lord, has a form, which is pure bliss and consciousness. His power is concealed within Himself through His *māyā*. He causes creation through *māyā*'s *guṇas*.
24. Because of all this, show kindness and friendliness to all living beings. Give up the demoniac mind-set of the *asuras* so that Viṣṇu might be pleased.
25. When the unlimited original Being is satisfied, what remains unattained? What is the use of the four goals of life, *dharma*, etc., which accrue of their own accord [due to past *karma*] through the permutations of His *guṇas*? What is the use of the liberated state beyond the *guṇas*, even though it is so desired, to us who are singing about His lotus feet and relishing their blissfulness?
26. What use is the group of three prescriptions outlined in the sacred texts, *dharma*, *artha*, and *mokṣa*; spiritual knowledge; study of the three Vedas; logic; polity and justice; and the various livelihoods? I consider the truth of all of these and of everything in the sacred texts to be the dedication of oneself to the Supreme Person. It is He who is one's true friend.
27. In actual fact it was Nārāyaṇa, the friend of living beings, who spoke to Nārada this very same knowledge. It is free from error and hard to obtain. This knowledge is meant for those whose bodies are smeared with the dust of the lotus feet of *Bhagavān*—those who have given up everything and are exclusively devoted to Him.
28. This pure *Bhāgavata dharma* combines knowledge with experienced realized wisdom. I heard it from Nārada, who always has visions of Lord Viṣṇu."
29. The sons of the *daityas* said:
"Prahlāda, you, just like us, do not know any *guru* other than the two sons of Sukrācārya, the *guru* of the *daitya* demons. They are the masters of us boys.

30. Association with a great soul [like Nārada] is difficult to attain for a young boy like you who has always resided in the inner chamber of the palace. [So how could you have been taught by him?] Remove this doubt of ours with some evidence so as to gain our confidence, O gentle Prahlāda."

Book VII, Chapter 7

1. *Śrī* Nārada said:
"Questioned in this way by the sons of the *daityas*, the great *asura* devotee of *Bhagavān* replied to them, smiling, as he remembered what I had previously told him.
2. *Śrī* Prahlāda said:
'After our father Hiraṇyakaśipu had departed to perform austerity (*tapas*)[14] on Mount Mandara, the celestials undertook a major expedition against the demons.
3. Indra and the celestials were saying: "By good fortune, this sinful person, the scourge of the universe, has been devoured by his own sins, like a snake devoured by large black ants."
4. After observing the enormous expedition against them, the army commanders of the demons fled in all directions, terrified of the gods. They were being slaughtered.
5. Desperate to stay alive, all of them in their desperate haste turned their backs on wives, sons, wealth, friends, homes, livestock, and possessions.
6. The immortals ransacked the king's residence, intent on victory. Then Indra seized the king's queen, my mother.
7. By chance, the sage of the celestials, Nārada, happened there and saw her being carried away, trembling in fear, like a *kurarī* osprey bird.
8. Nārada said:
"Indra, you are chief of the gods and blessed with good fortune. You should not take this innocent woman, given in marriage to another man. She is a chaste woman: release her, release her!"
9. *Śrī* Indra replied:
"In her womb lies the semen of the enemy of the gods, who [will become] unconquerable. Let her remain [with us] until she gives birth, then I will release her, once I have accomplished my intention [of killing the child]."

10. *Śrī* Nārada replied:
"This child is sinless, and he is a great and eminent devotee of *Bhagavān*. As a powerful devotee of the unlimited Viṣṇu, he will not meet his end by your hand."
11. Addressed in this way, Indra obeyed the words of the celestial sage and released her. He respectfully circumambulated her out of devotion for the dear devotees of the unlimited Lord Viṣṇu, and returned to the celestial realm.
12. Then the sage brought my mother to his own *āśrama* hermitage. "Stay here safely, child, until the return of your husband," he said.
13. "I will do so," she said, and lived in the safekeeping of the divine sage with no fear from any quarter until the Lord of the demons had fulfilled his fierce austerities (*tapas*).
14. That chaste pregnant lady served the sage with utmost devotion for the protection of her embryo and for [the boon of being able to] give birth when she herself so desired.
15. The powerful sage was very kindhearted and bestowed upon her both these wishes. He imparted knowledge and the truth of *dharma* to her and also to me [within her womb].
16. Due to the long time that has elapsed since then . . . my mother's memory has not retained those instructions. But, since I was blessed by the sage in this regard, mine has not been lost up till today.
17. If you have faith in my words it may come to pass that you will also gain insight into Truth, just as happened to me, who had faith, and as it can happen to women or children.
18. The six transformations consisting of birth, existence, growth, change, dwindling, and death are visible in the body—just as they are in the fruits of a tree. This is because of Time, a manifestation of *Īśvara*. But they do not occur in the *ātman*.
19. The *ātman* is eternal, undecaying, pure, individual, the knower of *prakṛti*, the support, changeless, self-conscious, the cause, and the pervader. It is autonomous and uncovered [by *māyā*].
20. Through [understanding] these twelve characteristics of the *ātman*, a wise person should renounce unreal notions pertaining to the body such as "I," and "me." These are born from ignorance.
21. Just as an expert goldsmith can attain gold from rocks in the fields through various processes, so a knower of the *ātman* attains the goal

of *brahman* from the body in the field of *prakṛti* through the processes of *yoga*.

22. The great teachers have spoken of eight *prakṛtis*, the three *guṇas* [underpinning them], and sixteen transformations. But there is one entity [soul] alone, who underpins them all.[15]

23. The collection of all these together comprise the bodies of living beings. These are of two kinds: moving and non-moving. It is from within the body that the *puruṣa* is to be sought through eliminating that which is different from it: "It is not this, It is not this."[16]

24. Through the process of positive and negative concomitance;[17] through discrimination; through a keen mind; and through mature reflection on the processes of birth, maintenance, and destruction, [the *ātman* is to be sought].

25. The states (*vṛttis*) of the intelligence (*buddhi*) are said to be wakefulness, dream, and deep sleep.[18] The one who is beyond these—the witness by whom these states are perceived—is the *puruṣa*.

26. Just as one becomes aware of the air by means of the smells that pervade it [even though the pure air molecules are different from the smells that pervade it], so, in the same way, one should become aware of the presence[19] of the *ātman* by means of the various intelligences covering it [even though the pure *ātman* is different from the intelligence it pervades]. These various intelligences function in differing ways in accordance with the three *guṇas*.

27. The bonds of action produced by the *guṇas* are the gate of *saṁsāra*. These are without reality and are the root of ignorance, like a dream superimposed on a person [when asleep].

28. Therefore, you should uproot the seeds of *karma*, which are products of the three *guṇas*. *Yoga* is the means to stop the outward flow of the intelligence.

29. Of the thousands of methods [of *yoga*], the one spoken by Nārada is the one by which love for *Īśvara*, *Bhagavān*, quickly arises.

30.–31. [This love is achieved] by serving the *guru*, by *bhakti*, by offering all that one attains, by association with *sādhu* saints and *bhakta* devotees, by worshipping *Īśvara*, by faith in the narrations about Him, by the glorification of His deeds and qualities (*kīrtana*), by meditation on His lotus feet, and by worshipping His deity forms.

32. Hari, *Bhagavān*, is the *Īśvara* within all living beings. Thinking in this way, one should wish all beings well in one's mind, along with their aspirations.
33. In this way, one should perform *bhakti* to *Īśvara*, *Bhagavān*, Vāsudeva, with the group of six—lust, anger, greed, illusion, pride, and envy—under control. It is in this way that love [for *Īśvara*] is attained.
34. When one hears of the deeds, incomparable qualities, and heroic feats performed in the bodies *Īśvara* assumes for his *līlā* pastimes, then, with head held high, one dances, shouts, and sings in a voice broken up with tears, and with hair bristling in ecstasy.
35. In this state, as if possessed by a spirit, one sometimes laughs, sometimes weeps, sometimes meditates, and sometimes offers respect to people. Breathing heavily, with one's mind absorbed in the *ātman* and without any inhibitions, one repeatedly cries out, "Hari," "Lord of the Universe," "Nārāyaṇa."
36. In this state, a person is freed from all bondage. Through meditation, one's body and mind are in complete accord with the will of *Īśvara*. The reactions of all seeds of *karma* are burned through complete dedication to *bhakti*, and one is then united with Kṛṣṇa (Adhokṣaja).
37. The end of the cycle of *saṁsāra* occurs for the embodied being whose mind has become purified from connection with Kṛṣṇa (Adhokṣaja). The wise know this as the bliss of *brahman-nirvāṇa*. Therefore, worship in your heart *Īśvara*, the Lord of the heart.
38. Is it really such a great effort to worship Hari, O sons of *asuras*? He is one's very self, existing in one's heart as a friend, like space [exists within everything]. What is the use of acquiring the objects of the senses, which are so commonly available to any living being?
39. Wealth, wife, livestock, sons and daughters, homes, land, elephants, treasuries, power, and all objects of desire are fleeting. What joy can these bring to a mortal whose life can be shattered in an instant?
40. The same is true of those celestial worlds, which are attained by the performance of Vedic ritualistic sacrifices: although superior [to this world], they are not perfect, since they are also subject to destruction. Therefore, to attain the *ātman*, worship *Īśvara*, the Supreme Being, by means of the *bhakti* that has been described—no faults have ever been perceived or heard of in *Īśvara*!

41. For the sake of sense enjoyment in this world, a person, thinking himself knowledgeable, performs actions, but he or she invariably obtains the opposite outcome [suffering].
42. The intention of one engaged in action is to attain happiness and avoid distress in this world—but one always ends up miserable because of desire. One is fully content, on the other hand, when free of desire.
43. Motivated by desire, a person desires objects of desire for this body. But this body actually belongs to others [that is, the elements]. Being perishable, it comes and goes [changing from life to life].
44. How much more, then, things separate from the body such as children, wife, home, and wealth, etc.? And not to mention kingdom, treasury, elephants, ministers, servants, and friends? All of these perpetuate the ego.
45. What is the value to the *ātman* of these trifling things, along with the perishable body? The *ātman* is an ocean of eternal relishable bliss. These things are useless, even though they take on the guise of being desirable.
46. Anyone who bears a material body should reflect carefully on the nature of true self-interest in this world given that one is suffering in various conditions since one's insemination in the womb because of deeds performed in the past, O *asuras*.
47. Because of lack of insight (*viveka*), an embodied being engages in activities with the body according to the dictates of the mind, but then must accept future bodies and minds as a consequence of those activities.
48. Therefore, even though wealth, desire, and *dharma* are dependent on *Īśvara*, Hari [and thus easily available to His *bhaktas*], worship Him without desire. He is the [Supreme] desireless *Ātman*.
49. Hari is *Īśvara*, the friend of all beings. The bodies of all beings are created by the five great elements, and these are created by Him. He is known as [existing within] the *jīva*.
50. Whether one is a celestial, a human, a *yakṣa*, or *gandharva*, one will become auspicious by worshipping the lotus feet of Mukunda [Kṛṣṇa], just as I have become.
51. O sons of the *asuras*! Being a *brāhmaṇa*, or celestial, or sage is not sufficient to please Mukunda; nor is virtuous conduct or great knowledge.

52. Nor is wealth, or austerity, or cleanliness, or vows. Hari is pleased by pure *bhakti*. Anything else is just show.
53. Therefore, O descendants of Danu, perform *bhakti* to *Bhagavān*, Hari, who is the *Īśvara* of the *ātman* of all beings, by [considering] everyone to be equal to your own self.
54. It is [in this way] that the *daityas*, the *yakṣas*, and *rākṣasas* (demons), women, villagers, birds, beasts, and sinful beings have attained the liberated state.
55. It is this that has been recorded in the *Smṛti* sacred texts as the supreme self-interest of a person in this world: exclusive devotion to Govinda [Kṛṣṇa], which consists of seeing Him in all beings and in all things.' "

Book VII, Chapter 8

1. *Śrī* Nārada said:
"After hearing the teaching delivered by Prahlāda, all the sons of the *daitya* demons accepted it, because of its faultless nature. But they did not accept what was taught by their other teachers.
2. At this, seeing them absorbed in one-pointed meditation [upon Hari], the son of Śukrācārya became alarmed and immediately informed the king of the situation.
3. His limbs trembling due to being possessed by rage, Hiraṇyakaśipu made up his mind to kill his son. He hurled abusive words at Prahlāda, who did not deserve this.
4. Hiraṇyakaśipu was cruel by nature; hissing like a snake struck by a foot, he cast a sideways glance with his sinful eyes and spoke to his son. Prahlāda was standing meekly in a humble bowed posture with his hands joined in respect.
5. Hiraṇyakaśipu said:
'Hey, you ill-mannered stupid fool. You are ruining my family name! You have disobeyed my order, you obstinate wretch, and so I will today dispatch you to the abode of Yama, god of death.
6. On what authority have you transgressed my command without fear, you fool? The three worlds along with their deities tremble when I am angry.'
7. *Śrī* Prahlāda replied:
'It is He who is the strength of the strong, and not only of my strength, but of yours too and of all others, O king. All these moving

and non-moving living entities, whether high or low, are being moved by His control.

8. He is Viṣṇu, *Īśvara*. He is Time. He is the essence of the senses, strength, the mind, power, and vitality (*ojas*). It is He indeed who is the Supreme Being who creates, impels, and destroys this universe by means of His own powers. He is the Lord of the three *guṇas*.

9. You should give up this demoniac mentality of yours: there are no enemies other than the one of a mind that has become uncontrolled by being situated on the wrong path. Fix your mind in equanimity. It is this equanimity that is the greatest act of worship to the unlimited Lord.

10. Some think that they have conquered the ten directions,[20] even though, to begin with, they have not even conquered the six plunderers—the mind and five senses. Who can be an enemy to a saintly person who has controlled his mind, who is wise, and who sees all embodied beings equally? 'The creation of enemies is nothing other than one's own illusions.'

11. *Śrī* Hiraṇyakaśipu said:

'It is obvious that you are eager to die. You speak without any restraint, you foolish fellow: your confused words are clearly words of those who wish to die.

12. The one of whom you spoke—who is [supposed to be] the *Īśvara* of the universe rather than me—where is he? If he is everywhere, then why is he not to be seen in this pillar here?

13. I will sever your head from your body even as you brag. Let him, this Hari, protect you now, he from whom you have sought shelter.'

14. Furiously and repeatedly berating his son, a great devotee, with these cruel words in this manner, the great demon, who was immensely powerful, sprang up from his splendid throne. Then he grasped his sword and struck the pillar with his fist.

15. At that very moment, a terrifying sound emanated from that pillar, which rent asunder the shell of the universe. Upon hearing that sound, which reached as far as their abodes, Brahmā and the other celestials thought it to be the destruction of their realm, my dear Yudhiṣṭhira.

16. As he was striding forth desiring to brutally murder his son, Hiraṇyakaśipu heard that incredible unprecedented sound, which terrified the leaders of his armies, who are the enemies of the celestials. But he could not locate its source in the inner chambers of the palace.

17. In order to fulfill what His devotee had declared—to establish [the fact of] His pervasion of all living entities—Hari manifested Himself from the pillar in the palace, assuming a most amazing form which was neither beast nor human.
18. As he was looking all around, Hiraṇyakaśipu [beheld] that creature emerging from the pillar: 'This incredible thing is neither a beast nor a man,' he exclaimed. '*Aho!* What is this form of a Man-Lion?'

[*We can recall from VII.7.2. that Hiraṇyakaśipu had gone off to perform austerities, seeking immortality from Brahmā. Although Brahmā was unable to grant this, being himself mortal, Hiraṇyakaśipu was granted boons that aimed to circumvent death in all conceivable ways. One of these was that he be killed by neither man nor beast, hence Viṣṇu's appearance as half lion half man to thwart this boon while still honoring Brahmā's word.*]

19. As he was deliberating in this way, the form of Nṛsiṁha, the Man-Lion, appeared before him. It was absolutely terrifying.
20. He had ferocious eyes of burnt gold. His jaws were gaping and he had a dazzling mane of hair. He had gaping fangs, a tongue with a razor sharp tip waving to and fro like a sword, and a fearsome frowning face.
21. His ears were motionless and erect. His nostrils and mouth were open and resembled majestic mountain caves. His gaping jaws were terrifying and his body touched the heavens. His waist was slim, and He had a short muscular neck and broad chest.
22. He was flecked with body hair as white as moon rays, had hundreds of rows of arms from all sides, and was armed with claws. He was unassailable, and caused the demons and enemies of the celestials (*daityas* and *dānavas*) to flee on account of his extensive invincible weaponry, some of it particular to Him (the discus) and some common to others.[21]
23. 'Hari has extensive *māyā* powers of illusion: probably this entity has been conjured up by him for my destruction. But what is the use of this type of fanfare?' Muttering this, that elephant of a demon rushed roaring toward Nṛsiṁha armed with his club.
24. Just as an insignificant moth falls into the fire, so was that demon [consumed] in the effulgence of Nṛsiṁha. There is nothing par-

ticularly remarkable about this for Hari: after all, formerly [at the time of creation] He consumed the primordial *tamas* by means of His own effulgence.[22] His own abode is pure *sattva*.

25. After charging, that great demon furiously struck Nṛsiṁha with his club with great force. Hari, withstanding his blow, seized him along with his club as he attacked, just like Garuḍa the son of Tārkṣa, Viṣṇu's eagle carrier, seizes a serpent.

26. As he was being toyed with like Garuḍa toys with a snake, that demon slipped out of Nṛsiṁha's grasp. The immortal celestials, who were hiding in the clouds [witnessing all this], thought this was a bad sign, O Yudhiṣṭhira descendant of Bharata. Although they were rulers over all the realms of the universe, their abodes had been seized [by Hiraṇyakaśipu].

27. Freed from His grasp, the great demon's tiredness from the fight dissipated. He took up his sword and shield and threw himself once more with force at Hari Nṛsiṁha, thinking Him to be afraid of his prowess.

28. With the speed of a hawk, the demon was brandishing his sword up and down, along with his shield, which was decorated with a hundred moons, leaving no opening. Hari, who was extremely fast, emitted a loud laugh—a rough and resounding sound—and seized the demon, whose eyes were wide open.

29. Hari placed him on His thighs at the doorway, just as a snake captures a mouse. Tormented by His grip, Hiraṇyakaśipu was quivering in every limb. Then, even though Hiraṇyakaśipu's skin could not be pierced by Indra's thunderbolt, Nṛsiṁha effortlessly tore him apart with His nails just as Garuḍa pierces a highly venomous serpent.

30. Nṛsiṁha's eyes were wide open and difficult to look at because of their fury. His face and mane were red and sprinkled with drops of blood, and He was licking the sides of His gaping jaws with His tongue, just like a lion wearing a garland of intestines after killing an elephant.

31. Nṛsiṁha cast aside Hiraṇyakaśipu, whose lotus of a heart had been torn out by the tips of His nails. He then slaughtered all his followers who had raised their weapons, with His claws, weapons, and nails. There were thousands of the demon's men, but Nṛsiṁha had numerous arms.

32. The water-bearing clouds, disrupted by His mane, became scattered, and the planets had their luster obscured by His glare. The oceans, pounded by His breath, became agitated, and the elephants at the cardinal points[23] experienced terror at His roar.
33. The heavens were filled with celestial vehicles scattered about by His mane, and the earth, pressured by His foot, was pulled off its axis. From the force of that Being, mountains sprang up. The sky and the quarters of the heavens could not shine because of His effulgence."

[*The celestials then attempt to appease Lord Nṛsiṁha.*]

Book VII, Chapter 9

1. *Śrī* Nārada said:
"With all this, Nṛsiṁha was extremely difficult to approach because of His furious countenance, and so all the celestials and heavenly beings, with Brahmā and Śiva at the forefront, were unable to come near Him.
2. Even Śrī, the Goddess of Fortune, who had been sent by the celestials, after witnessing that incredibly wondrous form, became fearful and could not approach Him. The form had never been seen or described before.
3. Then Brahmā summoned Prahlāda, who was standing near him: 'My dear boy, please go and pacify the Lord, who has been enraged by your father.'
4. 'I will do so,' said the boy. That great devotee slowly approached, O king, and, with hands folded [in humility], offered obeisance with his body on the ground.[24]
5. The Lord, seeing that boy fallen at the soles of His feet, was overwhelmed with kindness. He raised Prahlāda up and placed His lotus hand on his head. That hand bestows fearlessness on those whose minds are fearful of the serpent of Time.
6. All Prahlāda's impurities were cleansed from the touch of that hand, and as a result a vision of his supreme *ātman* was revealed to him. Ecstatic, he placed the lotus feet of Nṛsiṁha in his heart. His body thrilled with bliss, his eyes filled with tears, and his heart melted.
7. With gathered composure and mind completely fixed on Hari, Prahlāda offered Him praise in a voice choked up with love, his eyes and heart completely dedicated to Him.

8. *Śrī* Prahlāda said:
'Just now Brahmā and the other celestial beings—the host of gods, the sages, and the perfected beings—were not able to worship Hari with streams of words rich in poetic qualities—and their nature is pure *sattva*. How is it possible that He allows Himself to be pacified by me, of savage birth?
9. It seems to me that the practice of *yoga*, intelligence, strength, influence, power, virility, study of sacred texts, austerity, beauty, lineage, and wealth are unhelpful in the worship of the Supreme Person. It was through *bhakti* that *Bhagavān* was satisfied by the king of the elephants.[25]
10. And it seems to me that a dog-eater whose life, resources, endeavors, words, and thoughts are devoted to *Bhagavān* is better than a *brāhmaṇa* endowed with the twelve characteristics of the *brāhmaṇa* caste,[26] who is averse to the lotus feet of Hari with the lotus navel. Such a devoted person purifies his lineage; not so one who thinks himself to be important.
11. The Lord is fully complete in His own attainments; it is certainly not for His own personal self that He accepts worship from ignorant people, but out of compassion. Whatever worship is offered to *Bhagavān* is ultimately for one's own benefit, just as beautifying the face is for the benefit of the face reflected back [in the mirror].
12. Because of ignorance I have entered the creation of the *guṇas* (*saṁsāra*) into a low birth. Therefore, freed of my anxiety, I will proclaim the greatness of *Īśvara* to the best of my understanding with my whole being. By such glorification, a person becomes purified.
13. You are the abode of *sattva*, yet all these celestials headed by Brahmā, who, unlike us [demons], are upholders of Your orders, are frightened, O Lord. Surely the pastimes of *Bhagavān* in the form of His delightful incarnations are supposed to give happiness, welfare, and prosperity.
14. The demon has now been killed by You, therefore restrain Your anger. Even a saintly person rejoices in the killing of a snake or scorpion. All the worlds have now attained peace of mind and are all waiting [for You to restrain Your wrath]: let the people remember the form of Nṛsiṁha without feeling fearful.
15. I am not afraid of this terrifying form, with its formidable horrible fangs, frowning brows, eyes like the orbs of the sun, tongue, and

horrific mouth. Nor of this garland of entrails, nor this bloody mane, ears [erect] like posts, roar which terrifies the elephants from the cardinal points, and nail tips, which tear apart enemies.

16. But I am afraid of the sufferings of the cycle of *saṁsāra*, which are so horrible to endure. I am bound by my *karma* and so have been cast among those who devour others [owing to my demon birth]. O wonderful being, You are compassionate to Your offspring: when will You be pleased to summon me to Your lotus feet, the abode of liberation?

17. I am scorched [with suffering] in all kinds of bodies because of the fire of misery encountered in life. This is caused by losing pleasant things and encountering unpleasant things. Even the [so-called] remedy for suffering is yet [more] suffering. I am wandering around this cycle of *saṁsāra* because of my identification with what I am not [that is, with the mind and body]. O master, please tell me about the *yoga* of service to You.

18. Nṛsiṁha, You are the Supreme Lord and dear friend! Glorifying the pastimes and stories recited by Brahmā about You, I will be freed from the *guṇas* and easily cross over all dangers in the company of the great swanlike devotees absorbed in meditation on Your feet.

19. O Nṛsiṁha! In this world, the parents are not the [real] refuge for the child, nor medicine for the afflicted, nor a boat for a person drowning in the ocean. For those embodied beings who are averse to You, whatever remedy is advised for a person suffering in this world has only limited value.

20. Any being, whether higher or lower, who, according to his or her distinct nature, is inspired to create or transform anything into something else, by means of something, through something, from something, because of something, for something, in whatever manner, at any time—all of that is nothing other than a form of Your Lordship.

21. Triggered by the Time factor of the Supreme Being, *māyā* creates the mind by means of the *guṇas*. The mind, which is formed in accordance with *karma*, is very strong. It is inclined toward the ritualistic activity of the Vedas.[27] It is also the wheel of *saṁsāra*, which consists of sixteen spokes [the mind, five organs of cognition and five of action, and the five subtle qualities of the senses, sound, and so forth]. These are created by ignorance.[28] Who can overcome the mind, other than by Your grace, O unborn One?

22. You always keep the *guṇas* under Your personal control by Your own powers. You are Time, the power by which causes and effects are supervised. I have been cast by ignorance into the wheel with sixteen spokes, and am being crushed. Bring me near to You, O Lord; I am a devoted soul.
23. Most people desire such things as the power, opulence, and longevity of lords in all the abodes of the celestial realms, O Lord. But I have seen how these celestials were thrown into disarray by my father's eyebrows, contracted in scornful laughter. And even he has been dispatched by You.
24. I know the [fleeting nature] of these boons sought by embodied beings, and so I do not desire longevity, beauty, power, or sensual indulgence, even up to those possessed by Brahmā the creator. These are all thrown into disarray by You in the form of all-powerful Time. Rather, please accept me into the ranks of Your personal servants.
25. What are these boons, these pleasures described in the Vedic ritualistic texts?[29] They are essentially mirages! What is this body, really? It is the womb of so many diseases. And yet even though people know all this, they do not become discouraged but attempt to satisfy the [unquenchable] fire of lust with little drops of honeylike [sense pleasures], which are anyway so difficult to attain.
26. What is my reality, O Lord, but that of a person with a nature in *rajas*, born in this family of demons where *tamas* predominates? And what is the nature of Your compassion [in contrast]? You offered Your mercy by placing Your lotus hand on my head, but did not do so on that of Brahmā, Śiva, or even Śrī, the Goddess of Fortune!
27. This mentality living entities have of "inferior" and "superior" [toward others] does not exist in Your Lordship: You are the intimate friend of the entire world. Rather, Your grace, like the wish-fulfilling tree of the celestials,[30] is bestowed based on people's worship. It manifests in accordance to service rendered, not based on notions of superior or inferior.
28. Indeed, chasing desires and pleasures, people have fallen into the snake pit of birth (*sāṁsāra*). And, by their association, I too was falling headlong into it. But I was saved, O Lord, by Nārada, the sage of the celestials, who took me under his wing. I am that person [he addressed in the womb]. So how can I ever abandon the service of Your devotees?

29. I think that the killing of my father was enacted to save my life, O Unlimited One, as well as to honor the word of Your sage devotee (Nārada). Intent on wickedness, my father seized his sword and said: "That *Īśvara* of yours who is supposedly superior to me, let him defend you now as I sever your head."
30. It is none other than You alone, who are this universe. It is You alone who remain at its beginning, middle, and end. You create this universe—this permutation of the *guṇas*—through Your own *māyā*, and then You enter it. You manifest Yourself through those *guṇas* as the variegation of the universe.
31. You, O Lord, are this universe of cause and effect, and yet Your Lordship is also different from it. This notion of "this is mine" and "that is another's" is surely meaningless illusion. When something takes its birth, maintenance, manifestation, and cessation from something else, then it is surely nothing other than that other thing, just as a tree is nothing other than its seed, which in turn is the same as the earth and its qualities.
32. You withdraw this universe into Your own Self. Then You lie in the middle of the waters of dissolution,[31] free of all desires, experiencing the bliss of Your own Self. Absorbed in rest within Your own Self through the power of *yoga*, with closed eyes, You are situated in the fourth state of consciousness,[32] unassociated with *tamas* or the *guṇas*.
33. This universe is His—that is to say, Your[33]—body, concealed within Yourself. You manifest forth the *guṇas* of *prakṛti* through the power of Your quality of Time. At the end of Nārāyaṇa's *samādhi* state, as He was lying on the waters on Ananta,[34] the great lotus manifested from His navel, like a banyan tree from its seed.
34. The sage Brahmā could not see anything apart from the lotus from which he was born. He determined that You were the seed manifested both inside himself and also outside. But he could not find You, even though he searched for a hundred years while he was immersed in the waters. After all, after the sprout has grown, how can it perceive its seed?!
35. Seated on the lotus, he became amazed at this. Then the self-born Brahmā's mind became purified by severe austerities performed over a very long time and he perceived that You, O Lord, pervaded his very self, which consists of mind, senses, and gross matter, as the most

subtle essence of all, just as the quality of smell pervades the element of earth.[35]

36. Thereafter he saw the Great Being (*mahā-puruṣa*) endowed with thousands of faces, feet, heads, hands, thighs, noses, ears, eyes, ornaments, and weapons. This form, composed by *māyā*, was arranged with its [differing parts] manifesting [in different portions] of the universe.[36]

37. Your Lordship assumed the form of the horse-headed incarnation,[37] and killed the two enemies of the Vedas, known as Madhu and Kaiṭabha,[38] who were [manifestations of] *rajas* and *tamas*, and then returned the collection of Vedas to Brahmā. [The sages] honor this most beloved form of Yours as pure *sattva*.

38. In this way, You appear in the universes through Your human, animal, sage, celestial, and fish incarnations. You destroy the enemies of the universe and protect *dharma* according to what is appropriate for each *yuga* age.[39] In the fourth age of Kali You are concealed, and because of not being visible then, You are known as Triyuga, the Lord of the three *yugas* (world ages).[40] You are that same Person, O Supreme Being.

39. This mind of mine does not take delight in narrations about You, O Lord of Vaikuṇṭha; it is sinful, contaminated, inauspicious, impetuous, and overset by lust. Moreover, it is afflicted by happiness, distress, fear, and desire. With such a mind, how is a wretch like me to contemplate Your nature?

40. My tongue, which is never satiated, drags me in one direction, O infallible Acyuta [Viṣṇu], and my genitals in another. My flesh, stomach, and ears pull me somewhere else, my sense of smell, somewhere else again, and my restless eyes to yet another place, and so it is with the many powers of my various organs. These are all like many co-wives who demolish the husband [with their various demands].

41. Just see the people of this world: because of their *karma*, they have fallen in the *Vaitaraṇī* river of *saṁsāra*,[41] and are terrified by repeated birth, death, and anxiety over sustenance. They exhibit friendship to bodies related to their own, and enmity to others. You are on the other side [of the river of *saṁsāra*]. Please deliver them today from their foolishness.

42. O *Bhagavān*, *Guru* of everyone, what effort is it for you in such deliverance? After all, You are the cause of creation, maintenance,

and destruction of this universe! Indeed, compassion by the great for the foolish [is fitting], and You are the friend of the lowly. But for us who are the servants of Your beloved devotees, such deliverance is unnecessary [we are already fully satisfied in service].
43. In fact, I am not even disturbed by the *Vaitaraṇī* river of *saṁsāra*, because my mind is absorbed in the wonderful nectar gained from chanting about Your prowess, O Supreme Being! [Deliverance] is for the ignorant whose minds are averse to this, and who are bearing the burden of [chasing after] the happiness of *māyā*.
44. Often, O God, sages, desirous of their own liberation, cultivate silence in a solitary place; they are not concerned with the welfare of others. But I have no desire for liberation for myself alone, abandoning these unfortunate souls. Other than You, I see no other refuge for one wandering [in *saṁsāra*].
45. The happiness of sex and other such pleasures of those attached to the household is meager; it bears frustration upon frustration, like the scratching of an itch with one's hands. Lusty people are never satisfied in this world, but simply experience repeated unfillment. A wise person tolerates [the arising of desires], which are simply products of the mind, just like one tolerates an itch.
46. O Supreme Person, the means of liberation—silence, vows, study of sacred texts, austerity, meditation, performing one's duty, teaching the scriptures, solitude, *japa* (*mantra* repetition), and full concentration of the mind—these often become mere means of making a living for those whose senses are not controlled. And those who are haughty cannot even succeed in doing this.
47. The two forms of cause and effect (*sat-asat*) proclaimed in the Vedas, which are like seed and sprout, are nothing other than You. Those whose minds are fixed, can, through the practice of *yoga*, perceive You directly here in this world in both these forms, just like fire can be perceived in wood. There is no other way to do so, as You have no material form.
48. You are the elements of air, fire, earth, ether, and water. You are the life airs (*prāṇa*); the senses, the heart, the mind, and the ego. Everything, whether with qualities or without qualities, is You alone, O Lord. There is nothing other than You that can be expressed by thought or word.
49. Neither these *guṇas*, nor the deities presiding over the *guṇas*, nor anything composed of the *guṇas* such as *mahat* (intelligence) and all

the other evolutes beginning with the mind,[42] along with gods and humans who have beginnings and ends, know You. Those with pure intelligence reflect on this, and desist from studying the Vedas, O Viṣṇu.

50. You are the goal of the highest order of ascetics (*paramahaṁsa*), O most worthy One. Therefore, how can people attain devotion to You without worshipping You through the six processes: performing worship (*pūjā*) through rites, composing verses, honoring with respect, offering one's actions, remembering Your lotus feet, and hearing Your narrations?' "

51. *Śrī* Nārada said:

"Although He is beyond all qualities, when His qualities had been extolled with devotion in this way by His devotee Prahlāda, the Lord became pleased and His anger restrained. He replied to Prahlāda.

52. *Śrī Bhagavān* said:

'My dear Prahlāda, may all auspiciousness be upon you. I am pleased with you, O best of the demons. I fulfill all desires of men: choose any boon you wish.

53. O long-lived one, a vision of Me is very difficult to attain for one who has not pleased Me. But having seen Me, a living being never experiences personal hardships anymore.

54. I am the Lord of all blessings. Saintly people with sober minds who seek to fulfill the highest satisfaction, therefore try to please Me with all their hearts.' "

55. Śrī Nārada said:

"Although he was enticed in this way by the highest allurements in the world, because of his exclusive devotion to *Bhagavān*, that best of the demons Prahlāda did not want anything."

Book VIII

The Tale of the Elephant *Bhakta*: Surrender to Viṣṇu

Yoga Blueprint

If the Bhāgavata *has time and again stressed that age, gender, social status, and birth are all irrelevant to eligibility for performing* bhakti, *this story goes even further by stretching the accessibility of approaching* Īśvara *to even the animal kingdom. Other than this, the main theological message of this narrative, typical of all theistic traditions, is that when one finds oneself trapped in a situation from which one cannot extricate oneself by any means or resources at one's disposal, one can always turn to God.*

Book VIII, Chapter 2

1. *Śrī* Śuka said:
"There was an enormous mountain known as Trikūṭa (three-peaked), O king, surrounded by the milk-ocean. It was very beautiful, and ten thousand *yojanas* in height.
2. It extended the same amount in width in all directions right up to the ocean of milk, and illuminated the sky and all directions with its three peaks made of gold, silver, and iron.
3. And it illuminated all the regions of the celestial realms with other peaks made of assorted gems and minerals. These were covered by an assortment of trees, creepers, and bushes, and resounded with the sounds of water from mountain cascades.

4. Since its feet were washed on all sides by the waves of milk, Trikūṭa made the earth dark colored on account of its stones of green emeralds.
5. Its valleys were enjoyed by the sporting of celestial beings: *siddhas*, *cāraṇas*, *gandharvas*, *vidādharas*, great serpents, *kinnaras*, and *apsaras*.
6. The caves there resounded with [their] music, and proud lions roared furiously, suspecting [the noise to be from] other lions.
7. It was adorned with valleys thronging with swarms of various wild animals. The sweet sounds of birds filled its manifold trees and celestial gardens.
8. It contained streams and lakes with crystal clear water, which had beaches with gems for sand. The breeze from the water was fragrant with the scent of the consorts of the celestials bathing there.
9. In one of its valleys is a park called Ṛtumat belonging to the noble great-souled Varuṇa. This is a leisure ground for the consorts of the celestials (*suras*).
10.–14. It was beautified and covered everywhere with celestial trees whose fruits and flowers were always blooming. These included *mandāra, pārijāta, pāṭala, āśoka, campaka, cūta* mango, *piyāla, panasa, āmra* mango, plums, *kramuka,* coconut, date, *bījapūraka, madhuka, śālatāla, tamāla, asana, arjuna, ariṣṭa, uḍumbara, plakṣa,* banyan, *kiṁśuka,* sandalwood, neem, *kovidāra, sarala, suradāru,* grapes, sugarcane, plantain, *jambu, badarī, akṣa, abhaya, āmala, bilva, kapittha, jambīra,* and *bhallātaka*. And on that mountain, there was a vast lake, gleaming with golden lotuses.
15. It looked spectacular with its blooming lotuses—such as the red *kumuda*, white *kahlāra*, and day-blooming *śatapatra* types—and reverberated with the humming of bees and warbling of *śakunta* birds.
16.–19. Its waters were filled with the pollen of lotuses swayed by the swimming of tortoises and fish. It was filled with swans and *kāraṇḍa* birds, as well as with *cakra* birds and cranes. The cooings of flocks of waterfowl, and *koyaṣṭi* and *dātyūha* birds resounded there. It was surrounded by *kadamba* flowers, and such plants as *vetasa, nalanīpa, vañjulaka, kunda, kurubaka, aśoka, śirīṣa, kūṭajeṅguda, kubjaka, svarṇayūthi, nāga, punnāga, jāti, mallikā, śatapatra, mādhavī, jālaka*. It was beautified by these and other all-season trees and plants growing on its banks.

20. One day, the leader of a herd of elephants who dwelled in the forests of that mountain was roaming about in a thorny place full of large thickets of *kīcaka* and *veṇu* bamboos and reeds, trampling down the trees there.
21. Even from just the scent of that beast, other elephants; lions; tigers and other wildcats; rhinoceroses and vicious horned animals; and huge snakes fled away in terror, as did black-and-white *sarabhas* and yaks.
22. [On the other hand,] wolves, boar, buffalo, bear, porcupine, jackals, *gopuccha* monkeys, *markaṭa* monkeys, and other weaker animals—deer, rabbits, etc.—were able to roam about without fear by the grace of the elephant.
23.–24. Making the mountain tremble on all sides by his weight, the elephant was surrounded by male and female elephants and followed by young elephant cubs. Afflicted by the heat, he was emitting rut, and so he was followed by swarms of bees who were consuming the rut. Smelling the breeze from the lake, fragrant with the scent of lotus pollen, and surrounded by his herd, which was afflicted by thirst, he quickly arrived near that lake, his eyes wavering from the intoxication of honey.
25. After plunging in, the elephant drank to his satisfaction the clear, nectarlike water of the lake, fragrant with the pollen of cool blooming lotuses. Refreshed, he bathed himself with water drawn up by his own trunk.
26. Being good-natured, the elephant was encouraging the female elephants and elephant cubs to drink and showering them with water spray drawn up with his trunk—just like a householder. The arrogant wretched creature could not perceive the calamity [that was approaching] by the *māyā* of the Unborn Lord.
27. Then, directed there by Fate, O king, a powerful alligator angrily seized his leg. The mighty elephant, fallen into this calamity by chance, tried to free himself with all his strength.
28. The female elephants, their minds perplexed [by seeing] the leader of the herd fallen into that predicament and being dragged about by that powerful force, trumpeted in alarm. The other bull elephants, grasping him from behind, were not able to free him.
29. While the elephant and the alligator were fighting in this way, dragging each other in, then out [of the water], a thousand years passed

by, O Lord of the earth. The immortal celestials thought it incredible that they both still remained alive.
30. Eventually, the vigour, strength, and mental state of the elephant leader became greatly depleted after that long period of time, and he became exhausted from being dragged into the water. The opposite was the case for the aquatic beast [who was in his natural element]: he became invigorated.
31. In this way, the elephant found himself helpless and in danger of his life due to the workings of Fate. Not able to rescue himself after so much time, he reflected, and came to this understanding:
32. 'These bull elephants of the herd were not able to free me from this calamity—not to mention the female elephants. Although I am caught by the bonds of Providence in the form of this alligator, I will approach someone who is Supreme, and the ultimate resort of all.
33. That Being is the Supreme Lord. From the fear of Him Death himself flees. He gives protection to anyone surrendered to Him who is greatly fearful of the powerful serpent of Death, who is in pursuit with ferocious intensity. I seek shelter from Him.' "

Book VIII, Chapter 3

1. *Śrī* Śuka said:
"After resolving in this way, the elephant fixed his mind in his heart and recited the supreme *mantra* (*japa*), which he remembered from his previous life.
2. *Śri* Gajendra (the elephant leader) said:
'*Oṁ namo bhāgavate*; I offer homage to *Bhagavān*. I meditate on Him who bestows consciousness into this world. He is the Ultimate Person, the primordial seed, and the Supreme Lord.
3. I surrender to that self-manifest One! From Him this world manifests, and by Him [it is maintained]. He is Himself this universe, but yet He is transcendent to it, and also to that which is beyond it.
4. This universe, which is sometimes manifest and sometimes unmanifest [at the times of its creation and eventual dissolution], exists in Him, created by His *māyā* potency. He is beyond sense perception, and the witness of both cause and effect. May that Person, who is the root of the *ātman* and the Ultimate transcendent Being, protect me.
5. In the due course of time, when the universes along with their celestial guardians, as well as all causes and effects, have completely

dissolved into the five gross elements,[1] then deep dense *tamas* remains. He, the transcendent Lord, shines forth beyond that.
6. The gods and sages do not know His nature—so then how is a beast [like me] qualified to attain or even speak about it? His ways are hard to fathom. He is like a dancer, acting in different roles. May He protect me.
7. Those who wish to see His most auspicious abode follow extreme vows in the forest without deviation—such as sages and eminent *sādhus* who are free from all attachments and see the *ātman* within all beings. He is the best friend and He is my goal.
8. Birth and *karma* do not exist in Him, nor, certainly, the faults of the *guṇas*, nor name and form (*nāma-rūpa*).[2] Nonetheless, when the time is appropriate, He engages these by His own *māyā* for the manifestation and dissolution of the worlds.
9. He has no form, and yet He has many forms. His deeds are amazing. Reverence to Him, the Supreme Lord, *Brahman*, who has unlimited powers (*śakti*).
10. Reverence to Him who is the Witness, the illuminator of the *ātman*, and the Supreme *Ātman*. Reverence to Him who is completely beyond words, mind, and thought.
11. Reverence to Him who is attained by the wise through *sattva* and detachment from the fruits of action. Reverence to Him who is the Lord of liberation, and the experience of the bliss of *nirvāṇa*.
12. Reverence to Him who is peaceful, fierce, and dull (i.e., *sattva*, *rajas*, and *tamas*) and the support of the *guṇas*. Reverence to Him who is beyond all material characteristics, who is equal to all, and who is full of knowledge.
13. Reverence to You[3] who are the knower of *prakṛti*,[4] the Controller of everything, and the Witness. Reverence to You the Supreme Person, the source of the *ātman* and of *prakṛti*.
14. Reverence to You, the Seer of the objects of all the senses, and the cause of all endeavor. You are the Truth that manifests as a reflection in the non-Truth.[5]
15. Reverence, reverence to You who are the cause of everything, who are Yourself without cause, and who are the cause of wondrous things. You are the ocean of all the Vedas and sacred texts (*āgama*). Reverence to You who are liberation (*apavarga*), and the shelter of the saints.

16. I offer homage to You, who are the fire lying concealed in the kindling wood of the *guṇas*, and who manifest Your will through their agitation. You reveal Yourself to those who have renounced the ritualistic parts of the Vedas[6] by freeing their minds from attachment to the fruits of work.

17. I am devoted to You. I offer homage to You who are Yourself free, and who can easily free a beast like me from bondage, as You are very compassionate. I offer homage to You, *Bhagavān*. You are *Brahman*. You are known as the inner Seer of the mind of all embodied beings by means of one of Your partial manifestations.[7]

18. You are impossible to attain for those who are attached to their bodies, offspring, relatives, homestead, wealth, and friends; but, for the liberated souls, You are the object of their heart's contemplation. Your nature is pure knowledge, devoid of any influence of the *guṇas*. I offer reverence to You, *Īśvara*, *Bhagavān*.

19. Those who desire righteousness, economic well-being, sensual enjoyment, and liberation (*dharma, kāma, artha, mukti*)[8] attain their desired goal. In fact, He bestows other benedictions—even an eternal body [in Vaikuṇṭha].[9] May that munificent Being grant me release.

20. The devotees of *Bhagavān* do not desire any material goal, but are dedicated exclusively to Him. Immersed in an ocean of bliss, they sing about His amazing, auspicious activities.

21. I worship that Supreme imperishable *Brahman*, the Ultimate Lord. He is unmanifest, transcendent, beyond the senses, subtle, unlimited, primeval, and absolutely complete. He is very hard to attain, but approachable through *yoga*.

22. The celestial beings headed by Brahmā, the worlds, and all moving and non-moving things distinguished by name and form (*nāma-rūpa*), are created by one of His insignificant partial expansions.[10]

23. Just like the flames of fire are sunbeams of Savitṛ the sun god, and they emanate and pervade forth from his effulgence, so in the same way, the flow of the *guṇas*—intelligence, mind, *karma*, the senses, and the multitude of bodies—emanates from Him.

24. Glories to Him. He is not a god, demon (*asura*), mortal, or animal. He is not female, neuter, male, or beast. He is not *guṇa*, *karma*, cause, or effect—He is what remains when these are negated, and yet He is the totality of everything.

25. I do not wish to live [if freed from the clutches of this alligator], as what is the use of this birth as an elephant, with its internal and external coverings [of the gross and subtle bodies]? I desire liberation from the layers that cover the presence of the *ātman*. These are not destroyed even after much time [without Your grace].
26. I bow to Him who is the Supreme destination, *Brahman*. He is the unborn Creator of the Universe. He both is the universe and simultaneously transcends the universe. He knows the entire universe and He is the Soul of the Universe.
27. The *yogīs*, whose activities have all been dedicated to *yoga* practice, perceive the Lord of *yoga* in their hearts. The heart can manifest Him [after being purified] by *yoga*. To Him, I bow.
28. Reverence, reverence to You, whose three powers (*śaktis*—the *guṇas*) are irresistibly potent. You are the intelligences of all beings, which are distinguished in accordance to their *guṇas*.[11] You are the Protector of those dedicated to You. Your powers are insurmountable, and the path to You is inaccessible to those whose senses are uncontrolled.
29. This person, overcome by *Īśvara*'s powers (*śakti*) in the form of the ego, does not know his own *ātman*. I take refuge in *Bhagavān*, whose majesty is overwhelming.' "
30. *Śrī* Śuka said:
"Gajendra's description [of the Supreme Being] remained unspecified,[12] but after he had finished, Brahmā and the other gods did not approach him. They were subject to their own egos, which were distinct one from the other according to their different personal characteristics. So Hari, who is the sum of all the immortals and the celestial gods, appeared there. He is the Soul of everything.
31. After hearing Gajendra's prayers and understanding the nature of his plight, the mind of the Lord of the Universe was satisfied. Transported by his eagle carrier, Garuḍa, who is the embodiment of the Vedic hymns, He speedily approached the place where Gajendra was, bearing his *cakra* weapon. He was accompanied by the celestials.
32. Gajendra had been seized with great force inside the water, and was in severe distress. When he saw Hari upon Garuḍa in the sky bearing the *cakra*, he raised up his trunk holding a lotus flower. With great difficulty, he spoke these words: 'Reverence to you Nārāyaṇa, the *Guru* of everything.'

33. The Unborn Viṣṇu, upon seeing the distressed Gajendra, immediately dismounted, and out of compassion quickly dragged him along with the alligator from the water. Then Hari severed the head of the alligator with his weapon, and released Gajendra while the celestials were all looking on."

Book VIII, Chapter 4

1. *Śrī* Śuka said:
"Then, the gods, sages, and *gandharva* celestials headed by Brahmā and Śiva released showers of *kusuma* flowers while praising that deed of Hari.
2. Divine *dundubhi* drums resounded, and the *gandharvas* danced and sang. The sages, *cāraṇa* celestials, and perfected *siddhas* offered hymns to the Supreme Being.
3. The being who had taken birth as that alligator then assumed an incredibly marvelous form. He was Hūhū, an eminent *gandharva*, who had now been released from the curse of Devala.[13]
4. Bowing his head, he offered respect to the Supreme imperishable Lord, and recited the pure narrations and praiseworthy qualities of that Abode of Glory. Viṣṇu's praises are supreme.
5. Being blessed by the Lord, Hūhū circumambulated Him, offered obeisance, and then, freed from all sins, returned to his abode as the celestials watched.
6. By being touched by *Bhagavān*, Gajendra was liberated from the bonds of ignorance. He attained the same form as *Bhagavān*—four armed and yellow garbed.[14]
7. He had previously been an eminent Pāṇḍya king from the south known as Indradyumna, dedicated to the vows of Viṣṇu worship.[15]
8. [After renouncing the kingdom,] the king became self-controlled, wore matted locks, and took up residence at an *āśrama* in Kulācala, where he took a vow of silence. One day, at the appropriate time for worshipping *Īśvara*, Hari, he was in the middle of conducting his adoration absorbed in thoughts of Acyuta, the infallible Lord.
9. By chance, a sage of great renown arrived there surrounded by crowds of disciples. Seeing the king seated in a secluded place in silence, without offering tokens of welcome, the sage became angry.
10. He directed this curse against Indradyumna: 'This uncivilized person is a wicked fellow of mean intelligence, as he has disrespected

a *brāhmaṇa*. Let him be cast into a state of deep *tamas*, like that of an elephant, who has dull intelligence.' "

11. *Śrī* Śuka said:

"After cursing him in this way, the great sage Agastya departed along with his followers. The sage-king, for his part, regarded this as the decree of Fate.

12. He was thus degraded into the womb of an elephant, but his personal memory was not nullified. Because of the potency of his worship of Hari [in the previous birth], even though he was in the state of being an elephant, he was able to recall the past.[16]

13. After he had liberated the elephant herd leader, the Lord with the lotus navel[17] bestowed upon Gajendra the liberated position of being his personal attendant. Accompanied by Gajendra, He then departed, mounted on Garuḍa. He returned to his personal abode, while this amazing deed was glorified by the *gandharvas*, *siddhas*, and other celestials.

14. Thus, O great king, I have described to you the glory of Kṛṣṇa in the form of the story of the liberation of the elephant king. Those who listen to it attain the celestial realm, renown, the eradication of the sins of the age of *Kali*, and the elimination of bad dreams, O best of the Kuru dynasty.

15. The pure, twice-born *brāhmaṇas*, who desire their own best interests, recite this story diligently after rising early in the morning, in order to pacify bad dreams.

16. Hari comprises everyone and is omnipresent. Being pleased, He spoke as follows to Gajendra while everyone was listening, O best of the Kuru dynasty:

[. . .]

24. 'Those who rise at the end of the night and remember My manifestations with concentrated and devoted minds are liberated from all sins.' "

Book IX

The Tale of King Ambarīṣa: The Consequences of Offending *Bhaktas*

Yoga Blueprint

The main theological message imparted by this narrative is the danger of offending the bhaktas *of Kṛṣṇa, even if, precisely because they are humble* bhaktas, *they themselves do not perceive the offense.*

Note the various ways bhakti *can be performed in verses 4.18–20: as we know, in contrast to Patañjali's system, where the activities of the mind and senses are completely curtailed, in* bhakti *they are completely engaged in a variety of modes in worship of Viṣṇu. Additionally, in an interesting series of comments in 4.63ff., Viṣṇu declares that He is under the control of His* bhaktas. *As discussed in* "Rāgānugā Bhakti," *love is reciprocal and God Himself becomes bound by it.*

Book IX, Chapter 4

13. *Śrī* Śuka said:
"From Nābhāga was born Ambarīṣa, a virtuous man and a great *bhāgavata* devotee. Even the curse of the *brāhmaṇa* could not touch him, despite the fact that such a curse has never been countered.
14. The king said:
'A *brāhmaṇa*'s punishment is impossible to evade, O lord! I wish to hear about that wise sage-king against whom it could not prevail after it had been uttered.' "

15. *Śrī* Śuka said:
"Ambarīṣa was greatly privileged: he was the ruler of this earth with its seven continents. He had attained unlimited wealth and incomparable power on earth.
16. But he considered all of this—which is so difficult for men to attain—as no better than a dream. He understood the [eventual] disappearance of opulence, and that a person enters into *tamas* because of it.
17. He had such utter devotion in *Bhagavān* Vāsudeva, and also in his *bhakta* devotees as well as the *sādhus*, that he considered this universe to be no different from a clod of earth.
18. He engaged his mind in [meditating on] the lotus feet of Kṛṣṇa, his words in describing the qualities of Vaikuṇṭha, his hands in such activities as cleaning the temple of Hari, and his ears in hearing the beautiful stories of Acyuta [Kṛṣṇa].
19. He engaged his eyes in seeing the temples and deities of Mukunda [Kṛṣṇa], the limbs of his body in touching the bodies of His servants, his sense of smell in the fragrance of the beautiful *tulasī* plant [offered to] the Lord's lotus feet, and his sense of taste in [the food] offered to Him.
20. He used his feet in frequenting the places touched by the feet of Hari, and his head in offering obeisance to the feet of Hṛṣīkeśa [Kṛṣṇa]. He channeled his desire in service rather than in the fulfillment of sensual desires. He did this to develop affection for those who have taken shelter of Viṣṇu, whose glories are supreme.
21. In this manner, he ruled over this earth, guided by *brāhmaṇas* who were devoted to God. With all his mind, he always dedicated all of his actions to *Bhagavān*, Adhokṣaja, the Supreme enjoyer of sacrifices.
22. He worshipped *Īśvara*, the enjoyer of sacrifice, with *aśvamedha* (horse) sacrifices,[1] conducted with massive pomp and appropriate remunerations for the priests. They were performed by sages such as Vasiṣṭha, Asita, and Gautama in the desert facing the flow of the *Sarasvatī* river.
23. In his sacrifices, the officiating priests, participants, and people were gorgeously attired and appeared as beautiful as the celestials—indeed, they did not blink![2]
24. His citizens did not seek the celestial realm, which is dear to the immortals.[3] They were content hearing and reciting the activities of Viṣṇu, whose glories are supreme.

25. Perceiving Mukunda [Kṛṣṇa] within their hearts and absorbed in the effulgence of their inner selves, they did not hanker after desires which are so difficult to fulfill even for *siddha*, perfected beings.
26. In this manner, pleasing Hari by means of *bhakti yoga* combined with austerity (*tapas*) and the performance of his *dharma*, the king gradually gave up all desires.
27. He developed the insight of perceiving the illusory nature of his palaces, wives, sons, relatives, exceptional elephants, chariots, and steeds, and of his priceless gems, ornaments, and garments, etc., as well as of his unlimited treasury.
28. Pleased by his mood of exclusive *bhakti*, Hari graced him with His *cakra* disc weapon, which protects the devotees and strikes fear in the opposing army.
29. Desiring to worship Kṛṣṇa, the hero undertook the *dvādaśī* fasting vow[4] for a year. He was accompanied in this by his queen, whose character was equal to his.
30. At the conclusion of the vow, in the month of *Kārtika*, the king fasted for three nights. Then he bathed and worshipped Hari in Madhuvan forest on the banks of the *Kālindī* river for one day.
31.–32. He ritually bathed the deity of Keśava [Kṛṣṇa] with the great *abhiṣeka* ceremony,[5] performed with all the requisite utensils according to the customary rites, and with clothing, ornaments, perfumes, garlands, and other choice items. With his mind fixed on Kṛṣṇa internally, he then worshipped Him externally with great devotion. He also worshipped the meritorious *brāhmaṇas*, who were fully accomplished (*siddhas*).
33.–34. He bestowed vast numbers[6] of cows in charity to the *sādhus* and *brāhmaṇas*. They had golden horns, silver hooves, and nice cloth. They were milk-bearing, with calves in tow, young, beautiful, and furnished with the requisite paraphernalia. He then fed the *sādhus* and *brāhmaṇas* choice foodstuffs.
35. Once everyone's appetite had been satisfied, the king was preparing with their permission to break fast himself. But then the great sage Durvāsā himself happened there as an unexpected guest.
36. The king honored this guest by standing up and offering him a seat and other items. Then he approached his feet and requested him to take food.

37. Gladly accepting that invitation, the sage first went to perform his prescribed duties. He immersed himself in the auspicious waters of the *Kālindī* river, meditating on *Brahman.*
38. Since only half an hour remained in which to terminate the *dvādaśī* fast [or its benefits would be wasted], the king, who knew the codes of *dharma* [that one should not eat before feeding one's guests], consulted with the twice-born *brāhmaṇas*:
39. 'There is fault in offending a *brāhmaṇa*, but also fault in not terminating the *dvādaśī* fast at the correct time. Which course of action should I follow, such that I will not be tainted by the sin of *adharma*, but rather gain merit?
40. The *brāhmaṇas* have stated that the drinking of water constitutes both having eaten as well as having not eaten; therefore I will take only water to break my fast.'
41. Thus, the sage-king consumed water, thinking of Acyuta [Kṛṣṇa] in his mind. He then awaited the return of the *brāhmaṇa*, O best of the Kurus!
42. Eventually Durvāsā, who had completed his ritual duties, returned from the banks of the *Yamunā.* He understood, through his power of intuition, the act of the king, who was welcoming him.
43. His face twisted with arched eyebrows, his limbs shaking with anger, and consumed by extreme hunger as well, Durvāsā spoke to the king, whose hands were joined in respect:
44. '*Aho!* Just see the transgression of *dharma* by this wicked man who has become intoxicated with his opulence. He is not a *bhakta* of Viṣṇu—he thinks that he himself is lord!
45. I came as an unexpected guest, and after welcoming me with the appropriate hospitality, he then ate food without offering me any. I will immediately demonstrate the consequences of this to him.'
46. Inflamed with anger, Durvāsā then pulled out a lock of his matted hair and created from it a female demon, who was like the blazing fire at the end of Time,[7] [to kill] the king.
47. Seeing her rushing toward him blazing with sword in hand, and making the earth tremble with her steps, the king did not move from his spot.
48. But the *cakra* disc, which had been entrusted earlier by the Supreme Being with the protection of His servant, incinerated that demon, like a fire burns up an angry serpent.

49. Seeing his effort had been fruitless and that the discus was now hurtling toward him, the terrified Durvāsā ran in all directions, desperate to save his life.
50. The discus pursued him, just as flames whipped up by a forest fire pursue a snake. Seeing it so close on his heels, the sage, desperate to distance himself from it, fled to a cave on Mount Meru.
51. He went in every direction—the sky, the earth, and the space between; the oceans, the celestial spheres along with their celestial guardians; and the three realms—the heavens, earth, and subterranean regions. But wherever he fled, he saw the *cakra*. It was impossible to tolerate, or even to look upon [because of its glare].
52. Seeking refuge but unable to find any protector anywhere at all, Durvāsā approached Lord Brahmā, his mind petrified. He said: 'O self-born creator! Please protect me from the effulgence of Viṣṇu, the Unconquerable.'
53. *Śrī* Brahmā said:
'Viṣṇu is the soul of Time. At the end of his pastimes—a period known as *dviparārdha*[8]—when He desires to burn up the universe, it will be dissolved along with my own abode by the simple knitting of His eyebrows.
54. I myself, Śiva, and prominent beings such as Dakṣa and Bhṛgu, as well as the primary lords of progeny, the lords of beings, and the lords of the *asura* demons, all of us are surrendered to Viṣṇu's law. We carry it placed upon our heads for the well-being of the world.'
55. Turned down by Brahmā, Durvāsā, still scorched by Viṣṇu's disc, sought shelter from Śiva, who resided on Mount Kailāsa.
56. *Śrī* Śaṅkara [Śiva] said:
'We also cannot prevail over the Supreme Being, my dear son! He is the Supreme. In Him, these universes filled with embodied souls, which are like the bodily coverings of Brahmā, and thousands of others too similar to this one, become manifest and then, in Time, return to unmanifestation. We are just wandering about within them.
57.–58. I, Sanat-Kumāra, Nārada, Lord Brahmā, Kapila, Apāntaratama, Devala, Dharma, Āsuri, and other perfected *siddhas* headed by Marīci, none of us understand His *māyā* since all of us are covered by it.
59. This weapon of the *Īśvara* of *Īśvaras* is insurmountable, even for us. So go to Him for refuge. Hari will grant you safety.'

60. Disappointed, Durvāsā then went to the abode of *Bhagavān*, known as Vaikuṇṭha, which is presided over by Śrīnivāsa [Viṣṇu] along with Śrī (Lakṣmī).
61. Scorched by the flames of the invincible weapon, he fell at the feet of Viṣṇu trembling and said: 'O Acyuta, Ananta, Master, beloved by the righteous. I have performed a sin: please protect me, O Lord of the Universe.
62. Because I was not aware of Your supreme power, I committed an offense against someone dear to You. Please nullify this offense, O Controller. Upon reciting Your name, even a person in hell is released!'
63. *Śrī Bhagavān* said:
'O *brāhmaṇa*! I am under the control of my *bhaktas*—it is as if I have no independence. My heart has been captured by the saints (*sādhus*) and *bhaktas*, and I, in turn, am dear to the *bhakta* community.
64. Without My *bhaktas* and the *sādhus*, I do not desire even My own self, O *brāhmaṇa*, nor Śrī, the Goddess of Fortune, who is very intimate to Me. I am the supreme goal for them.
65. They have renounced spouse, home, sons, great wealth, and even their own life and approached Me for shelter. How am I capable of rejecting them?
66. The *sādhus* see all beings with equal vision and have their hearts bound to Me. They control Me with their devotion, just as a chaste wife controls a true husband.
67. Satisfied by My service, they do not even desire the four types of liberation,[9] which are all available through service, to say nothing of any other temporal thing.
68. The *sādhus* are My heart, and I am the heart of the *sādhus*. They do not know anything other than Me, and I can barely think of anything other than them.
69. Now I will tell you the remedy for your predicament, O *brāhmaṇa*: pay heed to it.
Go to that person against whom you unleashed this curse, sir. Force directed against the *sādhus* results in harm against the one who is the instigator.
70. Austerity (*tapas*) and knowledge both bring benefit to the *brāhmaṇas*. But they bring the opposite results to the agent who is of bad character.

71. O *brāhmaṇa*! You should go to King Ambarīṣa, son of Nābha, and seek the pardon from that great devotee; then you will find peace, O son.' "

Book IX, Chapter 5

1. "When he was advised in this way by *Bhagavān*, Durvāsā, still afflicted by the disc weapon, approached Ambarīṣa and clasped his feet in misery.
2. Seeing Durvāsā struggling, Ambarīṣa was ashamed at the touching of his feet. Feeling greatly aggrieved, he prayed to Hari's weapon with compassion.
3. Ambarīṣa said:
'You are the fire, the master, the moon, and the lord of all luminaries. You are water, you are earth, ether, and air, and the qualities perceived by the senses.
4. Obeisance to you, Sudarśana of a thousand spokes! You are dear to Viṣṇu. Let there be well-being for the *brāhmaṇa*, O lord of the earth.
5. You are *dharma*, you are *ṛta* (cosmic harmony), you are truth, you are the sacrifice (*yajña*) as well as the consumer of the sacrifice. You are the protector of the worlds and the soul of everything. You are the energy of the Supreme Being.
6. Obeisance to you! Your effulgence is pure, you have a beautiful hub, and you are the upholder of *dharma*. You are the protector of the three worlds, but a blazing comet for the *asuras* (demons) and those who do not follow *dharma*. I offer homage to you, who perform amazing deeds at the speed of mind.
7. *Tamas* has been dispelled by your potency, which is composed of *dharma*, and *sattva* has been upheld for the *mahātmās*. You are unfathomable. You are the master of speech. This universe, with its causes and effects and higher and lower forms, is your form.
8. O unconquerable one! When you are discharged by Viṣṇu, you penetrate the army of the demons and sever their arms, bowels, feet, and necks incessantly. Your potency is supreme.
9. You have been appointed by Viṣṇu, the wielder of the club, who is all-tolerant, to destroy the miscreants and to protect the universe. Bestow your grace on this twice-born *brāhmaṇa* for the sake of our family tradition. This will be a favor upon us.

10. If we have ever properly performed a sacrifice, given charity, or conducted our *dharma*, and if our lineage is one that considers *brāhmaṇas* to be gods, then let this twice-born one be freed from distress.
11. If *Bhagavān*, the sole source of all qualities, is pleased with us, due to our attitude of seeing the *ātman* in all beings, let this twice-born one be free of distress.' "
12. *Śrī* Śuka said:
"When it was entreated in this way by the king, Sudarśana, Viṣṇu's disc weapon, which had been scorching the twice-born *brāhmaṇa*, became completely pacified by the king's supplication.
13. Upon being freed from the heat of the fire weapon, Durvāsā regained his composure. He then praised the king, bestowing the highest blessings upon him.
14. Durvāsā said:
'*Aho!* Today I have witnessed the greatness of the servants of Viṣṇu! Although an offense was committed to you, O king, you nonetheless endeavored for our welfare.
15. What is impossible for the *sādhus* to accomplish? What is impossible for the *mahātmās* (great souls) to renounce? *Bhagavān*, Hari, the Lord of the *Sātvata* lineage, has been won over by them.
16. What needs do they have, the servants of Viṣṇu, whose feet are places of pilgrimage? Merely by hearing His name, a person becomes purified.
17. I am most fortunate, O king—you are an extremely compassionate soul. You overlooked the offense committed by me, and saved my life.'
18. The king, who had himself not taken any food because of awaiting Durvāsā's return, clasped the sage's feet, satisfied him, and fed him.
19. After he had eaten the food that had been brought with great care and hospitality, and which had satisfied all his needs, the sage was fully satisfied. He then said to the king very respectfully: 'Now you please eat.
20. I am very pleased. I have been favored by seeing, touching, and conversing with you, a *bhāgavata*, and by receiving hospitality and spiritual wisdom.
21. The celestial ladies will constantly sing about this pure deed of yours, and the entire world will praise your supremely auspicious glories.' "

22. *Śrī* Śuka said:
"Durvāsā praised the king in this manner and then, fully satisfied, bade Ambarīṣa farewell. He then departed through his mystic power via the sky to the abode of Brahmā.
23. A whole year had elapsed since the sage had gone off [to take his bath] without returning, yet during this time the king had remained without eating, desiring to see him.
24. After Durvāsā had departed, Ambarīṣa ate the pure remnants of the *brāhmaṇa*'s food.[10] Thinking over the sage's plight and subsequent release, he determined that his own power was but the potency of the Supreme.
25. In this manner, the king, who had so many good qualities, performed *bhakti* to Vāsudeva, who is *Brahman*, the Supreme *Ātman* through all of his activities. As a result, all destinations in *saṁsāra* [devoid of *bhakti*], even up to the highest abode of Brahmā, appeared like hell to him.
26. Eventually, Ambarīṣa fixed his mind and handed over the kingdom to his sons, who all had his same qualities, and entered the forest. There he absorbed his mind in Vāsudeva, the Supreme *Ātman*, and the flow of the *guṇas* ceased for him.
27. By glorifying and contemplating this pure narrative about the emperor Ambarīṣa, O king, one becomes a *bhakta* of *Bhagavān*."

The Tale of Saubhari: Suppressed *Saṁskāras*

Yoga Blueprint

*The short Tale of Saubhari illustrates that even though one may renounce the world radically—*Saubhari *went so far as to meditate underwater in his attempt to completely distance himself from sense objects—*saṁskāras *of desire never fully disappear but remain latent. They can be triggered at any moment—in his case, simply by witnessing two fish mating. This narrative feeds into the* Bhāgavata's *overall insistence that only through* bhakti *can the desires themselves be burned. Other processes can remove the* karmic *consequences of past actions, and suppress the desires that cause them, but not eliminate them. The story also strongly underscores the perception that desires, even if fulfilled in abundance, can never fulfill.*

39.–40. *Śrī* Śuka said:
"Saubhari was submerged in the waters of the *Yamunā*, disciplining himself with severe austerities. There, under the water, desire was kindled in him after he saw the king of fishes happily engaging in sex. As a result, the *brāhmaṇa* [gave up his practices] and then requested the king for one of his maiden daughters. The king replied: 'You may take a maiden, O *brāhmaṇa*, at her choice in a *svayaṁvara* ceremony, [where the maiden chooses her own husband].'
41. Saubhari thought to himself: 'I am gray and wrinkled, and my head shakes. I am in fact being spurned [by the king] as I am old and unattractive to women and so will not be chosen.'
42. So the [*yoga*] master resolved: 'I shall perfect my body such that it becomes desirable even to celestial women, not to mention mortal princesses.'
43. After doing this, the sage was then admitted by the guard into the opulent inner quarter of the palace reserved for maidens. There, although he was a sole suitor, Saubhari was selected as husband by all fifty princesses!
44. Because their minds had all become drawn to him, great dissent broke out between the maidens, and their affection [for each other] was broken: 'This man is fit for me, not you,' they all said.
45.–46. Saubhari was well versed in the *Ṛg-Veda* [and thus skilled in *mantra* incantations]. He enjoyed with those princesses without interruption in palaces furnished with the most exquisite and priceless opulence [created by] his austerities.[11] They were filled with costly garlands, foodstuffs, ointments, bathing places, ornaments, garments, sitting places, and beds, and they were attended by beautifully adorned male and female attendants. They had fragrant groves, streams with crystal waters, and a variety of garden parks with birds, bees, and bards celebrating in sound.
47. The ruler of the seven continents, Māndhatā, was so astounded at seeing Saubhari situated in his householder life that he gave up the pride that accompanied his own universal opulence.
48. But, absorbed in sense gratification in his palaces and stimulated by varieties of pleasures, Saubhari was still not satisfied, just as fire is not extinguished by drops of ghee.[12]

49. One day, that great master of the *Ṛg-Veda*, while sitting down, realized his compromised condition, caused by his own self, which had all come about because of the mating of fish.
50. '*Aho!* Just look at my downfall, me, an ascetic performer of austerities, who had taken a vow of acting in Truth! [My absorption on] *brāhman*, cultivated for such a long time, was derailed because of the mating of fish underwater!
51. One desirous of liberation must renounce all association with those who are dedicated to sex. With all one's heart and soul, one must not let the senses flow outwardly. Living alone in a secluded place—or perhaps in the company of *sādhus* who have taken the same vows—one should engage one's mind on the unlimited Lord.
52. I was a lone ascetic performing *tapas* underwater, but because of associating with fish, I have become fifty [as it were]—without even mentioning my five hundred offspring! I can find no satisfaction for my desires for this world or the next—they demand never-ending indulgence. My mind has been overwhelmed by the *guṇas* of *māyā*, and my consciousness has sense objects as its goal.'
53. Living in this way in his household for some time, Saubhari eventually became averse to it. Once he had become fixed in renunciation, he eventually went to the forest. His wives followed him, considering their husband to be their lord.
54. There, with controlled mind, Saubhari performed intense austerities. It is through these that the *ātman* is revealed. Then, along with the sacred fires, he joined his *ātman* with the Supreme *Ātman*.
55. The wives, seeing that their husband had attained the supreme destination, followed him by dint of his potency, just as flames [become extinguished], when a fire has become extinguished, O great king."

PART III

Śrī Kṛṣṇa's Incarnation

Book X[1]

Kṛṣṇa's Birth

Bhāva Blueprint

Since Kṛṣṇa's birth parents are aware of His divinity in this passage, we find a rather formal bhāva *in this section, in contrast with the intimacy we will encounter in the next sections. Indeed, both Vasudeva and Devakī eulogize Kṛṣṇa in the standardized and technical rhetoric of the Vedānta and Sāṅkhya philosophical traditions. Nonetheless, we see his parents are fearful that Kaṁsa will harm Kṛṣṇa, and we will recall from* "Rāga, Bhāva, *and* Rasa" *that one of the characteristics of* vātsalya rasa *is the conviction that Kṛṣṇa is dependent on the protection of the* bhakta.

Of interest here are the incredible past-life austerities performed by Vasudeva and Devakī to attain Kṛṣṇa as their son. We note that Kṛṣṇa first appears in His Viṣṇu form, then transforms into the two-armed Kṛṣṇa form. Additionally, III.21 points to the "official" reason for Kṛṣṇa's incarnation.

[*Preamble: Kaṁsa, the brother of Kṛṣṇa's birth mother, Devakī, has been informed by a celestial voice that the eighth child of his sister will be the cause of his death. So he imprisons her in his capital city of Mathura along with her husband, Vasudeva, and slaughters their first six children. The seventh appears to be a miscarriage, but in actual fact he is Balarāma, who is transferred by* yogamāyā *into the womb of Rohiṇī, Vasudeva's co-wife, who is residing in the forests of nearby Vraj under the protection of Nanda. Hence, Balarāma is Kṛṣṇa's elder brother. The scene is thus in Kaṁsa's prison house at the birth of the eighth child, Kṛṣṇa. Vasudeva transfers Kṛṣṇa to Vraj and switches Him with Yaśodā's newborn girl. Hence, it appears Devakī has given birth to a female, and Kṛṣṇa grows up with His foster parents, Nanda and Yaśodā, who are unaware that He is not their child.*]

[*The reader will have noted that I have up to now used capital letters for pronouns referring to Kṛṣṇa as God, following the conventions of biblical scholarship and to underscore the point that Kṛṣṇa is perceived as God in this same sense. In this part 3, in a somewhat clumsy attempt to coordinate these pronouns with the workings of* yogamāyā, *I use capitals only when the participants in the narrative are aware of Kṛṣṇa's majesty, but not when they are unaware of it or only partly aware of it and thus participating in one of the selected* bhāvas of sakhya, vātsalya, *and* madhurā.]

Book X, Chapter 3

1. In due time, an extremely auspicious moment endowed with all good qualities arrived. At the time of [Kṛṣṇa's] birth, the constellations and the stars were all favorable. The constellation was Rohiṇī, which is presided over by Brahmā.
2. The directions were clear and the sky covered with clusters of visible stars. On the earth there was a happy abundance of mines, pastures, villages, and towns.
3. The rivers contained crystal-clear water and the ponds were beautiful with lotuses. Lines of trees offered eulogies with the loud sounds of bees and birds.
4. A fresh breeze blew in that region, pleasing the senses and bearing pleasant scents, and the sacred fires of the *brāhmaṇas* blazed forth, undisturbed.
5. The minds of the ascetics and the celestials were peaceful, and kettledrums resounded in unison at the moment of birth of the unborn One.
6. The celestial *kinnaras* and *gandharvas* burst into song, the *siddhas* and *cāraṇas* offered prayers, and the *vidyādharas* joyfully danced along with the *apsarās*.

7. The sages and demigods, overflowing with happiness, showered flowers, and the clouds rumbled gently, resonating with the ocean.
8. At midnight, when deep darkness had fallen, Janārdana [Kṛṣṇa] was born. Viṣṇu, who dwells in the heart of everyone, appeared in Devakī, who resembled a goddess, like the full moon appearing in the eastern direction.
9.–10. Vasudeva[2] saw that amazing, lotus-eyed child, His four arms wielding the weapons of the conch, club, lotus, and discus.[3] He bore the mark of *śrīvatsa*, and the *kaustubha* jewel was radiant on His neck. Clad in a yellow garment, He appeared beautiful as a dark rain cloud. He was resplendent with a magnificent belt, and arm and wrist bracelets, and His profuse locks were encircled with a lustrous helmet and earrings made of valuable *vaidūrya* gems.
11. Upon seeing His son, Hari, Vasudeva was overwhelmed by the auspicious occasion of Kṛṣṇa's incarnation. His eyes were wide with amazement. Overcome with joy, he bestowed ten thousand cows on the *brāhmaṇas*.
12. Vasudeva understood that this was the Supreme Being illuminating the birth chamber with His radiance, O Parīkṣit, descendant of Brahmā. Realizing His majesty, Vasudeva's fear was dispelled. He praised Kṛṣṇa with body bowed, hands joined in supplication, and concentrated mind.
13. Vasudeva said: "It is clear that You are *Bhagavān*, God Himself, the Supreme Being beyond the material world. You are the knower of the minds of everyone. Your form is pure bliss and majesty.[4]
14. It was You, in the beginning, who created this world, comprising the three *guṇa* qualities, out of Your own nature. Then, although not actually entering into it, You nonetheless make it seem that You have entered it.
15.–16. This is like these material elements: although full of potency, they do not produce form when existing separately. Yet, when they combine and interact together, they produce the manifold universe with all its forms. They appear to enter into this world, but actually this is not the case since they existed beforehand.
17. In the same way You exist, along with the *guṇas*. These can be perceived by their characteristics, which are recognizable by the intelligence. You, however, cannot be perceived by these *guṇas*, due to being concealed. There is no inside and outside of You.

18. You are the universal soul of everything, and the essence of the soul. One who considers the external manifestation of the *ātman* [soul] in the form of the *guṇas* [the body] to have existence separate from oneself is foolish. Such an analysis is incorrect and without foundation. Consequently, such a person accepts a view that has been refuted.
19. O all-pervading Lord, they say that the origin, maintenance, and destruction of this world is from You. Yet You do not exert effort, are devoid of the *guṇas*, and are not subject to transformation. But this is not contradictory for You—You are *Brahman*, the controller, and all this is performed by the *guṇas* under Your auspices.
20. Through Your divine potency, You, the Lord, produce from Yourself a white color for the maintenance of the three worlds [Viṣṇu], then a red color infused with power for creation from *rajas* [Brahmā], and then a black color for the dissolution of all creatures from *tamas* [Śiva].
21. O Lord of everything and omnipresent One, desiring to protect this world You have incarnated in my house. You will destroy the armies arrayed for battle with millions of demoniac leaders masquerading as kings.[5]
22. But when the barbaric Kaṁsa heard that Your birth was to be in our house, he murdered all Your brothers born before You. Hearing the reports of Your incarnation from his servants, he is rushing here even now, weapons in hand."
23. *Śrī* Śuka said:
"Then, Devakī, seeing this son of hers displaying the characteristics of the Supreme Being, went toward Him in great astonishment. She was afraid of Kaṁsa.
24. *Śrī* Devakī said:
'That form which they call *Brahman*, unmanifest, original, the light, devoid of the *guṇas*, unchanging, pure being, undifferentiated, and devoid of activity is You. You are Viṣṇu Himself, the light of the self.
25. When, through the force of time, the universe is destroyed at the end of two *parārdhas*,[6] when the great elements have entered into their elemental matrix, and when the manifest has withdrawn into the unmanifest,[7] Your Lordship alone remains. You are known as all-inclusive.

26. O Supreme spirit and friend, they say that this Time factor of Lord Viṣṇu, from the twinkling of an eye up to the period of a year, is Your activity. As a result of it, this universe acts. I surrender to You, who are that mighty controller, O refuge.
27. Mortal beings, fearful of the serpent of mortality, do not attain fearlessness, despite escaping to all corners of the world. But now, after serendipitously obtaining Your lotus feet, they can sleep peacefully. Death escapes from them.
28. You are He, the Lord. Protect us from Kaṁsa, the fearsome son of Ugrasena. We are terrified. But do not reveal this form as the Supreme Being, the object of meditation, to ordinary sight.
29. Let that sinful one not know about Your birth in me, O Madhusūdana [Kṛṣṇa]. My mind is disturbed and I am trembling with fear of Kaṁsa on account of You.
30. O Lord of the Universe, withdraw that transcendent form. It has four arms and is adorned with the splendor of lotus, club, disc, and conch.
31. That Supreme Person who, at the appropriate occasion at the end of Brahmā's night,[8] bears this entire universe within His own body, is Your Lordship, the same person who has entered my womb. How wonderful is this imitation of the human [ways] of the world.'
32. *Śrī Bhagavān* said: 'You, in a previous creation, during the era of Svāyambhuva Manu,[9] were Pṛśni, O chaste lady, and this Vasudeva was a faultless *prajāpati* called Sutapā.
33. After you were both instructed by Brahmā in the creation of progeny, you restrained your senses and underwent extreme ascetic practices.
34. You endured the various features of the seasons—heat, cold, sunshine, wind, and rain. The impurities of your minds were removed by breath control.
35. You endeavored to worship Me, desiring benedictions from Me, your minds appeased by a diet of wind and fallen leaves.
36. In this way, absorbed in Me and performing extreme and very arduous disciplines, ten thousand divine years passed by for you both.
37. Then, fully satisfied with your continual austerity, faith, and devotion, I manifested in your heart in this form, O sinless one.
38. Being asked to choose a boon, you requested a son like Me. So I, the Lord of boon givers, have become manifest out of a desire to satisfy your desire.

39. You were childless as husband and wife, and had not indulged in sexual intercourse. Deluded by My divine *māyā*, you did not choose liberation.
40. After I had departed, you received the blessing of a son such as Me. Having fulfilled your heart's desire, you enjoyed the pleasures of sexual intercourse.
41. Not finding anyone else in the world who was My equal in the qualities of magnanimity and virtue, I became your son, known as Pṛśnigarbha, born of Pṛśni.
42. As Upendra, I was again born from both of them—that is, you both—of Kaśyapa in the womb of Aditi. Because I was a dwarf, I became known as Vāmana [the dwarf].[10]
43. In this third appearance, I have now again taken birth from you both through that same form [of Viṣṇu]. I have stated the facts, O chaste lady.
44. This form was shown to you to remind you of My previous birth. Otherwise, because of My appearance as a mortal, knowledge of My real nature would not arise.
45. Both of you, constantly thinking affectionately of Me in my nature as *Brahman*, as well as in My nature as a son, will attain My supreme destination.'
46. After speaking in this way, Lord Hari [Kṛṣṇa] fell silent and immediately changed into an ordinary child through His *yogamāyā* power of illusion while His parents were watching.
47. Vasudeva, the son of Śūra, removed his son from the room of the birth, as had been directed by the Lord. Then, just at the time that he wanted to leave, Yogamāyā[11] was born to the wife of Nanda [in Vraj].
48.–49. As Vasudeva approached carrying Kṛṣṇa, all the entrances, which had been securely shut with huge doors and iron bolts and chains, opened of their own accord through *yogamāyā*'s influence, just as darkness [disappears] before the sun. Meanwhile, all of the doorkeepers and citizens slept, their consciousness and all their functions overcome [by sleep]. The clouds, rumbling mildly, showered rain. Śeṣa followed, warding off the water with his hoods.[12]
50. While Indra was pouring down rain incessantly, the *Yamunā* river, younger sister of Yama, the Lord of death,[13] foaming with the force of waves from its mass of deep water, became agitated with hundreds of fearful whirlpools. But she gave passage, as the ocean did to Rāma, the husband of Sītā, the Goddess of Fortune.[14]

51. On reaching Nanda's Vraj, Vasudeva found all the cowherd men there fast asleep. Putting his son down on Yaśodā's bed and picking up her daughter, he again returned home.
52. Vasudeva then put the infant girl down on the bed of Devakī, refastened his leg-shackles, and remained as he was before.
53. Afterward, Yaśodā, Nanda's wife, aware of the birth but exhausted, and with her memory stolen by sleep, could not recall the gender of the child."

Vātsalya Bhāva: Kṛṣṇa as Mischievous Child

The Vision of Kṛṣṇa's Cosmic Form

Bhāva Blueprint

In these beautiful passages we feature the vātsalya bhāva, *where the participants assume a parental relationship with Kṛṣṇa. This* bhāva *is not just limited to Kṛṣṇa's actual (foster) parents, but pertains to all the elder* gopas *and* gopīs *of Vraj. The defining feature of this* bhāva *is that it is God who is perceived as dependent on His* bhaktas *for protection and well-being! The passage begins with sage Garga implying that Kṛṣṇa is Viṣṇu and has had numerous previous incarnations. However, the main feature of this passage, in addition to giving a sense of the delightful nature of this type of parental relationship with Kṛṣṇa, is that it provides an excellent example of the workings of* Yogamāyā. *Notice how Yaśodā's intimate mothering of Kṛṣṇa is shattered when* Yogamāyā *lifts her spell and Yaśodā realizes who Kṛṣṇa actually is: her* vātsalya bhāva *is destroyed. It is replaced by the formal Vedānta-type rhetoric uttered by Kṛṣṇa's birth parents when He was born. It is only when the spell is again recast that Yaśodā can again reenter into the intimacy of this* bhāva.

[*Preamble: Kṛṣṇa and Balarāma are now toddlers scurrying around Vraj.*]

Book X, Chapter 8

1. *Śrī* Śuka, said:
"On being invited by Vasudeva, Garga, the *purohita* [family priest] of the Yadus, went to Nanda's Vraj, O king. He was a very austere person.

2. Seeing him, [Nanda] was overjoyed, considering him to be [equal to the Supreme Lord] Adhokṣaja [Viṣṇu]. Nanda rose up to greet him with folded hands, and worshipped him by falling down in full obeisance.
3. The sage was comfortably seated and given a hospitable reception. After pleasing him with agreeable and honest words, [Nanda] said: 'What arrangements can we make for one who is already fully complete, O *brāhmaṇa*?
4. The wanderings here and there of great souls, O Lord, are for the ultimate benefit of the common people, who are householders and poor in spirit. They never have any other purpose.
5. That knowledge of astrology, the movement of the stars, has been composed by yourself, sir, and is beyond sense perception.[15] By this knowledge, a person becomes aware of both imminent and distant events.
6. You are certainly the most eminent of the knowers of *Brahman*. You should please perform the purificatory rites of these two boys. *The brāhmaṇa* is the *guru* of men, by birth.'
7. *Śrī* Garga said:
'I am well-known everywhere on the earth as the spiritual preceptor of the Yadus. If your son is consecrated by me, He will be revealed to be the son of Devakī.
8.–9. Kaṁsa has a sinful mind. He has heard the words of Devakī's daughter, and his suspicions are aroused. After deliberating on your friendship with Vasudeva, and on the fact that the eighth pregnancy of Devakī was not supposed to be a female he will kill [your son]. This might, therefore, be a bad course of action for us.'
10. *Śrī* Nanda said:
'Perform the purificatory rites of the twice-born and utter words of blessing in this cowpen in secret. It will not be observed even by my own relatives.' "
11. *Śrī* Śuka said:
"Appealed to in this way, the *brāhmaṇa*, unrecognized, secretly performed the name-giving ceremony of the two boys. He had in any case wanted to perform it personally.
12. *Śrī* Garga said:
'This one, the son of Rohiṇī, gives pleasure [*rama*] to His loved ones by His qualities, and so will be known as Rāma. Because of His ex-

cessive strength [*bala*], He will be known as Bala, and, because of His association with the Yadus, He will also be named Saṅkarṣaṇa [the uniter].

13. Bodies of three different colors, according to the *yuga*—white, red, and then yellow—were accepted by this other one.[16] Now He has come with a black (*kṛṣṇa*) complexion.

14. Previously, this son of yours was born of Vasudeva, and that is why the learned refer to Him as beautiful Vāsudeva.[17]

15. There are many names and forms of your son, according to deed and quality. I know them, but common people do not.

16. This boy, who is the delight of Gokula and the *gopas*, will bring good fortune. Because of Him, you will all easily overcome every obstacle.

17. Previously, O lord of Vraj, in times of anarchy, the righteous were harassed by bandits. Protected by Him, they were strengthened and conquered the bandits.

18. People who are very fortunate place their affection in this boy. Enemies cannot overpower them, just as the demons cannot overpower those who have Viṣṇu on their side.

19. Therefore, O Nanda, this son of yours is equal to Nārāyaṇa in qualities, splendor, fame, and authority. Protect Him with great diligence.' "

20. *Śrī* Śuka said:

"After he had been instructed about himself in this way and Garga had gone to his own home, Nanda was filled with joy. He considered himself full of good fortune.

21. After a short time had passed, Balarāma and Keśava [Kṛṣṇa] roamed about Vraj, crawling around on Their hands and knees.

22. The two of Them crawled in the dust of Vraj like snakes, dragging Their legs, which [from Their anklets] gave off sweet sounds and tinkling noises. They delighted in that sound, and so They followed people, but then scurried back to Their mothers as if frightened and confused.

23. Their two mothers, whose breasts were seeping milk from affection, picked their two boys up in their arms. The boys looked adorable with the mud smeared on Their bodies. After offering their breasts and gazing at Their faces and Their tiny teeth as they suckled, the mothers fell into a blissful state.

24. When the women found the boys' childhood *līlā* worth watching, the ladies of Vraj would leave their households and enjoy themselves, looking and laughing as the two were dragged hither and thither by the calves whose tails They had grasped.
25. The two boys were very active and Their play [sometimes] took Them out of bounds. When their mothers could not safeguard their sons from horned or fanged animals, fire, swords, water, winged creatures, and thorns, nor even perform their household duties, they became very anxious.
26. After a short time, O kingly sage, Balarāma and Kṛṣṇa were walking easily in Gokula and no longer had bruised knees.
27. Thereafter, *Bhagavān* Kṛṣṇa, along with Balarāma, played with the boys of Vraj of the same age, arousing rapture in the women of Vraj.
28. Observing the delightful childish activity of Kṛṣṇa, the *gopīs* gathered and spoke tongue in cheek as follows [in the presence] of His mother, who was listening:
29. 'Sometimes, he releases the calves at the wrong time, and laughs when cries [of protest] are raised. Moreover, he eats the tasty milk and whey that he steals by means of his thieving devices. He divides [the curds and whey] and feeds the monkeys. If he does not eat, he breaks the pot. When there is nothing available, and he leaves angry with the household, he blames the children.
30. When he cannot reach, he devises a system [to get things] by arranging benches and rice-husking mortars. Knowing what has been placed inside the pots hanging on rope slings, the cunning boy [makes] a hole [in them] at that time of day when the *gopīs* are absorbed in household chores. His own body, which bears clusters of precious jewels, functions as a light in the dark house.
31. While he is engaged in such audacities, he passes urine and other things in our houses. Although his deeds are carried out by theft, he outwardly appears virtuous.' In this way, these affairs were related by the women as they gazed at Kṛṣṇa's beautiful face with its fear-stricken eyes. With a smile on her face, Yaśodā did not want to scold Kṛṣṇa.
32. Once, when Balarāma and the other cowherd boys were playing, They complained to mother Yaśodā: 'Kṛṣṇa has eaten mud.'
33. Yaśodā was concerned for His welfare, and scolded Kṛṣṇa, whose eyes seemed to be full of fear. Grasping Him in her hand, she said to Him:

34. 'Why have you secretly eaten mud, you naughty boy? These young friends of yours are saying so, and so is your elder brother.'
35. 'Mother, I didn't eat any mud. They are all spreading false accusations. if you think they are speaking the truth, then you look into my mouth yourself.'
36. 'If that is the case, then open wide,' she said. Lord Hari [Kṛṣṇa], whose supremacy cannot be constrained, but who is God assuming the form of a human boy for play, opened wide.
37.–38. Yaśodā saw there the universe of moving and non-moving things; space; the cardinal directions; the sphere of the earth with its oceans, islands, and mountains; air and fire; and the moon and the stars. She saw the circle of the constellations, water, light, the wind, the sky, the evolved senses, the mind, the elements, and the three *guṇa* qualities.[18]
39. She saw this universe with all of its variety differentiated into bodies, which are the repositories of souls. She saw the time factor, nature, and karma. Seeing Vraj as well as herself in the gaping mouth in the body of her son, she was struck with bewilderment:
40. 'Is this actually a dream? Is it a supernatural illusion, or is it just the confusion of my own intelligence? Or is it, in fact, some inherent divine power of this child of mine?
41. Therefore, I offer homage to His feet, which are the support of this world. From them, and through their agency, this world manifests. Their true nature cannot be known by the senses nor by reason. They are very difficult to perceive by thought, words, deeds, or intellect.
42. He is my refuge. Through His illusory power arise ignorant notions such as: "I am me; he over there is my husband; and this is my son; I am the virtuous wife, protectress of all the wealth of the ruler of Vraj; and all the *gopas* and *gopīs*, along with the wealth derived from the cattle, are mine." '
43. Then the omnipotent Supreme Lord cast His *yogamāyā* [divine power of illusion] in the form of maternal affection over the *gopī*, who had come to understand the truth.
44. Immediately, the *gopī*'s memory was erased. She sat her son on her lap and returned to her previous state of mind, with her heart full of intense love.
45. She considered Hari [Kṛṣṇa], Whose glories are sung by the three Vedas, the Upaniṣads, Sāṅkhya *yoga*, and the Sātvata sages, to be her very own son."

46. The king said:
"O supreme *Brahman*, what did Nanda do to obtain such great fortune? And what did the greatly fortunate Yaśodā do, that Hari drank from her breast?
47. His mother and father did not fulfill their desire of experiencing the wonderful childhood activities of Kṛṣṇa. These can eradicate the sins of the world. Even to this day, sages sing of them."
48. *Śrī* Śuka said:
"Once, previously, Droṇa, best of the Vasus, accompanied by his wife, Dharā, said to Brahmā: 'I will follow the orders of Lord Brahmā.
49. When we are born on earth, supreme *bhakti* [devotion] to Hari, the Lord of the Universe, and the Supreme God on earth, will flourish. Through this *bhakti*, one can easily overcome the miseries of this world.'
50. 'Let it be so,' was the reply. He, the greatly fortunate Droṇa, of wide renown, was born in Vraj and became known as Nanda, and she, Dharā, became Yaśodā!
51. Thereafter, O Parīkṣit, descendant of Bharata, eternal devotion to Lord Janārdana [Kṛṣṇa], who had become their son, was manifest in the husband and wife and in the *gopas* and *gopīs*.
52. In order to fulfill the order of Brahmā, Lord Kṛṣṇa resided in Vraj together with Balarāma, and enchanted them by His *līlā*."

Kṛṣṇa's Favor to the *Gopī* Yaśodā

Bhāva Blueprint

This passage continues the vātsalya bhāva. *Here we find God in the mood of a naughty child, fearful because of His mischief, and Yaśodā in that of a loving, chastising parent. Despite Yaśodā's failed attempts to bind Kṛṣṇa with all the rope in her household, she still remains unaware that anything is untoward in the nature of her child. Such is the power of* yogamāyā. *The passage ends with Kṛṣṇa becoming compliant in His own binding:* bhakti *is reciprocal, and from His side, Kṛṣṇa is just as committed to succumbing to His devotees as they are to succumbing to Him.*

Book X, Chapter 9

1. "One time, when the house servants were busy with other chores, Yaśodā, the wife of Nanda, churned the milk herself.
2. Remembering the songs about the activities of her child, she sang them while she was churning yogurt.
3. Yaśodā churned, swaying back and forth. Her bracelets were moving on her arms, which were tired from pulling the rope, and her earrings were swinging to and fro. *Mālatī* [jasmine] flowers dropped from her hair, and her face, with its beautiful eyebrows, was sweating. She wore a linen cloth bound by a girdle on her broad, sloping hips, and her quivering breasts were leaking milk out of affection for her son.
4. Hari approached His mother as she was churning, desiring to drink her breast milk. Grasping the stirring stick, He obstructed her, demanding her love.
5. He climbed on her lap. Looking at His smiling face, she allowed Him to drink from her breast, which was leaking milk from affection. But before He was satisfied she put Him down in a hurry and rushed off when the milk that had been on the fire boiled over.
6. Furious and biting His quivering red lower lip with His teeth, Kṛṣṇa broke the butter-churning pot with a stone. With false tears in His eyes He went inside to a hiding place and ate the freshly churned butter.
7. Yaśodā removed the boiling milk and came in again. Noticing the broken vessel, she saw what her son had done. Not finding Him there, she laughed.
8. She spied Him standing on top of the base of a rice-husking mortar. He was wantonly giving fresh butter to a monkey from a hanging pot, looking anxious on account of His thieving. She approached her son stealthily from behind.
9. Seeing her with stick in hand, Kṛṣṇa hastily climbed down from there and fled, as if in fear. The *gopī* ran after Him whom the minds of *yogīs*, directed by the power of asceticism, are not able to reach.
10. The slender-waisted mother chased Kṛṣṇa, her progress slowed by the burden of her broad, moving hips. A trail of flowers falling from her loosened plait in her wake, she seized Him.
11. Grasping His arm, she chastised Him, scaring Him. Looking up with eyes agitated with fright, the guilty boy was crying and rubbing His eyes, smearing the mascara with His hands.

12. Yaśodā was fond of her child, and so threw away the stick when she realized her son was frightened. Unaware of the power of her son, she wanted to bind Him with a rope.
13. Kṛṣṇa has no beginning and no end, no inside and no outside. He is the beginning and end and inside and outside of the universe. He is the universe.
14. The *gopī* tied Him with a rope to the mortar as if He were a common being. She considered Kṛṣṇa, who is the unmanifest truth beyond sense perception in the form of a human, to be her own son.
15. The rope for binding her guilty child was short by two fingers. So the *gopī* joined another one to the first.
16. When that also was too short, she joined another one to it, but however many ropes she brought out, they were always two fingers lacking.
17. In this way, while all the *gopīs* chuckled with amusement, Yaśodā joined together all the ropes in her household. Smiling, she was struck with wonder.
18. Seeing the efforts of His mother, whose limbs were sweating and whose wreath of flowers had fallen from her hair, Kṛṣṇa became compliant in His own binding.
19. Indeed, by this act, dear Parīkṣit, the quality of submission to [His] devotee was demonstrated by Hari [Kṛṣṇa] despite the fact that He is only constrained by His own free will. By Him this universe, along with those who control it, is controlled.
20. Neither Brahmā, nor Śiva, nor even Śrī, the Goddess of Fortune, despite being united with His body, obtained the benediction which the *gopī* obtained from Kṛṣṇa, the giver of liberation.
21. God, this son of the *gopī*, is not attained as easily in this world by embodied beings, nor by the wise, nor by the knowers of the self, as He is by those who have devotion."

The Killing of the Calf Demon

Bhāva Blueprint

In our final vātsalya bhāva *passage, we again see a variety of delightful examples of Kṛṣṇa reciprocating with His beloved* bhaktas, *submitting out of love to their control "like a wooden puppet."*

Book X, Chapter 11

[Preamble: In the previous chapter, after numerous attempts on Kṛṣṇa's life by various demons, Yaśodā had tied Kṛṣṇa to a mortar for His safekeeping. Kṛṣṇa then dragged the mortar between two trees. It wedged between them and eventually uprooted both trees as He kept crawling. Two celestial beings emerged from these trees: owing to their inappropriate behavior, they had been cursed by Nārada to take birth as trees, but blessed that these trees would be in Nanda's courtyard, where they would be liberated by Kṛṣṇa.]

1. *Śrī* Śuka said:

"After hearing the thundering sounds of the falling trees, all the *gopas*, headed by Nanda, approached the place full of fear of an earthquake, O Parīkṣit, best of the Kurus.

2.–3. There, they saw the pair of *arjuna* trees fallen on the ground. They were bewildered, unable to understand the cause of their fall even though it was in plain view—the child, bound by a rope and dragging the rice-husking mortar. But they were doubtful, saying: 'Whose [work] is this? How has this amazing calamity come about?'

4. The boys said: '[It was done] by Kṛṣṇa over there as he was going through, dragging the mortar, which then fell crossways. And we also saw two beings.'

5. The *gopas* were unable to accept what was said: 'That could not have happened,' they declared. Some found it incredible that such an uprooting of the trees could be caused by the small boy.

6. Naturally, after seeing His own son bound and dragging the mortar by a rope, Nanda, smiling, freed Him.

7. Applauded by the *gopīs*, *Bhagavān* Kṛṣṇa would sometimes dance like a child, and sometimes sing innocently. Like a wooden puppet, He was controlled by them.

8. Sometimes, on command, He would carry a stool, measure, or slippers, or He would sometimes throw His arms about, arousing the love of His relatives.

9. For those who could understand, *Bhagavān* Kṛṣṇa manifested the condition of [submitting] himself to the control of His dependents in this world. Truly, He brought joy to the residents of Vraj by His childhood activities.

10. [Once], upon hearing, 'Hey! Come and buy fruits!' Acyuta [Kṛṣṇa], the bestower of all fruits, grabbed some grains [as exchange] and rushed out, desiring fruit.
11. As the grain was falling from His hands, the woman fruit-seller filled both of Acyuta's [Kṛṣṇa's] hands with fruit, and Kṛṣṇa filled the fruit container with jewels.
12. [On another occasion] Kṛṣṇa, who had shattered the trees, went to the bank of the river and was absorbed in playing with the boys. After some time, Queen Rohiṇī called both Him and Balarāma.
13. The two boys did not present themselves when called, because of their absorption in the game. So Rohiṇī sent Yaśodā, who had great affection for her son.
14. Yaśodā called her son, who, along with his elder brother, was still playing with the boys even though Their time for play had run out. Her breasts were leaking milk out of love for her son:
15. 'Kṛṣṇa, lotus-eyed Kṛṣṇa, my young one, come, drink from my breast. Enough games! You are hungry and exhausted from playing, O son.
16. Hey, Balarāma, my son, the darling of the family, come quickly with your younger brother. You have had only breakfast early in the morning, so you must eat.
17. O Dāśārha [Kṛṣṇa], the chief of Vraj is waiting for you, wishing to eat. Come, bring us both your love. Boys—return to your own homes.
18. Your body is black with dust, my son. Come and take your bath. Today is your birthday; clean up and donate cows to the *brāhmaṇas*.
19. Look, look at the boys your age—they are scrubbed clean by their mothers and adorned beautifully. You, too, should enjoy yourself after you are bathed, nicely adorned and well fed.'
20. In this way, Yaśodā, her mind bound by affection, considered Kṛṣṇa, who is the Absolute Truth, to be her son. Grasping Acyuta [Kṛṣṇa] along with Balarāma by the hand, she led Them to Their own compound, and then performed the rites for prosperity."
21. *Śrī* Śuka said:
"After experiencing the great disturbances in Bṛhadvana, the great forest (Gokula),[19] the elders of the cowherd men, led by Nanda, gathered together and deliberated on the affairs of Vraj.
22. In that gathering, a *gopa* by name of Upananda, who was advanced in age and knowledge, spoke up. He was a well-wisher of Kṛṣṇa and

Balarāma, and someone who understood time, place, and the cause of things:

23. 'We, who desire the welfare of Gokula, should depart from this place. Major calamities are on their way here aimed at the destruction of the boys.

24. Somehow or other, that boy was saved from the child-slaughtering demoness.[20] What is more, by the grace of God, the cart did not fall on top of him.

25. Then he was whisked up to disaster in the sky by the demon in the form of a whirlwind.[21] He fell on a rock over there, but was saved by the powerful demigods.

26. That this boy or someone else was not killed after finding himself between the two trees is also owing to the protection of Acyuta [Viṣṇu].

27. For as long as such calamitous misfortunes overrun Vraj, let us take the boys away from here and go somewhere else along with our followers.

28. There is a forest called Vṛndāvana, which is fit for habitation by the *gopas*, *gopīs*, and cows. It has fresh groves, plants, grass, and sacred mountains.

29. Therefore, if this is pleasing to you all, let us go there this very day. Yoke the carts without delay. Our herds of cows should set out and go in front.'

30. When they heard this, the *gopas* unanimously declared: 'Well said! Well said!' They fastened together their respective cowpens and set out, laden with their domestic chattels.

31.–32. After placing the elderly, the children, women, and chattels on the carts, and with their cows in front, the cowherd men set out with their priests, O king. Fully alert with bows in hand, they blew their horns in every direction and made loud trumpet sounds.

33. Seated on the carts, the *gopīs* looked beautiful. Dressed attractively with golden ornaments at their necks, and with fresh *kuṅkuma* powder on their breasts, they took pleasure in singing about Kṛṣṇa's *līlā*.

34. Yaśodā and Rohiṇī were seated on the same cart. They were delighted by Kṛṣṇa and Balarāma, and eager to hear those narrations.

35. They entered Vṛndāvana, and set up their cowherd camp there, with their carts arranged like a half-moon. It was a place that brings happiness in all seasons."

Sakhya Bhāva: Kṛṣṇa as Playful Friend

Bhāva Blueprint

The sakhya bhāva *featured in the next passages is characterized by a mood of equality between* bhakta *and* Bhagavān. *While there are various forms of friendship, those featured in the Vraj* līlā *are of very young boys playfully whiling away their days in fun and frolics in the forests of Vraj as they graze their cows.*

Book X, Chapter 11 (continued)

36. Seeing Vṛndāvana, Mount Govardhana, and the sandbanks of the *Yamunā* river, Balarāma and Mādhava [Kṛṣṇa] experienced great joy.
37. The two boys became, in time, caretakers of the calves, amusing the residents of Vraj with Their childish antics and unformed words.
38. Accompanied by the cowherd boys and [equipped] with paraphernalia for different games, They grazed the calves nearby, in the land of Vraj.
39.–40. Imitating the animals with Their cries, They roamed like two mortals. Sometimes They played flutes, sometimes They let fly with slings, sometimes [They played] with Their feet, Their ankle bells [jingling], and sometimes, acting like bulls with other pretend bulls and cows, They fought each other, roaring.
41. One time, a demon came to the banks of the *Yamunā*, intending to kill Kṛṣṇa and Balarāma while They were grazing Their cows with Their young friends.
42. Seeing the demon, in the form of a calf, enter the herd of calves, Hari slowly approached, pretending to be unaware, while pointing him out to Balarāma.
43. Seizing him by his rear legs and his tail, Kṛṣṇa whirled him around and hurled him lifeless to the top of a *kapittha* tree. Assuming a huge body, the demon fell, along with the *kapittha* trees, which he brought crashing down.
44. Seeing that, the boys were amazed and praised Kṛṣṇa: "Well done! Well done!" The celestials, showering Them with flowers, were all delighted.
45. The two boys, the sole keepers of the whole universe, became keepers of calves. Taking Their breakfast with them, They roamed here and there, grazing the calves.

The Killing of the Demon Agha

Bhāva Blueprint

The fun and frolics of the gopa *boys in this passage give an excellent sense of the intimate nature of* sakhya bhāva. *The mood of this* bhāva *is that the* bhakta *sees God as an equal. We can note here that despite the seeming equality of the boys with Kṛṣṇa, all their games and activities are undertaken with their focus fully centered on Him, the indispensable element of* bhakti. *We see here, too, the boys' simple but unbreakable faith in Kṛṣṇa even in the jaws of death. Also of interest is that even Kṛṣṇa Himself is surprised at the marvelous workings of His power of* yogamāyā.

Book X, Chapter 12

1. One day, Hari decided to have breakfast in the forest. After arising at dawn and waking up His *gopa* friends with the pleasant sound of His horn, he set out, herding the calves in front.
2. Thousands of comely boys, equipped with flutes, bugle horns, staffs, and slings, joined Him. Accompanied by thousands of calves, the boys, each driving his own before him, set out merrily.
3. Joining their own calves with the numberless calves of Kṛṣṇa, the cowherd boys diverted themselves in *līlā* while they grazed their cows here and there.
4. Although they were decorated with gold, jewels, *guñjā* berries, and crystals, the boys adorned themselves with minerals, peacock feathers, bunches of flowers, young shoots, and fruits.
5. They stole each other's slings and various objects and, when detected, threw them at a distance, from where others then threw them farther still. Eventually they returned them, laughing.
6. If Kṛṣṇa went far off to view the beauty of the forest, they would enjoy themselves by [running up and] touching Him, saying: "I was first, I was first!"
7. Some played their flutes, some blew their horns, others hummed with the bees, and still others cooed with the cuckoos.
8. They chased the shadowless birds, moved gracefully with the swans, seated themselves with the cranes, and danced with the peacocks.
9. Tugging at the young monkeys, they climbed the trees with them. Then, imitating them, they joined them in swinging through the trees.

10. Jumping about with the frogs, they got soaked by splashes from the river. They laughed at their own shadows and hurled abuse at their echoes.

11. Thus, those boys who had accumulated an abundance of merit roamed about joyfully with Kṛṣṇa. He is the experience of the bliss of *Brahman* for the wise, the Supreme Deity for those who are dedicated to His service, and the child of a human being for those who are absorbed in ignorance.

12. Although the dust of His feet is not obtained by *yogīs* with disciplined minds, even after many births undertaking ascetic practices, He has personally become an object of vision for the people of Vraj. How, then, can their fortune be described?

13. At that time, a great demon named Agha rushed out. Wanting to protect their own lives, the immortals constantly longed for his death, even though they had drunk the nectar of immortality. Agha could not tolerate the sight of the boys' happy games.

14. The demon Agha was the younger brother of Baka and Bakī [Pūtanā], and had previously been dispatched by Kaṁsa [to kill Kṛṣṇa]. He saw that the boys were led by Kṛṣṇa: "This is undoubtedly the one who brought destruction to my siblings. I will kill him, with his friends, as retribution for those two [siblings] of mine," he said.

15. "When they have been made into sesame and water [as oblations] for my kinsmen, then the residents of Vraj will be as good as finished. When the vital airs have left, what need is there to worry about the body? Children are the very breath of all beings that possess vital airs."

16. After thus resolving, the evildoer assumed the spectacular body of a huge boa constrictor. It extended for one *yojana*,[22] was as dense as a mountain, and had a mouth like a gaping cave. Agha then lay on the path in the hope of swallowing [the children].

17. His lower lip was the ground, and his upper lip the clouds. The inside of his mouth was a cave, his teeth the peaks of mountains, and there was darkness inside his jaws. His tongue was an extended highway, his breath a pungent wind, and the glow of his glare was like fire.

18. After seeing this thing there in such a form, everyone thought it to be one of Vṛndāvana's attractions, and playfully imagined that it resembled the mouth of an extended boa constrictor.

19. "Hey, friends, say: Does this heap of a creature lying ahead resemble the mouth of a snake stretched out to devour us, or not?
20. In truth, the cloud reddened by the sun's rays is like its upper jaw, and the bank, copper colored by its reflection, is like its lower jaw.
21. Look: the two mountain caves on the left and the right resemble the corners of its mouth, and even these high mountain peaks resemble its teeth.
22. Moreover, this highway in length and breadth seems like a tongue, and this darkness within it is like the inside of a mouth.
23. Look—this pungent air, hot with fire, seems like breath, and this foul odor of burnt creatures is just like the smell of dead flesh inside it.
24. Will it devour us as we enter it? If so, it will be destroyed in an instant by Kṛṣṇa as Baka was." Thinking thus, the boys glanced at the beautiful face of Kṛṣṇa, the enemy of Baka, and ventured in, laughing and clapping their hands.
25. *Bhagavān* heard the discussion among the boys about this spurious [creature]—even though they were unaware of what it actually was. Since He is situated in the hearts of all creatures, He knew that it was really a demon pretending to be what it was not, and so decided to hold His friends back.
26. Meanwhile, however, the boys, along with their calves, had already entered the belly of the demon. But they were not devoured by him since he, remembering his intimate friends who had been killed by Kṛṣṇa, the enemy of Baka, was awaiting Kṛṣṇa's arrival.
27. Kṛṣṇa, who bestows fearlessness on everyone, saw that the poor boys, who knew no Lord other than Him, had slipped beyond His control and were like grass in the fire of the stomach of death. He was surprised at the workings of Fate, and was filled with compassion.
28. But what was to be done in this situation? Kṛṣṇa wondered how two purposes could be achieved—how to kill the wicked one without harming the innocent boys. He deliberated, made a decision, and entered that mouth.
29. At this the celestials, hiding in the clouds, exclaimed, "Alas! Alas!" from fear, but the corpse-eating demon friends of Agha, such as Kaṁsa, were filled with joy.
30. When He heard this, the imperishable *Bhagavān* swelled up in the throat of the demon, who was intent on crushing Him as well as the boys and calves.

31. At this, the vital airs of the demon's huge body were blocked, and filled the interior of the body; but the outlets were stopped up, and so the eyes popped out and rolled here and there. Then the vital airs burst out of the hole in the top of the head, and escaped outside.
32. As all the vital airs were seeping out, *Bhagavān* Mukunda [Kṛṣṇa] brought His dead friends and the calves back to life with His glance. Then He reemerged from the mouth, together with them.
33. An amazing great light rose up from the thick coils of the snake, illuminating the ten directions with its splendor. It waited in the sky for the Lord to emerge, and then entered into Him before the very eyes of the residents of the celestial realms.[23]
34. Everyone was overjoyed at this, and they all offered worship with their own particular activities—the celestials with flowers, the celestial *apsarās* with dance, those who sang beautifully with songs, musicians with instrumental music, the *brāhmaṇas* with hymns of praise, and the crowds with the sound of "Victory (*jaya*)!"
35. The unborn Brahmā heard those many celebrations of wonderful hymns, beautiful music, songs, and [sounds of] "Victory!" and hastened there from his abode, which was nearby. Seeing the greatness of the Lord, he was struck with wonder.
36. The amazing dry skin of the boa became an amusement-cave in Vṛndāvana for the residents of Vraj for many months.
37. This deed—Hari's escape from death by the serpent—occurred during the *kaumāra* period of life [one to five years]. Yet the boys who had seen it related it in Vraj during the *paugaṇḍa* period [six to sixteen years].
38. There is nothing in this that is astonishing for Kṛṣṇa. By His *māyā* potency, He [appeared] as a small human boy, but He is the supreme creator of both the highest and the lowest. Even Agha had his sins cleansed by Kṛṣṇa's touch, and achieved *ātmasāmya*[24] liberation—attaining the same form as God—which is very difficult for the sinful to achieve.
39. Kṛṣṇa bestows the devotional path [to one who] once internalizes a mental image of Kṛṣṇa's body. Such a person is completely freed from *māyā*, and experiences the eternal happiness of the *ātman*. What is there to say, then, when [the Lord] has entered inside a person?

40. *Śrī* Śuka said:
"In this way, O *brāhmaṇas*, Parīkṣit heard about the wonderful activities of His benefactor.[25] With his mind focused, he again asked Vaiyāsaki [Śuka] about Kṛṣṇa's purifying activities."
41. The king said:
"How can something relating to a particular period of time be performed in another period of time, O *brāhmaṇa*? That which the boys related in the *paugaṇḍa* period was performed by Hari in the *kaumāra* period.
42. Tell me this, O great *yogī*. I am extremely curious, O *guru*. Surely this must be nothing other than the *māyā* of Hari?
43. Although we only pose as *kṣatriyas*, we are in fact the most fortunate people in the world, because we continually drink the purifying nectar of the stories [about Kṛṣṇa] from you."
44. *Śrī* Śuka said:
"When he was questioned in this way, O most eminent of devotees, Śuka, son of Bādarāyaṇa, lost the functions of all his senses in remembering Ananta [Kṛṣṇa]. He then regained awareness of his surroundings with difficulty, and slowly replied to the king."

Kṛṣṇa Manifests as the Calves and Cowherd Boys

Bhāva Blueprint

In this extraordinary passage, Kṛṣṇa becomes each and every cowherd boy and calf for an entire year in order to satisfy the secret bhāva *aspirations of the other elder* gopīs *and* gopas, *as well as the cows, who had always hankered to have Kṛṣṇa as their very own child and offspring. The plot is subtle: the original cowherd boys and calves are placed in a dormant state and are unaware of this entire episode. We can also note an important theological message imparted by this tale: even the most intelligent Being in the entire universe, Brahmā, the secondary creator, is utterly incapable of understanding the nature of Kṛṣṇa; what, then, of common mortals?!*

Book X, Chapter 13

1. *Śrī* Śuka said:
"You have raised an appropriate question, O greatly fortunate Parīkṣit.

Although we hear the narrations of the Lord repeatedly, you make them fresh, O best of devotees.
2. This is the natural mentality of saintly persons who cultivate only the essence [of truth]; their minds, ears, and voices are used only for that purpose. This is because pure discussion about Acyuta [Kṛṣṇa] always seems fresh, just like discussion about women is always fresh for debauchees.
3. Listen attentively, O king, and I will tell you, even though it is confidential. Actually, *gurus* explain even confidential things to their affectionate disciples.
4. After saving the calf-keepers from death in the mouth of Agha, *Bhagavān* Kṛṣṇa led them to the sandy bank of the river, and spoke as follows:
5. 'Hey, friends, the sandy beach is really delightful and covered with soft, clear sandbanks for our play. It is filled with trees reverberating with the sounds and echoes of birds, and of bees attracted by the scent of lotuses in flower.
6. The day is advanced: we should eat our meal here. The calves, who are hungry, may graze at leisure nearby, after they have drunk water.'
7. 'Let's do it,' the boys said. After the boys had watered the calves, they climbed onto the grassy place, opened their sling bags, and enjoyed their meal, together with the happy *Bhagavān* Kṛṣṇa.
8. The boys of Vraj sat in many rows encircling Kṛṣṇa, with their faces turned toward Him. Their eyes were wide with joy, and they glowed like petals round the pericarp of a lotus flower.
9. Some of them made plates from petals and flowers, and others used shoots, sprouts, fruits, slings, bark, and rocks; then they ate.
10. All of them showed one another the different samples of the things they each were eating. Laughing and making one another laugh, they ate their food along with the Lord.
11. While the residents of *svarga* [the celestial region] looked on, Kṛṣṇa, the enjoyer of sacrifices, took pleasure engaging in childish play. He carried a flute in the garments around His stomach, and a horn and a staff in His belt. In His left hand was a tender morsel of food, and in His fingers were pieces of fruit. Standing in the middle of His circle of intimate friends, He made them laugh with His games.
12. However, O Parīkṣit, descendant of Bharata, while the keepers of the calves, whose very soul was Acyuta [Kṛṣṇa], were eating in

this fashion, the cows wandered far into the forest, tempted by grass.

13. Seeing the boys struck by fear, Kṛṣṇa, who is the fear of the fears of this world, said to them: 'Do not stop eating, friends. I will fetch the calves back myself.'

14. Having said this, *Bhagavān* Kṛṣṇa, a morsel of food in His hand, went off to look for their calves in mountains, caves, groves, and thickets.

15. Meanwhile, the lotus-born Brahmā came to see yet another pleasing wonder of the Lord who had become a boy by His *māyā*. Previously he had been greatly astonished after descending from the celestial realms and seeing the liberation of Aghasura by the eminent Kṛṣṇa. He led the calves and calf-herders away from there to some other place, O best of the Kurus, and then disappeared.

16. Failing to find the calves after some time, or, after going to the riverbank, the calf-herders either, Kṛṣṇa searched thoroughly for both in the forest.

17. Needless to say, not finding the calves and the calf-keepers anywhere inside the forest, Kṛṣṇa, the knower of the universe, immediately understood everything that had been done by Brahmā.

18. Thereupon Kṛṣṇa, the Lord and maker of the universe, transformed His own self into both [the calves and the boys] in order to give pleasure to the mothers of those [calves and calf-herders] as well as to Brahmā.[26]

19. He took the form of as many little bodies of calves and calf-herders as there were calves and calf-herders, with as many hands and feet and bodily parts. He assumed the shape of as many staffs, horns, flutes, petals, slings, ornaments, and garments, and adopted as many behaviors, qualities, names, appearances, and ages, and as many playful personalities. The unborn One, who is the form of everything, became as if an affirmation of the saying 'Everything is the *māyā* of Viṣṇu.'[27]

20. Then Kṛṣṇa took care of His calves, who were His own self, by Himself in the form of the calf-herders. The Self of everything entered Vraj, playing games with Himself [in the form of the calves and boys].

21. After leading each and every one of the calves separately, Kṛṣṇa made them enter into their respective cowsheds and He then entered into each and every house. He existed as each and every entity, O king.

22. Their mothers hastily rose up at the sound of the flutes, picked [the boys] up in their arms, and embraced them profusely. Thinking the Supreme *Brahman* to be their sons, they then made Them drink the nectar of their breast milk, which was flowing from love.
23. Thus Mādhava [Kṛṣṇa], after engaging in the regular schedule of the day, came to the evening, O king, giving joy with His activities. He was then tenderly attended to with massage, a bath, the application of scents, ornaments, protective mantras, sacred clay, food, and other things.
24. Meanwhile the cows hurried toward the cowsheds and suckled their respective calves, who had assembled there, summoned by the sounds of the cows' mooing. The cows licked the calves repeatedly, milk flowing from their udders.
25. The motherliness of the cows and the *gopīs* toward Kṛṣṇa was just the same as [it had been for their own calves and sons] previously, except that now there was an increase in affection, and the filial behavior of Hari toward them was the same [as that of the real calves and sons], except without the illusion.
26. The affection of the people of Vraj for their own sons grew gradually, like a creeping plant, day by day throughout the year. It was not the same as before; it was without limits, just as it had been for Kṛṣṇa.[28]
27. In this way, Kṛṣṇa, the Supreme Soul as a cowherd boy, herded Himself by means of Himself through the assumed forms of the calves and calf-herders, and sported in the forests and cow pastures for an entire year.
28. On one occasion, when five or six nights remained to complete the year, the unborn Kṛṣṇa, who was grazing the calves with Balarāma, entered the forest.
29. At that time, the cows, who were grazing on the grass at the top of Mount Govardhana, saw the calves grazing far away near Vraj.
30. On seeing them, the cows were overcome with love for their calves. Forgetting themselves, they hastened along on two [pairs of] legs by a path that was hard going even for their own keepers. Their heads and tails were raised, their necks were [stretched back] onto their humps, they were making lowing sounds, and their milk was flowing.
31. After meeting the calves below, the cows made them drink milk from their own udders, even though they possessed calves [of their own]. They also licked their limbs as if they were going to swallow them.

32. The *gopas* were furious with embarrassment at the failure of their efforts to prevent them. They approached by the same arduous route with difficulty, and saw their sons with the calves.
33. Their hearts were overwhelmed by a loving surge of *rasa* at seeing them. Affection was kindled and their anger was dispelled. They lifted up the boys, embraced them with their arms, and experienced the highest ecstasy by smelling their heads.
34. After this, the adult *gopas* departed slowly and with difficulty. Their minds were happy from embracing their children and tears welled up at the memory of them.
35. Balarāma noticed the Vraj community's constant longing for their offspring because of this increase in love, even though these offspring had been weaned. Not knowing the cause, He thought:
36. 'What is this amazing thing? The love of the community of Vraj, and of Myself, for the children is growing as it never has before, as if it were for Vāsudeva, the soul of everything.
37. Who is this being [who has caused this] and why has she created this condition? Is she a divine being, a woman, or even a demoness? In all probability it is the *māyā* [illusion] of My Lord Kṛṣṇa. There is no other entity that can bewilder even Me.'
38. Thinking this, Balarāma understood with the eye of knowledge that the calves and all the companions as well were Kṛṣṇa, the Lord of Vaikuṇṭha.
39. 'These are not lords of the demigods, nor are they sages; it is You Yourself, O Lord, who are manifest in these individual forms. Tell Me briefly—how did their separate existence come about?' Balarāma eagerly absorbed the turn of events from the Lord whom He had addressed in this way.
40. Meanwhile, Brahmā, the self-generated god, returned after a period of time which, by his standards, was merely an instant. He saw that Hari had been playing throughout the year with Himself transformed [into the forms of His companions] just like before:
41. 'However many boys and their calves there were in Gokula, that same number are all sleeping in the bed of my *māyā*. To this very day, none of them has reawakened.
42. So where do these boys who have been playing here together with Viṣṇu for one year come from? They are different from those there [in the hiding place] who are bewildered by my *māyā*, although they are certainly the same in number.'

43. After pondering thus on these differences for a long time, the self-generated Brahmā was not able to understand in any form or fashion which of the two [sets of boys and calves] was real and which not.
44. Thus, in causing illusion for Viṣṇu, who is free from illusion and who deludes the whole universe, even the unborn Brahmā was in fact himself deluded by his very own *māyā*.
45. Inferior *māyā* used on a superior person destroys the power of the person invoking it, just like the darkness of fog is destroyed in the night, or the light of a glowworm in the day.
46. Meanwhile, as the unborn Brahmā was watching, all the calves and herders suddenly became dark as rain clouds and appeared wearing yellow silk garments.
47. They had four arms and held the conch, disc, club, and lotus in Their hands. They wore helmets, earrings, pearl necklaces, and garlands of forest flowers.
48. They were adorned with the *śrīvatsa* [tuft of hair], arm-bracelets, and two jeweled conch bangles and bracelets on Their wrists. They glittered with foot-bracelets, arm-bracelets, belts, and finger rings.
49. Their bodies were covered from head to toe with soft garlands of fresh *tulasī*,[29] which is offered by those who excel in piety.
50. With radiant, moonlike smiles, and glances from the reddish-colored corners of Their eyes, They looked like the creators and protectors of the needs of Their devotees by means of *sattva* and *rajas*.
51. They were venerated in various ways by many forms of worship. These included singing and dancing by all moving and non-moving embodied entities—from the first being, Brahmā, down to the clump of grass.
52. They were surrounded by the mystic powers such as *aṇima* [the ability to become minute]; the potencies such as that of *māyā*; and the twenty-four elements such as the *mahat*.
53. They were worshipped by Time, nature, the *saṁskāras*, desire, *karma*, and the *guṇas*, and so forth, all of them possessing form. Their greatness was eclipsed by the personal greatness of Viṣṇu.
54. The forms were only of one *rasa*, essence: truth, knowledge, and unlimited bliss.[30] Their unlimited glory had not been experienced even by the seers of the Upaniṣads themselves.
55. In this fashion, Brahmā, the unborn one, saw everything simultaneously as the personal self of the Supreme *Brahman*, from whom

the appearance of everything in this world, moving and non-moving, manifests.

56. Then Brahmā, the unborn one, opened his eyes wide with amazement, his eleven senses[31] stunned, and fell silent before that majesty. He was like a doll before the local goddess of a town.

57. Thus he was unable to understand that [Absolute Truth], which is beyond reason, which is self-manifest, which stands in its own glory, and which is established in the principal Vedic texts by the elimination of that which it is not.[32] 'What is this?' he thought. When Brahmā, the lord of Irā [Sarasvatī], was bewildered in this way, Kṛṣṇa, the transcendental, unborn, Supreme Being, understood and instantly concealed His *māyā*.

58. Then, Brahmā, who had regained his material vision, stood up like a corpse [that had come back to life]. Opening his eyes with difficulty, he saw the entire universe, along with his own self.

59. Immediately looking around in all directions, he saw Vṛndāvana in front of him. It was spread with trees, which afford a livelihood for the inhabitants, and with other desirable things.

60. In Vṛndāvana, those who by nature live in enmity, such as man and deer, lived together like friends. Craving and anger, and other such negative qualities, dissolved in the abode of Ajita [Kṛṣṇa].

61. There, Brahmā, the supreme deity, saw Kṛṣṇa, the absolute *Brahman*, continuing to act as a child in the family of cowherd folk. The one Supreme eternal Being, who is without a second, and whose knowledge is without limit, was searching all over for His friends and His calves, with a tasty morsel in His hand, just as before.

62. Seeing this, Brahmā quickly got down from his vehicle, and prostrated himself upon the ground like a golden rod. He touched Kṛṣṇa's two feet with the crest of his four crowns[33] and worshipped Him with a bathing ceremony performed using auspicious tears of joy.

63. He continued rising repeatedly and then falling at the two feet of Kṛṣṇa for a long time, remembering again and again the grandeur that he had just seen.

64. Then, getting up slowly in humility and wiping his eyes. Brahmā gazed at Mukunda [Kṛṣṇa]. Stammering and trembling he worshipped Kṛṣṇa with a stream of prayers, his neck bent in submission, his hands folded in supplication, and his mind intent."

Bhāva Blueprint

Continuing in the mood of sakhya, *we see in this passage that* bhāva *is not unidirectional: Kṛṣṇa is just as keen to please His devotees and satisfy their wishes as they are to please Him. Also, we can note that since Balarāma, Kṛṣṇa's elder brother, is a manifestation of Viṣṇu, He is addressed as such in the opening verses.*

Book X, Chapter 15

1. *Śrī* Śuka said:
"Thereafter, when They had attained the age of *paugaṇḍa* [six to sixteen years], the two boys were approved as cowherd men in Vraj. Herding the cows along with Their friends, the two made Vṛndāvana sacred with Their footprints.
2. At that time, looking for sport, Mādhava [Kṛṣṇa], accompanied by Balarāma and with His cows in front, entered a forest that was suitable for cattle and covered with flowers. He was playing His flute and was surrounded by *gopas* telling of His glories.
3. Seeing the forest full of the delightful sounds of bees, deer, and birds, *Bhagavān* turned His mind to pleasure. The forest was enticing, abounding as it did with ponds whose water was as clear as the minds of great souls, and [swept] by a wind scented by hundred-petaled [lotuses].
4. Kṛṣṇa, the original person, saw the forest trees, beautiful with reddish buds, their tops [bent down] to touch His two feet everywhere through the weight of their abundant flowers and fruits. Smiling a little with delight, He spoke to His elder brother.
5. *Śrī* Bhagavān said:
'Just see, O best of Gods! After gathering offerings of jasmine flowers and fruits, these trees are bowing down their heads to Your lotus feet, which are worshipped by immortals. This is in order to terminate their birth as trees, which was attained through ignorance.
6. These bees are singing of Your glories, which are the subject of veneration for the whole world. As they pursue You along the way, they are worshipping You, O original Person! They are mostly the hosts of sages, Your most fervent devotees [from past lives]. Although

deep in the forest, they do not abandon the Lord of their heart, O One without sin.
7. The forest-dwellers are truly fortunate. These peacocks are dancing, O praiseworthy One, and the does are joyfully soliciting Your affection with glances as if they were *gopīs*. The flocks of cuckoos [welcome] You with Vedic hymns, since You have come to their home. Such is the greatness of the nature of saints.
8. Fortunate is the earth, today: the grass and plants have been touched by Your feet and the trees and creepers have been brushed by Your nails. The rivers and mountains, birds and animals, [have been embraced] by Your merciful glances, and the *gopīs* have [been enfolded] in Your two arms, which are desired even by Śrī, the Goddess of Fortune.' "
9. *Śrī* Śuka said:
"In this way Kṛṣṇa enjoyed beautiful Vṛndāvana, happy in spirit, grazing the cows on the mountain river banks together with His friends.
10. Sometimes when the bees sang, blinded with intoxication, Kṛṣṇa, whose deeds are sung, would sing along the way with His followers. He was accompanied by Saṅkarṣaṇa [Balarāma].
11. Sometimes He would honk in imitation of the honking swans. Sometimes He would dance in imitation of the dancing peacocks, giving rise to laughter.
12. Sometimes, in a voice that was pleasing to the cows and cowherd boys and was as deep as the rumbling of a cloud, He would call by name the cows who had strayed far off.
13. He would imitate the sounds of birds such as the *cakora*, *krauñca*, *cakravāka*, *bhāradvāja*, and peacock, as if afraid of the tigers and lions from the animal kingdom.
14. At other times He would give relief to His elder brother by personally massaging His feet, etc., as Balarāma, fatigued from playing, used the lap of a *gopa* as a cushion.
15. Sometimes, holding hands and laughing, the two boys would urge on the cowherd boys in their dancing, singing, jumping about, and wrestling with each other.
16. Sometimes, exhausted from the effort of wrestling, Kṛṣṇa would lie down on a bed of buds. Taking shelter at the base of a tree, He would use the lap of a *gopa* as a pillow.

17. Some great souls would massage His feet and others, whose sins had been eradicated, cooled Him with fans.
18. Others, their hearts moved with love, would softly sing songs for that great Soul that were appropriate to the occasion and pleasing to the mind.
19. In this way, Kṛṣṇa concealed His personal nature by His own *māyā*, and imitated the nature of the son of a cowherd man by His activities. Although He can conduct Himself as the Supreme Lord, and His budlike feet are caressed by the Goddess of Fortune, He can nonetheless enjoy Himself like a villager in the company of villagers.
20. [Once], the cowherd boy called Śrīdāmā, a friend of Balarāma and Keśava [Kṛṣṇa], and of the *gopas* such as Subala and Stokakṛṣṇa, spoke lovingly as follows:
21. 'O Balarāma, Balarāma! O mighty-armed Kṛṣṇa, scourge of miscreants! Not far from here is a huge forest full of rows of *palmyra* trees.
22. Abundant fruits have fallen and keep falling there, but they are guarded by that evil soul Dhenuka.
23. O Balarāma! O Kṛṣṇa! He is an extremely powerful demon who has assumed the form of a donkey! He is surrounded by many other kinsmen whose strength is equal to his.
24. The forest is not frequented by humans and herds of cows because they are terrified of him, O destroyer of enemies—he has devoured human beings. It is even shunned by the flocks of birds.
25. Fragrant fruits that have never before been eaten are found there. In fact, this all-pervading fragrance [of the fruits] can be detected at this moment.
26. Obtain those fruits for us, Kṛṣṇa—our minds are disturbed by their smell. Our desire is great, Balarāma, so, if you like, let us go.'
27. After hearing those words from Their friends, the two Lords laughed. Surrounded by Their friends, They went to the *palmyra* forest, desiring to please them.
28. Balarāma entered and then, with strength like an elephant, shook the *palmyra* trees with His arms, making the fruit drop.
29. When he heard the sound of the falling fruit, the donkey demon came rushing up, making the surface of the earth, as well as its mountains, quake.

30. Encountering Balarāma, that mighty one turned around and struck Him on the chest with two of his legs. The wicked fellow circled Balarāma, making a *kā* sound.
31. The enraged ass attacked again. Rump-first, it kicked furiously at Balarāma with its two hind legs, O king.
32. Balarāma seized the donkey by two legs and whirled him around with one hand. When the donkey had died from the whirling, Balarāma hurled him to the top of a palm tree.
33. Struck by the donkey, the great *palmyra* tree with its huge top trembled, causing its neighboring tree to shake. This latter tree broke and made the next tree shake, and that tree did likewise to another.
34. Thus, struck by the dead body hurled effortlessly by Balarāma, all the trees shook as if agitated by a great wind.
35. This is not remarkable for *Bhagavān*, who is, after all, the unlimited Lord of the Universe. By Him, this universe is woven lengthwise and crosswise, like a cloth on threads, my dear Parīkṣit.[34]
36. Then all the donkeys of Dhenuka rushed toward Kṛṣṇa and Rāma, furious that their relative had been slain.
37. Kṛṣṇa and Rāma seized each one of them by their rear legs as they came hurtling forward, and threw them effortlessly into the palm trees, O king.
38. The ground was colored with heaps of bodies of dead demons, tops of trees, and fruit strewn about. It resembled the surface of the sky colored by clouds.
39. When they heard of the pair's marvelous feat, the celestials released a shower of flowers, played instruments, and offered eulogies.
40. Thus, people ate the fruit of the palm trees and the cows grazed in the forest of the dead Dhenuka without fear.
41. After this, lotus-eyed Kṛṣṇa returned home to Vraj to the praise of His followers, the *gopas*. Hearing and reciting about Him are means to purification.
42. The *gopīs* came forward in a body, their eyes hungry for a sight of Him. Smeared with the dust of cows, Kṛṣṇa had a charming smile and delightful eyes. Forest flowers and a peacock feather were attached to the locks of His hair. He was playing His flute and His glories were being sung by His followers.
43. After drinking the honey of Mukunda's face with their beelike eyes, the women of Vraj cast off their fever born of separation during

the day. After accepting that welcoming reception, conveyed from the corners of the *gopīs'* eyes with modesty, giggles, and bashfulness, Kṛṣṇa entered the cow compound.

44. Yaśodā and Rohiṇī were affectionate toward their boys, and heaped their best blessing for the occasion upon their two sons, to their hearts' content.

45. At home, the boys' weariness from the road was removed by bathing and massage, and so forth. They then dressed in beautiful clothes and were adorned with lovely garlands and scents.

46. The two pampered boys ate the food offered to Them by Their mothers, lay down on the best-quality beds, and went happily to sleep in the land of Vraj.

47. Kṛṣṇa *Bhagavān* wandered around Vṛndāvana in this way, O king."

The Killing of the Demon Pralamba

Bhāva Blueprint

The mood of equality between Kṛṣṇa and His beloved gopa *friends is further highlighted in this passage. Additionally, the landscape of Vraj described here gives a good sense of the actual nature of Goloka, the kingdom of God in the* Brahman *realm, for the Kṛṣṇa traditions.*

Book X, Chapter 18

1. *Śrī* Śuka said:

"One day, surrounded and glorified by his relatives, who were in a joyful mood, Kṛṣṇa entered Vraj. It was picturesque with herds of cows.

2. While the two boys were sporting in Vraj in the *māyā* guise of cowherd boys, the summer season came, a season that is not very pleasant for embodied beings.

3. However, because of the special features of Vṛndāvana—*Bhagavān* himself, Keśava [Kṛṣṇa], was there with Balarāma—it exhibited the qualities of spring.

4. In Vraj, the sound of waterfalls drowned the chirping crickets. Spray from these waterfalls constantly fell on groups of trees.

5. There were abundant pastures there, and the forest-dwellers did not experience the heat produced by the sun, fires, and summer. This was

because of the breeze from the waves of waterfalls, streams, and brooks that carried pollen from the blue lotuses, bowers, and water lilies.
6. The fierce rays of the sun, terrible as poison, did not drain everywhere, so the soil was saturated with waves from the shores of the deepwater rivers.
7. The forest was beautiful, full of flowers, and echoing with the sounds of various animals and birds, singing peacocks and bees, and the noises of cuckoos and cranes.
8. Preparing to play, *Bhagavān* Kṛṣṇa entered that forest vibrating His flute. He was accompanied by Balarāma and surrounded by the *gopas* and their cows, which were Their riches.
9. The *gopas*, led by Balarāma and Kṛṣṇa, were decorated with ornaments made from minerals, garlands, clusters of blossom, peacock feathers, and fresh leaves. They danced, wrestled, and sang.
10. While Kṛṣṇa danced, some *gopas* sang, some made sounds with horns and handclaps, while others applauded.
11. The gods, disguised as members of the cowherd clan, praised Kṛṣṇa and Balarāma, who had assumed the forms of cowherd men, like dancers praise [other] dancers, O king.
12. Sporting sidelocks, the two boys played by whirling, jumping, hurling, slapping, dragging, and sometimes wrestling.
13. And sometimes the two boys Themselves became the singers and players while others danced, O great king. They gave encouragement, saying: 'Bravo! Bravo!'
14. Sometimes [They played] with *bilva* fruits, sometimes with *kumbha* fruits, and sometimes with handfuls of *āmalaka* fruits. Sometimes They bound Their eyes, and [played] at not being touched, and other such games, and sometimes They pretended to be animals and birds.
15. Sometimes [They played] leapfrog or practical jokes, sometimes on swings and sometimes at acting as kings.
16. In this way, the two [played] games that were familiar to people. They wandered about the forest, rivers, mountains, valleys, bowers, woods, and lakes."

Madhura Bhāva: Kṛṣṇa as Amorous Lover

The Deliverance of the Wives of the Sacrificers

Bhāva Blueprint

This passage concludes our sakhya bhāva *section but includes* madhura *elements. We will save our comments on* madhura *for the following passage but alert the reader to note the difference in the reaction of the wives of the* brāhmaṇas *to Kṛṣṇa's instruction to them to return to their husbands from the reaction of the* gopīs *to the same instruction that will follow in the next section.*

Book X, Chapter 23

1. The *gopas* said:
"Balarāma, mighty-armed Balarāma! The annihilator of the wicked! Our hunger is really troubling us; please satisfy it."
2. *Śrī* Śuka said:
"*Bhagavān*, the son of Devakī, was feeling pleased with His devotees, the wives of the *brāhmaṇas*. When He was appealed to in this way, He spoke as follows:
3. 'Go to the sacrificial arena. Desiring to attain *svarga* [the celestial abode of the gods], the *brāhmaṇa* reciters of the Vedas are taking part in a sacrifice called *āṅgirasa*.
4. Go there and request some cooked rice, mentioning the names of the worthy *Bhagavān* Balarāma, and of Me Myself; say that you have been dispatched by Us.'
5. Directed thus by *Bhagavān*, the boys went and asked as suggested. They fell on the ground before the *brāhmaṇas* like sticks,[35] their hands cupped in supplication:
6. 'You are celestials on earth, please listen. May good fortune be with you. Please know that we *gopas* have been dispatched by Balarāma and come to you to execute Kṛṣṇa's instructions.
7. Balarāma and Acyuta have become hungry while grazing the cows not far from here, and desire cooked rice from you. You are distinguished in the knowledge of *dharma*, and if you have any respect for them, give them cooked rice. They entreat you, O *brāhmaṇas*.
8. The eating of food, even from a person who has been consecrated for the performance of sacrifice, is not defiling, O most noble ones,

the exception being during the consecration ceremony, the slaughter of the sacrificial animal, and the *sautrāmaṇi* sacrifice.'[36]

9. Although they heard *Bhagavān*'s request, the *brāhmaṇas* did not listen to it. They had petty aspirations. They thought themselves distinguished, but despite the fact that they performed numerous rituals, they were ignorant.

10.–11. Kṛṣṇa is *Bhagavān*, Adhokṣaja, the Supreme *Brahman* in person. The place, time, sundry utensils, *mantras*, Tantra rituals, *ṛtvik* priests, fires, gods, sacrificer, offering, and the results accrued [from the sacrifice] are constituted by Him. But the *brāhmaṇas'* intelligence was perverted; thinking their bodies to be their real selves, they did not show Him courtesy, perceiving Him to be a mortal.

12. When they did not respond with either a 'yes' or a 'no,' the *gopas* returned dejected and reported what had happened to Kṛṣṇa and Balarāma, O scorcher of enemies.

13. After listening to this, *Bhagavān*, the Lord of the Universe, laughed, pointing out the materialistic ways of the world. He then spoke again to the *gopas*:

14. 'Inform the wives that I have arrived, along with Saṅkarṣana [Balarāma]. They will give you as much food as you wish. They are affectionate, and their minds dwell in Me.'

15. So, the *gopas* went to the *patnīśālā* [women's quarter],[37] where they saw them sitting down, prettily bedecked. They humbly paid homage to the wives of the *brāhmaṇas* and spoke as follows:

16. 'Greetings to you, O wives of *brāhmaṇas*; please listen to what we have to say. We have been sent by Kṛṣṇa, who is passing by not far from here.

17. He has come from afar, and has been grazing the cows with Balarāma and the *gopas*. Please give food to him. He and his companions desire to eat.'

18. The women had always been eager for a glimpse of Acyuta, because they had been captivated by accounts of Him. When they heard that He had arrived nearby, they became flustered.

19. Taking along a great variety of the four types of food[38] in pots, they surged forth to meet their beloved, like rivers to an ocean.

20. [Although] they were obstructed by their husbands, brothers, relatives, and sons, their hopes [of meeting Kṛṣṇa] had long been sustained by hearing about Him. He is *Bhagavān*, who is praised in the best of hymns.

21. The women saw Kṛṣṇa surrounded by the *gopas* and wandering about with His elder brother in the grove on the *Yamunā*, which was a picturesque sight with fresh buds of *aśoka* trees.
22. He was dark blue in color, and wearing a golden garment. He was dressed like an actor with fresh shoots, minerals, a peacock feather, and a forest garland. One hand was placed on the shoulder of a companion, the other was twirling a lotus flower. His smiling lotus face had curls on the cheeks and lotuses behind the ears.
23. The women had heard so much about their beloved, and His celebrity had so filled their ears, that their minds had become absorbed in Him. Now, they drew Him into [their hearts] through the openings of their eyes. They embraced Him for a long time, and cast off their distress, just like false notions of the self are cast off after wisdom is embraced.
24. Kṛṣṇa is the seer who discerns everything, and so understood that they had arrived in this fashion, giving up all false aspirations out of a desire to see Him. He spoke to them, smiling.
25. 'Welcome. You are very fortunate women! Please be seated. What can I do for you? You have come desiring to see Us, which is certainly worthy of you.
26. There is no doubt that those who are learned and who understand their self-interest engage in selfless, uninterrupted *bhakti* to Me, because I am the one who is dear to their souls.
27. The vital airs, intelligence, mind, body, wife, children, wealth, and other worldly assets become dear because of contact [with Me]. Therefore, what else is there that is dear in actuality?
28. So, go to the sacrificial arena. Your *brāhmaṇa* husbands are householders, and can only complete their sacrifice with your participation.'[39]
29. The wives replied: 'You should not speak to us in such a cruel fashion, O lord! Abide by your own doctrine![40] We have transgressed against all our relatives and have arrived at your lotus feet to wear on our hair the *tulasī* garland discarded by your feet.
30. Our husbands, parents, sons, brothers, relatives, and friends, not to speak of others, will not accept us. We are souls who have fallen down at your lotus feet, so there can be no other destination for us. Therefore, grant [us your shelter].'

31. *Śrī Bhagavān* said: 'Neither your husbands, fathers, brothers, sons, nor other relatives, nor people in general, will be angry with you. Even the gods will approve, as they take shelter of Me.
32. Physical contact between people in this world does not [produce] joy or affection. Therefore, fix your mind on Me, and you will obtain Me without delay.' "
33. *Śrī* Śuka said:
"When they had been addressed in this way, the wives of the *brāhmaṇas* returned to the sacrificial enclosure. The [*brāhmaṇas*] were not displeased with them and completed the sacrifice with their wives.
34. One woman there, who had been impeded by her husband, embraced *Bhagavān* in her heart as she conceived of Him from what she had heard—and gave up her body, the product of *karma*.
35. So *Bhagavān*, Govinda, the Lord, fed the *gopas* with the four kinds of foodstuffs, and then He himself ate.
36. Imitating the world of men in a human body for the purpose of *līlā*, He brought pleasure to the cows, *gopas*, and *gopīs* through His deeds, words, and beauty.
37. Later, those *brāhmaṇas* repented in retrospect: 'We have committed an offense because we ignored the request of the two Lords of the universe. They are playing the role of mortals.'
38. Seeing the supreme devotion of the women to *Bhagavān* Kṛṣṇa, they lamented their own lack of it, and rebuked themselves:
39. 'Curses on that birth which is threefold,[41] curses on vows, curses on extensive learning, curses on our family lineage, curses on skill in rituals: we still remain averse to Adhokṣaja [Kṛṣṇa].
40. Truly, the *māyā* of *Bhagavān* bewilders even the *yogīs*. Because of it, we *brāhmaṇas*, the *gurus* of humanity, are confused about our own self-interest.
41. *Aho!* See the unlimited devotion of these very women to Kṛṣṇa, the *Guru* of the world. It has pierced the fetters of death under the guise of household life.
42. Neither the *saṁskāra* purificatory rites of the twice-born,[42] nor residence in the house of the *guru*, nor austerity, nor inquiry into the self, nor rites of cleanliness, nor auspicious rituals were [practiced] by these women.
43. Nonetheless, they were constant in devotion to Kṛṣṇa, the Lord of the lords of *yoga*, whose glories are renowned. This was not the

case with us, even though we have undergone the *saṁskāras* and other such rites.
44. *Aho!* Through the words of the *gopas*, Kṛṣṇa reminded us about the path of the virtuous, but we were deluded about our self-interest and heedless because of our domestic activities.
45. Otherwise, what was the purpose of this playacting with us by the Lord, the controller who grants blessings such as that of liberation? His own desires are fulfilled, but we are meant to be controlled [by Him].
46. His begging [for food] bewilders people, since the Goddess of Fortune, spurning others and relinquishing the faults of Her own nature,[43] worships Him constantly with the desire to touch His feet.
47. The place, time, sundry utensils, mantras, Tantra rituals, *ṛtvik* priests, fires, gods, sacrificer, offering, and the results accrued [from the sacrifice], are constituted by Him.
48. He indeed is *Bhagavān* Himself, Viṣṇu, the Lord of the lords of *yoga*, born among the Yadus. Although we had heard this, being fools, we did not understand.
49. *Aho!* How fortunate we are to have wives such as these! Their devoutness has given rise to unwavering devotion to Hari in us.
50. Homage to Him, *Bhagavān*, Kṛṣṇa, whose intelligence is ever fresh. We are wandering on the path of *karma*, our intelligence bewildered by His *māyā*.
51. He is the primeval person and so should graciously forgive our offense. Our minds are confused by His *māyā* and we are ignorant of His might.'
52. Reflecting on their offense in this way, the [*brāhmaṇas*], who had been contemptuous of Kṛṣṇa, desired to see Vraj; but they did not go, out of fear of Kaṁsa."

The Description of the *Rāsa* Pastime

Bhāva Blueprint

The following passages constitute the pañcādhyāya *(five chapters). More has probably been written about these, and the* madhura bhāva *they express, in the secondary literature of the Kṛṣṇa traditions that emerged in the sixteenth century than about all the other chapters and* bhāvas *of the* Bhāgavata *put together. They are also the most easily misunderstood theologically. We will be brief in our comments but can note that so intense is the* gopīs' *determination to be with Kṛṣṇa that in order to remain with Him, they reject Kṛṣṇa's direct instruction to return home to perform their* dharmas*—in contrast with the wives of the* brāhmaṇas *in the previous section. Just as, in the Abrahamic tradition, God tests Abraham to see if he will obey Him even by the performance of an abhorrent deed—the killing of his own son, Isaac—so the* gopīs' *devotion informs us that there is a higher principle than mere* dharma. *By ignoring their husbands, children, and other duties and risking social ruination by openly going to the forest at night to be with Kṛṣṇa without even giving a thought to the possible repercussions, the* gopīs *demonstrate that love of God trumps all social, cultural, or any other mundane considerations. Hence they are considered the greatest of all* bhaktas. *Thus the illiterate females born in a cowherding caste are the greatest of all* yogīs *in the* Bhāgavata, *thereby trumping the* brāhmaṇa *male dominance of normative Vedic culture. Once again, the text points to* bhakti *as transcendent to caste, gender, social status, and any and all other material considerations.*

Book X, Chapter 29

1. *Śrī* Śuka, the son of Bādarāyaṇa, said:
"Even *Bhagavān*, God Himself, beholding those nights, with autumnal jasmine [*mallikā*] flowers blossoming, called upon His divine power of *yogamāyā*, and turned His thoughts toward enjoying love.
2. At that time, the moon, king of the constellations, arose in the east, covering the face of the heavens with its copper-colored soothing rays. It wiped away the cares of the onlookers, like a lover who has been absent for a long time wipes away the cares of his beloved.
3. Seeing that full disk, herald of the white night-lilies, reddened with fresh vermilion powder, its splendor like the face of Lakṣmī, the Goddess of Fortune, and seeing the forest colored by its silky rays, Kṛṣṇa played [His flute] softly, capturing the hearts of the beautiful-eyed women.
4. The music aroused Kāma.[44] When they heard it, the women of Vraj, enchanted by Kṛṣṇa, came to their lover, their earrings swinging in their haste, and unknown to one another.
5. Some, who were milking cows, abandoned the milking and approached eagerly. Others had put milk on the fire, but then came without even removing [the milk or] the cakes [from the oven].
6.–7. Others interrupted serving food, feeding their babies milk, and attending to their husbands. Still others were eating but left their food.

Others were putting on makeup, washing, or applying mascara to their eyes. They all went to be near Kṛṣṇa, their clothes and ornaments in disarray.
8. Their hearts had been stolen by Govinda, so they did not turn back when husbands, fathers, brothers, and relatives tried to prevent them. They were in a state of rapture.
9. Some *gopīs*, not being able to find a way to leave, remained at home and thought of Kṛṣṇa with eyes closed, completely absorbed in meditation.
10.–11. [The *karma*] from their impious deeds was destroyed by the intense and intolerable pain of separation from their lover, and their auspicious deeds were diminished by the complete fulfillment resulting from the intimate contact with Acyuta that they obtained through meditation.[45] Their bondage was destroyed, and they immediately left their bodies made of the *guṇas*.[46] Uniting with the Supreme Soul, they considered Him their lover."
12. *Śrī* Parīkṣit said:
"O sage, they related to Kṛṣṇa as their supreme lover, not as *Brahman*, the Absolute Truth. So how did the flow of the *guṇas*, in which their minds were absorbed, cease for the *gopīs*?"
13. *Śrī* Śuka said:
"This was explained to you previously: in the same way as the king of the Cedis, Śiśupāla, attained perfection despite hating Hṛṣīkeśa.[47] What, then, of those dear to Adhokṣaja [Kṛṣṇa]?
14. God appears for the supreme good of humanity, O king. He is immeasurable and eternal. As the controller of the *guṇas*, He is beyond the *guṇas*.
15. Those who always dedicate their desire, anger, fear, affection, sense of identity, and friendship to Hari enter for certain into His state of being.
16. You should not show such surprise at Lord Kṛṣṇa. He is unborn and the master of all masters of *yoga*. From Him the whole universe attains liberation.
17. The Lord saw that the women of Vraj had arrived in His presence. Being the best of speakers, He addressed them, captivating them with the charm of His words:
18. 'Welcome—you are most fortunate. What can I do to please you? Is everything well in Vraj? Tell me the purpose of your coming.

19. This fearsome dark night is frequented by ferocious creatures. Go back to Vraj, O slender-waisted ones; this place is not fit for women.
20. Your mothers, fathers, sons, brothers, and husbands are worried because they cannot find you. Do not cause your relatives concern.
21.–22. You have seen the forest, adorned with flowers, colored by the rays of the full moon, and made beautiful by the blossoms of the trees quivering playfully in the breeze of the *Yamunā* river. Therefore hurry now to the cowpen and serve your husbands—you are chaste ladies. The babies and calves are crying; suckle them and milk them.
23. Or perhaps your hearts are captivated, and you have come out of love for Me. This is commendable of you—living beings delight in Me.
24. The highest *dharma* [duty] of a woman is to serve her husband faithfully, to ensure the well-being of her relatives, and to nourish her children.
25. A husband who is not a sinner, even though he be of bad character, ill-fated, old, dull-headed, sick, or poor, should not be abandoned by women who desire to attain heaven.
26. Without exception, the adultery of a woman of good birth does not lead to heaven. It is scandalous, fear-laden, worthless, fraught with difficulty, and abhorrent.
27. Love for Me comes from hearing about Me, seeing Me, meditating on Me and reciting My glories—not in this way, by physical proximity. Therefore, return to your homes.'
28. Hearing Govinda speak these unwelcome words, the dejected *gopīs* had their aspirations dashed and were inconsolable in their distress.
29. They stood silently, their red *bimba* fruit–colored lips faded by their sighs, and the vermilion powder on their breasts smeared by the mascara carried by their tears. Casting down their faces out of sorrow and scratching the ground with their feet, they were weighed down by extreme unhappiness.
30. Wiping their eyes, and having checked their tears somewhat, the *gopīs* spoke to Kṛṣṇa, their beloved, with voices faltering with agitation. They were utterly devoted, and had sacrificed all desires for His sake, but He had replied to them as if He were anything but their beloved:

31. 'You should not speak to us in such a heartless fashion, O Lord. Renouncing all enjoyments of the senses, we are devoted to the soles of Your feet. Reciprocate, you obstinate one, just as the Lord, the original being, reciprocates with those who desire liberation. Do not reject us.
32. You, the knower of *dharma*, have declared that the occupational *dharma* of women consists of attending to friends, husbands, and children. Then let this be our *dharma* when it comes to You, the source of this advice, O Lord—after all, You are the soul within all relatives. Indeed, You are the most dear of all embodied beings.
33. You are the eternal beloved, O soul of all, and so the learned place their affection in You. What is the use of husbands and children who simply cause problems? Therefore, O Supreme Lord, be pleased with us. Do not dash our hopes. They have been sustained by You for such a long time, O lotus-eyed one.
34. Our hearts, which were absorbed in our households, have been stolen away with ease by You, as have our hands from domestic chores. Our feet cannot move one step from the soles of Your lotus feet. How can we go to Vraj? And besides, what would we do there?
35. O beloved, pour the nectar of your lips on the fire dwelling in our hearts, which has been kindled by Your musical harmonies, Your glances, and Your smiles. If you do not, we will traverse the path to Your feet through meditation, our bodies consumed by the fire born of separation.
36. Lotus-eyed Kṛṣṇa, You are dear to the forest-dwelling hermits. Somewhere or other, for a moment, we providentially touched the soles of Your feet, which belong to the Goddess of Fortune. Alas, from that moment, instantly enamored of You, we became incapable of remaining in the presence of any other man.
37. The Goddess of Fortune aspires to the dust of those lotus feet, which is worshipped by Your servants, even though She has obtained a place on Your chest along with Tulasī.[48] Other gods, even, strive to attract Her personal glance. In the same way, we solicit the dust of Your feet.
38. It is You who banish distress—therefore be compassionate to us. In the desire to worship You, we have given up our homes and arrived at the soles of Your feet. Allow us, whose hearts are burning with

intense desire born from Your beautiful smiles and glances, to be Your servants, O ornament of men.

39. We have gazed on Your face covered with curls, with its smiles and glances, and on Your honeyed lips placed between Your cheeks made beautiful with earrings. And we have beheld Your two strong arms, which bestow fearlessness, and Your chest, which is the exclusive delight of the Goddess of Fortune. After this we have become Your servants.

40. Dear Kṛṣṇa, what women in the three worlds would not stray from the behavior proper to Āryans, when thrown into turmoil by the melodies of Your flute, which vibrates harmoniously? And what woman would not stray after seeing this, Your form, which brings good fortune to the three worlds and causes the hair of cows, birds, trees, and deer to stand on end with bliss?

41. It is clear that You have accepted birth to remove the tribulations and fears of Vraj just as the Lord, the primeval person, protects the denizens of heaven. Therefore, since You are the friend of the afflicted, place Your lotus hands on the burning breasts and heads of Your servants.' "

42. *Śrī* Śuka said:

"The Master of the masters of *yoga*, hearing their despairing words, laughed and engaged in amorous pleasures with them from kindness, even though His satisfaction is self-contained.

43. Kṛṣṇa, the infallible one, whose conduct is upright, shone forth with the assembled *gopīs*, who were dazzling with jasmine teeth and broad smiles. As the *gopīs'* faces blossomed from the glances of their beloved, Kṛṣṇa appeared like the moon surrounded by stars.

44. Praised in song, and singing loudly Himself, the Lord of hundreds of women, wearing a garland of *vaijayantī* flowers, frolicked in the forest, making it beautiful.

45.–46. Accompanied by the *gopīs*, Kṛṣṇa approached the bank of the river. Its cool sand was swept by a wind bearing the scent of *kumuda* flowers and refreshing from its contact with the waves. Arousing *kāma* in the young women of Vraj with jokes, smiles, and glances, playfully scratching their breasts, girdles, thighs, hair, and hands with His nails, and embracing them with outstretched arms, He gave them pleasure.

47. Such attention from Kṛṣṇa, *Bhagavān*, the Supreme Soul, made

the *gopīs* proud. Indeed, they thought themselves to be the best of women on earth.
48. Keśava saw their pride, which was born from the exhilaration of their good fortune, and vanished from the spot out of kindness, in order to moderate [their pride]."

Searching for Kṛṣṇa in the *Rāsa* Pastime

Bhāva Blueprint

This passage contains a good example of viraha bhakti, *love in separation from the beloved. The Gauḍīya tradition considers this form of love to be even more intense than that of union with the beloved. In their ramblings to the trees and plants, we gain some sense of the extent of the* gopīs' *devotional madness when Kṛṣṇa disappears from their midst. Their absorption in thoughts of Kṛṣṇa is revealed in the fact that everything reminds them of their departed beloved, in their reenactment of His* līlās *among themselves and in their obsessive conviction that Kṛṣṇa has gone off with someone else. The divine intoxication of the* gopīs *is not paralleled by any other* bhakta *in the text, thus again underscoring their devotional preeminence in the* Bhāgavata.

Book X, Chapter 30

1. *Śrī* Śuka said:
"When *Bhagavān* suddenly vanished, the women of Vraj were filled with remorse at His disappearance. They were like female elephants who had lost sight of the leader of the herd.
2. Intoxicated by the pleasing gestures, playfulness, and words, as well as by the quivering glances, smiles of love, and movements of Kṛṣṇa, the husband of Ramā, the Goddess of Fortune, their minds were overwhelmed. They acted out each of those behaviors, their hearts [dedicated] to Him.
3. Those beloved women were so bewildered by Kṛṣṇa's pastimes that their bodies imitated their darling in the way they moved, smiled, glanced, spoke, and so forth. With their hearts [dedicated] to Him, the women declared: 'I am He!'
4. Singing loudly in unison only about Him, they searched from grove to grove, like madwomen. They asked the trees about the Supreme Being who, like space, is inside and outside living creatures:

5. 'O *aśvattha* tree! O *plakṣa* tree! O *nyagrodha* tree! Have you seen the son of Nanda at all? He has stolen our minds with his glances and smiles of love, and has gone.
6. O *kurabaka*, *aśoka*, *nāga*, *punnāga*, and *campaka* trees! Has the younger brother of Balarāma [passed] by here? His smile steals away the pride of haughty women.
7. O auspicious *tulasī* plant, you who are dear to Govinda! Have you seen your most beloved, Acyuta, wearing you [as a garland covered] with swarms of bees?
8. O *mālatī* plant! O *mallikā* plant! O *jātī* plant! O *yūthikā* plant! Has Mādhava [Kṛṣṇa] passed by, awakening your love with the touch of his hand? Have you seen him?
9. O *cūta* [mango], *priyāla*, *panasa* [breadfruit], *asana*, *kovidāra*, *jambū* [rose-apple], *arka*, *bilva* [wood-apple], *bakula*, *āmra* [mango], *kadamba*, and *nīpa* trees, and those others which grow on the shore of the *Yamunā* river and which exist to benefit others! Point us to the path [taken] by Kṛṣṇa. We have lost our hearts.
10. O earth, you are beautiful in that the hairs of your body [the trees] stand up from the bliss of the touch of the feet of Keśava [Kṛṣṇa]. What ascetic practice have you performed? Is the cause of this these very feet [of Kṛṣṇa]? Or is it because of the step of Urukrama?[49] Or rather from the embrace of the body of Varāha?[50]
11. O wife of the deer, has Acyuta passed by here with his beloved, his limbs giving pleasure to your eyes? O friend, the scent from the jasmine garland of the lord of our group is wafting here—a garland colored with breast saffron contracted from the body of his lover.
12. O trees, did the younger brother of Balarāma wander here? Was he followed by swarms of bees, blinded with intoxication, on his *tulasī* [garland]? With his arm placed on the shoulder of his beloved, he [must have been] holding a lotus flower. And did he acknowledge with glances of love your bowing down?
13. Ask these creeping plants! Just see, although they are embracing the arms of the forest tree, they surely must have been touched by his fingernails, for they are bristling with ecstasy.'
14. The *gopīs*, [uttering] these crazed words, became perplexed in their search for Kṛṣṇa. With their hearts [dedicated] to Him, each of them imitated the *līlā* of *Bhagavān*.

15. One, who was acting as if she were Kṛṣṇa, suckled the breast of someone else, who was playing the part of Pūtanā.[51] Another became an infant, began crying, and then kicked another one, who was acting as a cart, with her foot.
16. After changing into a demon, one *gopī* kidnapped another, who was imagining herself to be the child Kṛṣṇa. Yet another crawled around, dragging her two feet, accompanied by the sounds from her jewelry.
17. Two *gopīs* enacted the roles of Kṛṣṇa and Balarāma, and others behaved as *gopas*. Yet another struck a *gopī* who had become Vatsa, the calf demon, while someone else there struck the *gopī* who was playing the role of Baka, the crane demon.
18. One called the cows who were far away, as Kṛṣṇa would have done. Others praised one *gopī* who was sporting and playing the flute in imitation of him: 'Bravo!'
19. Another, wandering about, placed her arm on someone else and said: 'There can be no doubt that I am Kṛṣṇa. Look at how gracefully I move.' Her mind was intent on him:
20. 'Do not fear the wind and the rain. I have arranged protection.' Saying this, one *gopī*, exerting herself, lifted up her garment with one hand.
21. Another *gopī* mounted and stepped on the head of another with her foot, O king, and said: 'Go, wicked snake! There is no doubt that I have undertaken birth as the chastiser of the wicked.'[52]
22. Someone there said: 'Hey, *gopas*, look at the terrible forest fire! Close your eyes, I will with ease arrange for your protection!'[53]
23. One slender-waisted *gopī* was tied to a mortar with a flower garland by another one. The former, her beautiful eyes afraid, covered her face and adopted a posture of fear.
24. Inquiring thus after Kṛṣṇa from the creeping plants and trees of Vṛndāvana, the *gopīs* noticed the footprints of the Supreme Soul in a certain part of the forest:
25. 'These footprints are certainly those of the great soul, the son of Nanda,' they said. 'They are recognizable from such marks as the flag, the lotus flower, the thunderbolt, the goad, and the barley.'[54]
26. Following Kṛṣṇa's tracks farther, footprint by footprint, the women noticed that they were clearly interspersed with the footprints of a young woman. They discussed this together in distress:

27. 'Whose footprints are these? She is going with the son of Nanda, his forearm placed on her shoulder, like a female elephant with a male elephant.
28. She has worshipped[55] *Bhagavān* Hari, the Lord. Consequently, Govinda was pleased, and so has abandoned us and led that *gopī* to a secluded place.
29. Just see, O friends, how fortunate are these particles of dust from the lotus feet of Govinda. Brahmā, Śiva, and the Goddess of Fortune, Ramā (Śrī), place them on their heads to remove their sins.
30. The footprints of that woman are causing us great distress because she alone of the *gopīs* is enjoying the lips of Acyuta in a secluded place.
31. Now, right here, her footprints are no longer visible: the lover has lifted up his beloved, whose feet with their delicate soles are bruised by the blades of grass.
31a.[56] Look, *gopīs*, at these deeper footprints of lusty Kṛṣṇa weighed down by carrying the young woman. And here the beloved has been put down by that great soul in order to [gather] flowers.
32. Look, here the lover plucked flowers for the beloved: these two footprints are incomplete because he stood on tiptoe.
33. Here, lusty Kṛṣṇa decorated that lusty woman's hair. Surely he sat here while making his lover a crown with those [flowers].' "
34. [*Śrī* Śuka said]:
"Kṛṣṇa took pleasure with that *gopī*, although He is complete, content within Himself, and delights in His own self. He was displaying the wretchedness of lusty men and women because of their depravity.
35.–36. The dispirited *gopīs* wandered about pointing [things] out in this way. The *gopī*, whom Kṛṣṇa had taken to the forest after abandoning the other women, then thought that she was the best of all women: 'Kṛṣṇa, my beloved, has abandoned the [other] *gopīs* who were impelled by Kāma and dedicated himself to me.'
37. Then, after going to a spot in the wood, the proud woman spoke to Keśava [Kṛṣṇa]: 'I am unable to walk any farther. Take me wherever your mind [desires].'
38. At this request, Kṛṣṇa told His beloved that she should climb on His shoulder, but then He disappeared. The young woman was filled with remorse:

39. 'O Lord, lover, dearest! Where are you? Where are you, mighty-armed one? Reveal your presence to me, friend—I am your miserable servant!' "
40. *Śrī* Śuka said:
"The *gopīs*, searching for the path of *Bhagavān*, saw a distressed girl not far away who was disorientated by the separation from her beloved.
41. Hearing her story of how she had first received respect from Mādhava [Kṛṣṇa], and then humiliation because of her bad faith, they were astounded.
42. After this, they went as far into the forest as the moon gave light. Then, seeing that darkness had descended there, the women returned.
43. Their minds absorbed in Kṛṣṇa, the *gopīs*' conversations focused on Him, their activities centered on Him, and they dedicated their hearts to Him. Simply by singing about His qualities, they forgot their own homes.
44. Meditating on Kṛṣṇa, they reached the bank of the *Kālindī* [*Yamunā*] river again. Gathering together they sang about Kṛṣṇa, longing for His arrival."

The *Gopīs'* Song in the *Rāsa* Pastime

Bhāva Blueprint

The gopīs' *love-induced pining for Kṛṣṇa in* madhura bhāva *continues.*

Book X, Chapter 31

1. The *gopīs* said: "Vraj has become preeminent because of your birth; indeed, Indirā [Lakṣmī] resides there permanently. O loved one, show yourself! Your devotees, whose lives are sustained in you, are searching for you everywhere.
2. You are taking our life, O lord of autumn; your glance excels in beauty the heart of a beautiful lotus perfectly born in autumn from a pool of water. We are your maidservants [and do not ask for] any payment. Isn't this killing us, O bestower of favors?
3. O bull among men, we have been continuously protected by you from destruction from the poisonous water, from the wicked demon, from the winds and rains, from fire and lightning, from the bull Ariṣṭa, from the son of Maya (Vyomāsura), and from fear from all sides.[57]

4. You are not, in fact, the son of a *gopī*. You are the witness of the inner self of all embodied beings. Being petitioned by Brahmā, You become manifest in the family of the Sātvatas, O friend, for the protection of the universe.
5. Place Your lotus hand on the head of those who have approached You out of fear of the material world, O foremost of the Vṛṣṇi clan. Your hand, which holds the hand of Śrī [Lakṣmī], bestows fearlessness and fulfills desires, O lover.
6. You are the hero of women, and you take away the pain of the people of Vraj! The pride of your devotees is annihilated by your smile! Accept your maidservants, friend! Show us your beautiful lotus face!
7. Place your lotus feet upon our breasts. Your feet have been placed on the hoods of the serpent [Kāliya] and follow the animals to the pasture. They are the abode of the Goddess of Fortune, Śrī, and they remove the sins of submissive embodied beings. Excise Kāma, who dwells within our hearts.
8. O hero, these women obedient to your will are stunned by your sweet voice, your charming words which please the mind and intelligence, and your lotus eyes. Reinvigorate us with the intoxicating liquid of your lips.
9. Those who repeat the sweetness of your words in this world are munificent. These words are praised by poets, spread abroad, and are auspicious to hear. They are life-giving for those who are suffering. They remove sins and bring good fortune.
10. Your bursts of laughter, pleasing looks of love, and pastimes are auspicious to contemplate. Those meetings in secret places touch our hearts, you cheater, and perturb us thoroughly.
11. When you go from Vraj grazing the animals, O lord, your feet, beautiful as lotuses, are troubled by blades of grass and corn stubble, and so we feel distress. You are our beloved.
12. You possess a lotus face, surrounded by blue locks of hair, which you constantly display covered with thick dust at the end of the day. You arouse Kāma in the heart, O hero.
13. O lover, place your most beneficent lotus feet on our breasts. They fulfill the desires of the humble and should be meditated upon in trouble, O destroyer of anxiety. They are worshipped by the lotus-born Brahmā, and are the ornament of the earth.

14. Bestow upon us the nectar of your lips, O hero, which have been thoroughly kissed by the flute as it plays music. It destroys sorrow, increases the pleasures of love, and causes men to forget other passions.
15. When you, Lord, go to the forest during the day, a moment becomes an aeon (*yuga*) for those who do not see you. He who created eyelashes is dull-witted, from the perspective of those beholding your beautiful face, with its curled locks of hair.[58]
16. Acyuta, you are the knower of [people's] movements. Bewildered by your song, we have thoroughly neglected our husbands, sons, family, brothers, and kinsfolk, and come before you. Who would abandon women in the night, you rogue?
17. We have become unsettled from contemplating your broad chest, the abode of Śrī, the Goddess of Fortune, as well as your looks of love, your smiling face, and the meetings in secret places which aroused Kāma. We long for you intensely all the time.
18. Your incarnation is for the good of the universe, and dispels the distress of the people of Vraj. Deliver a little of that [medicine] which removes the ailment from the hearts of your devotees to us. Our hearts yearn for you.
19. We gently place your tender lotus feet on our rough breasts with trepidation. You wander in the forest on them and our minds are disturbed: What if they have been hurt by small stones? Your Lordship is our life."

The *Gopīs'* Lamentation in the *Rāsa* Pastime

Bhāva Blueprint

After intensifying their love for Him by His absence, Kṛṣṇa reappears to satisfy His beloved gopīs. *The passage ends with even God Himself stating that He has no way to reciprocate with the extremes of their love for Him.*

Book X, Chapter 32

1. *Śrī* Śuka said:
"Thus, the *gopīs* sang and spoke incoherently in various ways. Longing to see Kṛṣṇa, O king, they wept loudly.
2. Kṛṣṇa, the descendant of Sūra, bewilderer of the mind of the mind-bewilderer Kāma himself, appeared in their midst, His lotus face smiling. He was wearing garments and bore a garland.

3. Seeing that their beloved had returned, the women, their eyes wide with love, sprang up simultaneously, as if the vital air of the body had returned.
4. One ecstatic woman caught hold of Kṛṣṇa's lotus hand in her folded hands. Another placed His arm, decorated with sandalwood paste, on her shoulder.
5. A slender woman accepted His chewed betel nut with folded hands. Another, burning [with desire], placed His lotus feet on her breast.
6. Yet another, trembling with the fury of love, was biting her lips with her teeth, her brows knitted in a frown. She glared at Kṛṣṇa as if she could strike Him with a look of rebuke.
7. Another woman dwelled on His lotus face with unblinking eyes. Although she drank it in with her eyes, she was not fully satisfied, just as a saint is not fully satisfied [by meditating on] Kṛṣṇa's lotus feet.
8. Some other woman, drawing Kṛṣṇa into her heart through the apertures of her eyes and then sealing them shut, stood embracing Him [in her heart], like a *yogī* immersed in bliss.[59]
9. All rejoiced at the wonder of seeing Keśava [Kṛṣṇa], and let go the distress they had felt at separation, just as people are joyful after encountering a wise man.
10. *Bhagavān*, Acyuta, surrounded by the women who had shaken off their sorrow, shone brilliantly, like the Supreme Being surrounded by His *śakti* powers.
11.–12. The Supreme Ruler took the women along and enjoyed Himself on the auspicious bank of the *Kālindī* [*Yamunā*]. There were bees with six legs and a breeze fragrant with blossoming jasmine and *mandāra* flowers. Its soft sands were lapped by waves that were like the hands of the *Kṛṣṇa* [*Yamunā*] river. The darkness of the night was dispelled by the full rays from the autumn moon.
13. The heartache of the *gopīs* had been assuaged by the bliss of seeing Kṛṣṇa, just as the Vedas attained the culmination of their hearts' desire.[60] The *gopīs* made a seat for the friend of their heart with their outer garments, which were smeared with the *kuṅkuma* powder from their breasts.
14. *Bhagavān*, the Lord, whose seat is fixed within the hearts of the masters of *yoga*, sat down there. He was worshipped as He sat in the company of the *gopīs*, and revealed Himself in a form that was a unique embodiment of beauty in the three worlds.

15. Those women worshipped that inciter of Kāma by massaging His hands and feet, which they had placed on their laps. They praised Him, their eyebrows quivering, with playful looks and laughter. Then they spoke, somewhat angrily.
16. The beautiful *gopīs* said: 'Some serve those who serve them. Some do the opposite of this [that is, serve those who do not serve them]. And some do not serve either. Can you explain this for us clearly?'
17. *Śrī Bhagavān* said: 'Friends, there are those who serve each other reciprocally, but their exchange is exclusively out of self-interest; there is no *dharma* or friendship there. Personal gain and nothing else is the motive.
18. Those, like mothers and fathers, who serve those who do not serve [them] are truly compassionate. There is perfect friendship and *dharma* in this, O slender-waisted ones.
19. Some do not serve even those who serve [them], let alone those who do not serve [them]. They include those who take pleasure in their spiritual self, those whose desires are fulfilled, the ungrateful and the *guru* haters.
20. I do not serve even those beings who serve Me so as to enhance their devotional state of mind, O friends. The case is like that of the poor man who is not conscious of anything else when the wealth that he had gained is lost, but continues to contemplate that wealth obsessively.
21. In this way, O women, when I disappeared from your presence—you who had abandoned relatives, the [injunctions of the] Vedas, and the world for My sake—it was really to further [your dedication] to Me. I was serving you. Therefore, beloved ones, you should not be displeased with your beloved.
22. You have broken the enduring shackles of the household, and have served me. You are full of goodness and without fault, and I am unable to reciprocate, even in the lifetime of a celestial. Therefore, let your reward be your own excellence.' "

The Description of the *Rāsa*[61] Pastime

Bhāva Blueprint

The rāsa *dance between Kṛṣṇa and the* gopīs *is the most famous episode in Kṛṣṇa literature as evidenced in Indian art, poetry, drama, and other cultural expressions. The passage ends with Parīkṣit asking the question most commonly raised about Kṛṣṇa from here in the text itself to colonial and missionary critiques of the tradition in the nineteenth and twentieth centuries: How can Kṛṣṇa, who is the propagator and exemplar of* dharma, *possibly transgress His own codes by cavorting with the wives of others? Śuka begins his answer, expectedly, with pointing out that Kṛṣṇa is the transcendent Godhead and not subject to mundane notions of* dharma. *But he continues with the more important* bhāva-*related answer: Kṛṣṇa, although self-fulfilled, satisfies His* bhaktas *according to their desires to be with Him and this trumps all mundane relationships and social considerations. Although the* Bhāgavata *strongly and unambiguously stresses* dharma *throughout all of its other eighteen thousand verses, the theological message of this short section on* madhura *is that the highest stages of pure* bhakti, *love of God, transcends all material expectations and obligations, including that of* dharma. Dharma *is relevant only to the sphere of* saṁsāra, *and this section of the text is dedicated to the highest and ultimate goal of human existence—pure love of God exclusive of all and every other consideration. Hence it is considered the apex of Kṛṣṇa devotion.*

Book X, Chapter 33

1. "Hearing the Lord's winning words spoken in this way, the *gopīs* relinquished their distress at separation, but their aspirations increased from touching His limbs.
2. Govinda [Kṛṣṇa] began the *rāsa* pastime there, in the company of those devoted jewels of women, who linked arms happily together.
3. The festival of the *rāsa* dance began, featuring a circle of *gopīs*. The Lord of all *yogīs*, Kṛṣṇa, inserted Himself between each pair of *gopīs*, and put His arms about their necks. Each woman thought He was at her side only. Meanwhile, the sky was crowded with hundreds of the vehicles of the celestials, who were accompanied by their wives and carried away with excitement.
4. Kettledrums resounded then, streams of flowers fell, and the chiefs of the *gandharvas* and their wives sang of Kṛṣṇa's spotless glories.
5. There was a tumultuous sound of bracelets, ankle-bracelets, and the bells of the young women in the circle of the *rāsa* dance with their beloved.

6. Kṛṣṇa *Bhagavān*, the son of Devakī, was radiant in their company, like a great emerald in the midst of golden ornaments.
7. The consorts of Kṛṣṇa, their braids and belts securely fastened, sang about Him with hand gestures and dancing feet. Their faces were sweating, their earrings rolling on their cheeks, and the garments on their breasts slipping. Their waists were bent, and they smiled, their eyebrows playful. They shone like lightning in a circle of clouds.
8. They were intent on amorous pleasure and overjoyed by Kṛṣṇa's touch. Their throats decorated with dye, they sang loudly as they danced, and the world reverberated with their songs.
9. One *gopī* led a duet in harmony with Mukunda. Kṛṣṇa was pleased and praised her: 'Well done! Well done!' Then she led the refrain and He heaped praises on her.
10. Another, tired by the *rāsa* dance, her *mallikā* [jasmine] flowers and bracelets loosened, laid her arm on the shoulder of Kṛṣṇa, the wielder of the club, who was standing by her side.
11. Kṛṣṇa placed His arm on the shoulder of one of the *gopīs*. Smelling it, fragrant as a blue lotus and smeared with sandalwood, she kissed it, the hairs of her body tingling with rapture.
12. Kṛṣṇa gave His chewed betel nut to another *gopī* as she placed her cheek, adorned with the glitter of earrings in disarray from the dancing, next to His cheek.
13. Yet another *gopī* who was singing and dancing, her belt and ankle-bracelets jingling, became fatigued. She placed the soothing lotus hand of Acyuta, who was at her side, on her breast.
14. The *gopīs* won their lover Acyuta, who is the exclusive beloved of Śrī, the Goddess of Fortune. Their necks encircled by His arms, they delighted in Him as they sang.
15. The *gopīs*, with glowing faces, cheeks adorned with locks of hair, and lotus flowers behind their ears, were beautiful. They danced with the Lord in the circle of the *rāsa* to the musical accompaniment of the bees complemented by the sound of their anklets and bangles. Wreaths of flowers fell from their hair.
16. Thus Kṛṣṇa, the Lord of Lakṣmī,[62] sported with the beautiful girls of Vraj with freely playful smiles, amorous glances, and with caresses and embraces. He was like a child enraptured by His own reflection.
17. The senses of the women of Vraj were alive with pleasure from the contact of His limbs. Their ornaments and garlands were awry,

and the women could not keep their garments or their hair or the cloth covering their breasts in order, O best of the Kuru dynasty.

18. The women of the celestial realm traveling in the air were stricken with desire at seeing Kṛṣṇa's pastimes, and became entranced. The moon and its entourage [the stars] were full of wonder.

19. Although content within Himself, the Lord became manifest in as many forms as there were *gopī* women, and enjoyed Himself with them in *līlā* pastimes.

20. With great compassion, Kṛṣṇa lovingly caressed with His very soothing hands the face of those *gopīs* who were exhausted from the pleasures of love.

21. The *gopīs* paid homage to their hero with sideways looks and honeyed smiles. Their beautiful cheeks glowed with locks of hair and the glitter of golden earrings. Thrilled by the touch of Kṛṣṇa's fingernails, they sang of His auspicious deeds.

22. When he tired, Kṛṣṇa went into the water with them. He was pursued by bees, who [sang] like *gandharva* chiefs, because of his garland. Crushed by contact with the limbs of the *gopīs*, it was stained with the *kuṅkuma* powder from their breasts. Kṛṣṇa was like the king of the elephants who had lost all inhibitions with his female elephants.

23. With looks of love, the young women around Him laughed and splashed Him vigorously, O king! Worshipped with showers of *kusuma* flowers by the celestial beings in their aerial chariots, Kṛṣṇa disported Himself like an elephant in *līlā* pastimes, even though He is content within Himself.

24. Later, He strolled in the groves of the *Yamunā* river, surrounded by groups of young women and bees. The farthest corners of the river, both on land and on the waters, were pervaded by a wind bearing the fragrance of flowers. He was like an elephant exhilarated by the company of His female elephants.

25. Kṛṣṇa's desires are always fulfilled, and His propensity for enjoyment is fulfilled within Himself, but during all those nights He participated in this way in the company of throngs of young women. Such nights, brilliant with the rays of the moon, are the setting for *rasa* in both poetry and prose that describe autumn."

26. Parīkṣit said:

"God, the Lord of the Universe, has descended into the world along with His expansion [Balarāma] for the establishment of *dharma*, and for the suppression of *adharma*, non-*dharma*.[63]

27. He is the original speaker, exemplar, and protector of the injunctions of *dharma*. How could He behave in a manner contrary to *dharma*, O *brāhmaṇa*, by touching the wives of others?
28. The Lord of the Yadu dynasty, who is content within Himself, has performed an abhorrent deed. What was His purpose? You who are true to your vows, please take away our doubt."
29. *Śrī* Śuka said:
"Just as fire consumes everything [without being polluted], so it is seen that the blatant transgressions of *dharma* by the more powerful of rulers are not faults.
30. One who is not a powerful being should certainly never behave in that fashion, not even in his mind. Otherwise, acting out of foolishness, he will be destroyed; just as one who is not Śiva will be destroyed [by drinking] the poison churned from the ocean.[64]
31. The words of powerful beings are truth, and so is whatever is performed by them. The wise will act in accordance with their words.
32. O master, those who are devoid of personal ego do not accrue benefit for themselves through appropriate behavior, nor undesirable results through its opposite.
33. What, then, of the applicability of auspiciousness and inauspiciousness to the Supreme Being of all Supreme Beings and of all living entities, whether celestial, human, or animal?
34. Satisfied by worshipping the dust of Kṛṣṇa's lotus feet, even the sages act according to their own free will. The bondage of all their *karma* has been destroyed through the power of *yoga*, and so they are never bound. How, then, can one speak of bondage for Kṛṣṇa, who accepts forms according to His own will?
35. He lives within the *gopīs*, their husbands, and all living beings. He is the supreme witness who has assumed a form in this world for the purpose of sport.
36. Manifest in a human form, He indulges in such pastime as a favor to the devotees. Hearing about these, one becomes fully devoted to Him.
37. Confused by His power of illusion, the menfolk of Vraj were not resentful of Kṛṣṇa; each thought his own wife was present at his side.
38. The *gopīs* held the Lord dear. When the duration of Brahmā's night had expired,[65] they went home unwillingly with the approval of Vāsudeva.

39. The sober person who is endowed with faith should hear and describe these pastimes of Viṣṇu with the maidens of Vraj. Achieving supreme devotion to the Lord, one quickly frees oneself from lust, the disease of the heart."

The Vision of Kṛṣṇa

Bhāva Blueprint

We conclude part 3 with this passage on Kṛṣṇa's flute. (We break the sequence of the chapters in the tenth book here.) While the narrative prioritizes the madhura bhāva, *we see here that the entire landscape of Vraj bristles with ecstasy merely from hearing the sound of Kṛṣṇa's flute. The animals and plants noted here and in the previous passages experience an expression of* sānta bhāva, *which, as discussed in* "Rāga, Bhāva, *and* Rasa," *is a nonactive state of ecstatic absorption in Kṛṣṇa. In this regard, the passage points to the Vaiṣṇava understanding of Vaikuṇṭha and Goloka as realms made of pure consciousness, where even the flora, fauna, and natural landscape are conscious beings immersed in an eternal, ecstatic state of rapture in communion with God in accordance with their respective* bhāvas. *Nothing is inanimate. This passage thus gives a glimpse at what constitutes the eternal postmortem Kingdom of God and ultimate goal of Kṛṣṇa devotion for the liberated* bhaktas.

Book X, Chapter 21

1. Thus, Acyuta entered the [forest of Vṛndāvana] with the cows and cowherders. Its waters were clear because it was autumn, and it was cooled by breezes bearing the pleasant scents of lotuses.
2. Kṛṣṇa, the chief of the Madhu dynasty, along with the cowherding boys, penetrated deep into [the forest] while grazing the cows. Its mountains, rivers, and lakes reverberated with the sounds of flocks of birds and of restless bees in the flowering trees. Kṛṣṇa played His flute.
3. The women of Vraj heard that flute music—music which incites Kāma. Some of them described Kṛṣṇa to their confidantes in private.
4. Remembering the activities of Kṛṣṇa, they began to describe them, but their minds became so agitated with the power of Kāma that they were unable [to continue], O king.

5. As his glories were being sung by the band of *gopas*, Kṛṣṇa entered the forest of Vṛndā, which was pleasantly transformed by [the touch of] His feet. His form was that of a superb dancer. He wore a peacock feather head ornament, pericarps of lotus flowers on His ears, garments of a reddish-gold color, and a *vaijayantī* garland. The nectar of His lips filled the holes of His flute.
6. The sound of the flute steals the minds of all living things, O king. After hearing and describing it, the women of Vraj embraced each other.
7. The beautiful *gopīs* said: "We do not know of any higher reward for those who have eyes than this [sight of] the faces of those two sons of the chief of Vraj as they, with their companions, make the animals follow them, O girlfriends. With their two flutes their faces are enchanting, and they cast loving glances which are absorbed by those [who have eyes].
8. Dressed in a variety of garments twined about with garlands of lotuses, lilies, clusters of blossoms, peacock feathers, and mango tree sprouts, they are unmistakable as they shine amid the assembly of cowherders. They are like two actors sometimes singing on a stage.
9. O *gopīs*, what auspicious deed did this flute perform? It personally enjoys the *rasa* nectar from Dāmodara's [Kṛṣṇa's] lips—which should belong to the *gopīs*; whatever flavor is left over is all that remains [for us]. The rivers manifest bliss through their surfaces, and the trees shed tears, just like noble Āryan people.
10. O girlfriends, Vṛndāvana, which has acquired the riches of the lotus feet of the son of Devakī, is spreading the glories of the earth. All other living beings are stunned after seeing the ecstatic peacocks from the mountain ridges dance to Govinda's [Kṛṣṇa's] flute.
11. These female does are lucky, even though they are in an ignorant birth. When they hear the flute playing of the beautifully dressed son of Nanda, they, along with the spotted antelopes, offer worship with glances of love.
12. Kṛṣṇa's nature and form are a delight for women—the celestial women became captivated when they saw it and heard the distinctive tunes played on his flute. The flowers from their braids dropped out, and the belts from their waists slipped off as they went about on celestial air-vehicles, their hearts agitated by Kāma.
13. The cows, their ears pricked, were also drinking the nectar of the flute music coming from Kṛṣṇa's mouth. The calves stood transfixed

with their mouths full of milk from the dripping udders. Shedding tears, in their hearts they caressed Govinda with their eyes.

14. It is a wonderful thing, O mother! In all probability, the birds in this forest are sages. They fly up to the branches of the trees that are covered with sweet fresh leaves, and, with unblinking eyes, listen to the melodious tunes of the flute coming from Kṛṣṇa. They make no other noise.

15. The rivers found their force disrupted by their state of mind after hearing the sound of Mukunda's flute, as could be seen from their whirlpools. Bearing offerings of lotus flowers, they grasped the two lotus feet of Murāri [Kṛṣṇa] and embraced them closely with their arms in the form of waves.

16. The water-bearing cloud saw Kṛṣṇa playing the flute as He was herding the animals of Vraj with Balarāma and the *gopas* in the heat. Bursting with love, it ascended with streams of flowers [in the form of rain], and with its own body spread out a large umbrella for its friend.

17. The *pulinda* women experienced the pain of Kāma from seeing Kṛṣṇa. Taking up from the grass the beautiful *kuṅkuma* powder that had decorated the breasts of the women and was red from the lotus feet of Urugāya [Kṛṣṇa], they smeared it on their faces and breasts, let go of their distress and became enchanted.

18. Look at this mountain, O women. It is overjoyed to be touched by Balarāma's and Kṛṣṇa's feet! It is the best of the servants of Hari because it honors those Two, as well as the herds of cows, by [gifts] of radishes, caves, good pasturage, and water.

19. O girlfriends, when those Two, conspicuous by Their cords and ropes for tying cows, lead the cows and cowherd boys into nearby forests, those embodied beings who are capable of movement are made motionless by the sounds of that renowned flute with its sweet harmonies. The trees bristle with ecstasy—it is a wonderful thing."

20. Discussing in this way the pastimes of *Bhagavān*, who was wandering around in Vṛndāvana, the *gopīs* entered into a state of complete absorption in Him.

PART IV

Caitanya's *Śikṣāṣṭakam*

The Eight Verses of Instruction

*While Caitanya imparted extensive teachings to Rūpa and Sanātana Gosvāmī, which are essentially the new revelations underpinning the specifics of the Gauḍīya theology outlined in part 1, he himself wrote only these eight (*aṣṭha*) verses of instruction (*sikṣā*).*

The first verse is highly embellished in terms of the literary ornamentations, alaṅkāra, *of Sanskrit poetics,* kāvya *(that is, replete with similes and metaphors), which aesthetically frame in a poetic manner the theological points imparted.*

1. May Kṛṣṇa's *saṅkīrtana* be supremely triumphant. The chanting of the names of Kṛṣṇa cleanses the mirror of the heart. It extinguishes the great forest fire of *saṁsāra*. It bestows moonlight on the white night-blooming lotus of supreme benefit.[1] It gives life to the young bride of wisdom. It increases the ocean of bliss. It bestows the taste of the highest nectar at every step. It cleanses the mind completely.

2. You have manifested many names and invested them with all Your potency. There are no restrictions as to when to chant them, the only criterion is absorbing the mind in them. Despite this grace of Yours, O *Bhagavān*, my misfortune is such that I was born in this world without any attraction for them.

3. The name of Hari should always be chanted while considering oneself lower than a blade of grass, and while being more tolerant than a tree. One should be free from any desire for personal respect, but yet one should offer respect to others.

4. I do not desire wealth, followers, beautiful women, or poetic virtuosity, O Lord of the Universe. I wish only for *bhakti* for You, *Īśvara*, that is without any motive, birth after birth.
5. O son of Nanda. Please consider me to be Your servant who has fallen into the dangerous ocean of *saṁsāra*. Consider me to be like a speck of dust attached to Your lotus feet.
6. When will streams of tears pour from my eyes from chanting Your name? When will my voice clog up and falter with emotion? When will my body appear with its hairs bristling in ecstasy?[2]
7. In the absence of Govinda, the blinking of an eye seems like an entire *yuga* aeon, the eyes behave like the rainy season, and this entire universe appears empty.
8. I am devoted to Kṛṣṇa's feet. He may embrace me, or crush me. Or He may pierce my heart by not appearing before me. That flirt may do as He pleases, but only He and no one else will remain the Lord of my life.

PART V

The *Nārada Bhakti Sūtras*

Athāto bhaktiṁ vyākhyāsyāmaḥ
1. Now we will explain *bhakti* in detail.

Sā tv asmin parama-prema-rūpā
2. In this matter, the nature of *bhakti* is supreme love.
or:
The nature of *bhakti* is supreme love for Him *(Bhagavān)*.

Amṛta-svarūpā ca
3. And its nature is eternal nectar.

Yal labdhvā pumān siddho bhavati amṛto bhavati tṛpto bhavati
4. When a person attains *bhakti*, he or she becomes perfected, he or she becomes immortal, and he or she becomes fully satisfied.

Yat prāpya na kiñcid vāñchati na śocati na dveṣṭi na ramate notsāhī bhavati
5. After attaining it, a person does not desire, lament over, hate, enjoy, or show enthusiasm for anything else.

Yaj jñātva matto bhavati stabdho bhavati ātmārāmo bhavati
6. Once one knows it, one becomes mad with love, one becomes overwhelmed with ecstasy, and one finds bliss in the self.

Sā na kāmayamānā nirodha-rūpatvāt
7. It is not caused by lust; its nature is cessation.

Nirodhas tu loka-veda-vyāpāra-nyāsaḥ
8. "Cessation" means the renouncing of all Vedic (that is, mundane ritualistic) and worldly activities.

Tasminn ananyatā tad-virodhiṣūdāsīnatā ca
9. And also exclusive devotion to *Īśvara* and disinterest in everything contrary to that.

Anyāśrayāṇāṁ tyāgo 'nanyatā
10. "Exclusive devotion" means relinquishing any other refuge [other than *Īśvara*].

Loka-vedeṣu tad-anukūlācaraṇaṁ tad-virodhiṣūdāsīnatā
11. "Disinterest to everything contrary to that" means engaging [only] in activities favorable to that goal, whether in everyday or in Vedic duties.

Bhavatu niścaya-dārḍhyād ūrdhvaṁ śāstra-rakṣaṇām
12. Even after becoming fixed in one's commitment [to *Bhagavān*], the injunctions of scripture should be respected.

Anyathā pātitya-śaṅkayā
13. Otherwise there is danger of falling [from the spiritual path].

Loko 'pi tāvad eva bhojanādi-vyāpāras tv āśarīra-dhāraṇāvadhi
14. And in everyday duties, too, there should be activities such as eating and the like, to the extent necessary for maintaining the body for its duration of life.

Tal-lakṣaṇāni vācyante nānāmata-bhedāt
15. The sages describe the characteristics of *bhakti* variously, in accordance with different points of view.

Pūjādiṣv anurāga iti pārāśaryaḥ
16. Vyāsa says *bhakti* is love of doing *pūjā* and other such devotional activities.

Kathādiṣv iti gargaḥ
17. Garga says *bhakti* is love of *kathā*—hearing about the narrations of *Bhagavān*'s activities and incarnations.

Ātma-raty-avirodheneti śāṇḍilyaḥ
18. Śāṇḍilya says it is that which does not obstruct delighting in the *ātman*.

Nāradas tu tadarpitākhilācāratā tad-vismaraṇe parama-vyākulateti
19. But Nārada says it is offering all acts to God and feeling extreme anguish upon not remembering Him.

Asty evam evam
20. It is just like that, it is just like that.

Yathā vraja-gopikānām
21. Just as was exemplified by the *gopīs* of Vraja.

Tatrāpi na māhātmya jñāna-vismṛty apavādaḥ
22. In their particular case, there is no fault in the *gopīs* not being mindful of God's greatness.[1]

Tad-vihīnaṁ jārāṇām iva
23. [Normally] without such mindfulness, love is just like that of mundane lovers.

Nāsty eva tasmin tat-sukha-sukhitvam
24. In such mundane love, happiness is not from the *happiness* of the beloved [as is the case with the divine love of the *gopīs* but is self-centered].

Sā tu karma-jñāna-yogebhyo 'py-adhikatarā
25. *Bhakti* is superior to ritualistic activity, knowledge, and the practice of *yoga*.

Phala-rūpatvāt
26. Because it is the [ultimate] fruit [of all of these].

Īśvarasyāpy abhimāni-dveṣitvāt dainya-priyatvāc ca
27. God is averse to the proud and fond of humility.[2]

Tasyā jñānam eva sādhanam ity eke
28. Some say that only knowledge is the means to *bhakti*.

Anyonyāśrayatvam ity eke
29. Some say that the two are interdependent.

Svayaṁ phala-rūpateti brahma-kumāraḥ
30. Nārada, the son of Brahmā, says *bhakti* is its own self-manifesting fruit.

Rāja-gṛha-bhojanādiṣu tathaiva dṛṣṭatvāt
31. This can be understood from the examples of a king's palace or of food.

Na tena rājā paritoṣaḥ kṣuc-chāntir va
32. The king is not satisfied by knowledge [about a theoretical palace], nor is hunger appeased by knowledge [of food].

Tasmāt saiva grāhyā mumukṣubhiḥ
33. Therefore only *bhakti* should be accepted by those desiring liberation.

Tasyāḥ sādhanāni gāyanty ācāryāḥ
34. Great teachers sing about the means of attaining *bhakti*.

Tat tu viṣaya-tyāgāt saṅga-tyāgāc ca
35. It comes from renouncing sense objects and renouncing attachments.

Avyāvṛtta-bhajanāt
36. It comes from unceasing worship.

Loke 'pi bhagavad-guṇa-śravaṇa-kīrtanāt
37. And it comes from chanting and hearing about the qualities of *Bhagavān*, even while one is engaged in worldly duties.

Mukhyatas-tu mahat-kṛpayaiva bhagavat-kṛpāleśād vā
38. But primarily, it comes from the compassion of the great saints or from a drop of *Bhagavān*'s compassion.

Mahat-saṅgas tu durlabho 'gamyo 'moghaś ca
39. The association of great saints is hard to achieve, difficult to understand, and infallible.

Labhyate 'pi tat kṛpayaiva
40. And it too is attained by the grace of *Bhagavān.*

Tasmins taj-jane bhedābhāvāt
41. Because there is no difference between Him and His devotees.

Tad eva sādhyatāṁ tad eva sādhyatām
42. Seek that association only, seek that only.

Duḥ-saṅgaḥ sarvathaiva tyājyaḥ
43. Bad association should be completely given up.

Kāma-krodha-moha-smṛti bhraṁśa-buddhi nāśa-sarva nāśa-kāraṇatvāt
44. Because it is the cause of lust, anger, illusion, confusion of memory, loss of intelligence, and the loss of everything.

Taraṅgāyitā apīme saṅgāt samudrāyanti
45. Although these are like waves, from association, they become like an ocean.

Kas tarati kas tarati māyām? yaḥ saṅgaṁ tyajati yo mahānubhāvaṁ sevate nirmamo bhavati
46. Who crosses over, who crosses over *māyā*? The one who gives up attachment, the one who serves a great devotee, and the one who becomes free from ego.

Yo vivikta-sthānaṁ sevate yo loka-bandham unmūlayati nistraiguṇyo bhavati yoga-kṣemaṁ tyajati
47. The one who resorts to a solitary place, who uproots all worldly

connections, who transcends the three *guṇas* (*sattva*, *rajas*, and *tamas*), and who renounces all clinging to security.

Yaḥ karma-phalaṁ tyajati karmāṇī sannyasyati tato nirdvandvo bhavati
48. The one who gives up the fruit of work and renounces activity and thereby transcends duality.

Yo vedān api sannyasyati kevalam avicchinnānurāgam labhate
49. One who gives up even the Vedas, attains exclusive and unceasing devotion.

Sa tarati sa tarati sa lokāṅs-tārayati
50. It is such a person who crosses over *māyā*, it is such a person who crosses over; and such a person causes others to cross over.

Anirvacanīyaṁ prema-svarūpam
51. The essence of love is beyond the ability of words to describe.

Mūkāsvādanavat
52. Like taste is beyond the ability of words to describe for a mute person.

Prakāśyate kvāpi pātre
53. It is revealed wherever there is a worthy vessel.

Guṇa-rahitaṁ kāmanā-rahitaṁ pratikṣaṇa-vardhamānam avicchinnaṁ sūkṣmataram anubhava-rūpam
54. It takes the form of a very subtle experience that is transcendent to the *guṇas*, devoid of all desires, uninterrupted, and ever-increasing.

Tat prāpya tad evāvalokayati tad eva śṛṇoti tad eva bhāṣayati tad eva cintayati
55. After obtaining it, one sees only *Bhagavān*, hears only about *Bhagavān*, speaks only about *Bhagavān*, and thinks only about *Bhagavān*.

Gauṇī tridhā guṇa-bhedād ārtādi-bhedād vā
56. Inferior *bhakti* is of three kinds, depending on the three *guṇas* or depending on the differences in material needs and other such things.

Uttarasmād uttarasmāt pūrva-pūrvā śreyāya bhavati
57. Each of these is successively higher than the previous one in terms of the ultimate goal.[3]

Anyasmāt saulabhyaṁ bhaktau
58. It is easier to attain success in *bhakti* than through other [paths].

Pramāṇāntarasyānapekṣatvāt svayaṁ pramāṇatvāt
59. It does not need to be proved by any other means, because it is its own proof.

Śānti-rūpāt paramānanda-rupāc ca
60. This is because its essence is peacefulness and its essence is supreme bliss.

Loka-hānau cintā na kāryā niveditātma-loka-vedatvāt
61. There should be no concern about the loss of worldly things, because Vedic and worldly things and one's very self have been dedicated [to God].

Na tat siddhau loka-vyavahāro heyaḥ kintu phala-tyāgas tat-sādhanaṁ ca kāryam eva
62. As long as *bhakti* has not been achieved, worldly and Vedic duties should not be abandoned; however, the fruits of action should be renounced, and devotional practices should be maintained.

Strī-dhana-nāstika-caritraṁ na śravaṇīyam
63. One should not listen to topics that are atheistic or related to wealth or sex.

Abhimāna-dambhādikaṁ tyājyam
64. Pride, arrogance, and other such things should be renounced.

Tad-arpitākhilācāraḥ san kāma-krodhābhimānādikaṁ tasminn eva karaṇīyam
65. All one's activities should be offered to *Bhagavān*, and even if desire, anger, pride, and the like are present, even they also should be offered to Him alone.

Tri-rūpa-bhaṅga-pūrvakaṁ nitya dāsya-nitya kāntā-bhajanātmakaṁ prema kāryaṁ premaiva kāryam.
66. The three types of *bhakti* noted previously should be transcended, and one should engage in love, one should engage only in love, in the devotional mood of the eternal servant or the eternal lover.[4]

Bhaktā ekāntino mukhyāḥ
67. The foremost devotees are those who are exclusively devoted.

Kaṇṭhāvarodha-romāñcāśrubhiḥ parasparaṁ lapamānāḥ pāvayanti kulāni pṛthivīṁ ca
68. Conversing with one another with tears in their eyes and their hair standing on end and their voices choking in ecstasy, they purify their family lineages and the whole world.

Tīrthīkurvanti tīrthāni sukarmīkurvanti karmāṇi sac-chāstrīkurvanti śāstrāṇi
69. It is they who make holy places holy, it is they who make ordinary activity into pious activity, and it is they who make teachings into true scripture.

Tanmāyāḥ
70. They are completely absorbed in *Īśvara.*

Modante pitaro nṛtyanti devatāḥ sa-nāthā ceyaṁ bhūr bhavati
71. [Because of their presence], the forefathers rejoice, the celestial beings dance, and this earth feels cared for.

Nāsti teṣu jāti-vidyā-rūpa-kula-dhana-kriyādi-bhedaḥ
72. Among these devotees, there is no discrimination based on birth, learning, beauty, family lineage, wealth, or occupation.

Yatas tadīyāḥ
73. This is because they belong to *Bhagavān.*

Vādo nāvalambyaḥ
74. Philosophical debate should not be relied upon.

Bāhulyāvakāśatvād aniyatatvāc ca
75. Because it is inconclusive and because there are so many points of view.

Bhakti-śāstrāṇi mananīyāni tad-bodha-karmāṇī karaṇīyāni
76. Scriptures on *bhakti* should be followed, and activities that awaken *bhakti* should be performed.

Sukha-duḥkhecchā-lābhādi tyakte kāle pratīkṣamāṇe kṣaṇārdham api vyarthaṁ na neyam
77. Not even half a moment should be wasted, as one passes one's time free of happiness and distress, desire, and gain.

Ahiṁsā-satya-śauca-dayāstikyādi cāritryāṇī paripālanīyāni
78. Nonviolence, truthfulness, cleanliness, compassion, and faith are the behaviors that should be upheld.

Sarvadā sarvabhāvena niścintair bhagavān eva bhajanīyaḥ
79. God alone should always be worshipped with all one's heart and without any worry.

Sa kīrtyamānaḥ śīghram evāvirbhavaty anubhāvayati bhaktān
80. Being glorified, God quickly manifests to the devotees and gives them direct experience.

Trisatyasya bhaktir eva garīyasī bhaktir eva garīyasī
81. From the three Truths,[5] *bhakti* alone is the highest truth, *bhakti* alone.

Guṇa-māhātmyāsakti-rūpāsakti-pūjāsakti-smaraṇāsakti-dāsyā-sakti-sakhyāsakti-vātsalyāsakti-kāntāsakty ātmanivedanāsakti-tanmayatāsakti-paramavirahāsakti-rūpaikadhā api ekādaśadhā bhavati
82. Although it is one, *bhakti* has eleven forms: attachment to the glories of *Bhagavān*'s qualities, attachment to His beauty, attachment to His worship, attachment to remembering Him, attachment to being His servant, attachment to being His friend, attachment to being His parent, attachment to being His lover, attachment to surrendering

one's whole being to Him, attachment to being one in essence with Him, attachment to feeling separation from Him.

Ity evaṃ vadanti jana-jalpa-nirbhayā eka-matāḥ kumāra vyāsa śuka śāṇḍilya garga viṣṇu kauṇḍinya śeṣoddhavāruṇi bali hanumad vibhīṣaṇādayo bhaktyācāryāḥ
83. So say all with one opinion irrespective of public opinion, the great teachers of *bhakti*: the Kumāras, Vyāsa, Śuka, Śāṇḍilya, Garga, Viṣṇu, Kauṇḍinya, Śeṣa, Uddhava, Āruṇi, Bali, Hanumān, Vibhīṣaṇa, and others.

Ya idaṁ nārada-proktaṁ śivānuśāsanaṁ viśvas iti śraddhate sa bhaktimān bhavati saḥ preṣṭhaṁ labhate saḥ preṣṭhaṁ labhate iti
84. One who believes with faith these teachings of Nārada, becomes endowed with *bhakti*; such a one attains the beloved, such a one attains the beloved.

APPENDIX I

APPENDIX II

GLOSSARY

NOTES

BIBLIOGRAPHY

Appendix I

Establishing the Authority of the *Bhāgavata Purāṇa* in the Vedic Tradition

On what grounds does the Gauḍīya Vaiṣṇava tradition authenticate its elaborate theology of Kṛṣṇa *bhakti*? It recognizes a number of *pramāṇas*, sources of knowledge, from which, like the *Yoga Sūtras* (I.7), it prioritizes sense perception, inference, and sacred texts. Since the senses and human reason are subject to defects and the limitations of human error, it also adopts the Vedānta stance that sacred testimony is the only fully reliable source of knowledge in those areas, such as the nature of God, that lie beyond the empirical domain (*Vedānta Sūtras* I.1.3). But is all sacred text qualitatively the same? The Gauḍīya Vaiṣṇava theology rests on the authority of the *Bhāgavata Purāṇa*, which it deems the paramount scripture. But what makes the *Bhāgavata* preeminent in the first place? By considering Jīva's arguments prioritizing the epistemological superexcellence of the *Bhāgavata* on the textual landscape of his time, we will encounter an example of traditional Vedānta hermeneutics.

Let us start at the beginning. The backdrop to the Purāṇa literatures is the Vedic culture. The oldest preserved literatures in India are the four Vedas (typically dated from the fifteenth to the twelfth century B.C.E.), which primarily contain hymns recited in the ritualistic context of the ancient Vedic sacrificial cult of the Indo-Aryans. To these Vedas, prose instructional manuals were later appended called the Brāhmaṇas (the term applies to the texts as well as the caste specialists who transmitted and enacted their rituals). In addition to these, the Vedic corpus includes two other strata or genres of literatures: the Āraṇyakas, which, overlapping in subject matter much of the material contained in the older Brāhmaṇa texts, on the one hand, and the later fourth stratum, the Upaniṣads, on the other, do not have a distinctive characteristic of their own and thus need not detain us; and the Upaniṣads. It is in the Upaniṣads that material clearly matriarchal to what comes to be associated with "Hinduism," both philosophical and devotional, is rooted. In other words, it is in the Upaniṣads, seminal to the later classical schools of Indian philosophy as well as to the contemporary devotional traditions in the Purāṇas, that the origins of *bhakti yoga* are to be found.

The four Vedas, fixed at a very early stage by various mnemonic devices,[1] along with the other three strata constituting the Vedic corpus, are considered *Śruti,* "that which is heard," eternally existent divine revelation. In contrast with these, the Purāṇas, along with all other pan-Indic classical texts such as the epics, are considered *Smṛti,* "that which is remembered," or indirect revelation, divine in origin but composed through human agency (albeit an agency usually associated with a divine figure). While they are considered sacred and authoritative, there are much more flexible expectations associated with the Purāṇas, which transmit information for the general public, and thus adjustments according to the day and age are not viewed askance. On the one hand, they recognize the need to preserve and transmit faithfully the ancient sacred material intact. But, on the other, they claim to clarify, expand upon, and even supersede the contents of previous scriptures by revealing secret truths not contained either in the Vedas or in other Purāṇas (in fact, they expand on and supersede the contents of the *Śruti* enormously). They are ongoing revelation. Such fluidity is inherent in the claim made by most Purāṇas of presenting the "essence" of the Veda according to time and place, as we shall see.

Nonetheless, and very important for our purposes, in Vedānta circles, the *Smṛti* such as the Purāṇas is considered authoritative only when it does not contradict the *Śruti.*[2] The old Vedic corpus thus retains a sense of authority in later times, even when the rituals that are the central feature of the latter had long fallen into disuse (or been radically reconfigured). The important point here is that, considered not of human authorship (*apauruṣeya*) by all Vedic schools,[3] these *Śrūti* texts were deemed infallible revelation, even as much of their content was being viewed dismissively and superseded in the later traditions such as the Purāṇas, as noted above. But (officially, at least) the status of *Śruti* retains its aura of paramount infallibility in comparison with the later texts that emerged on the religious landscape of India. What this means is that any later school wishing to consider itself "Vedic," howsoever nominally, and thus be accepted as bona fide, had to develop hermeneutical strategies to somehow locate its theology and soteriology somewhere in the four Vedic strata—unlike, for example, Buddhism and Jainism, which simply jettisoned the Vedic corpus and established new traditions (albeit with their own claimed lines of preexisting authority).

But how do they accomplish this? Although it certainly has some clear proto-roots in the old Vedic corpus in many areas, how does a text like the *Bhāgavata* locate itself in the *Śruti*, when it contains in other areas a theology, ontology, cosmology, soteriology, set of sociocultural specificities, sense of historicality, and, in short, entire worldview with, at best, tenuous Vedic connections and, in other areas again, no Vedic precedents whatsoever? One need only consider the fact that there is simply no reference to the Kṛṣṇa of the *Bhāgavata*, the summum bonum of the entire text, in any Vedic (*Śruti*) text other than a solitary dubious passage in the *Chāndogya Upaniṣad* (indisputable references to Kṛṣṇa as a Divine Being do not occur in significant numbers of Sanskrit textual sources until the fifth and fourth centuries B.C.E. and then soon thereafter also in early Greek, as well as archaeological, sources).[4] How does an exegete of a sect-specific Purāṇic tradition for whom Vedic pedigree is indispensable deal with this?

Since we have selected Jīva as our lens into traditional hermeneutics and guide to the text, let us consider how he goes about resolving this dilemma of authenticating the *Bhāgavata* as a bona fide scriptural source of knowledge, upon which the entire edifice of Kṛṣṇa *bhakti* rests. Since Jīva's *Sandarbhas* are essentially commentaries on the *Bhāgavata*, in order for them to be taken seriously as a source of knowledge, he must first of all establish sacred scripture in general as a valid episteme,[5] then make a case for the Purāṇic genre as a serious scriptural source, and finally indicate why he is devoting his exclusive attention to the *Bhāgavata* rather than any other Purāṇa.

Accordingly, Jīva briefly situates himself within the Vedānta epistemological tradition that accepts scripture as the highest source of knowledge. As heir to this tradition, he need not reformulate the extensive and well-known argumentation honed within the *pūrva mīmāṁsā* and *uttara mīmāṁsā* (Vedānta) lineages over the centuries.[6] Indeed, scriptural authority is accepted by all Vedic-derived "Hindu" traditions,[7] so discussions between schools revolved around which source of knowledge should be awarded primary status and which secondary and supportive, especially between scripture (*āgama/śabda*) and the two other primary alternative modes of knowing: knowledge acquired through the senses (*pratyakṣa*, empiricism) and through inferential reasoning (*anumāna*, logic).[8] For Jīva and the Vedāntins, while the latter two sources are important epistemes, they are subject to four human defects: the imperfection of the senses themselves, and human subjectivity to delusion, error, and the cheating propensity. Besides, the senses cannot be expected to provide knowledge of that which lies beyond their sphere of perception. As for inferential reasoning derived from (and dependent upon) the senses, "Logic cannot establish anything conclusively" (*Vedānta Sūtras* II.1.11), so "one should not try to employ logic for that which lies beyond the sphere of thought" (*Mahābhārata, Bhīṣma Parva* V.22; quoted in the *Tattva Sandarbha anu* 11). For such reasons, for the Vedānta traditions that by Jīva's time had long been prominent in intellectual circles across India in general,[9] the Vedas (and here they primarily intend the Upaniṣads) are the only source of knowledge for transempirical, transrational topics, as they are deemed trans-human revelation handed down intact via lineages, the *paramparās*[10] (*Tattva Sandarbha anu* 10).

So Jīva's claiming the primacy of scripture was not a particularly controversial thing to do, even as other schools prioritized other sources of knowledge. But there are now several steps missing between the *Śruti* as universally recognized scripture par excellence, the Purāṇas in general, and the *Bhāgavata* in particular. Here, too, Jīva has long-established Vaiṣṇava and Śaivite forerunners, as these traditions had long and thoroughly (throughout two millennia) permeated the intellectual landscape of India by the sixteenth century. So Jīva is able to avail of two well-known verses from the *Śruti* itself: one, from the *Bṛhadāraṇyaka Upaniṣad*, stating: "The *Ṛg-Veda, Yajur-Veda, Sāma-Veda, Atharva-Veda,* Itihāsa [epics], and Purāṇa were breathed out by the great Being" (II.4.10); the other, from the *Chāndogya Upaniṣad*, where the Itihāsa and Purāṇas are called "the fifth Veda" (VII.1.2). These are echoed by statements from another *Śruti*, the *Taittirīya Āraṇyaka*,[11] as well as the widely accepted *Smṛti* text, the *Mahābhārata*,[12] all bestowing authority on the epics and Purāṇas as the fifth Veda and as augmenting the Vedas. Thus he has invoked the *Śruti* itself to promote the Purāṇas as authoritative scriptural sources on a par with *Śruti*. Even better, he then quotes a statement "*pūraṇāt purāṇam*: the Purāṇas [are so called] because they complete,"[13] to argue that these texts are in fact indispensable for understanding the very Vedas themselves.[14]

Having done this, and with the authority of the Purāṇas as a genre now legitimated by the *Śruti*, Jīva next produces numerous quotes from the other Purāṇas themselves as to the preeminence of the *Bhāgavata* within the *Purāṇic* corpus—the verses quoted previously in "*Īśvara*, Pure *Bhakti*, and Motivated *Bhakti*" from the *Matsya Purāṇa* and *Padma Purāṇa*, dividing the eighteen Purāṇas according to *guṇas* with the *Bhāgavata* in the *sattva* category.[15] With this established, Jīva feels that he can now quote the *Bhāgavata* itself to bolster its indispensability as a tool to understanding the *Vedas*, without needing to further demonstrate its credential as a source of knowledge. We will return to this shortly.

In Purāṇic narrative, as we will see in the Tale of Vyāsa, the hymns of the Vedas, along with the Purāṇic stories, were transmitted orally through the first three of the four *yugas*, or world ages—the *satya*, *tretā*, and *dvāpara yugas*. Then, with a view to preserving the material from the ravages of time heralded by the beginning of the present degenerate fourth world age of *Kali yuga*,[16] the great sage Vyāsa ("the divider") divided the originally single ur-Veda into the four.[17] Additionally, he is held to have composed the *Vedānta Sūtras*, which was written to clarify the seemingly contradictory nature of the Upaniṣads.[18] Vyāsa then compiled a *Purāṇa Saṃhitā*, or singular ur-Purāṇa text, from the tales, lore, anecdotes, and teachings that had been handed down through the ages. This original Purāṇa text was then further divided by his disciples into the eighteen known to later tradition.[19] In addition to his role as divider of the Vedas and compiler of the Purāṇas, Vyāsa is the traditional author of the enormous one-hundred-thousand-verse *Mahābhārata* epic (composed, like the Purāṇas, for those who had no access to the Veda owing to social restrictions, *SB* I.4.25). As compiler of both the Vedic corpus and the Purāṇic one, Vyāsa is thus deemed by the *Bhāgavata* to be the foremost authority on both the *Śruti* and the *Smṛti* (and tradition even assigns him the role of author of the primary and canonical commentary on the *Yoga Sūtras*, the Vyāsa *bhāṣa*).

We will see in the *Bhāgavata* (I.5.iff.) that Vyāsa remained unfulfilled even after this massive and prolific output of knowledge, until his *guru*, sage Nārada, confirmed his suspicion that the cause of his despondency was that he had not yet described the ultimate goal of knowledge—he had thus far covered only lesser mundane topics concerned mostly with material well-being. This diagnosis resulted in the composition of the *Bhāgavata*, the *galitam phalam,* the ripened fruit of the Vedic tree (I.1.3), the essence of all the Vedas, Purāṇas, and Itihāsa epics (I.2.3; I.3.42). Here we see an excellent example of how a Purāṇa positions itself as superseding the Vedas, but the point in all this is that the *Bhāgavata* depicts Vyāsa, the author and composer or systematizer of just about all the most important sacred texts associated with the Vedic and late Vedic period and thus the ultimate authority on the *Śruti* and *Smṛti*, as himself acknowledging the primacy of the *Bhāgavata* among all other scriptures. Additionally, the *Bhāgavata* was mystically revealed to him, as we will see, making Vyāsa an experiential authority in addition to being a scriptural savant. Jīva has now arrived at a point where the *Bhāgavata* is a defensible and indeed preeminent source of knowledge in its own right.

From an academic text-critical historical point of view, there is little doubt that some of the material in the Purāṇas does go back to the earliest Vedic age. Many of the Vedic hymns assume common knowledge of bygone persons and events to which they briefly allude and which would have been remembered through tradition, and some of these are fleshed out and reworked over time in the Purāṇas.[20] As early as the *Atharva-Veda* of circa 1000 B.C.E., there are references to "the" Purāṇa[21] and numerous references to it in the later Vedic texts. Thus, while the present Purāṇas contain later material, as well as references to events in historical time, they also contain ancient narratives and anecdotes reworked from the earliest period of protohistory in southern Asia. (And it is for such reasons that it is futile to speak of absolute dates for any Purāṇa as a whole, since one would have to speak of the age of individual sections within particular Purāṇas; one can venture to estimate the final date of a Purāṇa's composition only in its extant form.)[22]

And as far as the Kṛṣṇa co-relatable to the *Bhāgavata* Kṛṣṇa is concerned, although He does not surface on the historical landscape of ancient India as derived from (academically dated) textual and archaeological sources until a few centuries prior to the Common Era, there is at least one point of overlap between traditional knowledge sources prioritizing the authority of *Śruti* and *Smṛti* and our modern ones prioritizing empirico-deductive methods. One point common to all sources is that Kṛṣṇa appears at the end of some sort of age—be it the late Vedic age as construed by Indological historiography or the very end of the *dvāpara-yuga* third age as proposed by traditional bodies of knowledge such as the epics and Purāṇas. And there is agreement that Kṛṣṇa is pivotal in the inauguration of a new age—the rise of the *bhakti* movements prior to the turn of the Common Era that swept across the subcontinent, relegating the old Vedic rites to quasi-redundant, or radically reconfigured, forms as documented by historians and the beginning of the *Kali yuga* in traditional epic and Purāṇic narrative, which is held to do similar sorts of things, by tradition.

Jīva still has much hermeneutical work left to do. Not only must the *Bhāgavata*'s essential message be tailored to embody and also supersede those of the Vedas, but the specifics of the Kṛṣṇa theology of his sixteenth-century lineage must also be accommodated within the *Bhāgavata*. This latter task is accomplished fairly effortlessly, that is to say organically, for much of the material that occupied the concern of this volume, *bhakti yoga*, but already by the end of part 1 (in the chapter "The Practices of Bhakti"), where we encountered the more advanced stages of *rāgānugā* and *rāgātmikā bhakti*, Jīva and Rūpa entered into transcendent domains that are nowhere to be explicitly found even in the *Bhāgavata*. Even from a traditional exegetical point of view, these must be acknowledged to be as implicitly "concealed" in the *Bhāgavata* as is Kṛṣṇa Himself in the *Śruti*. In fact, Jīva's tradition itself lays claim to transmitting hitherto unrevealed Truths imparted by Caitanya to the *Gosvāmīs*, especially Rūpa and Sanātana. And Caitanya is deemed to be an incarnation of Kṛṣṇa by this tradition (again on the basis of verses scattered throughout the Purāṇas),[23] which is the basis upon which his teachings are considered authoritative in turn. So while in effect we are dealing with new revelation, traditional exegesis is uncomfortable with the idea of "new" revelation, as Truth is eternal; so it cannot be newly created, even as it may be revealed fully or partially according to time and place. So Jīva and the *Gośvamīs* set out to anchor Caitanya's teachings to the larger *Śruti* and *Smṛti* corpus in similar sorts of ways as the *Bhāgavata* is legitimized. Following them in this endeavor would take us too far afield, but hopefully this brief overview of how the *Bhāgavata* itself has been authenticated has afforded some sense of the world of Vedānta exegesis.

Given its well-established roots on the Indian subcontinent, and its recent exportation to the West,[24] we thus find in the tradition of Gauḍīya Vaiṣṇava Kṛṣṇa *bhakti* an excellent example of a "living" tradition, with its tensions and resolutions in matters of epistemological authoritativeness, its periodic revelatory "updates," and its ongoing dialogue with its ever-evolving greater intellectual context, all of which lie at the very core of the phenomenon of religion in general, and certainly of the vibrant and variegated Hindu *bhakti* traditions.

Appendix II: Sāṅkhya Chart

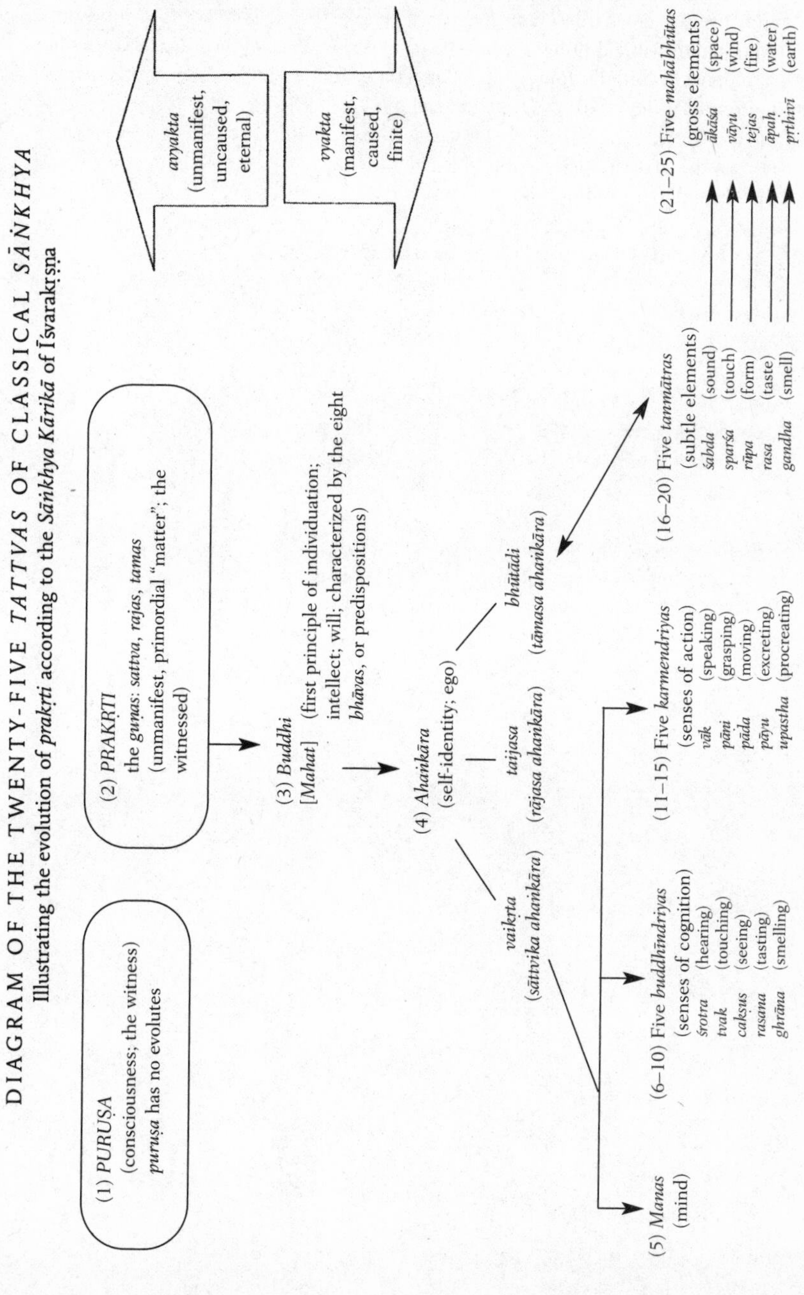

Glossary

Acyuta, name of Viṣṇu/Kṛṣṇa (one who never falls down; the infallible Lord).
Adhokṣaja, name of Viṣṇu/Kṛṣṇa.
advaita, philosophy of nondualism.
aho!, an exclamation in Sanskrit, with various meanings from alarm and despair to surprise or appreciation, depending on context.
aṁśa, partial incarnation of Viṣṇu or Kṛṣṇa.
ānanda, bliss.
Antaryāmī, form of Viṣṇu who pervades the *ātman* and all reality.
anuccheda (*anu*), a section of a *Sandarbha*.
apsarā, a type of celestial being.
artha, prosperity; one of the traditional four goals of human life (*puruṣārthas*).
Ārya, a follower of civilized Vedic culture.
asamprajñāta, final stage of *samādhi*; consciousness absorbed in its own nature.
āsana, bodily poses; third of the eight limbs of *yoga*.
āśrama, one of the progressive stages of life (student, householder, religious retiree, solitary ascetic); also, an ascetic's hermitage, usually in the forest.
asura, demoniac being; enemy of the celestials.
ātman, the soul, also known as *puruṣa*.
avatāras, divine descents of Viṣṇu into the world.
avidyā, ignorance of the *ātman*.
Balarāma, Kṛṣṇa's brother (often simply referred to as Rāma).
Bhagavad Gītā, episode of the *Mahābhārata* epic that has become a quintessential Sanskrit scripture; Kṛṣṇa's discourse to Arjuna.
Bhagavān, name for God.
bhāgavata, devotee of *Bhagavān*; *bhakta*.

Bhāgavata (*Purāṇa*), the primary scripture for the Kṛṣṇa traditions.
bhakti, devotion to *Bhagavān*.
Bhārata, traditional term for India; named after Bharata, a great devotee who retired to the forest.
bhāva, devotional state of mind in a specific relationship with Kṛṣṇa.
Brahmā, the secondary creator, functions like an engineer, manipulating the *prakṛtic* stuff to create the specific forms of the universe.
brahmacārya, the period up to the age of twenty-five, when students would study Vedic knowledge systems under the tutelage of the teacher.
Brahman, name for the Absolute Truth in the Upaniṣads.
brāhmaṇa, teaching/priestly caste.
Caitanya, sixteenth-century Kṛṣṇa ecstatic, considered an incarnation of Kṛṣṇa by his followers.
cakra, Viṣṇu's discus weapon.
cāraṇa, type of celestial being.
citta-vṛtti-nirodha, stilling of all states of mind; definition of *yoga* in the *Yoga Sūtras*.
daitya, demoniac being; synonymous with *asura*.
dāsya, one of the five *bhāvas*, servitorship.
deva, celestial being.
dharma, used variously; in Vedic culture, the variegated duties incumbent on embodied beings; one of the traditional four goals of human life.
dīkṣā, initiation into a Vedic or *yogic* lineage.
dveṣa, aversion; one of the five *kleśas*, obstacles to *yoga* in the *Yoga Sūtras*.
Gajendra, the elephant *bhakta*.
gandharva, celestial being, renowned for musical as well as martial skills.
Garuḍa, Viṣṇu's eagle carrier.
Gītā, see *Bhagavad Gītā*.
Goloka, divine *brahman* abode of Kṛṣṇa.
Govinda, name of Kṛṣṇa, "Lord of the cows."
gṛhastha, householder.
guṇa, one of the three metaphysical strands formative of *prakṛti*.
guru, teacher.
Hari, name of Kṛṣṇa.
Hiraṇyakaśipu, demon father of Prahlāda.
Indra, warrior chief of the celestials.
Īśvara, term for God.
jīva, embodied soul.
Jīva Gosvāmī, one of the six principal followers of Caitanya in the sixteenth century; wrote the *Sandarbhas*.
jñāna, knowledge; sometimes used as a synonym for consciousness.
jñānendriyas, instruments for attaining knowledge: hearing (ears), touching (skin), tasting (tongue), smelling (nose), seeing (eyes).
kaivalya, liberation; the autonomy of the *ātman* from *saṁsāra*.

Kali yuga, last and most degraded of the four ages; the current age.
kāma, material enjoyment; one of the traditional four goals of human life (*puruṣārthas*).
Kaṁsa, Kṛṣṇa's evil uncle, king of Mathurā.
karma, action; every action breeds a corresponding reaction.
karmendriyas, five working senses: speaking (mouth), grasping (hands), locomotion (feet), excreting (anus), procreation (genitals).
kaustubha, gem worn by Kṛṣṇa.
kīrtana, the chanting of the names and deeds of *Īśvara*.
kleśa, the five obstacles to yoga in the *Yoga Sūtras* (II.4): ignorance (of the *ātman*), ego, desire, aversion, clinging to life.
kṣatriya, warrior/administrative cast.
Kuru, royal dynasty of both the Pāṇḍavas and their cousins in the *Mahābhārata* epic.
līlā, pastimes, particularly used in the *Bhāgavata* to point to Kṛṣṇa's loving pastimes with His beloved devotees.
madhura, one of the *bhāvas*; amorous mood.
Madhva, thirteenth-century theistic philosopher of Vedānta; founder of the *dvaita* lineage.
Mahābhārata, great epic of the story of the descendants of Bharata; features the strife of the Pāṇḍavas and their cousins and their subsequent saga culminating in the great war between them.
mahābhūtas, the ultimate elements of Sāṅkhya metaphysics: earth, water, fire, air, ether.
mahant, saintly person or great soul.
Maitreya, sage who delivers teachings to Vidura at various places in the *Bhāgavata*.
māyā, illusion covering the *ātman* causing it to misidentify with its gross and subtle coverings; a negative function (see also *yogamāyā*).
Mīmāṁsā, a school of Indian philosophy concerned with Vedic ritualism.
mokṣa, liberation from *saṁsāra*.
Mokṣadharma, a section of the *Mahābhārata* that is particularly philosophical in nature.
mukti, liberation from *saṁsāra*.
Nanda, Kṛṣṇa's foster father.
Nārada, a traveling sage and preeminent *bhakta*.
Nārāyaṇa, the supreme *Īśvara*, Viṣṇu.
nirbīja, contentless awareness absorbed in its own nature; the final state of *yoga*.
nirodha, cessation; used primarily to refer to meditative states.
Nṛsiṁha, Man-Lion incarnation of Viṣṇu.
Nyāyā, school of Indian philosophy specializing in inferential debate.
Pāṇḍava, five sons of Pāṇḍu.
paramahaṁsa, literally "great swan"; final of the four stages of *sannyāsa*, the renounced order of life.

pāramārthika, highest reality compared with conventional reality (see *vyāvahārika*).
Paramātman, form of Viṣṇu pervading the *ātman*; synonymous with *Antaryāmī*.
Parīkṣit, king who receives the teachings of the *Bhāgavata* from Śuka; grandson of Arjuna.
Patañjali, author of the classical text on the practice and goal of *yoga*.
Prācīnabarhis, king to whom Nārada delivers the allegory of King Purañjana.
Prahlāda, great child *bhakta*, son of the demon king Hiranyakaśipu.
Prajāgara, the serpent protector in the Purañjana allegory.
prāṇa, life airs.
prāṇāyama, control of the breath in *yoga* practice; fourth of the eight limbs of *yoga*.
prema, love; in *bhakti*, love of God.
pūjā, worship, usually of a deity, involving items such as ghee lamps and incense.
Purāṇa, genre of ancient literature focusing on the forms of *Īśvara*.
Purañjana, the king in the allegory Nārada delivers to King Prācīnabarhis.
Purañjanī, Purañjana's wife in the allegory.
puruṣa, synonym for *ātman*; innermost consciousness.
puruṣa-arthas, the four conventional goals of life: *dharma*, performance of duty; *artha*, attainment of prosperity; *kāma*, fulfillment of desires; *mokṣa*, liberation from all these.
rāgānuga, a *bhakta* immersed in *rāgānugā bhakti*.
rāgānugā, spontaneous form of *bhakti*.
rāgātmika, eternally perfected and liberated *bhakta*.
rajas, one of the three *guṇas*: energy, power, desire, and so forth.
Rāma, incarnation of *Īśvara*.
Rāmānuja, eleventh- to twelfth-century Vedānta theologian; founder of Śrī Vaiṣṇavism.
rasa, experience of *bhakti*.
rāsa, Kṛṣṇa's dance with the gopīs.
Rūpa Gosvāmī, one of the six *Gosvāmī* followers of Caitanya and prolific author.
sādhu, ascetic.
Śaivite, devotee of Śiva.
sakhya, one of the five *bhāvas*: friendship.
Śākta, follower of a form of the Goddess.
śakti, power.
samādhi, final stages of *yoga* culminating in awareness becoming immersed in its own pure nature; the eighth of the eight limbs of *yoga*.
samprajñāta, penultimate *samādhi* state.
saṁsāra, cycle of birth and death.
saṁskāra, memory imprint.
Sanātana Gosvāmī, one of the six *Gosvāmīs* of Vṛndāvana.
Sandarbha, one of the six treatises by Jīva Gosvāmī establishing the philosophical and theological basis for the Gauḍīya Vaiṣṇava Vedānta tradition.

Śaṅkara, eighth- to ninth-century Vedānta theologian.
Sāṅkhya, school of metaphysics.
sannyāsa, full ascetic renunciant.
sat-cit-ānanda, qualities of *brahman*: being, consciousness, and bliss.
satsaṅga, association of saints.
sattva, one of the *guṇas* of *prakṛti*, characterized by qualities such as wisdom, detachment, lightness, and peacefulness.
Sātvatas, a community devoted to Kṛṣṇa.
siddha, perfected being.
Śiva, a primary form of *Īśvara*.
smaraṇa, retaining sacred narratives and teachings in mind.
Smṛti, sacred text posterior to the Vedas, but with links thereto.
śravaṇa, hearing from sacred texts.
śrī, an honorific, used as an appellative of respect before a person's name.
Śrī, the Goddess of Fortune.
Śrīmad Bhāgavata Purāṇa, also referred to as the *Śrīmad Bhāgavata*, or just *Bhāgavata*; most important of the Purāṇas and dedicated to Kṛṣṇa *bhakti*.
śrīvatsa, tuft of hair on Kṛṣṇa's chest.
Śruti, sacred text; the Vedic corpus.
śūdra, the employed as well as artisan caste.
Śuka, the principal speaker of the *Bhāgavata*, which he relates to King Parīkṣit.
sūra, celestial; synonymous with *deva*.
Sūta, attended Śuka's discourse to Parīkṣit and then repeated the *Bhāgavata* to the sages at Naimiṣa.
tamas, one of the three *guṇas*, characterized by ignorance and laziness.
tanmātras, subtle qualities of the great elements, which later spring from them.
tapas, austerity.
tattva, literally "the nature of that-ness," in Sāṅkhya; refers to all or any of the evolutes from *prakṛti*.
tulasī, plant sacred to Kṛṣṇa.
Uddhava, survivor of the great war who receives instruction from Kṛṣṇa in the form of the *Uddhava Gītā* in book 11. Most of book 3 is in the form of sage Maitreya's instructions to him.
Upaniṣads, ancient late Vedic mystic-philosphical texts.
Uttamaśloka, name of Viṣṇu: "He whose praises are supreme."
Vaikuṇṭha, the divine *Brahman* abode of Viṣṇu.
vaiśya, merchant/landowning caste.
Vallabha, sixteenth-century contemporary of Caitanya; a great theologian who founded the school of *puṣṭi-mārga*.
vānaprastha, third stage of life when husband and wife begin to practice celibacy, detach themselves from the household, and retire to sacred places to pursue *yogic* practices.
Vasudeva, father of Kṛṣṇa.
Vāsudeva, Kṛṣṇa, son of Vasudeva.

vātsalya, one of the primary *bhāvas*; parental relationship with Kṛṣṇa.
Veda, one of the four most ancient texts in Sanskrit.
Vedānta, school of hermeneutics stemming from the Upaniṣads.
Vedānta Sūtra, primary text of the Vedānta tradition.
Vidura, half-brother of Dhṛtarāṣṭra, who receives teachings from sage Maitreya at various places in the *Bhāgavata*.
viśiṣṭādvaita, Vedānta school stemming from Rāmānuja.
Viṣṇu, form of *Īśvara*; Creator of the universes.
Vraj, area around Vṛndāvana.
Vṛndāvana, the forest where Kṛṣṇa spent his childhood; present-day holy town.
Vyāsa, an incarnation of Viṣṇu and the legendary composer of the *Mahābhārata* epic, compiler of the Purāṇas, and divider of the one Veda into four.
vyavahārika, conventional reality.
yajña, Vedic rites involving oblations into a fire sacrifice.
Yamunā, river in Vraj, central to Kṛṣṇa's *līlā*.
Yaśodā, Kṛṣṇa's foster mother.
yogamāyā, divine illusion, one of the functions of which is to cover Kṛṣṇa's majesty such that His devotee can interact with Him as a child, friend, lover, and so forth.
Yoga Sūtras, classical text on the practice and goal of *yoga*; written by Patañjali.
yojana, distance, considered variously as two, four, five, or nine miles.
Yudhiṣṭhīra, eldest of the five Pāṇḍavas.
yuga, one of the four world ages.

Notes

Introduction to the Volume

1. The term *purāṇa* will be defined more precisely below.
2. The term "history" has now long been associated not merely with textual narrative, but with empirical disciplines such as archaeology, linguistics, numismatics, and so on. Clearly the Purāṇa literature such as the *Bhāgavata* dealing with Kṛṣṇa's incarnation is not subject to this type of empirical scrutiny. On the other hand, a term such as "myth" indicates that the stories have no factual basis at all. Epistemology is the branch of philosophy that deals with what constitutes a valid source of knowledge (for instance, empiricism, reason and inference, sacred scripture, and the like), and different epistemologies have been and are prioritized by intellectuals at different points in history and in different contexts and domains. So taking a position that the stories are purely "myths" would be an imposition of epistemological presuppositions and beliefs derived from the post-Enlightenment West upon the worldviews and convictions of countless millions of devotees over a period of two millennia and thereby would run contrary to the stated purpose of this volume, which is precisely to attempt to represent a sense of such beliefs. The term "legend," in contrast, remains neutral as to the truth content of the stories, indicating simply that these stories present themselves as truth and have been handed down as such, without taking any further stance as to their veracity. We discuss such problems further in the chapter "Concluding Reflections."
3. As is by now well-known, "Hinduism" is not a term found in Indic texts prior to the sixteenth century, as it was appropriated from the immigrants and invaders who had introduced it into India. We retain it now for practical purposes, given its de facto intractable usage to refer to the vast array of beliefs and practices that retain some form of nominal allegiance to the old Vedic texts.

4. Jīva and Rūpa quote the *Bhāgavata* abundantly, since as traditional commentators they strive to exemplify each theological point with a quote from the primary text in order to substantiate and authorize the devotional principles they are organizing into a system in their expositions. So by following Jīva and Rūpa, we will likewise be quoting profusely from the *Bhāgavata* itself in part 1 also.
5. We must note, of course, that there are many expressions of Gauḍīya Vaiṣṇavism, and we are featuring its more elite—in the sense of erudite and scholastic—canon-forming tradition, imparted by the lineage's founding figurehead, Caitanya, to Rūpa, whose work we feature, and other followers.
6. The term "Indic" refers to anything written in ancient Sanskrit (the linguistic name for which is Indo-Aryan), but I use it primarily when I wish to refer to commonalities in thought between Vedic, Buddhist, Jain, and other such traditions.
7. Thus, we begin with some delimiters: the goal of this volume is not to attempt to lay out some of the prominent features or personages of the diachronically and synchronically variegated landscape of *bhakti* by tracing its historical, geographic, social, or cultural roots from early historical sources through its growth into its numerous branches past and present. These are all essential projects in their own rights, but they are not the focus of interest in this volume.
8. As filtered through the subjective understanding of this author, needless to say: we claim no privileged access to any authorial intention underpinning these texts. However, we have tried to minimize our own filter by dint of translating the sources themselves, but, naturally, what we have selected and what omitted reflect our own subjective dispositions.
9. I note also, for my colleagues in the academy, briefly and perhaps simplistically, that it is my position that one way to navigate around the postcolonial, post-Orientalist impasse as to how to represent non-Western traditions such as those of *bhakti yoga*, without perpetuating the Eurocentric attitudes and stereotypes as well as the Christian presuppositions and biases of the founders and predecessors of our field of the study of religion, is precisely to at least endeavor to allow these traditions to speak in their own voices, using their own intellectual concepts and terminologies. In other words, to attempt to consider these traditions' own theologies, practices, metaphysics, epistemologies, and worldviews in their own right, without being filtered either through the religious vocabularies and assumptions of our Western religious traditions or through the theoretical categories and secular presuppositions of our modern Western post-Enlightenment academies. To explicitly or implicitly assume they have so little to offer in their own terms that they require the imposition of Western categories of knowledge and theoretical analysis is, to say the least, a remarkable act of hubris that has long extended its shelf life. This is not to deny that such texts have their own ideologies and attempt to normalize and impose their own structures of power, such as caste and the like. But

so much attention has been directed to this aspect of *brahmanical* Sanskrit culture that we have chosen to direct our own focus on the aspects of the *Bhāgavata* that concern theology, soteriology, and praxis (we do, however, make some comments on *bhakti* and *dharma* in part 1; see "*Bhakti* and *Dharma*").

10. I use the somewhat problematic term "classical" to refer to transregional Veda-acknowledging texts that reached their completion by or shortly after the Gupta period from the fourth to the sixth century C.E. (as I have argued is the case with the *Bhāgavata*; Bryant 2002).
11. Of course, numerous preexisting ingredients that Patañjali was systematizing in his *Sūtras*, such as the eight limbs of practice and various other elements, surface or are appropriated in numerous distinct sectarian contexts, Jain, Buddhist, Vaiṣṇava, Śākta, Śaiva, and so forth.
12. Although the view that Vyāsa was Patañjali himself writing a commentary on his own *Sūtras* has recently resurfaced with the dedicated work of Philipp Maas (2010).
13. Thus while, for example, the sixteenth-century commentator Vijñānabhikṣu may quibble with the earlier commentator Vācaspati Miśra, and introduce a good deal of Vedānta-related issues, there is no disagreement on the essential metaphysics of Yoga or on the nature of its mental states, practices, or goals (see discussion in Bryant 2009, xxxix).
14. Thus, from the various topics the *Bhāgavata* claims to comprise (noted later), part 2 is concerned with *mukti*, the attainment of liberation from suffering through the practice of *bhakti*.
15. From its stated list of topics, Kṛṣṇa is the *Bhāgavata*'s tenth and final subject matter, the substratum (*āśraya*) or goal of everything else.
16. See Bryant (2003) and, for the most comprehensive academic study on the Purāṇas as a genre, Rocher (1986).
17. Based on Bryant (2003, ixff.).
18. Even the non-Vedic Buddhist and Jain traditions partly defined themselves in contradistinction to the Vedic one.
19. For instance, see *Kūrma Purāṇa, Pūrva* 52.19–20; *Padma Purāṇa, Uttara-khaṇḍa* 236.18–21.
20. There are, of course, other texts, such as the *Āgamas* and *Pañcarātras*, that provide much information pertaining to the minutiae of ritual and theological technicalities, but they are of interest primarily to ritual specialists and theologians.
21. In addition to the eighteen *mahā* (great) Purāṇas, there are a further eighteen *upa* (minor) Purāṇas, which are just as extensive in scope but deemed less authoritative, being later in composition and much less widespread.
22. See *Matsya Purāṇa* 53.9–11; *Śiva Purāṇa* VII.1.1.37–38.
23. Brahmā is more of an engineer than a creator in the classical sense, since he creates the forms of the universe from preexisting matter. But in texts such as the *Bhāgavata*, matter itself emanates from Viṣṇu, who is thus the primary

creator. Śiva is assigned the same status in the Śaiva Purāṇas, but Brahmā is never the supreme creator God in this ultimate sense.

24. *Gītā* (VIII.17) points to Brahmā's life span.
25. The Goddess (Śākta) traditions tend to be monistic, rather than strictly monotheist, a distinction we will discuss in part 5.
26. See the papers in Gupta and Valpey (2013) as well as Beck (2005) for some sense of this. See also the papers in "Vaishnavism and the Arts" in *Journal of Vaishnava Studies* 21, no. 2 (2013).
27. Much of this explosion of interest in the text stems from our featured sixteenth-century Caitanya tradition, of which Jīva is a follower.
28. See Sharpe (1985, 83ff.) and Davis (2015) for some sense of this.
29. There are actually several thousand verses fewer than eighteen thousand, but traditional exegetes factor in the extra length of prose passages, as well as colophons and the like, to justify the traditional number (see Satyanārāyaṇa Dāsa 1995, 80n1) for discussion.
30. These were initiated by influential charismatics such as Caitanya and Vāllabha, whom we will encounter within.
31. This is mostly on the grounds that neither the later dynasties nor later famous rulers such as Harṣa in the seventh century C.E. are to be found in the king lists contained in the texts.
32. Bryant (2002).
33. A number of the other Purāṇas clearly mention the *Bhāgavata* along with some mention of its subject matter (*Skanda Purāṇa*, *Prabhāsa-khaṇḍa* 7.1.2.39–42; *Agni Purāṇa* 272.6–7; *Padma Purāṇa*, *Uttara-khaṇḍa* 22.115, 198.30, and elsewhere; *Matsya Purāṇa* 53.20–22; these and other references from Satyanārāyaṇa Dāsa 1995). However, in contradiction to this, as we will see in the Tale of Vyāsa, the *Bhāgavata* places itself as being written by the despondent Vyāsa shortly after the completion of the other Purāṇas. Also, we need not concern ourselves with the controversy raised by the followers of the *Devī Bhāgavata*, that these references to the *Bhāgavata Purāṇa* in the other Purāṇas refer to their *Devī* text, not that of the Vaiṣṇavas (for which see Mackenzie Brown 1983; and Dāsa 1995, 88ff.).
34. See, for discussion, Preciado-Solis (1984).
35. See appendix 1 for discussion on the *Śruti* and *Smṛti* genres of sacred text.
36. For example, see III.8.7–9.
37. These are *sarga*, creation of the universe; *visarga*, secondary creation of forms within the universe; *vṛtti*, maintenance of the living entities; *rakṣā*, protection of living entities; *manvantara*, governance of the various Manu dynasties; *vaṁsa*, dynasties of great kings; *vaṁsānucarita*, activities of the kings in these dynasties; *saṁsthā*, annihilation of universe; *hetu*, motivation; and *apāśraya*, the Supreme shelter (*Īśvara*) (XII.7.9–10). Earlier in the text, these are labeled somewhat differently: *sarga*, primordial creation; *visarga*, secondary creation; *sthāna*, maintenance; *poṣaṇa*, sustenance/grace; *ūti*, desire; *manvantara*, periods of the Manus; *Īśānukathā*, stories of *Īśvara*'s

incarnations; *nirodha*, annihilation of the universe; *mukti*, liberation; and *āśraya*, ultimate shelter (II.10.1–2). According to other Purāṇas, there are only five topics: *sarga*, *pratisarga* (destruction), *Manv-antarāṇi*, *vaṁsa*, and *vaṁsanucarita* (*Matsya Purāṇa* 53.65).

38. *Tattva Sandarbha* (*anuccheda* 58).
39. The name used here is Uttamaśloka, literally "verses about whom are supreme."
40. Book 11, in fact, is mostly devoted to Kṛṣṇa's instructions to Uddhava, sometimes called the *Uddhāva Gītā*. It covers a vast range of subject matter, including social and civic duties as well as all manner of *yogic* and religious practices, all culminating in *bhakti*.
41. The Indian painting collection at the Brooklyn Museum is a good example of this.
42. In point of fact, Vṛndāvana is the town that has developed since the sixteenth century in the place where a number of Kṛṣṇa's pastimes took place, where Vraj includes but also extends beyond this to a much larger area touching the outskirts of Delhi.
43. See Haberman (1994b) and Entwhistle (1987).
44. See *Caitanya Caritāmṛta*, *Madhya-līlā* 20.
45. Jīva Gosvāmī credits the directive to write his six *Sandarbhas* to his uncle Rūpa but acknowledges that Gopāla Bhaṭṭa Gosvāmī compiled the original version of the *Sandarbhas*, based on the works of older Vaiṣṇava theologians, which he is systematizing and completing (*anu* 3–5).
46. A verse of unknown origin, quoted from Baladeva Vidyābhūṣaṇa by Dāsa (*Tattva* 13).
47. We will also be representing arguments from the first *Sandarbha*, the *Tattva,* in appendix 1.
48. The Vedānta tradition stems from the ancient Upaniṣads, the oldest mystic-philosophical texts in Sanskrit. By locating itself as a Vedānta tradition, the Gauḍīya theologians are laying claim to representing the Ultimate Truths of the ancient Vedic heritage, the oldest Sanskrit and Indo-European texts (see the chapter "The Object of *Bhakti*: *Īśvara*, *Bhagavān*, *Brahman*, and Divine Hierarchies" and appendix 1).
49. Jīva adopts a fourfold schema in conceptualizing the contents of the Sandarbhas: the subject (*viṣaya*), who is Kṛṣṇa; the relationship (*sambandha*) between Him and His *śaktis*, "energies," such as the *jīvas*, living beings; the process for attaining Him (*abhidheya*, that which is to be spoken of); and the ultimate purpose or goal to be acquired (*prayojana*), which is love of God, *prema*.
50. Satyanārāyaṇa's Dāsa's erudite Sanskrit edition and translation of the *Bhakti Sandarbha* is available, and at the time of this writing, he has completed the translation of and is preparing all six *Sandarbhas* for publication (see www.jiva.org for status). Rūpa Gosvāmī's *Bhaktirasāmṛtasindhu* is also worthy of more robust consideration for anyone with a serious interest in Kṛṣṇa *bhakti*, for which Haberman (2003) has produced an excellent annotated English

translation. I made use of both of these translations to determine which passages to select for part 1 of this work, but all Sanskrit translations are my own. Similarly, owing to the extensive amount of Sanskrit materials involved, I availed myself of the translations of the *Bhāgavata* noted in the next note, in order to determine which tales and teachings to extract for part 2, and then used the Chowkambha Sanskrit edition of the text for my own translations of these sections.

51. Here, Bhaktivedānta Swāmī's multivolume translation and commentary is the easiest available in numerous languages—as is his version of the *Bhaktirasāmṛtasindhu* as well as his trademark rendition of the tenth book of the *Bhāgavata* under the title *Kṛṣṇa* (all of which can be downloaded for free at www.vedabase.com). Being written by a preeminent devotee of *Śrī* Kṛṣṇa, the founder of ISKCON, the Hare Krishna Movement, these devotionally laden editions underscore the spiritual appeal of *bhakti* as what we will call in "Concluding Reflections" a "living tradition." This author's own lifelong dedication to studying the traditions of Kṛṣṇa *bhakti* stems from encountering these books in the late 1970s. There is a highly recommended accessible edition with the Gauḍīya commentary of Viśvanātha by Bhanu Swami (2008–11), where one receives both text and verse-by-verse exegesis. Other than this, for those with access to Indian publishing houses, the Motilal Banarsidass edition translated by Tagare (1976–78) is excellent, as is the translation by Gosvami C. L. (n.d.). Additionally, we ourselves have published a literal annotated translation of the tenth book under the title *Krishna: The Beautiful Legend of God* (2003), and the stories of Kṛṣṇa in part 3 consist of extracts from this.

Definition of *Bhakti*

1. For example, see *Yoga Sūtras* II.15–16, and the definition of *yoga* itself as "freedom from suffering" in *Gītā* VI.23.
2. The Cārvāka-related philosophies (which left no formal school or body of literature of their own) accepted neither an *ātman* nor *Īśvara* (see Bhattacharya 2011 for a compilation of sources from other schools on these traditions).
3. The first time the term *viveka*, insight, is used in the *Yoga Sūtras* is in relation to the realization by a wise person that all is suffering. This *viveka* is then developed by the practices of *yoga* (II.28) and reaches its zenith as that which removes *avidyā*, ignorance, and bestows liberation (II.25–26).
4. Jīva calls this taking of shelter *śaraṇāpatti*. He quotes the Vaiṣṇava Tantra: "There are six elements in *śaraṇāpatti*: the determination to act favorably, the avoidance of unfavorable actions, the belief that '*Īśvara* will protect me,' the conscious acceptance of *Īśvara* as one's protector, the submission of the self, and humility" (*anu* 236, reference not given). The fourth item from this list, according to Jīva, consciously accepting *Īśvara* as one's protector, is especially associated with *śaraṇāpatti*, with the other five serving as *aṅgas*, limbs.

5. In the words of the *Bhāgavata*: "O Lord! For one afflicted by the threefold suffering in the terrifying fire of *saṁsāra*, I see no other shelter than your lotus feet, which are like an umbrella raining down nectar" (XI.19.9).
6. For the *Gītā*, see VII.7, X.8, and throughout.
7. The great monotheistic deities are, in fact, almost always accompanied by their consorts: Rādhā-Kṛṣṇa, Lakṣmī-Nārāyaṇa, Śiva-Parvatī, Sītā-Rāma, and so on.
8. There are many names for Kṛṣṇa, and the one used here is Hṛṣīkeśa, "the Lord of the senses." I am standardizing these alternatives here for ease of reference, but on occasion I retain them in parts 2 and 3, as the choice of names reflects specific associations that are being invoked according to context.
9. *Nārada Pañcarātra*, quoted in *Bhaktirasāmṛtasindhu* Eastern Quadrant I.12, exact reference not given. Tradition associates this text, too, with the epic sage Nārada (see *Bhāgavata* I.3.8).
10. *Bhakti* is a nominal form of the verbal root *bhaj*.
11. *Garuḍa Purāṇa* (*pūrva kaṇḍa* 227.3). However, the first line of Jīva's verse does not appear in the Nag edition of this Purāṇa. The verse adds instead that the *bhaktas* engage in reciting the names and deeds of the Lord of the Universe.
12. According to Jīva, this eliminates other forms of meditation on Kṛṣṇa, such as hatred (as in the case of Kṛṣṇa's enemies, Kaṁsa, Śiśupāla, or Pauṇḍraka, indicated in *Bhāgavata* X.29.13, 66.24, and 87.23), which can also award liberation and are discussed in "Meditation in Hate and Lust."
13. We will elaborate on *bhakti* motivated by a desire for *jñāna* or *karma* in "*Bhakti* Mixed with Attachment to *Dharma* and *Jñāna*."
14. These are: residing in the same abode as Viṣṇu (*sālokya*), having the same opulence as Him (*sārṣṭi*), being close to Him (*sāmīpya*), having the same form as Him (*sārūpya*), and merging into Him (*sāyuja*/*ekatvam*). They are discussed in "The Liberated *Bhakta*: Different Types of *Mokṣa* in the *Bhāgavata*."
15. These are: "*bhakti* destroys all obstacles (*kleśas*); it brings auspiciousness; it minimizes [interest in] *mokṣa* (liberation); it is very difficult to attain; it has a special intense bliss bestowing nature; and it attracts Śrī Kṛṣṇa" (*Upadeśāmṛta*, 17).

The Practices of *Bhakti*

1. We can recall that Rūpa divides his *Bhaktirasāmṛtasindhu* (*Ocean of the Nectar of the Experience of* Bhakti) into four "quadrants," from which we will mostly be quoting the Eastern Quadrant.
2. The relationship between Viṣṇu and Kṛṣṇa will be discussed in the chapter "The Object of *Bhakti*: *Īśvara*, *Bhagavān*, *Brahman*, and Divine Hierarchies." They are the same Supreme Being, manifest in different forms to accomplish different purposes.

3. The *Maitrī Upaniṣad* (VI18), for example, speaks of six limbs, and there were various other variants (see Bryant 2009, xxiff.).
4. *Śravaṇa, manana, nidhidhyāsana*, hearing about, reflecting, and concentrating on the *ātman,* have their roots in the *Bṛhadāraṇyaka Upaniṣad* (II.4.5). In later texts, a fourth is added, *samādhi*, absorption of consciousness in its own ultimate nature (see Sadānanda's *Vedāntasāra* I.4.128).
5. As a technical aside, in Vedānta (and *Mīmāṁsā*) hermeneutics, the placing of items first (and last) on a list reflects their importance with relation to other items listed.
6. "Some do not desire liberation, O Lord. Freed from all distress they immerse themselves in the great nectarean ocean of stories about the forms you have assumed in order to teach Truth about the self" (X.87.21).
7. Sarvabhāvāna Dāsa translation, 238–39.
8. "Dishonesty" is here understood as any scriptural teaching promoting bodily, mental, or worldly (that is, temporal and nonultimate) gain as its goal (rather than imparting teachings about the soul or God).
9. These are the miseries caused by one's own body and mind, by other living entities, and by the environment.
10. The *kalpa-taru* is a tree in the celestial realm that offers anything requested of it.
11. The passage adds, "The *Bhāgavata* is permeated with the nectar flowing from the mouth of sage Śuka." Śuka, the speaker of the *Bhāgavata*, also means "parrot." The poetic implication (*dhvani*) here is that as the parrot will choose the sweetest fruit with its beak, so Śuka has spoken the highest and most relishable of scriptures with his mouth.
12. *Aho!* is a common exclamation.
13. The passage appeals to the connoisseurs "of poetic experience (*rasa*) and experts of poetic moods (*bhāva*)." These terms will be discussed in "*Rāga*, *Bhāva*, and *Rasa*" in the context of the *Bhāgavata*'s appropriation of them. Their origins lie in Indian aesthetics, where *rasa* refers to the aesthetic experience felt by the audience in, say, a well-performed drama, and *bhāva* the mood it invokes.
14. The *Mahābhārata* epic does in fact contain descriptions of the adult Kṛṣṇa, as does the *Harivaṁśa* appendage to it, which includes narratives from the youthful portion of Kṛṣṇa's life. Similarly with some of the Purāṇas, especially the Viṣṇu and Padma. But the *rasa* and *bhāva* elements of such centrality to the *bhakti* of the sixteenth-century Kṛṣṇa theologians are much less discernible in those literary sources.
15. These are four *puruṣārthas*, goals of human life.
16. The passage adds: "But that composition, even if its every verse is improperly composed, destroys the sins of people if it contains [the sacred] names denoting the glory of the unlimited Lord. Saints hear, recite, and glorify them."
17. "The chanting of the name of Hari has been prescribed for those *yogīs* who are disinterested [in material enjoyment] and who desire freedom from fear" (II.1.11).

18. At least, in the Indic context, this is partly true according to the Nyāya school of philosophy, although this school would hold that meaning is assigned by *Īśvara*. The followers of the school of Mīmāṁsā, in contrast (along with the Grammarians), would posit that Vedic words and their designations are eternal, based on their belief that the Vedas are eternal, and hence so are the words they contain. In fact, other philosophical schools, including perhaps Patañjali's Yoga tradition (see Rukmani 1975; Bryant 2009, 106ff.), also hold that Sanskrit words and their denotations are eternal, and thus language is not conventionally derived.
19. We will discuss below how Kṛṣṇa's form is made from pure *Brahman*, consciousness (*caitanya*).
20. The famous *cintāmaṇi* is a gem found in Viṣṇu's *Brahman* realm of Vaikuṇṭha, which can fulfill any wish posed to it.
21. The "etc." here applies to the vision of Kṛṣṇa, as also any contact with Him through the other senses.
22. While other monotheistic traditions tend to prioritize the notion of "visions" of God, *bhakti* traditions, while also featuring visions, prioritize sonic presence. See Beck (1993) for a problematizing of assigning higher epistemic value to the visual. In fact, from a philosophical perspective (for example, the school of Vaiśeṣiká), if form and sound are both qualities that reveal their substances, why should the form of a substance be prioritized as somehow more authentically true of the existence of that substance than any other quality such as sound? Since both require a sense organ to be perceived by consciousness (the *ātman*), what determines that the eye is a more reliable implement than the ear? Applied to *Īśvara*, then, why should *Īśvara* manifest as form be deemed more authoritative or authentic a spiritual experience than *Īśvara* manifest as sound?
23. Quoted from Dimock 2000, 899.
24. For the *kleśas*, ignorance, ego, desire, aversion, and fear of death, see *Yoga Sūtras* II.2ff.
25. *Saṁsāra* is the cycle of birth and death.
26. For example, see *Viṣṇu Purāṇa* VI.2.17.
27. As is evident in the quote, in each *yuga*, epoch, humankind is prescribed a particular type of devotional activity in the Purāṇas. In the present and most degenerate age, the *Kali yuga*, *kīrtana* is prescribed, as it is the most easily accomplished for the misfortunate people born in this age. The *Bhāgavata* even states that people in previous *yugas* aspire to take birth in *Kali* because of this ease (XI.5.38).
28. See also XI.5.32.
29. Ārya is an ancient Sanskrit term denoting a civilized person, or one who follows the righteous codes of conduct outlined in late Vedic texts.
30. The prefix *saṅ* here indicates communal *kīrtana*.
31. In early *Brāhmaṇa* texts, *japa* refers to the soft repetition of Vedic *mantras* by priests. See *Bṛhadāraṇyaka Upaniṣad* I.3.28, VI.3.6; *Chandogya Upaniṣad* V.2.6.

32. See, for example, *Māṇḍūkya Upaniṣad*.
33. For instance, *Yoga Sūtras* I.27–28 and *Gītā* VII.8.
34. See VII.8, IX.17.
35. The traditional day in Hinduism is divided into eighteen *muhūrtas*, out of which seventeen are considered to be dominated by the lethargic energy of the *guṇa* of *tamas* or agitating energy of that of *rajas* (the three *guṇas* will be discussed in the chapter "The Object of *Bhakti*: *Īśvara*, *Bhagavān*, *Brahman*, and Divine Hierarchies"). In only one *muhūrta* is the peaceful and content *guṇa* of *sattva* dominant—the *muhūrta* before sunrise.
36. This mood is how *bhaktas* might interpret "keeping its meaning in mind," *tad-artha-bhāvanam*, in Patañjali's verse on how one should perform *japa* on *oṁ* (I.27–28).
37. The worship of the *tulasī* plant, sacred to Kṛṣṇa, is discussed later.
38. ISKCON has by now both spawned a variety of offshoots and set the stage for other branches of the Gauḍīya Vaiṣṇava tradition to also propagate the Kṛṣṇa *bhakti* of the Caitanya tradition (see Bryant and Ekstrand 2004).
39. Hence the phrase "Kṛṣṇa Consciousness." This phraseology was foundational to the language adopted by Bhaktivedānta Swami, founder of the Hare Krishna Movement, who was responsible for the transplanting of Kṛṣṇa *bhakti* all around the world in the 1960s.
40. See also chapter 9 and the sequencing of practices in XII.1–12, and of *yogīs* in VI.46–47.
41. As a very interesting aside, and while this is beyond the scope of this work, it would be interesting to trace what I suspect to be the progressive "caucasianization" of Kṛṣṇa from paintings depicting Him in art prior to the colonial period to the chronological production of art thereafter (one of our undergraduate students did, in fact, undertake a cursory study of paintings in the Brooklyn Museum collections that did point to this phenomenon). Be this as it may, both Kṛṣṇa and Shyāma (a very popular appellation for this deity) mean black. The color, when described, is that of a dark monsoon cloud.
42. Even as one can fix the mind on any object "according to one's inclination" (*Yoga Sūtras* I.39), *Īśvara* is prioritized by dint of heading the list of *ālambanas*, objects upon which the mind can be fixed in concentration, which according to traditional (*Mīmāṁsā*) hermeneutics indicates preeminence. Additionally, *Īśvara* as *ālambana* receives eight verses where other suggested *ālambanas* receive only one each. Moreover, only *Īśvara* can bestow liberation, where other objects cannot (II.45). Hence Patañjali is discreetly and nonassertively, but nonetheless clearly, prioritizing this form of practice. (See commentary to I.44 in Bryant 2003, 152–53, for an application of *Īśvara* meditation in the context of Patañjali's *samādhi* sequencing.)
43. This metaphor is also found in the *Yoga Sūtras* commentaries. The commentaries to *Yoga Sūtras* III.1–3 highlight the difference between *dhāraṇa* and *dhyāna* by comparing a dripping water tap with the thick, unctuous flow of oil. The drips from a tap have identical drops of water punctuated by gaps,

paralleling the mind focusing on its support, interspersed with periodic distractions, as in *dhāraṇa*. The pouring of oil, which flows without drips, is comparable to the undeviating flow of the mind when it has reached a stage of undistracted one-pointedness, as in *dhyāna*.

44. See, for instance, *Yoga Sūtras* I.17 and 42–46 and commentaries.
45. This is sometimes referred to as *sa-guṇa Brahman, Brahman* with qualities, but the term *guṇa*, in this case, refers not to the *guṇas* of *prakṛti*, but rather to the Nyāya-Vaiśeṣiká sense of quality.
46. This account and the vision of Kṛṣṇa obtained by Nārada in I.6.18 are narrated in part 2.
47. Dimock 2000, 960–61. See also *Antya-līlā* 14.81–106.
48. This is a cultural renactment of *Bhāgavata* X.83 and the main religious festival in the East Indian state of Orissa.
49. Service to the *tulasī* plant is also included in this category of *bhakti*: "One should worship the Lord with pure water, garlands of forest flowers, roots and fruits, etc., freshly cut sprouts and stems, and with the *tulasī* plant, which is dear to the Lord" (IV.8.55). Although there is little explicit reference to worshipping *tulasī* in the *Bhāgavata* (see X.13.49), traditionally, a *tulasī* is typically grown and worshipped in Vaiṣṇava households, and certainly in temples. In prescriptive Kṛṣṇaism, food is offered to the Deity (discussed in the next process) before consumption, in the form both of lavish offerings in temples and at the modest family meal of the Vaiṣṇava householder prior to the family partaking of it, and one leaf of *tulasī* is placed on each item of foodstuffs. *Tulasī*'s sanctity is further underscored by the fact that practicing Kṛṣṇa *bhaktas* can be recognized by the necklace of *tulasī* wood beads worn around their necks (as can Śaivites, by *rudrākṣa* beads).
50. See "The Liberated *Bhakta*: Different Types of *Mokṣa* in the *Bhāgavata*."
51. Verse number not given.
52. See Holdredge (2013) for an excellent analysis of divine embodiment in Gauḍīya Vaiṣṇavism.
53. The *śālagrāma* is a sacred stone found in the *Gaṇḍakī* river of Nepal that does not require ritualistic installation to invoke the Deity, as *Īśvara*'s direct presence is deemed eternally present within it.
54. This is a form made of eternity (*sat*), pure consciousness (*cit*), and bliss (*ānanda*), rather than matter (*prakṛti*). But it is a form.
55. The *guṇas* are discussed in "*Prakṛti* and the Three *Guṇas*: *Sattva*, *Rajas*, and *Tamas*."
56. Of course, present *karma* reflects choices made in the past.
57. "Other agency" can include partial incarnations such as Vyāsa.
58. Literally "Joy of the king of Vraj," Kṛṣṇa's father.
59. This refers to the *Pañcarātra* genre of texts, which are the source for most of the ritual aspects of the Vaiṣṇava traditions.
60. Thus in Gauḍīya worship, twelve names of Kṛṣṇa (such as *oṁ Keṣavāya namaḥ*, *oṁ Govindāya namaḥ*) are consecutively invoked in *nyāsa*, each one

specific to one of twelve bodily parts touched in a circular fashion (forehead, belly, chest, throat; then waist and arm on the right side; then shoulder on the right; then waist, arm, and shoulder on the left side, followed by top of the back, and, last, lower back.

61. This "root" *mantra* is typically received from the *guru* and is sect-specific.
62. Thus, Nandi, Śiva's bull carrier, for example, is also worshipped in Śiva *pūjā*, as is Hanumān, the monkey *bhakta*, in Rāma worship, and so on.
63. Thus, *oṁ namo Śivāya*, for Śiva; *oṁ namo Bhāgavate Vāsudevāya*, for Kṛṣṇa; and so forth.
64. We will see later that the *ātman* is an *aṁśa*, or partial manifestation, of *Īśvara* (who is everything, including the individual *ātman*) and, in this sense, "made of Him."
65. The household Deity is typically moved from its altar in order to bathe and dress it and so forth and is returned upon completion of the worship. Temples with large immovable deities typically have a small Deity also invested with divine presence that can be moved and bathed and so on: "The Deity can be established in the temple in two ways: movable and non-movable; when worshipping a non-movable Deity, the *āvāhana* (invoking) and *udvāsa* (bidding farewell) are not necessary" (XI.27.14).
66. Jīva notes, in terms of the very personal meditation accompanying the rituals, that in order to cultivate love, "when one offers food, one should contemplate the Lord's beaming face" (*anu* 296).
67. This entire section contains more ritualistic specifics, elaborating on those quoted previously in XI.3.
68. Tantric here refers to the aforementioned Sanskrit textual sources that deal with the prescriptive details of deity worship, the *Āgamas* and *Pañcarātras*. Note the different but possibly overlapping usage of the term *kriyā yoga*, the path of acts, in *Yoga Sūtras* II.1.
69. These are the four monsoon months, a period when itinerant ascetics (*sādhus*) are allowed to remain in one place.
70. *Ekādasi* is "the eleventh" day of the full moon and of the new moon. Vaiṣṇavas fast from grains or from all foodstuffs on these two days of the month.
71. Vaiṣṇavas wear sacred markings made from paste from the clay of the *Gaṅgā* or *Yamunā* rivers on the twelve parts of the body mentioned previously as part of *nyāsa*.
72. In fact, by worshipping the Deity, the defect of disrespecting others can be curbed (*anu* 290). According to the *Bhāgavata*, it was in the third of the four *yugas* (world ages), the *Tretā* age, that deity worship was introduced, after strife entered into human affairs (one might assume so as to bring people together for a higher common purpose): "After perceiving the nature of strife between people in the age of *Tretā*, the deity worship of Hari was established by the sages" (VII.14.37).
73. I have reversed the order of the verses, here, placing 39–40 before 37–38.
74. See *Gītā* V.18.

75. As always, Jīva illustrates this practice from the *Bhāgavata*: "One who offers obeisance to you with heart, words, and body; contemplates Your compassion; and accepts the ripened fruits of personal *karma* that have been accumulated receives Your mercy and lives in a state of liberation" (X.14.8).
76. In Hinduism, 108 is a sacred number. Reasons given for this are as numerous as the sects that provide them. But, for example, the *japa mālā* (rosary) has 108 beads.
77. See Bryant 2009, xxiiiff.
78. This was composed by Gopal Bhaṭṭa Gosvāmī, one of the six *Gosvāmīs* of Vṛndāvana noted earlier. Drawing from the South Indian *Pāñcarātrika Āgamas*, it is the authoritative text on the full detailed universe of *vaidhī bhakti* for the Gauḍīya tradition.
79. In the final three verses of the *Upadeśāmṛta*, Rūpa assigns gradations to the various holy places associated with Kṛṣṇa, such as Mathurā.
80. These are typically listed as cleanliness, contentment, austerity, study of scripture, and devotion to *Iśvara* (for example, see *Yoga Sūtras* II.32). Rūpa would have assumed and intended the *yamas* as well.
81. These are also known as *niśkāmā bhakti*, devotion performed with no desire for any personal gain, and *sakāmā bhakti*, devotion performed for the fulfillment of self-centered desire. The former is also known as *akiñcanā bhakti*.
82. "Even pure knowledge [of the *ātman*] free of attachment to the fruits of action does not shine forth if devoid of devotion for Kṛṣṇa; let alone action, which is always inferior when not offered to *Īśvara*" (I.5.12, repeated verbatim in XII.12.53).
83. See Coleman (2010) and the bibliography therein for critiques of the text in this regard. For an analysis and critique of the efforts of a modern Gauḍīya Vaiṣṇava expression, ISKCON (the Hare Krishna Movement), attempting to reestablish the *varṇāśrama* social order and gender dynamics in its communities based on the founder's reading of the *Bhāgavata*, see the articles in part 5 of Bryant and Ekstrand (2014).
84. The term *dharma* in fact has numerous usages: in Nyāya, it is the property of a substance; in Buddhism, the teachings of the Buddha; and so forth.
85. This is explicit in *Bhāgavata* VII.2.31 and 35; and arguably implicit in *Gītā* IV.13.
86. The cluster of *dharmas* incumbent on an *ātman* taking birth as a *kṣatrīya* female in one birth, for example, will be quite different from those the same *ātman* encounters in a subsequent birth as, say, a *brāhmaṇa* male, and completely different again from those in any birth as a dog (which also has a *dharma*, or inherent nature and place in the grand scheme of things), and so on. Even in one life, youthful *dharmas* might differ from elderly ones.
87. See, for instance, II.47ff. Even the *Gītā* acknowledges that *karma yoga* was innovative for its day and age (IV.2–3), as the expectation surrounding the practice of *yoga* at the time was that it involved the cessation of all actions so

as not to perpetuate *karmic* reaction and subsequent *saṁsāra*. Hence, in the older texts, including the *Gītā*, *yoga* is associated with asceticism, typically in the forest.

88. See, for example, IX.27.
89. See, for example, VII.11–14 and XI.17–18.
90. See, for example, XVIII.66.
91. See *Mīmāṁsā Sūtras* IV.2.
92. We will discuss the differences here more fully in the chapter "The Object of *Bhakti*: *Īśvara*, *Bhagavān*, *Brahman*, and Divine Hierarchies."
93. See *Muṇḍaka Upaniṣad* I.7–11; *Gītā* II.42–45; *Yoga Sūtras* I.15.
94. The normative goal of Vedic *dharma*, the conventional religiosity of the time, was material gain in this world and the attainment of the celestial realms in the next (see *Gītā* II.42–46 for a deprecatory dig at such attitudes).
95. Indeed, the text has extensive passages outlining the *dharma* duties of the various castes, especially in the eleventh book.
96. These are listed in the *Mahābhārata* (V.43.12) as knowledge, truthfulness, control, tranquillity, freedom from malice, modesty, tolerance, freedom from envy, charity, performance of sacrifice, austerity, and sacred learning.
97. See also III.33.7.
98. According to the commentator Śrīdhara, the threefold birth is that from the parents, that pertaining to initiation into the *brāhmaṇa* caste, and that pertaining to initation for performing a sacrifice.
99. Since those arguing for caste based on birthright do so on the authority of statements made in sacred texts, a number of Hindu apologists and spokespersons agitating against such notions of birthright have countered such claims by reference to contrary statements in other sacred texts (or passages in the same texts). The *Bhāgavata* is thus relevant to such enterprises.
100. For an important and well-argued critique of the view (including statements made by this author) that such subversion has potential relevance to the real world of gender or other social power dynamics, see Coleman (2010). Coleman, in fact, sees the *Bhāgavata* as consciously reasserting male patriarchal dominance. Nonetheless, where women were excluded from other forms of religiosity at the time, such as Vedic ritualistic recitation and active performance at the sacrificial rites, or orthodox Vedānta study, the fact that the *Bhāgavata* not only includes female participation, but extols it as preeminent, is not trivial.
101. These are all tribes outside of the Vedic fold, some of them foreign to the subcontinent, most famously the *yavana*, a reference to the Greeks (a Sanskritization of the term "Ionian").
102. For a discussion of the social innovativeness of the *Bhāgavata*, see Hopkins (1966).
103. See *Bhāgavata* V.19.21ff. for the celestials musing about how, from the perspective of *yoga*, they would have been better off being born on the earth.
104. See Doniger and Smith (1991) and Olivelle (1999).

105. These are also referred to *puṇya* vs. *apuṇya* in the *Yoga Sūtras* (II.14–15) and *karma* vs. *vikarma* in *Gītā* (IV.17). The *Gītā* here also speaks of *akarma*, "in-action."
106. Of course, *samādhi* (*asaṁprajñāta*) in the *Yoga Sūtras* refers to the ultimate reimmersion of the *ātman* in its own nature (I.3, II.20), which is not of interest to Jīva's *bhakti* as we will see later.
107. Jīva exemplifies *bhakti* performed to satisfy personal desires through the example of sage Kardama, who, desiring offspring, "worshipped through *samādhi yoga* and *kriyā yoga* Hari, who fulfills the desires of those devoted to Him" (III.21.7). He notes that Kardama's case is exceptional, however, in that he was ordered to beget progeny by Brahmā and thus dutifully adopted this desire in order to comply with this request, not out of any personal inclination (*anu* 225).
108. The sense here is that because of poor deeds performed in the past, a person's intelligence is limited or deluded as a consequence and confounded even in his or her motives for approaching *Īśvara*.
109. Jīva in fact introduces a further tripartite schema in the *Bhakti Sandarbha* consisting of three divisions of "devotion mixed with *karma*" (*karma-miśrā bhakti*). In addition to *sa-kāmā bhakti*, and *kaivalya-kāmā bhakti*, he mentions *bhakti-mātra kāmā*, the adoption of *karma* or *jñāna* practices, but now with a desire for devotion alone. This third group, which performs a mixed type of devotion, *bhakti-mātra kāma*, also mixes *karma* or *jñāna* elements with its *bhakti*, but unlike the other two performers of *bhakti*, this third group does so with the intention of developing pure devotion and not for the standard fruits associated with *karma* or *jñāna*. Jīva exemplifies this with a passage, which we will find in the Teachings of Lord Kapila, where we see practices associated with *karma* and *jñāna* mixed in with some of the nine processes of *bhakti* (III.29.15–19).
110. This type of *bhakti* is exemplified by Jīva with the following prescription: "Residing in an isolated place, with mind made pure by contemplating Me, the sage should meditate on that non-dual *ātman* as being non-different from Me" (XI.18.21).
111. See, for instance, *Gītā* (VI.45).
112. As Rūpa notes in *Bhaktirasāmṛtasindhu* Eastern Quadrant II.309, Vallabha was a contemporary of Caitanya, and his followers established a lineage extant today as the Vallabha *saṁpradāya*.
113. This is a reference to one of the five types of liberation, *sārūpya*, that will be discussed in the chapter "The Object of *Bhakti*: *Īśvara*, *Bhagavān*, *Brahman*, and Divine Hierarchies."
114. See *Brahma Saṃhitā* 43 and Sanātana Gosvāmī's *Bṛhad-Bhāgavatāmṛta*.
115. This has some overlap with Plato's analogy of the cave.
116. The inference here is a cause-and-effect argument: whatever is present in the effect must be present in the cause; living beings, who are effects of some cause, have personalities, qualities, and forms, therefore it is at least logically

defensible to propose that their cause must also have a personality, qualities, and form. In Indian philosophy, this is called the *satkarya* principle, typical of Sāṅkhya metaphysics, but also of Vedānta, albeit differently construed. (There are schools, however, that refute these principles: Nyāya, Vaiśeṣiká, and Mīmāṁsā, upholding an *a-satkaryavāda* metaphysics: effects are distinct entities, the products of numerous causes.)

117. In particular, the sixteenth-century lineages stemming from Caitanya and Vallabha, as also the earlier Vaiṣṇava theologian Nimbārka.
118. A curt mention is made that Kṛṣṇa is worshipped there by the Vedic hymns.
119. We can contrast this with the term "sport" or even "game," which might contain a suggestion of drivenness or competition. The term *līlā* first surfaces in literary sources in the *Vedānta Sūtras* II.1.33, where we find the author addressing an opposing atheistic view that if there really were a God who is in possession of everything, He would not need to create, because people create in order to attain possession of something they do not already have. The *Sūtras*' response to this is that "just as [one finds] in the world, it [creation] is merely *līlā* (play)." The commentators on this verse compare God with a king who, although completely fulfilled, plays as an act of spontaneity, simply from fullness of spirit and not out of some unfulfilled need.
120. See X.23.37, X.45.44, X.52.36, and X.58.37.
121. Nevertheless, X.33.23 tells us that although Kṛṣṇa is *svarati*, "one whose pleasure is self-contained," He still takes pleasure from His *līlā*, as do those devoted to Him—the residents of Vraj, including the livestock (X.23.36); the cowherd boys who accompany Him on His adventures in the forests (X.12.3); and the elderly *gopīs* who enjoy themselves watching and laughing at His childhood antics (X.8.24).
122. See X.14.44, X.51.46, and X.70.28.
123. See, for example, X.40.23; *Gītā* VII.14. As in Hindu philosophical discourse in general, the bonds of illusion are typically articulated in terms of attachment to one's body, home, wealth, spouse, and offspring (X.4 8.27, X.60.52, and X.63.40).
124. See X.11.2ff., X.16.14, X.20.2, X.42.22, and X.61.2.
125. See X.12.27–28, X.70.47, and X.77.23, 28.
126. Kṛṣṇa does the same to His real parents, Vasudeva and Devakī, after they too become aware of His supremacy (X.45.1).
127. See the poetry of the sixteenth-century Sūr Dāsa for masterful juxtapositions of *līlā* with periodic reminders as to His majesty (Hawley 2009).
128. The partial exception is some of the left-handed Tantra traditions, touched upon later.
129. See *Muṇḍaka Upaniṣad* III.2.2; *Yoga Sūtras* II.12–15; *Gītā* V.22 and throughout.
130. For an earlier expression of this directed toward Śiva, see *Śvetāśvatara Upaniṣad* VI.21–23.

131. Since *saṁskāras* are made of the *sattva guṇa*, discussed later, which also underpins not only the psychic makeup of an individual (the *citta*), but all gross physical objects, along with the other two *guṇas*, *rajas* and *tamas*, Yoga psychology is also, in a sense, metaphysics. There is no duality between the mind and matter in terms of their ultimate constitution (the dualism in Yoga and Vedānta is between consciousness on the one hand and mind and matter on the other, not, as with the Greco-Christian or Cartesian model, between consciousness and mind on the one hand and matter on the other).

132. We can note here that any form of recognition of an object requires that the object be already known and, hence, a memory. Thus, to recognize, in our example, the chocolate in the shop window in the first place, one must already have a preexisting *saṁskāra* of the chocolate—a prior experience of it. That *saṁskāra* may have positive or negative valences associated with it. If pleasant, the *saṁskāra* can morph into *rāga*, and if unpleasant, *dveṣa* (*Yoga Sūtras* II.8).

133. See introduction, note 49, for Kṛṣṇa as *viṣaya* (sense object).

134. Technically, *rāgānugā* imitates *rāgātmikā*, discussed below (Eastern Quadrant II.270).

135. This verse is in fact spoken by the incarnation Kapila, whom we will encounter within.

136. Rūpa defines *bhāva* somewhat technically "as a special state of pure *sattva*, which softens the mind with a taste [for Kṛṣṇa], like a ray of the sun of love (*prema*)" (III.1). The word for "taste" here is *ruci*, which is more or less synonymous with *bhāva*, which in turn is synonymous with *rati*, "attraction" (*Bhaktirasāmṛtasindhu* Eastern Quadrant III.13).

137. *Mamatā*. In this state of "my-ness," the *bhakta*'s intimate absorption in intense thoughts of God causes a feeling that one belongs exclusively to God, and God to oneself as "my" son, "my" friend, and so on.

138. *Anarthas* (which are the equivalent of Patāñjali's *kleśas*).

139. Rūpa uses the term "taste" (*ruci*) here, which he associates with *bhāva* in *Bhaktirasāmṛtasindhu* Eastern Quadrant III.2. (Given this, I substituted *bhāva* so as to avoid overloading the reader with a plethora of Sanskrit terms and synonyms.)

140. See *Bhaktirasāmṛtasindhu* Eastern Quadrant III.6. "After appearing in the mind's activities (*vṛttis*), *bhāva* follows the natural inclination of the mind. It appears as if it has been manifest [by the mind], but it is actually self-manifesting" (*Bhaktirasāmṛtasindhu* Eastern Quadrant III.4; see Haberman 2003 for discussion following Jīva's commentary on Rūpa). Kṛṣṇa's various *śakti* powers are an extensive esoteric topic beyond the scope of this discussion.

141. *Bhāva* can also be the product of past-life *saṁskāra* (*Bhaktirasāmṛtasindhu* Southern Quadrant V.38). On a related note, *prema* can be experienced either with awareness of *Īśvara*'s majesty or in the form of what Rūpa calls *kevalā bhakti*, "exclusive devotion" devoid of such awareness (that is, thinking of Kṛṣṇa as one's friend, child, or lover, under the influence of *yogamāyā*; *Bhaktirasāmṛtasindhu* Eastern Quadrant IV.11). The former is generally for

those following the path of *vaidhī*, and the latter corresponds to the mind-set of the *rāgānugā bhaktas* (*Bhaktirasāmṛtasindhu* Eastern Quadrant IV.14).

142. See *Bhaktirasāmṛtasindhu* Eastern Quadrant III.2.
143. See *Bhaktirasāmṛtasindhu* Eastern Quadrant IV.17.
144. The usage of the term *rasa* in a *yogic* context goes back to the brilliant Kaśmīr Śaivite theologian Abhinavagupta (see Haberman 1988 for discussion).
145. There are also seven other secondary *rasas*, outlined in the *Bhaktirasāmṛtasindhu* (*Bhaktirasāmṛtasindhu* Southern Quadrant fifth wave), which need not detain us here.
146. *Kaivalya-kāmā bhakti*.
147. The term here is *asamprajñāta samādhi*. See *Yoga Sūtras* I.18 for *asamprajñāta samādhi*, also known as *nirbīja* (I.51), the state where consciousness is immersed exclusively in its own nature, devoid of any and all other objects (I.3).
148. Reference not given. Here the term *nirvikalpa* is used as a synonym of *asamprajñāta samādhi* and *nirbīja samādhi*. Still other terms include *kaivalya*, *ātma-jñāna*, and the more generic terms *mokṣa* and *mukti*.
149. See, for instance, *Gītā* X.12 and IX.27 in conjunction with XII.16–18.
150. These terms are all synonyms, and there are numerous other terms for the generic-liberated state, which are less frequently encountered (*nirvāṇa* was a term used by all the *mokṣa* traditions in the earlier period, such as in *Gītā* V.26 and VI.15, even as it became associated with Buddhism in later times).
151. In Patañjali's terms, *draṣṭuḥ svarūpe 'vasthānam*, "the seer abiding in its own nature" (*Yoga Sūtras* I.2).
152. He states this in his commentary to this verse of his uncle's work.
153. See Haberman (1994).
154. For a good accessible secondary source on *madhura bhakti*, see Schweig (2005).
155. We noted previously that the residents of Vaikuṇṭha and Goloka have bodies and forms made of *Brahman* rather than of the *guṇas* of *prakṛti*; this includes the minds of the inhabitants: these too are made of *Brahman* (see X.13.54 in part 3). This will be discussed further later.
156. Therefore, when *rāgātmika bhaktas* engage in any of the nine processes of *vaidhī bhakti* such as hearing, chanting, or remembering, they do so spontaneously and naturally and not in the form of a prescribed discipline or cultivated practice.
157. These *bhaktas*, of course, possess the requisite attainments from past-life *bhakti* practices in this material realm.
158. As we will see, Kṛṣṇa is born in a cowherding community.
159. For an excellent discussion of this phenomenon, see Haberman (1988).
160. The text would have been heard orally in premodern times rather than read. Prior to the advent of the printing press, the *Bhāgavata*, as with the entire Purāṇa tradition, would have been orally transmitted. Only a relatively few *brāhmaṇa* scholars would have had access to costly written manuscripts, reproduced individually by hand, often under the patronage of a king.
161. The verse states that the *yamas*, moral principles, are *sārva-bhaumā*, "universal," which is an absolute term that needs no further qualification. That

Patañjali proceeds to qualify them by specifying birth, place, time, and condition as nongrounds for anyone angling for exceptions is redundant and therefore out of place and technically anomolous in the curt minimalism of the *sūtra* genre. It therefore represents emphasis, unusual for Patañjali but underscoring his commitment to the indispensability of *yama* practices.

162. It is only left-handed Tantra that proposes socially taboo behavior can be undermined in spiritual practice. But even then, this is done in a highly ritualized and meditative environment that seeks to transcend individualized notions of selfhood and the dualities of good and bad perceived through that egoistic, individualized state. Such environments quickly weed out those adopting the practice to enjoy mundane sensuality predicated on misidentifying with the ego (*ahaṅkāra*) that classical Tantra also seeks to transcend, just like all other *yoga* traditions. Much of what is being peddled and consumed under the name of Tantra in the modern West is, from the perspective of the premodern textual Tantra traditions, simply foolishness.
163. For an examination of this recondite area of philosophy, free will, and agency in various Indic philosophical traditions, including that of the Gauḍīya tradition, see Dasti and Bryant (2014).
164. There are five types of liberation listed in Vaiṣṇava sources such as the *Bhāgavata*, one of which is *sāyūjya*, "merging," also known as *sāmyam*, the fourth type of liberation. *Sāyūjya* is not, in fact, acceptable to *bhaktas*, as it does not accommodate service. There are two types of *sāyūjya*, *brahma-sāyūjya* and *Bhagavat-sāyūjya*, described in the *Prīti-sandarbha* (*anu* 15). In *Bhagavat-sāyūjya*, the *ātman* enters into Kṛṣṇa's body and remains there, relishing the bliss of Kṛṣṇa's body, as is the case with Agha here. Jīva does not approve of either type of *sāyūjya*, as they do not accommodate service, but considers *Bhagavat-sāyūjya* the worse of the two because one is trying to enjoy *Bhagavān* rather than serve (my thanks to Satyanārāyaṇa Dāsa for this reference). On a related note, Rūpa comments that from the five types of liberation, those of the absorbed enemy and the loving *bhakta* are not actually identical: "The enemies of Hari usually merge into *Brahman*, but some, attaining a semblance of *sārūpya* liberation (achieving the same form as *Īśvara*), become immersed in happiness" (*Bhaktirasāmṛtasindhu* Eastern Quadrant II.279). He also adds that just as the sun ray resembles the sun but is a far lesser entity, so *Brahman* resembles Kṛṣṇa but is obviously quantitatively and qualitatively far inferior (Eastern Quadrant II.278). The verses indicating that the enemies and friends of Kṛṣṇa both attain the same destination are to be understood similarly.
165. Specifically, in this case, from the five types mentioned in the previous note, the type of liberation Kaṁsa attained was *sārūpya*, having the same form as the Lord.
166. *Bhāgavata* VII.1.15–25; *Gītā* VII.12–13; *Yoga Sūtras* I.25.
167. After all, our notions of our universe are nothing other than the range of our awareness of it (and hence this awareness of it keeps expanding as the instruments channeling our awareness become more sophisticated).

168. According to the *Gītā* (VIII.6), whatever state of mind one is absorbed in at the moment of death conditions the next life.
169. Jīva, and indeed the *Bhāgavata* itself, frequently uses this principle of *kaimutya*: "If *x* is the case, what then to speak of *y*" (which would be much more obviously the case).
170. The Soma ritual was one of the most important Vedic rituals (even as, long before the earliest extant commentator's Sāyaṇa's time in the fourteenth century, no one knew exactly what plant corresponded to the *soma* mentioned in the early texts). Lower castes such as dog-eaters would not normally have been permitted near the sacred sacrificial premises in pre-*bhakti* Vedic orthopraxy.
171. See note 29 in "The Practices of *Bhakti*" on Āryan.
172. Jīva finds this verse quoted by the Vaiṣṇava theologian Madhva (verse reference not given, *anu* 320).
173. This far surpasses the *Gītā*'s statement that women, normally marginalized in mainstream Vedic ritualistic orthopraxis, and excluded in Vedāntic textual studies, could also attain the "supreme destination" (IX.32), a statement that was itself radical for the time.
174. *Bhaktirasāmṛtasindhu* II.301–302. Reference not given.

The Practitioner of *Bhakti*, the *Bhakta*

1. There are twelve *mahājanas*, literally "great people," or exemplar *bhaktas* enumerated in the *Bhāgavata* (VI.3.20–21). Prahlāda, in this verse, is in fact behaving as an exemplar—posing as an everyday person overwhelmed by mental defects—since his mind was actually always fixed on Viṣṇu and transcendent to the base qualities he mentions here.
2. See XII.7 and XVIII.56, 58, 62.
3. See II.45, and as early as *Śvetāsvaṭara Upaniṣad* (III.20).
4. See also X.33.39.
5. Compare this with *kriyā yoga* "weakening" the *kleśas*, rather than completely eradicating them (*Yoga Sūtras* II.2).
6. See *Śvetāśvatara Upaniṣad* VI.21; *Mokṣadharma śānti parvan* 250.10 and 306.19–22; *Yoga Sūtras* I.3, III.55, and IV.34; *Gītā* II.29, IX.1–2, and XI.54.
7. *Bhagavat-tattva-vijñāna*.
8. *Daṇḍa-vat*, like a stick, is full prostrations on the ground, with arms extended in front full length.
9. *Kaṭha Upaniṣad* II.20.
10. Jīva states that from the three sources of knowledge accepted by most schools (for example, *Yoga Sūtras* I.7; *Sāṅkhya Kārikā* 4), the study of scripture removes the doubt about whether Truth can be realized; reason and argument, the doubts pertaining to opposing points of view; and personal experience, the doubt as to whether one is qualified to realize the Truth (*anu* 16).
11. There are numerous verses in this regard: "Bondage cannot exist after seeing *sādhus*, who see everything with equanimity and whose selves are dedicated

to Me [Kṛṣṇa], just as darkness cannot exist in the eyes of a person after seeing the sun" (X.10.41); and, again, "Let me always have the association of those great pure-hearted devotees, who are constantly immersed in devotion to You, O unlimited One. With this, I will become intoxicated with drinking the nectar of the narrations about You, and easily cross over the ocean of material existence, brimming with grave dangers" (IV.9.11).

12. As Prahlāda noted earlier, Nārada is another of the twelve *mahājanas*, the only twelve beings who fully understand *bhakti* (VI.3.20–22).
13. Ascetics eat one meal a day. Eating the remnants of their food, *prasādam*, is considered purifying, a reflection of the purity of saints.
14. For example, the Mīmāṁsā tradition established that one can determine the primary intention behind a text, even if it appears to contain conflicting or contradictory passages, by considering six criteria of the text: its opening and closing statements; its repetition of a subject; extraordinary statements made in it; results to be attained promoted by it; its glorification of a subject; and logical argumentation undertaken by the text to support some conclusion. Of course, as an aside, such criteria did not prevent profound differences in interpretation and the subsequent formation of numerous Vedānta lineages, as we will see.
15. Jīva here offers this *Bhāgavata* quote in support of those who experience spontaneous attraction: "From association with saints, realization of my power arises. These narratives of my activities become pleasing to the ears and the heart. By enjoying them, faith, love, and devotion quickly manifest consecutively on the path to liberation" (III.25.25). He contrasts this with the limitations of study: "Neither gods nor mortals, who have beginnings and ends, understand You, O most famous Lord. Considering this, those whose intelligence is pure abandon study of the Vedic texts" (VII.9.49).
16. Termed *sthita-dhī*, or *sthita-prajñā*, in the second chapter of the *Gītā*.
17. Arjuna's question in the second chapter, using the language of the Vedānta philosophical tradition, is raised again in chapter 14, using the language of Sāṅkhya, with essentially the same response reworded accordingly.
18. *Rati-rasa*.
19. See also I.18.13.
20. While this strikes us as a sexist comment in our modern day and age, as is the case with *Gītā* IX.32, we should remember that in Vedic orthopraxy, women were not allowed to study the sacred texts and could participate in Vedic rituals only in a secondary, passive role (Jamieson 1996), while laborers (*śūdras*) were barred from all such contexts. Likewise with formal lineage-embedded Vedānta study, traditionally an exclusive male preserve. *Bhakti* is thus an equalizer in gender as in social hierarchies and was socially revolutionary for its time (see *Bhāgavata* I.4.25 for an expression of this).
21. See Haberman (1994) for a premodern example of scandal in the Krishna tradition.
22. The *yamas* are listed and discussed in *Yoga Sūtras* II.30–45 as *ahiṁsā*, nonviolence; *satya*, truthfulness; *brahmacarya*, celibacy; *asteya*, nonstealing; and

aprarigraha, noncoveting. The *niyamas* are listed as *śauca*, cleanliness; *santośa*, contentment; *tapas*, austerity; *svādhyāya*, study and *mantra* recitation; and *Īśvara-praṇidhāna*, surrender to *Īśvara*.

23. Rūpa in verse 262 here is quoting the *Skanda Purāṇa*, reference not given.
24. For a critique of the *guru* culture in a modern Gauḍīya Vaiṣṇava expression, ISKCON (the Hare Krishna Movement), see relevant articles in Bryant and Ekstrand (2004). A few simple key word searches will bring up a plethora of scandals associated with numerous *guru* figures representing Eastern spirituality in the modern period.
25. *Sama-cittāḥ*. *Gītā* II.48 defines *yoga* itself with a form of the same adjective used here: *samatvam yogam ucyate*, *yoga* is equanimity.
26. Compare with *Yoga Sūtras* I.3.
27. Compare with *Gītā* V.8–9.
28. There are three types of *karma* accepted by the Yoga school: *sañcita*, already accumulated in the past and lying latent, awaiting its fructification in a future life; *sañcīyamāna*, ongoing (that is, being continuously accumulated in the present); and the type noted here, *prārabdha*. This latter category refers to *karma* that was activated at the moment of birth for this particular lifetime (the *jāti, āyur, and bhoga*, "family/species of birth, life span, and quality of life" of *Yoga Sūtras* I.13–14) and thus already set in motion. While the former two types of *karma* are annulled upon enlightenment, the *prārabdha* continues for the duration of that final life. In the *Sāṅkhya Kārikā*, the analogy of the potter's wheel is used to illustrate this already activated *karma*: even when the potter takes his or her foot off the wheel, it will not immediately stop spinning owing to the kinetic energy already invested in it (LXVII). Likewise, if a person becomes enlightened in the middle of a lifetime, the remnant of the *karma* already accrued for that lifetime will still run its course.
29. This is a reference to one of the implements Viṣṇu holds in His four arms, along with the conch shell, club, and lotus.
30. Although often associated with Buddhism, these were generic: the Buddhist *Saṁyutta Nikāya* and *Saṁyukta Āgama* acknowledge that these were followed by non-Buddhist schools (Bronkhurst 1993, 93).
31. This term was widely used by the *ātman* traditions before becoming associated in later times more exclusively with Buddhism (see, for instance, *Gītā* V.24–26 and VI.15).
32. As a point of fact, as we will discuss later, the Sāṅkhya tradition posits bliss not as an attribute of the *ātman*, but as an absence of suffering (which might appear blissful to one newly released from pain). But here, too, it is the intellect that quibbles over such things.
33. Although the *Vedānta Sūtras* limit this by noting that only *Īśvara* can create universes, the *ātman* cannot (IV.4.17); likewise, so do the *Yoga Sūtras* in the statement that *Īśvara*'s omniscience is unsurpassed (I.25). Thus, the liberated soul's omnipotency and omniscience cannot surpass that of *Īśvara*.
34. We will encounter several descriptions of these divine forms in part 2. For instance: "These attendants have brilliant dark hues, and lotus-petal eyes. They

wear yellowish garments and have extremely attractive and beautiful forms. They are effulgent and decorated with the choicest ornaments and medallions of brilliant flawless gems. Their complexions are of coral, gems, or lotus fiber. They wear dazzling necklaces, crowns, and garlands." (II.6.11)

35. Jīva in *Bhakti Sandarbha anu* 234 and Rūpa in Eastern Quadrant II.55.
36. Keeping in mind here that in Vaiṣṇavism the *ātman* is an eternal part, *aṁśa*, of the whole (*Gītā* XV.7 and references from the *Vedānta Sūtras* in I.4n81).
37. As we touched upon earlier, this latter possibility was the liberation attained by some of Kṛṣṇa's enemies in the tenth book. See, for instance, X.12.33, X.74–75, and X.78.9–10.
38. For an example of this, see Mārkanḍadeva's *Śiva-jñāna-bodha* XI; and Appayya Dīkṣita's *Śivādvaita-Nirṇaya* 3.2355. See also Law and Palmer, 56.
39. *Nija-iṣṭa*.
40. Gopīparāṇadhana Dāsa (2002). This section of the text recounts the travels of Gopa-Kumāra through various realms of the universe and then beyond, into the transcendent realms within *Brahman*.
41. For primary sources here, see the *Devī Gītā*, *the Devī Bhāgavata*, and the *Devī Mahātmya*; for secondary sources, Brooks (1990, 1992).
42. See *Gītā* XII.1–4, XIV.27, XV.16–20.

The Object of *Bhakti*: *Īśvara*, *Bhagavān*, *Brahman*, and Divine Hierarchies

1. See *Sāṅkhya Kārikā* I.1. Also see *Nyāya Sūtra* I.1.9 and 22; *Vaiśeṣiká Sūtras* V.16; *Gītā* VIII.15; and as early as the *Bṛhadāraṇyaka Upaniṣad* III.7.23 and IV.4.14. See Bryant 2003, 210ff., for the distribution of these four truths throughout chapter 2 of the *Yoga Sūtras*. They also occur elsewhere, including Āyurveda (there is disease, disease has a cause, there is a state free of disease, there is a means to attain this state free of disease).
2. While *duḥkham* is typically translated as suffering, it can mean any sort of mental in addition to physical suffering. I prefer to translate the term as "unfulfilling" since it is perhaps easier to recognize the lack of deep-level fulfillment as being *sarvam*—pertaining to everything one does (when in a state of ignorance of the true self).
3. I use the term "Vedic-affiliated" for schools, such as Yoga, Sāṅkhya, Vedānta, and the *bhakti* traditions, that lay claim to roots in the Upaniṣads, even though they are technically post-Vedic. I qualify the Vedic schools here because Buddhist traditions do not accept an autonomous *ātman* (with the possible exception of an early *pudgala* school). The problems with using the alternative term "Hindu" are well-known (it is a term introduced by invaders, rather than an indigenous label—as an aside, the first time the term surfaces in Indic sources is in the hagiography of *Śrī* Caitanya, Rūpa's own teacher). Nonetheless, the term "Hindu" can be used for ease of reference, given its by now irretractable prevalence.
4. The *ātman* is the innermost self, pure consciousness, distinct from both the psychic overlay of mind and its gross material embodiment.

5. For easily accessible primary sources on these basic points, see *Dhammapada* (for instance, 1, 3, 16, and throughout); *Yoga Sūtras* (chapter 2, especially II.2–26); and *Gītā* (II.62–66, V.22ff., and throughout).
6. See, for example, *Kaṭha Upaniṣad* II.22 and VI.13ff.; *Yoga Sūtras* II.29; *Gītā* VI.27–28.
7. As in the *Gītā* (IV.1–2, XV.15), Kṛṣṇa claims to be the origin of all these paths.
8. It may sometimes also lead to a motivated type of *bhakti* that will be discussed later, such as that associated with the role of *Īśvara* in the *Yoga Sūtras* (I.23–28). See the author's commentary on *Yoga Sūtras* I.23–24 for discussion.
9. See XV.16–20, XIV.27.
10. "Of what use are the sacred texts, austerities (*tapas*), the powers of speech, the control of mind (*citta-vṛtti*), keen intelligence, and strong senses? Of what use is the practice of *yoga*, or *sāṅkhya* (knowledge), the celibate vow of *sannyāsa*, or study of scripture and recitation of *mantra* (*svādhyāya*)? And what use are other attainments, unless they are offered to Hari [Kṛṣṇa]?" (IV.31.11–12).
11. The term *Īśvara* is already used five times by the *Atharva-Veda*, circa 1000 B.C.E., and has valences of lordship in the oldest texts. See Shastri (1935) for a history of the term with relation to theism.
12. From the classical schools of philosophy, the Mīmāṁsā school rejects the inferential necessity of positing an *Īśvara*. Sāṅkhya is typically (and hastily) assumed to be nontheistic, as the later *Sāṅkhya Kārikā* does not mention *Īśvara* (an assumption that can be brought into question—see, for instance, Edgerton 1924). But there were many schools of Sāṅkhya, most of which, preserved in the Purāṇas and *Mokṣadharma* section of the *Mahābhārata*, were in fact theistic (although the much later *Sāṅkhya Sūtra* is more explicitly nontheistic). There were thus both theistic and nontheistic Sāṅkhya strains, with—I would argue as others have done—the majority theistic.
13. See also *Bhāgavata* I.2.36 and III.24.32.
14. The *d* and *ta* endings on these two texts, respectively, reflect Sanskrit grammatical endings of the term *Bhagavān*, which is in the masculine, nominative case of the stem *bhagavat* (grammatically *bhaga* + *vat* possessive suffix = literally "one who possesses qualities"). *Bhaga* is an old Vedic term, used to refer to the share apportioned to the various gods in the Vedic *yajña*, sacrifice. By the Purāṇas, it becomes coupled with the possessive suffix and denotes the superexcellent qualities of a transcendent Being.
15. The terms can even, on occasion, be used figuratively for a powerful person (such as a sage like Nārada).
16. The term has earlier Vedic roots associated with the power of the sacrifice. The root is *bṛh*, to grow, increase, expand.
17. See, for example, *Kena Upaniṣad* I.1–6.
18. *Bṛhadāraṇyaka Upaniṣad* II.3.1–2. Since "being" is a present active participle (of the root *as*)—that is, a never-ending ongoing state—*sat* is often translated as "eternal."

19. See *Bṛhadāraṇyaka* 4.3.32; *Chāndogya* VI.2.1; *Taittirīya* II.2.1 and II.8; *Muṇḍaka* II.1.7. Also, as a technical aside, *advaita Vedānta*, in its radical nondualism, would not speak of the "qualities" of *Brahman*, as this implies a duality between qualities (*dharmas/guṇas*) and quality bearers (such as substances, *dharmins/guṇins/dravyas*). For this school, the inherent nature of *Brahman* is itself *sat-cit-ānanda*; it has no qualities.
20. See, for example, *Muṇḍaka* I.6–7.
21. See, for example, *Taittirīya* II.6; *Aitareya* I.1ff.; *Śvetāśvatara* I.8ff.
22. We will provide examples below.
23. Such schools point to verses such as the famous *sātmātattvam asi*, "you are that *ātman*," series of verses in the *Chāndogya* (VI.9ff.) and *Kaṭha*, "from death to death he goes, who sees here any kind of diversity" (IV.10–11; repeated from the *Bṛhadāraṇyaka* IV.4.19; these and translations in next note from Olivelle 1996).
24. Verses favored by such schools point to the *Śvetāśvatara*, such as I.6 and 9. Rāmānuja frequently quotes verses such as "The self of yours who is present within but is different from all beings, whom all beings do not know, whose body is all beings, and who controls all beings from within—he is the inner controller [*antaryāmin*], the immortal" (*Bṛhadāraṇyaka* III.7.21); "He had this desire, 'Let me multiply myself, let me produce offspring' " (*Taittirīya* II.6); and "It thought to itself, 'Let me become many' " (*Chāndogya* VI.2.3).
25. This can be readily seen by the *ṭilak*, sacred clay forehead marking, on pictures of Krishnamacarya, as well as on early photos of Iyengar, which denotes the school of *Śrī* Vaiṣṇavism, the formal name of Rāmānuja's lineage (the philosophical name is *viśiṣṭādvaita Vedānta*). I personally asked Iyengar, on his last tour to the West, whether he still identified with Rāmānuja's Vedānta lineage, *Śrī* Vaiṣṇavism, and whether he considered *Īśvara* to be Nārāyaṇa/Viṣṇu, as per the very specific theology of this lineage. He immediately and unambiguously replied in the affirmative. Since I was receiving a lot of requests to conduct *yoga* philosophy workshops in Iyengar *yoga* communities, I then asked him whether he wished for me to teach his students the *viśiṣṭādvaita Vedānta* position (which will be discussed later in this section) on fundamental Vedānta issues pertaining to *Iśvara*, *Brahman*, the *ātman*, and *bhakti*. He replied in the affirmative, then added that I should also teach them Śaṅkara's *advaita Vedānta* and all different points of view (personal communication in the Harvard Faculty Club, 2005). I very much appreciated this response.
26. This is especially central to the later Upaniṣads such as the *Śvetāsvatāra*, but emerging already in the earlier ones, too.
27. This is called *āgama*, as in *Yoga Sūtras* I.7, or, more commonly, *śabda* or *śruti/smṛti* (or just *śāstra*, as in *Vedānta Sūtras* I.I.3). Vedānta also employs reason and arguments secondarily, which occupy the second of the four chapters of the *Vedānta Sūtras*.
28. See *Yoga Sūtras* I.7 for a discussion of the three modes of gaining right knowledge according to Yoga, including *anumāṇa* and *āgama*. For an excellent

overview of Nyāya theism in both primary and secondary sources, see Dāsti (2010) and references therein, and Patil (2009).

29. For primary sources, see *Caitanya Caritāmṛta, ādi līlā*, chapter 10, and *Caitanya Bhāgavata, ādi khaṇḍa*, chapter 13; for secondary sources, see Ganeri (2011, chapter 4).
30. *Yoga Sūtras* I.24; *Gītā* 15.17.
31. This would be the Vaiṣṇava reading of, for example, *Gītā* XIV.27.
32. See I.4.20–22.
33. Or, with the Vedāntin Madhva (and also the Nyāya school), *Īśvara* is at least accepted as the overseer, sustainer, and support of *prakṛti*, which is not created but coeternal with Him.
34. As with the cluster of Yoga traditions, there were numerous variants of Sāṅkhya, amply attested to in the *Mahābhārata* epic (the Chinese Buddhist pilgrim Hsöen Tsang's disciple in the seventh century C.E. reports eighteen schools, and the *Bhāgavata Purāṇa* also refers to several). Only fragments quoted by other authors have survived from the works of the original teachers of the system. The later *Sāṅkhya Kārikā* of Īśvarakṛṣṇa, which scholars assign to the fourth to fifth century C.E., has by default become the seminal text of the tradition, just as Patañjali's *Yoga Sūtras* has become for the Yoga tradition, and represents its more developed, systematic form.
35. *Prakṛti* has been called "the undifferentiated plenitude of being" (Larson 1979, 167).
36. *Sat-tva* literally means "being-ness," from the root *as*, "to be." *Rajas* is from the root *rañj*, "to color" or to "redden." *Tamas* is from the root *tam*, "to choke, block, or stop."
37. Without *rajas*, for example, one could not even blink one's eyes, and without *tamas*, there would be no sleep or rest.
38. When the *guṇas* maintain what we might call an "equi-tension," *prakṛti* remains in a precreative state of dynamic potential called *avyakta*. Once the equilibrium is disrupted, however, creation takes place.
39. The analogy of milk holds good only in terms of the evolution of by-products. Where *prakṛti* differs from milk is that it and its evolutes maintain their own separate identities while simultaneously producing further evolutes, unlike milk, which is itself fully transformed when producing yogurt.
40. I have specified the Vedānta and Purāṇa traditions, as there are always exceptions to categories and terminologies: Nyāya, for example, would accept an eternal, primary, and nonderivatory *Īśvara*, but the earlier tradition would likely not use the term "personal" to depict Him. For this tradition, *Īśvara* as the nonreducible "individual" *ātman* who differs from other *ātmans* in being an omniscient Overseer would be a better way to demarcate this tradition from the monist understanding (although later Naiyāyikas were Śaivite and thus "personalists" in the sense I am using the term here).
41. We define "monotheism" here as one personal and transcendent God as supreme cause.

42. In his commentary of *Yoga Sūtras* I.24, the commentator Vyāsa, in support of one Supreme *Īśvara*, quips that if the various manifestations of *Īśvaras* were all exactly equal, and one says of an object "Let it be old" and the other says "Let it be new," the wishes of one of them will be thwarted (which would contradict the definition of *Īśvara*). And if their wishes never contradict, adds the commentator Vācaspati Miśra, then what is the point of having more than one *Īśvara* in the first place?!
43. Śaṅkara's *Upadeśasāhaśrī* is an excellent place to encounter accessible *advaita* teachings from its most famous exponent, all the more since it is a text attributed to Śaṅkara's own composition, in contrast with his other writings, which are commentaries on other preexisting Vedānta texts. For good secondary sources, see Deutsch (1969, 1971).
44. For the enlightened state while still embodied (*jīvan-mukta*) in Śaṅkara, see Fort (1996).
45. The twelfth-century commentator Madhva is a partial (and somewhat technical) exception here. Madhva does not accept *Īśvara* as the creator of *prakṛti*, although he accepts Him as the sustainer and support of both matter and the pluralist individual souls. Madhva's philosophy is one of dualism, *dvaita*, where, along the lines of the Nyāya school, God, the souls, and matter are all eternal coexistents (rather than the latter being emanational from the former). Nonetheless, *Īśvara* is unambiguously the Supreme Controller and Overseer in his very robust form of monotheism. See Sharma (1971) and Buchta (2013).
46. For good secondary sources on Rāmānuja, see Clooney (2007), Carmen (1974), Lipner (1986), and Cari (1998). For primary sources other than his commentary on the *Vedānta Sūtras* (the Śrī Bhāṣya) and *Gītā*, see Rāmānuja's *Vedārtha Saṅgraha*.
47. I thank Matthew Dasti for this conceptualization.
48. It is in fact listed in Mādhava's fourteenth-century doxography, the *Sarvadarśanasaṁgraha* (see Nicholson 2010, 148ff., for discussion on the Sanskrit doxographies).
49. While the notion of "six schools" surfaces frequently in the doxographies across the centuries, different schools were identified as comprising these six, or more than six were recognized. Additionally, sometimes the schools were differentiated differently—for instance, Yoga was not deemed separate from Sāṇkhya until later times. See Nicholson (2014) for discussion.
50. Glimpses of Śākta metaphysics can be read into the Upaniṣads, which these traditions—like all others—can then point to as their roots. All Vedic traditions needed to legitimate themselves by somehow or other locating themselves in the Ś*ruti*, as we will find in appendix 1 with Jīva himself. From this vantage point, later traditions could then claim to be the "real" or "hidden" or "higher" teachings of the Ś*ruti*. The *mokṣadharma* section of the *Mahabhārata*, which predated the Common Era, and various Purāṇas contain more explicit Śakta references, so these currents are ancient. And, of course, the *Śvetāśvatara Upaniṣad* (circa fourth century B.C.E.), despite being frequently quoted

by Vaiṣṇava theologians owing to its dualistic and theistic orientations, is explicitly Śaivite.

51. For excellent sources on Kaśmir Śaivism, see Muller-Ortega (1989), Lawrence (1999), and Dyczkowski (1987).
52. As noted earlier, so uncompromising is this form of *advaita* that even *sat*, *cit*, and *ānanda* are considered not "qualities" of *Brahman*, but its essence. A quality requires a quality bearer, or substance, in which the quality resides, hence creating a dualism between the quality and that in which it adheres. No such semblance of dualism or differentiation in *Brahman* is accepted by classical *advaita*.
53. Rāmānuja never mentions the *Bhāgavata*, prioritizing rather the *Viṣṇu Purāṇa*. We resist the proposal that this omission suggests that the *Bhāgavata* must have been written after Rāmānuja's time in the twelfth century. We prefer to see this as a theological neglect stemming from, precisely, discomfort with the *Bhāgavata*'s prioritization of Kṛṣṇa over Viṣṇu.
54. The Gauḍīya lineage traces its own pedigree (but not without contestation) to Madhva. This connection is not recognized by the orthodox Madhva tradition, however (see De 1986, 13ff.).
55. As in English negations like theist/atheist, an *a*- prefix negates the noun to which it is attached.
56. Where Rāmānuja tends to agree with Śaṅkara at least regarding the identification of the source Upaniṣadic text being referred to in any particular Vedānta *sūtra*, Madhva frequently identifies completely different source texts, even as his philosophy is very much closer to the former than the latter. See Adams (1993) for a comparative analysis of these three pivotal thinkers on the first chapter of the *Vedānta Sūtras*.
57. We take this usage from Dasgupta (1922, 246).
58. Madhva's ontology draws heavily from Nyāya categories.
59. The Nimbarka tradition has a commentary and calls its philosophy *dvaita-advaita*; Vallabha, a contemporary of Caitanya, did likewise for his *śuddha-advaita* philosophy; and most recently, the followers of the eighteenth-century Swami Nārāyaṇa tradition have just completed a commentary for the philosophy of their lineage, called *navya-viśiṣṭa-advaita*.
60. This trans-human status is irrespective of whether, as with Nyāya and the theistic traditions, the texts are authored and bestowed by *Īśvara* at the beginning of creation or, as with the nontheistic Mīmāṁsā school, the texts are authorless but nonetheless eternal.
61. Part of the Vedānta project, as an important aside, is to prove that the overarching primary subject matter of the Upaniṣads ultimately relates to *Brahman* rather than some other topic (I.3).
62. Like the *Yoga Sūtras*, many *sūtras* consist of only three or four words. They rarely indicate to which passage, section, or phrase in the Upaniṣads they refer and thus are completely inaccessible without commentary.
63. Precise labels are slightly problematic here since Śaṅkara could, in point of fact, be considered a type of Vaiṣṇava (even as some narratives place him as

an incarnation of Śiva), but along the lines noted above—in other words, he accepted in terms of conventional reality that the creator is Viṣṇu (in, for instance, his *Gītā* commentary), but that in ultimate reality both creation and creator are products of ignorance (see Nelson 2007 for an excellent discussion here). Moreover, since Rāmānuja's Vedānta school is called *viśiṣṭa-advaita*, "qualified nondualism," it has retained the term *advaita*, since everything is an expression of the one *Brahman*, but qualified it by positing differences within it, *viśiṣṭa*, along the lines noted previously. The terms "personalist" and "nonpersonalist" have similar sorts of problems.

64. This divisioning is seen in Mahāyāna Buddhism. Saṅkara's *param-guru*, Gauḍapāda, was either a Buddhist or heavily influenced by Buddhism (for discussion, see King 1995).
65. The standard primary Vedānta texts—the *prasthāna traya*, threefold corpus—consist of the Upaniṣads, the *Vedānta Sūtras*, and the *Gītā*.
66. The *Padma Purāṇa* states: "When *Īśvara* is described as *nirguṇa*, without qualities, what is meant is an absence of the *guṇas* connected with *prakṛti* like inferior objects" (*uttara-khaṇḍa* 255.39–40).
67. There are much less fundamental but still important variations, too, within post-Śaṅkara expresssions of *advaita*, as among the Vaiṣṇava schools (see Karl H. Potter, ed., *Encyclopedia of Indian Philosophy*, vol. 11: "Advaita Vedanta from 800 to 1200: From Vacaspati Misra to Citsuka." [Delhi: Motilal Banarsidass, 2006]).
68. The Swami Nārāyaṇa tradition, originating in Gujarat in the eighteenth century, has, at the time of this writing, recently completed its own commentary on the *Vedānta Sūtras* (Ahmedabad: Swaminarayan Aksharpith, 2009). This school calls its philosophy *navya-viśiṣṭa-advaita*, a "new" variant of Rāmānuja's philosophy (indeed, their monks are often trained in philosophy and logic by *viśiṣṭādvaita* Vaiṣṇava theologians).
69. Nyāya (the school of logicians) argues vigorously contra *advaita Vedānta* for both the *ātman* and *Īśvara* as eternally independent and individual "reals" (which they term *padārthas*, things that can be named because of having inherent existence), and as discussed, even the monistic Kaśmir Śaivite tradition rejects Śaṅkara's illusionism when it comes to the world of forms, which they hold to be real *citi-śakti*.
70. There are 150 dense pages in Thibaut's translation (1904). Madhva also vigorously opposed Śaṅkara, as did the great *bhakta* scholar and theologian Vallabha, a contemporary of Caitanya.
71. We can briefly touch upon one commonly encountered argument Jīva raises against the *advaita* position (so as not to burden here those less interested in Vedānta argumentation), in order to give a flavoring of this issue through Vaiṣṇava theological sensitivities. The first argument he introduces against the *advaita* position in his *Bhakti Sandarbha* is the most commonly encountered in anti-*advaita* argumentation and, as with so much else, can be traced back at least to the twelfth-century Vedānta theologian Rāmānuja. If it is true, as *advaita* holds, that there is in ultimate reality (*paramārthika*) only one

undivided *Brahman*, whose nature is *cit*, pure consciousness, but that owing to *māyā/avidyā* (ignorance), the *ātman* is erroneously perceived as different from it, when in fact it is nothing other than that same *Brahman*, then this is tantamount to suggesting that *Brahman* can fall under the influence of illusion. As Rāmānuja puts it: "*Kasyā avidyā,*" Whose is this ignorance? Where is its locus? Is ignorance somehow covering *Brahman*? This is constitutionally impossible, as *Brahman*'s very nature is *cit*, full awareness: it can never be unaware or subject to ignorance, any more than the sun can be unilluminated. So ignorance cannot exist in *Brahman*. But nor can it be located outside of *Brahman*, as that creates a situation of *dvaita*, duality (two distinct entities), which contradicts the nonnegotiable tenet of *advaita*—absolute nonduality. Nor can it be covering the individual *ātman* since the *ātman*'s individuality is itself caused by ignorance, hence this ignorance must have existed prior to its effect of individualization. Besides, for *advaita* metaphysics, ignorance cannot be within a part of *Brahman* of any sort, for the same reason—*Brahman* has no parts, once again, because, ex hypothesi, it must only be nondual. In fact, says Jīva, the latter possibility is actually the only coherent one: there must be some sort of difference between the part of *Brahman* under the spell of *māyā*—namely, the *jīva*—and the part of *Brahman* that can never be reduced to this condition but is, in fact, the wielder of ignorance (*māyā*)—namely, *Īśvara* (*Tattva Sandarbha anu* 35–40).

The basic *advaita* response to this dilemma (and the issue has been treated differently through the history of the tradition) is that an explanation of ignorance is beyond human comprehension (*anirvācanīya*). To be fair, the Gauḍīya Vedāntins do not hesitate to resort to a similar position of inconceivability (*acintya*) when discussing their own ontology. So all this points to the obvious limitations of the human intellect in capturing Truths that, by the definition of all Vedantins (and all *mokṣa* traditions), lie completely beyond it. Nonetheless, the debate remains an indispensable polemical mainstay of the various Vedānta communities to this day, since clearly, for Vaiṣṇavas, *bhakti yoga* requires an eternal *Īśvara* in devotional relationship with an *ātman* that is quantitatively distinct on the one hand, even as it is qualitatively the same on another (that is, also comprising *sat*, *cit*, and *ānanda*). Hence the perennial effort invested in relentlessly marshaling exegetical and philosophical methods in defense of these Truths.

72. *Bhajana*, in addition to its meaning discussed in the *kīrtana* section, is sometimes more broadly used as another term for *bhakti* practice.
73. For the *Bhāgavata*, nonduality indicates that everything emanates from *Bhagavān*—nothing has separate or independent existence. *Advaya* is a synonym of *advaita* but understood by the Vaiṣṇavas very differently from Śaṅkara.
74. *Paramātman*, Supreme *Ātmān*, is another term understood variously in the Vedānta schools. For the *Bhāgavata* and Vaiṣnava traditions, it generally refers to derivative forms of Viṣṇu involved in various levels of overlordship in

the matter of creation (see I.6.29), as well as the form that manifests to *yogīs*. Rūpa quotes a verse from the *Skanda Purāṇa* stating that "*Bhagavān* is called *Paramātman* by the followers of the eight-limbed *yoga* (*aṣṭāṅga*), *Brahman* by those who follow the Upaniṣads, and *jñāna* by the *jñāna-yogis*" (*Laghu-Bhāgavatāmṛta* I.196, reference not given; for a rearticulation of this verse, see *Bhāgavata* III.32.26).

75. See, for example, Rūpa in yet another of his publications: *Laghu-Bhāgavatāmṛta* (V.216).
76. Nyāya is an exception, here, positing that the *ātman* has consciousness as a quality, but that this quality is instantiated and manifest only when the *ātman* is coupled with a mind but remains latent when the *ātman* is liberated and uncoupled from the mind. Hence liberation for Nyāya (and its sister school, Vaiśeṣiká) is a not a state of pure consciousness.
77. Indeed, Sheridan (1983) reads an "*advaitic* theism" in this text. See also Bhattacarya (1960–62), Vyasa (1974), and Rukmani (1970) for other studies on the text's philosophy.
78. *Paramātman* in Vaiṣṇavism is the immanent aspect of the personal Absolute consciously active within His own power of *māya-śakti*, the material world of *prakṛti* and the *guṇas*. It is God as regulator of the universe and the selves within it. Specifically, it refers to the various Viṣṇu forms. For example, there is the Mahā-Viṣṇu (Kāraṇodakaṣayī), from whose pores unlimited parallel universes emanate (X.14.11, X.88.41). Unlimited derivative Viṣṇus are manifest from that Mahā-Viṣṇu and enter into each individual universe (the Kṣīrodakaśayī Viṣṇus), and it is from the navels of these Viṣṇus that the lotus grows upon which Brahmā, the secondary creator, finds himself (as we will encounter in the Tale and Teachings of Lord Brahmā). There is a further tertiary Viṣṇu who then enters into the hearts of all beings, as well as into every atom, the *Paramātman* or *Antaryāmin*. This ontology, derived from the *Pāñcarātrika* tradition, is outlined in various sources such as the *Paramātma Sandarbha*.
79. See also *Gītā* XIV.27 and VII.4–7ff.
80. *Draṣṭuḥ svarūpe 'vasthānam*, the seer abides in its own nature (*Yoga Sūtras* I.3), which is just pure consciousness (II.20).
81. *Aṁśa*, "part," in *Gītā* XV.7 and *Vedānta Sūtras* II.3.43; *bheda*, "difference," in *Vedānta Sūtras* I.1.17 and 21, I.2.20; and *viśeṣana*, "distinction," in *Vedānta Sūtras* I.20.22.
82. Written *Puruṣottama* for syntactical reasons.
83. Like the obtainment of an M.Phil. for one pursuing a Ph.D.!
84. Written *Paramātman*.
85. See, for a parallel discussion, the commentaries on the *vitārkas*, the unwanted impulses contrary to the *yamas* and *niyamas*, in *Yoga Sūtras* II.33–34.
86. Nyāya posits the liberated state as one free of suffering, rather than a more positive state of actual bliss.
87. Hence, "the poet-sages always engage in great ecstasy in *bhakti* for *Bhagavān* Vāsudeva, which satisfies the mind" (I.2.22).

88. *Draṣṭuḥ svarūpe 'vasthānam* (*Yoga Sūtras* I.3). The fifth limb of *yoga*, *pratyāhāra*, is precisely to withdraw consciousness from the senses and all sense objects, and the remaining three limbs of *dhāraṇā*, *dhyāna*, and *samādhi* to totally still the mind (*Yoga Sūtras* II.49, III.1–3).
89. See VII.8.42, X.16.37, X.87.21, XI.20.34, XI.14.14, and XII.10.6.
90. See III.4.15, III.25.34, III.29.13, V.14.44, VI.18.74, and IX.4.67.
91. See IV.9.10, IV.20.24, VI.18.74, and VII.6.25.
92. See VI.11.25.
93. The commentator Viśvanātha states here that if one's *bhakti* is not strong, one will become distracted by the mystic powers accruing from *yoga*. Like the *Yoga Sūtras* (III.37), the *Bhāgavata* considers such powers useless (XI.15.33), for reasons that should be obvious by now.
94. Although thinkers such as Madhva held that the Vedic gods were originally attributes of Viṣṇu, who became reified in their own right only after the degeneration of the ages (Madhva wrote a commentary on certain verses of the *Ṛg-Veda*). Dayānanda of the Arya Samaj was to argue something similar in much later times.
95. *Śivarātrī* has various stories associated with it.
96. Sectarian lineages are known as *saṁpradāya* or *paramparā* (for instance, see *Gītā* IV.2).
97. Sacred text is also called *āgama* (for example, in *Yoga Sūtras* I.7).
98. For instance, placing a *tulasī* leaf on all food offered to the Deity in Vaiṣṇavism.
99. The *Dina-Candrikā* was the last book published by Hari Dāsa Śāstrī, a prolific scholar and author, before he passed away in 2013 (Vṛndāvan: Śri Gadādhara Gaurhari Press, n.d.).
100. This term is not typically used for Lakṣmī but is employed here as a play on words to parallel Śiva's consort Umā with a view to emphasize the near identicality even in nomenclature of these *Īśvaras* and *Īśvarīs*.
101. It is for these sorts of reasons that the eighteenth-century Baladeva Vidyābhūṣaṇa wrote a commentary on the *Vedānta Sūtras* on behalf of the Gauḍīya tradition. Without this, no emerging school claiming to be representing the true teachings of the Vedas or Vedānta can be considered authoritatively grounded in the old *Śruti* (Vedic) texts (we have noted this is an ongoing expectation, with the Swami Nārāyaṇa tradition's most recent addition to the commentarial tradition).
102. See *Yoga Sūtras* I.7; *Sāṅkhya Kārikā* IV.
103. Despite the usually poorly informed references to the so-called Hindu trinity, Brahmā, the (nominal) third *Īśvara*, is a mortal being and so is never a genuine contender for the role of supreme transcendent *Īśvara*, as we will see from his tale within. Although there are Purāṇa stories where the three compete, the playful competition in the Purāṇas is between Viṣṇu and Śiva, which is resolved according to the sectarian nature of the different lineages. Brahmā, if he competes, as in the Atri story mentioned above, is merely a placeholder (see *Bhāgavata* X.89.1–20).

104. While these traditions are "later" in terms of the compositions of their textual traditions, in fact it is impossible to tell how old some of the stories they contain are or if they may have existed orally (especially if they did not feel compelled to engage in orthodox Vedic rituals or Vedāntic exegesis). In all probability they coexisted with the ancient Vedic corpus. See the *Devī Bhāgavata Purāṇa*, *Devī Māhātmyā*, or *Devī Gītā* as important "later" texts in the Goddess tradition.
105. For example, we have discussed how Śaiva schools follow similar bifurcations between, for instance, Kaśmir Śaiva and Śaiva Siddhānta expressions, as to whether the form of Śiva is ultimate and supreme or derived from a higher transpersonal Truth. Likewise, there are Vaiṣṇava Śākta traditions as well as Vaiṣṇava *advaita* adherents; and one can find Śaivite Vedāntins and the like. This can all be seen as reflecting the infinite and unlimited potentiality of the Divine from the Purāṇic perspective.
106. We need not concern ourselves with the Purāṇic references associated with Brahmā, which are considered of the nature of *rajas*, for reasons offered in note 103.
107. There are some differences among Purāṇa lists as to which Purāṇas constitute the eighteen.
108. Brahmā is associated with its creation, a quality of *rajas*, but as we have noted, he is a mortal being and not in the same category as Viṣṇu and Śiva.
109. As we will see, the *Vaiṣṇava Purāṇas* associate Śiva and Brahmā with religiosity that seeks material gain (or, at best, spiritual gain mixed with materialism, as in I.2.26–27, quoted later). Hence the statement here that the ultimate good—which was established in the opening verses of the *Bhāgavata* as being free of any such motives (I.1.2 and note)—is attainable only from Viṣṇu.
110. Vedic religiosity involves a highly elaborate, technical, and expansive set of rituals, for which fire, as consumer of the oblations, is central. The metaphor indicates that fire—as actual consumer of the offerings and a form of the god Agni—is more important than wood or smoke, even as these are intertwined and inseperable.
111. We reiterate that for the Vaiṣṇava traditions, Viṣṇu's form is made not of *prakṛti*, but of *Brahman*, the *viśuddha sattva* noted here.
112. The *Harivaṁśa* is another extensive account of Kṛṣṇa's life, added as an appendage to the *Mahābhārata* epic and generally taken by scholars to be an older rendition.
113. In the *Mahābhārata*, *Harivaṁśa*, and *Viṣṇu Purāṇa*, there is no doubt that Kṛṣṇa is an incarnation of Viṣṇu. The roles, for the most part, have been somewhat reversed in the *Bhāgavata*: while there are abundant passages in the text that relate to Viṣṇu without explicitly subordinating him to Kṛṣṇa, particularly in the books prior to the tenth, the general thrust of the tenth book, which takes up a quarter of the entire twelve books of the Purāṇa, prioritizes Kṛṣṇa. The *Gītā* can also be read as prioritizing Kṛṣṇa (see VII.6–7, X.8) but is obviously not viewed this way by Rāmānuja and Madhva.

114. Rūpa identifies four aspects unique to Kṛṣṇa that are not manifest in any other *Īśvara* form: "His *līla*, the unsurpassed love of His devotees, the sweetness of His flute, and His beauty" (*Bhaktirasāmṛtasindhu* Southern Quadrant 1.43).
115. See, for discussion, Sheth (1982).
116. *Mahāvākyas* are especially associated with Śaṅkara and the *advaita* tradition, for whom *tat-tvam-asi* ("you are that [*ātman*]," *Chāndogya Upaniṣad* VI.9–11) is the best known among four prominent in that tradition. Rāmānuja also has his equivalents of the *mahāvākyas*, such as "In the beginning, son, this world was simply what is existent—one only, without a second . . . and it thought to itself: 'Let me become many.' " (*Chāndogya Upaniṣad* VI.2.1–3; Lipner 1986, 82). See Goswami (2012) for a discussion about *Kṛṣṇas-tu Bhagavān svayam* as a parallel *mahāvākya* of the *Bhāgavata* and its derivative traditions.
117. This is a reference to *parama-Śiva*, the ultimate expression of Truth in Śaivite theology.
118. The text reminds us constantly that "Brahmā, Śiva . . . the Goddess of Fortune, Śrī, are only a fraction of a fraction of Him [Kṛṣṇa]" (X.68.37). Śiva discloses to his consort Parvatī that it is upon Viṣṇu that He meditated when He engaged in *yoga* for one thousand years (VIII.12.43–44). See also Śiva's eulogy of Viṣṇu's supremacy after being bewildered by the latter's female incarnation of Mohinī (VIII.12.4–13). *Śaiva Purāṇas* claim the same for Śiva, as we will see below.
119. Since *bhūta* can refer to "ghosts" (literally "one who has gone"), Jīva mentions Bhairava here, a particular form of Śiva that is the Lord of ghosts and other afflicted beings.
120. We can also mention here, from the *Bhāgavata*, Sudakṣiṇa (X.66.27ff.) and Saubha (X.76). Likewise, the story of Hiraṇyakaśipu, who attained near invincibility from the worship of Brahmā, is an important narrative of the *Bhāgavata* that we will encounter in part 2.
121. There are exceptions to just about everything in the Purāṇas!
122. The text adds here: "He is ego in its three divisions of *sattva*, *rajas*, and *tamas*. The transformations from this have resulted in the sixteen ingredients of the world."
123. See I.12.23, IV.4.15, and X.76.5.
124. "Who see all beings in the *ātman*."
125. However, it can be inferred from the Agha story in part 3 that one variant of *sāyūjya* involves an actual merging into Kṛṣṇa's body, which would entail, to all intents and purposes, becoming one with Viṣṇu (not a spiritual clone, so to speak, as is the case with *sārūpya*). This state is called *ātmasāmya* in X.12.38.
126. See Valaveetil (1996) for a brief discussion on this.
127. Consider, for example, this passage from the *Rūdrasaṃhitā* of the *Śiva Purāṇa*: "Śiva thought within Himself like this: 'Another being shall be created by Me. Let him create everything, protect it, and in the end let him dissolve it with

My blessing. Having entrusted everything to him, we two [Śiva and Śakti] . . . shall roam as we please, keeping only the prerogative of conferring salvation. We can stay happily . . . free from worries. . . .' Thereupon [after Śiva churns the ocean of His mind] a person came into being who was the most charming one in the three worlds, who was calm with Sattva Guṇa being prominent, and who appeared to be the ocean of immeasurable majesty. . . . He bowed to Śiva Parameśvara and said: 'O Lord, give me names and assign me my task.' On hearing it, Lord Śiva laughed. With words thunderlike in resonance, Lord Śiva addressed the person thus. Śiva said: 'You will be famous as Viṣṇu by name as you are all-pervasive. You will have many other names conferring happiness on devotees'" (6.33–43). Interestingly, Viṣṇu's association with *sattva* and his creatorship and dominion over everything are retained in this story but reworked into a very different relationship with Śiva. See also *Śiva Purāṇa, Vāyavīyasaṃhitā* 13.11–47. The most widely recounted story associated with Śiva's supremacy is the famous narrative where Viṣṇu (and Brahmā) is not able to find the limits of Śiva's *liṅga* (uniconic) form: *Śiva Purāṇa, Rudrasaṃhitā* 7–9; *Liṅga Purāṇa* I.17–19; *Skanda Purāṇa, Uttarārdha* 9–14. See also *Śiva Purāṇa, Vidyeśvarasaṃhitā* 5.28–29. Elsewhere, this text expresses an interesting arrangement whereby all three Lords get to be progenitors of the other two in different ages, albeit always as derivative entities born of the great Śiva (*Vāyavīyasaṃhitā* 13.2–26). All Puraṇas quoted here from the Motilal Banarsidass edition.

128. For an example from the Devī tradition, see the *Devī Gītā* I.14ff. and the *Devī Bhāgavata Purāṇa* 7.29.23–30.

129. See, for instance, *Gītā* II.62–62 and III.37; *Yoga Sūtras* II.12; *Kaṭha Upaniṣad* VI.14–15; *Mokṣadharma, Śānti Parvan* 251.7. Consider also the Second Noble Truth of Buddhism, the cause of suffering (that is, desire).

130. With some qualifications, in certain Tantra traditions it is not desire that must be renounced, since *prakṛti* is *citi-śākti*, the power of consciousness, and thus (for instance, in Kaśmir Śaivism) nondifferent from Śiva and therefore divine, not a negative entity to be renounced. So it is not the desire to enjoy *prakṛti*, but the illusion of enjoying as an entity imagined to be separate from Śiva that must be relinquished. Once that ignorance is removed, and one realizes one's own Śiva nature, then one can enjoy *śākti*. Nonetheless, the schools of right-handed Tantra do follow *yama* equivalents.

131. The *devas*, by the time of the *Gītā* and *Bhāgavata*, are depicted as beings in *saṁsāra* who, because of inordinately good *karma*, have attained highly *sāttvic* forms in celestial realms. However, they too reattain a human birth once this good *karma* has expired (*Gītā* VIII.10).

132. In fact, the *Gītā*'s comments pertaining to the Vedic texts parallels the discussion above of the *Bhāgavata*'s perception of other Purāṇas: "The subject of the Vedas is the three *guṇas*. Become free of the *guṇas*, Arjuna. Be situated always in *sattva* . . ." (II.45).

133. See also *Gītā* IX.23–24 and X.20–42.

Concluding Reflections

1. John in a vision saw God seated upon His throne (Revelation 4:1–3), and Daniel had a similar vision (Daniel 7:9–10), as did Isaiah (6:1–5). Similarly, we are told that Moses, Aaron, his sons, and the elders of Israel "saw the God of Israel" (Exodus 24:9–11). And Moses was permitted to see the back (but not the face) of God (Exodus 33:18–23). See also Ezekiel 1.40.2. See Williams (2009) for discussion and references to transcendent anthropomorphism in the Semitic traditions.
2. Colossians 1:15 and Timothy 1:17 indicate that God is invisible.
3. Certain sages recount how, despite performing intense austerities, when they arrived at Nārāyaṇa's abode within the universe called Śvetadvīpa in the hope of seeing the Supreme Being, they were blinded by His effulgence. Other great souls who resided there, however, were able to see Nārāyaṇa.
4. Thus, etymologically, the name Jupiter is cognate with Zeus pater and, in Sanskrit, Dyaus *pitṛ*. And functionally, Thor, Zeus, and Indra are all leaders of the other celestials, associated with rain, thunder, and lightning, and have a weapon that they hurl.
5. As is well-known, aspects of the old pre-Christian traditions are absorbed into Christianity (such as the appropriation of the birthday of Mithras on December 25).
6. Various texts speak of the *devas* as having forms made of expressions of *prakṛti* other than the gross matter of this realm, such as *tanmātra* (see Bryant 2009, 74, for references; the inhabitants of Śvetadvīpa mentioned in note 3 are one such example).
7. When compared with the sword-bearing archangel Gabriel, the warrior nature of the *gandharvas* enhances the comparison.
8. Of course, *Īśvara* is simultaneously also immanent given that *prakṛti* and the *ātmans* are a part of His manifestation and therefore nondifferent from Him.
9. Actually, in Gauḍīya theology there are unlimited Vaikuṇṭha realms, as God has unlimited manifestations.
10. The exception to this is the early Vedic religion as expressed in the four Vedas, at least as construed by academic Indological methods. There is no transcendent supreme deity explicitly revealed there, but rather a situation much closer to the other Indo-European pantheons, where, at best, we find a martial chieftain prominent in the form of Indra (performing the functional parallel role of Zeus or Thor) among ontologically equal celestials. Traditional Hindu theologians have reworked this potential problem in different ways. The thirteenth-century Vaiṣṇava theologian Madhva, for example, who wrote a commentary on forty hymns of the *Ṛg-Veda*, argued that these gods originally represented the various powers of the transcendent Viṣṇu that came to be considered separate autonomous entities only in later, more spiritually decadent times. Other revisionist reworkings can be found in nineteenth- to twentieth-century monotheistic exegeses of the Vedas by prominent Hindu apologists such as Dayananda and Aurobindo.

11. *Bhāgavata* I.4.14.
12. We resist the usual translation for *avatāra* as "incarnation" (etymologically, "to enter flesh"), since Vaiṣṇava theology holds that Kṛṣṇa descends in this *Brahman* (pure consciousness) body and not one made of matter (see Lipner 1976 for a discussion in Rāmānuja's lineage).
13. See, for example, from the most seminal thinkers, Freud as the externalization of subconscious forces; Durkheim as social forces; Tyler as primitive science; Weber as economic forces; Marx as related to the control of the modes of production; and others.
14. For instance, Max Muller, Mircea Eliade, the Theosophists, and other shades of perennialist thinkers.
15. For a good start on the construction of the category of religion triggered by the early European encounter with the non-Western world, see Halbfass (1988), King (1999), Masuzawa (2005), Oddie (2006), Pennington (2005), and Balagangadhara (2012).
16. There are a number of instances of this throughout the text, such as the *Virāṭ-rūpa* material form in the second book, which is explicitly described as being meditative rather than factual.
17. The *pratyakṣa* and *anumāna* in, for instance, *Yoga Sūtras* I.7.
18. The prioritizing of empiricism and reason is most noteworthy in the Cārvāka, Nyāya, and Buddhist traditions, but most schools incorporated rich intellectual argumentation into their theologies, and almost all in one way or another accepted the paramount nature of empiricism as the basis of other epistemes, other than in domains inaccessible to reason and sense perception.
19. See Halbfass (chapter 21), however, for resistance to the trump card of experience in certain conservative discourses such as the Mīmāṁsā, as in the writing of Śaṅkara.
20. The ultimate *vairāgya*, detachment, is *guṇa vaitṛṣṇyam*, disinterest in anything made of the *guṇas*.
21. The roots of the tension between mythos and logos in fact goes back to the pre-Socratics.
22. See references in previous citations.
23. Of course, aspects of the historical method are selectively appropriated by a certain genre of nationalists in such political contestations as that over Ayodhyā, the birthplace of Rāma in epic sources (Gopal 1992), and the Aryan invasion debate (Bryant 2001).
24. See Brown (2013) for an excellent discussion.
25. See Holdrege (2013) for discussion.
26. Shukavak Dāsa (1999).
27. Albeit for completely different reasons, here he appropriates part of the hierarchical schema of Śaṅkara noted earlier (himself following a Madhyāmakā Buddhist schema).
28. Raja Ram Mohan Roy, for example, the so-called father of modern India, had no place for Kṛṣṇa in his Christian Upaniṣadic mélange, institutionalized as

the Brahmo Samaj, and, indeed, lambasted him with no small measure of pre-Victorian-derived indignity. Like his successors in the Brahma Samaj, such as Devendranatha Tagore and Krishna Chandra Chaterjee, he was nonetheless a monotheist (as opposed to, say, a neo-*advaitin* such as Vivekānanda), but he espoused a monotheism that conceived of God in terms much closer to the Abrahamic models that influenced them so greatly than to those of the premodern Vaiṣṇava and Śaivite traditions. We can also place the influential Dayānanda, founder of the Ārya-Samaj, on this side of the monotheistic spectrum. Others, like the more devotional Bankim Chandra Chatterjee, set out to construct and propagate a righteous Kṛṣṇa as preserved in the *Bhagavad Gītā* by extricating him from what Bankim deemed centuries of Purāṇic accretions epitomized by the Kṛṣṇa of the *Bhāgavata*. Thus purged, the sterilized Kṛṣṇa could be set up as a superior role model for humanity to the Christ of the colonizers. There was a wide spectrum of monotheistic responses to the encounter with modernity on issues lying at the core of Hindu *bhakti* (see Sardella 2010, 2013, for discussion). The monistic neo-*advaita* response is an enormous topic in its own right, which lies outside the main concerns of this study. It has, in fact, received far more attention in both scholarly and popular circles than the monotheistic strains in Hinduism, for reasons that have arguably a lot more to do with Hindu nationalism in India and New Age spirituality in the West than any de facto reality of on-the-ground Hindu beliefs and practices past and present.

29. Note, for instance, Yaska's interpretation of Indra killing the Vṛtra demon, a pivotal Vedic and Purāṇic narrative, as the production of rain.
30. The historical accords with the traditional Vedic exegetes such as Sāyana; the mystical, which is his main focus, involves identifying hymns to various deities as actually denoting attributes of Viṣṇu; and the transcendent features the relationship between the *ātman* and *Brahman* (see Sharma 1971, 180ff., for discussion). One might wonder whether the nineteenth-century Dayānanda Sarasvatī was influenced by Madhva's approach.
31. See Edelmann (2013) for discussion.
32. For discussion and references, see Edelmann (2013). The astronomical traditions of the *Siddhāntas* and *Jyotiḥśāstra* in the period 500–1900 C.E. were willing to depart from Purāṇic cosmology without rejecting the Purāṇas themselves. Similarly, literary theory presents elaborate theoretical criteria pertaining to when a primary signification (*vācya*) of a text is to be superseded by secondary (nonliteral) readings, specifically indicated (*lakṣya*) and suggested (*vyaṅga*) meanings (briefly, wherever the primary meaning of scriptural passage is obstructed [*baddha*] by other knowledge, secondary meanings can be applied).
33. We should note, however, that Jīva would not call the mental absorption of the *asuras bhakti*, even as they might have attained some form of liberation. *Bhakti* requires a positive attitude toward *Īśvara* (see "Meditating in Enmity: Kṛṣṇa and the Demons").

34. *Gospel of Sri Ramakrishna*, 361, 743; Schiffman, 130.
35. *Autobiography of Swami Sivananda*, ix.
36. The record of this claim is buried in the organization's archives, which I was not able to access, but it is common knowledge and surfaces in the brochures and other literatures of the organization (such as the Grass Valley, California, *Guide to Programs*, 2014, 26).
37. Uttarapara speech, May 30, 1909.
38. This well-known anecdotal exchange is noted in, for example, the Inaugural Souvenir of the Ramamani Iyengar Memorial Yoga Institute, 1975.
39. Cornell (2001).
40. *Autobiography of a Yogi*, 399.
41. Muktānanda (1978), chapter 20. In Kaśmir Śaivism, blue is the color of pure consciousness.
42. For excellent historical excavations of the evolution of modern postural *yoga*, see DeMichelis (2004), Alter (2004), Singleton (2008, 2010), Straus (2005), Syman (2010), Sjoman (1996), and Jain (2015).
43. Western forms of dualism correlate the mind and cognition with the soul (*psyche*), whereas these are outer material coverings completely distinct from the *ātman*, in Sāṅkhya, Yoga, and Vedānta (but not in Nyāya and Vaiśeṣiká, where they are qualities of the *ātman* itself).
44. There are, of course, sections of the text dealing with the mystic powers that are obviously beyond the pale of scientific acceptability.
45. In terms of theological dialogue, see the excellent work of Goswami (2012; one can only lament the author's premature demise after laying such a substantial cornerstone for a Vaiṣṇava contribution to inter-religious dialogue). In terms of the interface between the science of the *Bhāgavata* and modern science, see Thompson (1981, 2006, 2007); Cremo (1993) for an antagonistic view; and Edelmann (2014) for an accommodative view. For an excellent discussion of the challenges posed to Hinduism in general by modern science and an analysis of some of the responses this has engendered, see Mackenzie Brown (2012).
46. At the time of writing this introduction, the author received a visit from Bhadresh Swami, a *sannyasī* of the Swami Nārāyaṇa tradition, who bestowed a copy of his recently completed commentary on the *Vedānta Sūtras*. Other than evidencing the continuation of the formal *Vedānta* commentarial tradition, the swami expressed great eagerness and commitment to improving his English, and in being exposed to the modes of the Western academic study of religion, in order to engage in dialogue with what we have been calling "modernity" in this field.
47. We follow here the Upaniṣadic usage of locating both the *ātman* and the *citta*, mind, in the heart (*Kaṭha* I.14, II.12, III.1, and IV.6–7; *Muṇḍaka* II.1.8 and 10, II.2.1, and III.1.7). Technically, according to Gauḍīya *siddhānta*, *bhāva* is bestowed by Kṛṣṇa as an act of grace (*Bhaktirasāmṛtasindhu* Eastern Quadrant II.233). It is a *śakti* power that permeates the *citta* (*antarāṅga śakti*).

48. We use the term "subject-centered" heuristically. More precisely, at this stage, all notions of subject and object dissolve.
49. See, for instance, *Kaṭha Upaniṣad* III.15, V.6; *Muṇḍaka Upaniṣad* I.1.6; *Gītā* II.11–30; and *Yoga Sūtras* II.5.
50. The Nyāya and Vaiśeṣiká traditions hold that consciousness is only an adventitious quality of the *ātman* when in conjunction with the mind and is not manifest in liberation. Mīmāṁsā holds a similar view, although earlier Mīmāṁsā was not committed to notions of liberation.
51. See, for example, *Yoga Sūtras* II.2–21; *Gītā* V.21–22. We focus on desires here, but this level of consciousness includes emotions and intellectuality—that is, all objects of the mind, ego, and intellect—in addition to the senses.
52. See *Kaṭha Upaniṣad* 1.24ff. and 2.1ff.; *Mokṣadharma* 177.16ff.; *Yoga Sūtras* II. 15–21; and *Gītā* II.64–65.
53. *Yoga Sūtras* I.3, 18.
54. *Taittirīya Upaniṣad* II.8.
55. Cārvāka and the Lokāyata traditions left no body of writing but must have been influential enough for not only most of the orthodox Hindu schools, but also the Buddhists and Jains to include (and, typically, initiate) their sections on *pūrva-pakṣa* (arguments against opposing schools), with refutations of "the materialists" (see Mādhava's *Sarva-darśana-saṅgraha* as an example of this). For an excellent compilation of all known Cārvāka sources, see Bhattacarya (2011).
56. See Vatsyāyana's commentary on *Nyāya Sūtras* I.1.22.
57. *Sāṅkhya Kārikā* 68.
58. *Sāṅkhya Kārikā* XI; *Yoga Sūtras* IV.34.
59. For example, *Sāṅkhya Sūtras* V.74. But see Bryant (2009, 182–83) for Yoga's possible difference with Sāṅkhya and its alignment with Vedānta on the issue of bliss in *mokṣa*.
60. *Sāndrānānda-viśeṣa*.
61. Contra Halbfass (1988), who in his superb tome argues that relying on *yogic* experience as a trump card for *yogic* realities in the face of opposing epistemologies is a modern phenomenon.
62. *Mahābhārata vana parva* 312.117. This often quoted verse appears in various renditions of the text in the section where Yuddhiṣṭhira answers the questions of the *yakṣa*, but it is not included in the BORI critical edition, where this exchange takes place in Book III, chapter 297. See also *Vedānta Sūtras* I.1.11 and the earlier *Kaṭha Upaniṣad* (II.9) for similar expressions of the limitations of rational thought.
63. See VII.13.8.
64. Here, too, Rūpa reflects the *Bhāgavata*: "He should not become attached to many disciples, he should not study many books, he should not become attached to lecturing, and he should not undertake major projects [like monasteries, say the commentators]" (VII.13.8).
65. See *Yoga Sūtras* II.18.

66. The Purāṇic tradition identifies 8.4 million species according to its system of differentiation as to what constitutes a species.
67. See *Yoga Sūtras* II.18; *Gītā* II.42, IX.20–21.
68. *Kaṭha Upaniṣad* II.2; *Yoga Sūtras* II.15; *Gītā* V.22 and VII.3.
69. *Gītā* VI.22; *Vaśeṣika Sūtras* V.16; *Nyāya Sūtras* I.1.9, 22.
70. *Sāṅkhya Kārikā* X–XI.
71. *Dṛṣi-mātra*, *Yoga Sūtras* II.20.
72. We use these terms heuristically, as dualities such as internal/external and subjective/objective become meaningless or, more precisely, transcended in this state.
73. For example, those where *Īśvara* is invoked as the bestower of liberation, such as the *Yoga Sūtras* II.45, versus those, such as the *Sāṅkhya Karikā*, where *Īśvara* is not mentioned.
74. *Samādhi siddhiḥ*, *Yoga Sūtras* II.45 (in Nyāya He is depicted as the bestower of the fruits of work, *Nyāya Sūtras* IV.1.362, following on the *Śvetāśvatara Upaniṣad* VI.16).
75. *Vedānta Sūtras* IV.4.10–14; and *Mahābhārata* (*Mokṣadharma* 196.21–22).
76. Rūpa identifies four qualities uniquely enticing about Kṛṣṇa: the sweetness of His *līlā*, the supremeness of His love, the sweetness of His flute, and the sweetness of His form (Southern Quadrant 1.209–15).
77. *Tattva Sandarbha anu* 6; and again in *Bhakti Sandarbha anu* 339.
78. The verb *kṛṣ* denotes to pull away, draw into one's power, pull toward oneself, overwhelm, and the like.

The *Bhāgavata Purāṇa*: Book I

1. *Janmādyasya yataḥ* is an exact duplication of *Vedānta Sūtras* I.1.2, where the phrase describes *Brahman*, the Absolute Truth of the oldest philosophical-mystical texts, the Upaniṣads. In doing so, the *Bhāgavata* is purposefully correlating Kṛṣṇa with *Brahman* as the ultimate highest Truth (as does the *Bhagavad Gītā*, for instance, in X.12, XIV.27). The commentators write their longest commentaries for this first verse, as it sets the theological parameters for understanding Lord Kṛṣṇa. In essence, the text is promoting Kṛṣṇa as the highest and ultimate Absolute Truth, God, a personal Supreme Being (see, in this regard, the Vaiṣṇava reading of the *Gītā* in XV.16–20, VII.6–7ff.).
2. Brahmā, the secondary creator, is not to be confused with *Brahman* (a more impersonal term to refer to the Absolute Truth). While Viṣṇu/Kṛṣṇa is the primary source creator of *prakṛti* (the primordial material stuff from which all material entities are constituted), Brahmā functions more like an engineer, manipulating the *prakṛtic* stuff to create the specific forms of the universe. His tale in this volume narrates part of his role.
3. See "*Prakṛti* and the Three *Guṇas*: *Sattva*, *Rajas*, and *Tamas*" for a discussion on these three *guṇas*, qualities, of *prakṛti*.
4. "Dishonesty" is understood here as any scriptural teaching promoting bodily, mental, or worldly gain as its goal. Since the *Bhāgavata* teaches that a being's

ultimate reality is not body, mind, or of this world, which are temporary coverings and locations, but *ātman*, an eternal spark of *Īśvara* (God), then texts promoting boons for the body or mind (specifically the older portions of the Vedic canon) are teaching only temporal truths, not the Ultimate Truth, and are in this sense dishonest.

5. These are miseries inflicted by one's own mind and body, by other living entities, and by the environment.
6. The *kalpa-taru* is a tree in the celestial realm that offers anything requested of it. The Vedic scriptures are likened to this, as they are vast and variegated in their offerings, reflecting the myriad types of desires pursued by different embodied beings owing to their situation under specific configurations of the *guṇas*.
7. Śuka, the speaker of the *Bhāgavata*, also means "parrot." The poetic implication (*dhvani*) here is that as a parrot will choose the sweetest fruit, so Śuka has spoken the highest and most relishable of scriptures.
8. An exclamation used repeatedly through the text. It corresponds to something like "I say!" in Victorian English.
9. See "*Rāga*, *Bhāva*, and *Rasa*" for a discussion of these terms.
10. See "The Divine *Brahman* Realms of Vaikuṇṭha and Goloka" for Viṣṇu's *Brahman* realm of Vaikuṇṭha.
11. In contrast with the highest *dharma* noted in I.1.2 and again in I.2.6, *dharma* in this context refers to the variegated duties incumbent on the social, gendered, civic, familial, and other responsibilities of embodied beings in Vedic culture. See I.2.9–13 and discussion in "*Bhakti* and *Dharma*" for the difference.
12. Vyāsa is the legendary compiler of the Purāṇas, composer of the *Mahābhārata* epic, and divider of the original one Veda into four. See appendix 1.
13. Śrīdhara's reading of *para-avara* is *Brahman* with form and without form. See "The Nature of *Īśvara* in Vedānta: Primary or Derivative?" for a discussion of the personal and nonpersonal characteristics of God and various ways of construing higher and lower notions of Truth.
14. There are four *yugas*, world ages, in Hindu cosmography, from which *Kali* is the last and most degraded. Taking birth in this age is a symptom of poor *karma* from a past life.
15. The sages are complimenting Sūta: the sacred rivers are considered sacred only by dint of the fact that saints such as he bathe in their waters.
16. *Kali*, the fourth and most degenerate of the four ages, has been ongoing since Lord Kṛṣṇa departed from this earth.
17. See "*Līlā* and *Yogamāyā*."
18. *Māyā* is the illusion covering the *ātman* causing it to misidentify with its gross and subtle coverings.
19. Uttamaśloka—literally "one the verses glorifying whom are the highest of verses."
20. See "*Rāga*, *Bhāva*, and *Rasa*."

21. Kṛṣṇa's brother is often simply named Rāma, but I translate this as Balarāma so as not to create confusion with the Rāma of the *Rāmāyaṇa*, who is an incarnation from a previous age (there is a third incarnation also sometimes called Rāma, Paraśurāma, whose narrative occurs in IX.15–16).
22. Vyāsa is an incarnation of Viṣṇu (I.3.21) and legendary composer of the *Mahābhārata* epic.
23. We can recall that there are eighteen Purāṇas, from which the *Bhāgavata* sees itself as "the succulent ripened fruit of the desire tree of the Vedic scriptures" (I.1.3).
24. Nara and Nārāyaṇa are incarnations of Viṣṇu who perform austerities together in the Himālayas. Kṛṣṇa and Arjuna are identified with them.
25. We find here the notion of *dharma* being reconfigured in the *Bhāgavata* to denote the cultivation of *bhakti*, rather than the mundane pursuit of prescribed activities as per the *Dharma sūtra* texts (see "*Bhakti* and *Dharma*").
26. We can recall here that the normative goal of Vedic *dharma*—that is, of the conventional religiosity of the time—was material gain in this world and the attainment of the celestial realms in the next.
27. For the *Bhāgavata*, nonduality indicates that everything emanates from *Bhagavān*—nothing has separate or independent existence (however, see "The Nature of *Īśvara* in Vedānta" for the ways in which the notion of nonduality is understood very differently in the various Vedānta traditions).
28. This is the all-important verse, where this three-level hierarchy within *Brahman*, distinctive of the Vaiṣṇava traditions, is expressed (see "A Three-Tiered Hierarchy of *Brahman*").
29. After the sacred-thread ceremony, *brāhmaṇas* are considered twice-born (once bodily, the other into the sacred realm of Vedic knowledge).
30. The Vedic socio-civic system is divided into four *varṇas*, professional occupations (*brāhmaṇa*, teacher and religious specialist; *kṣatriya*, warrior/administrator; *vaiśya*, merchant; and *śūdra*, general work assistant) and four *āśramas*, progressive stages of life (*brahmācarya,* student; *gṛhastha*, householder; *vanaprastha,* religious retiree; and *sannyāsa*, solitary ascetic).
31. *Kīrtana* consists of the chanting of the names and deeds of *Īśvara*. See "The Nine Practices of *Vaidhi Bhakti*."
32. See "The Object of *Bhakti*" for the three *guṇas* of *sattva*, *rajas*, and *tamas*, as the terms occur frequently throughout the text.
33. As in all *yoga* practice, the goal of *bhakti* is direct perceptual experience, in this case of *Īśvara*.
34. As discussed in part 1, from these three divine manifestations, the Purāṇas typically associate Hari/Viṣṇu/Kṛṣṇa with *sattva* and the maintenance of the universe; Brahmā with *rajas* and its creation; and Śiva with *tamas* and its destruction. The *Vaiṣṇava Purāṇas* associate Śiva and Brahmā with religiosity that seeks material gain (or, at best, spiritual gain mixed with materialism, as in I.2.26–27, below, and discussion in "*Bhakti* Mixed with Attachment to

Dharma and *Jñāna*"). Hence the statement here that the ultimate good—which was established in the opening verse (I.1.2) as being free of any such motives—is attainable only from Viṣṇu.

35. Vedic religiosity involves a highly elaborate, technical, and expansive set of rituals, for which fire, as consumer of the oblations, is central (see introduction).
36. Since *bhūta* can refer to "ghosts" (literally "one who has gone"), Jīva, in his commentary here, mentions Bhairava, a particular form of Śiva that is the Lord of ghosts and other afflicted beings.
37. The Manus are celestial progenitors. The present one is noteworthy for the *Dharma sūtra* texts that tradition associates with him, the *Mānava Dharmaśāstras* (also known as the *Manu Saṁhitā*).
38. *Aṁśa* (and its near synonym *kalā*) refers to derivative manifestations of a divine being that embody a partial but not full expression of the potencies and qualities of the source being.
39. This is an extremely important and seminal verse for Kṛṣṇa theologians and the cornerstone of their assertion that Kṛṣṇa is the source of Viṣṇu, rather than vice versa (see "Who Is the Supreme *Īśvara*?: The Purāṇic Context").
40. Indra is the martial leader of the celestials, and his *dharma* is to battle the *asura* demons (for an example of an *asura* whom Indra could not defeat, thus requiring the intervention of an incarnation, see the Tale of Child Prahlāda).
41. In the *yogic* language of this verse, the "seen" as body and mind are external coverings imposed upon the "seer," the *ātman*, which is pure consciousness, because of ignorance (*avidyā*). See *Yoga Sūtras* II.17.
42. The subtle body referred to here, *sūkṣma śarīra* (also known as *liṅga śarīra*, or *antaḥkaraṇa*), also a covering of the *ātman*, is made from the subtler (=more *sattva*) evolutes of *prakṛti* prior to the densification of the *guṇas* into the gross elements, *mahābhūtas* (=more *tamas*) of the gross physical body. The latter dissolves at death, but the former transmigrates with the *ātman*—which, as the true self, is distinct from gross and subtle bodies—birth after birth. So there are three layers of selfhood, only one of which, the *ātman*, is ultimate, essential, and eternal.
43. Since the subtle body contains the mind, desires, and *kleśas*, its decisions are causally responsible for the type of gross body or effects received in this and future lives (*Yoga Sūtras* II.1–15).
44. Kṛṣṇa is not explicitly mentioned in the Vedas.
45. These are enumerated in the *Viṣṇu Purāṇa* (VI.5.73–75) as *jñāna*, knowledge; *śakti*, power; *bala,* strength; *aiśvarya*, lordship; *vīrya*, power; and *tejas*, splendor. In the Purāṇas, the term *Bhagavān* comes to mean possessor of these qualities in fullness.
46. The sense of this phraseology is that just as one can smell a fragrance from a distance, so, since He pervades everything while yet simultaneously remaining distinct, the Lord in all beings experiences through the senses of all beings in a detached manner.

47. Viṣṇu's trademark weapon is the *cakra* disc.
48. While this phraseology seems strange to Western sensitivities, references to Kṛṣṇa's feet are ubiquitous throughout the text. The idea is that what might be considered the lowest part of a normal person's anatomy is a highly coveted source of bliss when it comes to *Īśvara*'s divine anatomy.
49. The *itihāsa* usually refers to the two epics, the *Mahābhārata* and the *Rāmāyaṇa*, but it is a term that can be used for any ancient narration or tale.
50. Knowledge systems in ancient India were transmitted by means of lineages, as we see in these verses (3.40–44; see also *Gītā* IV.1–2).
51. The idea is that the maidens could sense that Śuka had transcended any bodily distinctions, since he saw beyond physical and gendered differences to the universality of the *ātman* in all beings, and therefore they did not have to worry about being perceived as members of the opposite sex or sexual objects; this was not the case with his father, however.
52. The old capital of the Kurus was Hastināpura, "the city of elephants" (underscoring its imperial power), modern-day Delhi.
53. The idea here is that ascetics do not remain anywhere for long, especially the residences of householders, so as not to become attached. And when great saints do approach such residences, under the pretext of mendicancy, it is to bless the household.
54. Parīkṣit was the last remaining member of the entire Yadu dynasty while still in the womb. The story of the circumstances of his birth after the great *Mahābhārata* war is recounted in the *Mahābhārata* (10.16.5–10, 14.68.15–25) and, with variations, *Bhāgavata* (I.7, 12).
55. The Vedic hymns deal with mundane boons for temporary material prosperity and thus would have been of no interest to a *yogī* such as Śuka.
56. Each *yuga* sees a progressive decline in the principles of *dharma*.
57. *Divya cakṣus*. See *Gīta* XI.8, where Arjuna is bestowed "divine eyes" to see the cosmic form of Kṛṣṇa, for another instance of this.
58. In addition to the *hotṛ*, the other three ritual specialists are *udgātṛ*, *adhvaryu*, and *brāhmaṇa*, who recite hymns from the *Ṛg*, *Sāman*, *Yajus*, and *Atharvan Vedas*, respectively. The *brāhmaṇas* oversee the procedures, and the others recite hymns from their respective Vedas noted in the next verse.
59. Vyāsa is considered a partial incarnation (*aṁśa*) of Viṣṇu in V.21, below.
60. One of the symptoms of the present age, *Kali yuga*, is that people's memories decrease, hence the larger corpus was subdivided into manageable subunits, making it easier to retain.
61. In Vedic orthopraxy, women and *śūdras* were denied access to Vedic study or participation in the rituals (other than the passive token role played by the sponsor's wife). While the epic and Purāṇa traditions do not directly oppose these attitudes, they are innovative in undermining them and bypassing them, specifically in the context of the *Bhāgavata*, by allowing all living entities equal access to at least the teachings, practices, and goals of *bhakti*, even as the larger social-civic order is still promoted as ideal. (It is useful to

keep in mind our own Western social and gendered history up to as recently as the post–World War II period, when judging this.)

62. Defined in I.2.6–8, as that through which *bhakti* for Kṛṣṇa is born (see "*Bhakti* and *Dharma*").
63. Literally "great swan." Swans are believed to be able to separate milk from water, a metaphor for great saints who can distinguish illusion from Truth.
64. Note the term *āśrama* here, in the premodern period, refers to a humble hermitage of a sage, typically on the banks of a sacred river.
65. As noted in part 1, there are four *puruṣārthas*, goals of human life: *dharma*, the performance of one's duties; *artha*, the material prosperity that ensues from this; *kāma*, the access to sense indulgence that this, in turn, facilitates; and *mokṣa*, the quest for liberation when *kāma* proves to be unsatisfying.
66. For a similar reference, but using the language of two *prakṛtis*, see *Gītā* VII.4–5.
67. "For the most part" might allude to the fact that the *Mahābhārata* epic does contain some description of Kṛṣṇa, most extensively in the *Harivaṁśa* appendage to it (as do a number of Purāṇas, such as the *Viṣṇu* and *Padma*).
68. The *nāma-rūpa* of the Upaniṣads (*Bṛhadāraṇyaka* I.4.7) refers to the *asat*, temporal (literally "that which has no enduring being")—the permutations of *prakṛti* (that is, the forms that emerge and fade away, to which convention assigns names).
69. For example, that desire leads to suffering and that one should actually seek Truth.
70. See note to I.3.28.
71. These are listed in the Tale of Ajāmila (VI.3.20–21).
72. We have interrupted the sequence of the *Bhāgavata* here, as Nārada recounts his previous life in a later book to the one in which his story is given.
73. The *gandharvas* are warrior celestials, also renowned for their musical abilities.
74. *Apsarās* are celestials renowned for their dancing abilities.
75. During the four months of the rainy season, *caturmāsa*, wandering ascetics, who otherwise do not stay in one place for more than three nights, are permitted to remain in one location.
76. Ascetics eat one meal a day. Eating the remnants of their food, *prasādam*, is considered purifying, a reflection of the purity of saints.
77. The *kleśas* of *avidyā* and *asmitā*, ignorance and ego, cause one to consider the material body and mind to be the real self (*Yoga Sūtras* II.2–4). Nārada here by the grace of the sages has essentially gained a realization of his true *ātman* nature, accompanied by the realization that what he had previously thought himself to be—the body and mind—was in fact a mental fabrication.
78. The notion of threefold *tāpas*, sufferings, is widespread in philosophical literature (see *Yoga Sūtras* II.15 and commentaries). The three *tāpas* are *ādhyāt-*

mika, the miseries of the body and mind; *ādhibhautika*, the miseries inflicted by other entities; and *ādhidaivika*, the miseries caused by nature and the environment.

79. Actions performed out of desire produce seeds of reactions that perpetuate *saṁsāra* (*Yoga Sūtras* II.12–14). But the same actions, when performed as an offering of devotion to God, do not produce reactions (*Gītā* IX.27–28). They also burn up the latent seeds of previous actions that have yet to bear their fruit, *prārabdha karma*.
80. These names are of the four *vyūhas*, particular four-armed forms of Viṣṇu, each of which appears as a family member of Kṛṣṇa in His incarnation. In the teachings of Lord Kapila, they are associated with the first evolutes from *prakṛti* (*Bhāgavata* III.26).
81. Since Brahmā is the first embodied being, he is not begotten by parents, as is the norm for living entities. See the story of Brahmā in this volume for the narrative pertaining to his origin.
82. It is standard in Hindu texts for those who renounce the world in search of spiritual Truth to set out in the direction of the north—the Himālayas, where the great sages reside.
83. See "The Liberated *Bhakta*: Different Types of *Mokṣa* in the *Bhāgavata*" for the different types of liberation in the *Bhāgavata*.
84. This refers to some kind of lightning, possibly forked.
85. According to *Bhāgavata* theology, the *bhaktas* who attain full liberation through devotional methods attain a *Brahman* body with which to pursue their devotional relationships with Viṣṇu in Vaikuṇṭha, or Kṛṣṇa in His divine realm of Goloka (see "The Divine *Brahman* Realms of Vaikuṇṭha and Goloka"). Nārada chooses to travel between Vaikuṇṭha and the material world so as to enlighten others.
86. As touched upon in the *Gītā* (VIII.17ff.), in Hindu notions of time, there are four (sub-)ages, *yugas*: the *Satya yuga*, *Treta yuga*, *Dvāpara yuga*, and *Kali yuga*. A thousand of these is a *kalpa*. A *kalpa* corresponds to one day of Brahmā and another to his night. Thus, Brahmā sleeps for a *kalpa*, during which the manifest universe is withdrawn into the body of Viṣṇu and remains in a latent state. Brahmā then awakes and re-creates for another *kalpa*, then sleeps and so on for one hundred Brahmā years. Thus, according to this verse, Nārada also remained in a hibernating state along with Brahmā for the duration of one of Brahmā's nights.
87. Normally one needs the requisite *karma* to transit from one realm in *saṁsāra* to another, but Nārada is able to go to any realm at will. Moreover, he is able to go beyond *prakṛti* to the pure *Brahman* realms called Vaikuṇṭha, where Lord Viṣṇu resides.
88. *Tīrtha-pāda*. India is full of holy places associated with incarnations of Lord Viṣṇu, that is, places touched by His "feet" (*pāda*).
89. *Aho!* is the classic Sanskrit exclamation of wonderment and appreciation.
90. "The city of elephants," capital of the Kuru dynasty (see earlier note).

91. This refers to attempts on the Pāṇḍavas' lives before they underwent their thirteen-year exile in the forest, described in the great *Mahābhārata* epic (for instance, the burning of the house of lac in I.124).
92. This story refers to a series of events: sage Māṇḍavya was innocently impaled by a king, after he happened to be arrested with some thieves. After the king released him upon realizing his mistake, the sage went to Yama, the Lord of death, asking him why he had been subject to this experience, despite his innocence. Yama replied that Māṇḍavya had once impaled an insect in his childhood. Hearing this, the sage cursed Yama that he would be born as a *śūdra* for such disproportionate punishment. Yama thus took birth as Vidura, who was born from Vyāsa in the womb of a servant girl. During his absence, the celestial being Aryamā took his post as Lord of death (*Mahābhārata* 1.101).
93. Vyāsa, the great sage, was requested by his mother, Satyavatī, widow of the emperor Śantanu, to beget children in the wives of his dead brother, heir to the throne, so as to perpetuate the royal dynasty as per Vedic custom. When one of them saw the appearance of the sage, frightful from his austerities, with his matted locks, fierce eyes, unwashed body, and unkempt beard, the poor girl covered her eyes during the sexual act. As a result, the offspring of this union, Dhṛtarāṣṭra, was born blind.
94. This clinging to life is one of the five *kleśas* in the *Yoga Sūtras* (II.9).
95. After the war, Dhṛtarāṣṭra was residing in the palace of his nephews the Pāṇḍavas and surviving on their benevolence, even though his own sons had tried to kill them and almost destroyed the entire dynasty, with very little effort made from the part of the blind king to control them (*Bhāgavata* III.1.6ff. touches on a few of the king's weaknesses).
96. These episodes relating to the attempts made by Dhṛtarāṣṭra's sons to kill the Pāṇḍavas refer to some of the episodes mentioned in verse 8 above.
97. This is a reference to the Himālayas, the destination of those abandoning the mundane world to seek Truth exclusively.
98. An ancient king of the Puru dynasty.
99. Members of the *sannyāsa* order of life often carry a staff.
100. The idea here is that renunciants enjoy the challenge of tolerating the hardships and austerities of the Himālayas, just as warriors enjoy a good fight.
101. Gāndhārī's one hundred sons, the Kurus, all perished in the great war.
102. For the *guru* as helmsman, see X.87.33 (quoted in "*Satsaṅga* and the *Guru*").
103. This refers to Kṛṣṇa's official mission during His incarnation: to eliminate all the *asuras*, the enemies of the celestials, who had taken birth as demoniac kings and had become a disturbance on earth.
104. These sages are Marīci, Atri, Aṅgiras, Pulastya, Pulaha, Kratu, and Vasiṣṭha.
105. The *kṣetra-jña* is the *ātman* still bound by the subtle body.
106. This state of *turīya* ("the fourth") is that of pure consciousness, where consciousness is not aware of any object external to itself. Attaining this is the goal of generic *yoga* practice. The *Māṇḍūkya Upaniṣad* features the four states of consciousness (which it correlates with the segments of the sacred

syllable *oṁ*). The idea here is that Śamīka's consciousness was not externalized, and thus he was not aware of the king's presence or request for water.

107. For similar concerns about the negative consequences of caste intermixture, see *Gītā* I.39ff.
108. The horse sacrifice was performed on the coronation of kings wishing to establish their supremacy over neighboring kings (see, for instance, Yudhiṣṭhira after the great war in the *Mahābhārata*, book 14).
109. The dualities are happiness and distress, hot and cold, honor and dishonor, and so on. They essentially refer to all shades of sensual or mental experiences.
110. See *Gītā* II.38, 64.
111. This is a reference to the Vāmana incarnation, who traversed the universe with his step, which was then washed by the celestials. The water from this, according to the *Bhāgavata*, is the origin of the *Gaṅgā* river (VIII.21.3–4). On its way to the earth, it flows past the celestial realms, hence the reference to "both worlds."
112. The *tulasī* plant is sacred to Viṣṇu and found in the homes of all traditional Vaiṣṇavas. When food is offered to the deities in Vaiṣṇava devotional practices (*bhakti*), a *tulasī* leaf is placed on each item of foodstuff.
113. The idea here is that in conventional lore, one goes to a holy place to be purified in the sacred rivers and such of that place. But since the saints residing in such places always carry Viṣṇu in their minds, it is actually they who purify the holy places to begin with.
114. This is a statement of humility, as well as of honor for the sages: the water used for washing feet is normally considered contaminated and discarded at a distance, but Parīkṣit is saying that kings are even more contaminated than this, so they should be discarded far from even where the water used for washing the feet of the *brāhmaṇas* is deposited.
115. These placements are all considered auspicious, as is *kuśa* grass, used as a seat in Vedic rituals.
116. The idea here is that lesser kings bow down to the royal throne of the Kurus (thereby touching it with the helmets on their heads).
117. The etymological meaning of the word *vai-kuṇṭha* is "free of dullness."
118. The Vedas have divine personalities; they can manifest as texts or as celestial beings.
119. Kṛṣṇa's father, Vasudeva, was the brother of Kuntī, the wife of Pāṇḍu. Hence Kṛṣṇa is a cousin of the Pāṇḍavas (the sons of Pāṇḍu). He is thus Parīkṣit's granduncle (Parīkṣit is the grandson of Arjuna, one of the five Pāṇḍavas).
120. For *japa*, see *Yoga Sūtras* I.27; *Gītā* X.25; and "*Kīrtana* (Chanting)."
121. The idea here is that renunciants do not associate with worldly people. They may come to a household in the guise of begging some alms in the form of a draft of milk, in order to bless the householders and give them an opportunity to inquire about Ultimate Truths, but they do not tarry there.

The *Bhāgavata Purāṇa*: Book II

1. For Khaṭvaṅga's story, see *Bhāgavata* IX.9.44ff.
2. In the *Kaṭha Upaniṣad*, the intelligence is analogized as the driver of the chariot of the body, with the mind as reins, the horses as senses, and the *ātman* as the passenger.
3. This is a reference to the earlier ritualistic portion of the Vedic corpus, which provides provisions as to how to attain material prosperity in this life and the attainment of the celestial realm in the next. Texts such as the *Bhāgavata*, here and throughout, the *Gītā* (II.42–43), and *Muṇḍaka Upaniṣad* (1.7–13) decry those who follow such injunctions, since they simply perpetuate their cycle of birth and death, rather than seeking the ultimate goal of liberation.
4. Dreams are the activation of *saṁskāras*, the imprints of memories recorded during the waking state (see commentaries to *Yoga Sūtras* II.11).
5. Ascetics in the forest sometimes wore coverings made of bark (archaeological discoveries of a type of material made from pulped bark in ancient China may possibly point to the method employed in this regard).
6. According to the commentator Śrīdhara, the *Vaitaraṇī* river flows by the gate of Yama's realm of the dead.
7. This is drawing from the reference in the *Śvetāśvatara Upaniṣad* (III.13).
8. The meditational form referred to here as "grosser" is outlined in the previous chapter (verses 23ff., which we have not included in these selections). It visualizes various natural phenomena as construing the parts of *Īśvara*'s body—the sky as His eyes, day and night as His eyelids, and so on.
9. We find in this verse the exact wording of Patañjali's verse on *āsana* in II.46, *sthira-sukham āsanam*, which here clearly refers to an actual seat, as it does throughout *yoga* literature.
10. Texts such as *Gītā* VIII.23–27 speak of the most auspicious times to leave the body, and the advantages of dying in auspicious holy places are also promoted in numerous texts. This verse dismisses such considerations.
11. The *kṣetra-jña* is the *ātman* still connected to the subtle body.
12. This well-known Upaniṣadic phraseology points to one method of realizing *ātman*/*Brahman* by eliminating all temporal things that it is not—namely, the *ātman* is not the body, or the mind, and so forth (*Bṛhadāraṇyaka* II.3.6, III.9.26, IV.2.4, and IV.4.22).
13. Here the *Bhāgavata* describes a praxis typically associated with the Tantra traditions. While the *Bhāgavata* clearly accepts this process, it is not a method emphasized throughout the text. Also, the names of the *cakras*, and even the term *cakra* itself, are not used in the text, merely the associated locations.
14. Those with mystic powers can travel to any of the celestial (and such) realms within *prakṛti*, and some, such as Nārada or the four Kumāra sages, can even go beyond these and enter the *Brahman* realms of Vaikuṇṭha (*Bhāgavata* III.15). The performers of Vedic ritual also aspire to the celestial realms, based on the merit of performing sacrifices (*karma*) but at best can attain only one such realm in their next life.

15. While the *suṣumṇā* is connected with the primary *prāṇa* channel through which the *kuṇḍalinī śakti* arises in Tantric physiology, it is also a section of the universe in Hindu cosmology.
16. The commentator Madhva identifies this location as Mahar-loka.
17. In the *Gītā* (VIII.17), a *kalpa* is equivalent to one day of the highest celestial being, Brahmā, a period equal to a thousand cycles of the four *yuga* ages, or 4.32 million human years. Brahmā lives for a hundred years in this time frame, in accordance with his superexcellent merit, but is nonetheless mortal and subject to the laws of *karma*. The celestial bodies, prolonged life spans, and heightened enjoyments of the celestial residents referred to in this verse are similarly attained by those with exceptional pious merit. But in actuality they are nothing but the highest expressions of *jatī*, *āyur*, and *bhoga* (type of birth and duration and quality of life) outlined in *Yoga Sūtras* II.12–13. The *Bhāgavata* cosmography, with all its various realms, is described in the fifth canto.
18. We can recall that Patañjali is considered an incarnation of Śeṣa, the thousand-headed serpent expansion of Lord Viṣṇu, upon whom the latter reclines when emanating and withdrawing the unlimited universes in cycles of creative evolution and involution.
19. After this period, the universe is destroyed, reduced to its matrix of pure *prakṛti*, and withdrawn into Lord Viṣṇu for a further two *parārdhas*, after which it is again manifest forth, in a never-ending cycle of creation and dissolution.
20. This entire process involves an involution or reversal of the sequencing of the Sāṅkhya categories during the manifestation of the universe.
21. This is a reference to the two paths mentioned in the *Bṛhadāraṇyaka* (and in the *Gītā* VIII.26ff.), one leading to liberation, the other to rebirth. The commentator Viśvanātha here also mentions the *Kaṭha* II.3.14 as a reference to the direct path.
22. The inference is that if there are instruments of perception and objects of perception, there must be a perceiver, or seer, who utilizes them. Therefore, because of the existence of instruments and objects of perception, we can validly infer the existence of a seer. The basic principle of Hindu logic (*nyāya*) is that when making an inference about the existence of something unperceived, there must be invariable concomitance (*vyāpti*—that is, no known exceptions) between a perceivable "sign" or a known characteristic (*liṅga*) of that thing and the inferred object possessing that specific characteristic. Thus, from the characteristic, one can infer the existence of the unperceived substance or thing possessing that characteristic. So, using the standard *nyāya* example, wherever there is smoke, there is always fire as its cause—there are no exceptions to this (if an opponent can find an exception to the supposed *vyāpti*, the inference is invalid and the argument fails). So if one sees smoke, one can legitimately infer that fire must be present—even if the fire itself is not perceived (since smoke is an invariable characteristic of fire and

has no other known cause). So in the inference referred to in this verse, wherever there are instruments and objects, there must be an entity using the instruments to perceive the objects. The *buddhi* (intelligence) and so forth are instruments of perception, therefore they must have a perceiver, the *ātman*.

23. Verses 2–9, which were omitted here, outlined various worldly boons attainable from the worship of the celestial beings. The sense is that even if one's *bhakti* is mixed with mundane desires, as discussed by Jīva in "*Īśvara*, Pure *Bhakti*, and Motivated *Bhakti*," one should still worship *Bhagavān*.
24. See *Mahābhārata* XII.326.65, 337.60.
25. *Nāma-rūpa* refers to any perceivable object in existence, which by dint of having a form, *rūpa*, can be known and therefore can be assigned a name, *nāma* (*Bṛhadāraṇyaka Upaniṣad* I.4.7).
26. By performing *tapas*, Brahmā could not be the Supreme Being, as one performs *tapas* to attain something, indicating that one is lacking that thing, and also that one requires powers beyond one's natural powers to attain it.
27. The idea here is that people bewildered by *māyā* (*avidyā*) think of themselves as their bodies and minds (*asmitā*), instead of *ātman*, and thus think in terms of "I" and their bodies, minds, families, and possessions as "my" (see *Yoga Sūtras* II.3–6; *Gītā* III.27).
28. See *Gītā* VII.19.
29. These are philosophical terms: *dravya* are substances like the elements of earth, water, air, fire, and ether that underpin qualities; *karma* is action and its reactions; *kāla* is Time, understood to be the glance of Viṣṇu in this text; *svabhāva* is one's inherent personality, formed by *saṁskāras*, as also the inherent nature of material entities; and *jīva* refers to the *ātman* in *saṁsāra*.
30. The *guṇas* underpin everything and thus are the basis of the substances noted here (that is, the elements of Sāṅkhya, an expression of the *tamas* aspect of *prakṛti*); knowledge, which is a function of the *citta*, is here a reference to the *sattva* aspect of *prakṛti*; and action is a reference to the *rajas* aspect of *prakṛti*. Anything enacted by these entities are causes, which produce effects. Owing to illusion, the *jīva* thinks that it is the agent, when in fact all action is performed by the *guṇas* (*Gītā* XIII.21).
31. The idea, of course, is that *Īśvara* is everything.
32. In the *Bhāgavata,* the *Virāṭ* is a meditational form incorporating all material entities as various aspects of the Supreme (see, for example, II.5–6). Kṛṣṇa's cosmic manifestation in the eleventh chapter of the *Gītā* is also considered a type of *Virāṭ-rūpa* by the commentators.
33. *Kha-ga* could also be a reference to the realm of birds, but given the context here (and that birds are mentioned later in the list), it is more likely a reference to those who have attained the mystic power of transporting themselves through the ether (referenced in *Yoga Sūtras* III.42).
34. These are all various types of celestials, expert in song and dance—and, with the *gandhārvas*, martiality (see *Mahābhārata* 3.130).
35. These are all subterranean but nonetheless powerful beings. The *yakṣas* and especially the *rākṣasas* play significant roles in the *Mahabhārata* epic.

36. See discussion in "Definition of *Īśvara* in Vedānta."
37. In the Sāṅkhya system, there are five *karmendriyas* (instruments of action)—the hands, feet, organ of evacuation, organ of procreation, and tongue; and five *jñānendriyas* (instruments for acquiring knowledge)—the eye, ear, nose, and senses of taste and touch.
38. Among the features characterizing Viṣṇu is the *śrīvatsa*, a tuft of hair on his chest.
39. These are identified variously in the commentaries.
40. The term for opulence here is *bhaga*, an old Vedic term that once referred to the portion of the sacrifice that was reserved for a deity but, by the classical period, refers in Vaiṣṇava sources to the six opulences. They are supremacy, righteousness, fame, opulence, knowledge, and detachment. As discussed in "Definition of *Īśvara*, *Bhagavān*, and *Brahman*," the term *Bhagavān* refers to the one who possesses these in full, eternally and unlimitedly—and this indeed is one definition of God Almighty in Vaiṣṇavism, since, as noted in this verse, all other beings may only partially manifest some of these opulences temporarily and sporadically.
41. *Paramahaṁsa*, literally "great swan," refers to the most fully realized saints. The line refers to the path of *bhakti*, often summarized by worship of the lotus feet of Viṣṇu.
42. While the *Bhāgavata Purāṇa* deals with *yogī* exemplars, Hindu literature is replete with references to those who perform *tapas* so as to attain supernormal powers for materialistic or even demoniac purposes—Rāvaṇa, who kidnapped Sītā, in the *Rāmāyaṇa* comes to mind, as does Hiraṇyakaśipu in the *Bhāgavata* (see the Tale of Child Prahlāda in this volume). Hence, although Patañjali discusses them, he takes pain to note that real *yogīs* are not interested in them (*Yoga Sūtras* III.37).
43. The metaphor of the *ātman* being seated in the cave goes back to the Upaniṣads (*Kaṭha* I.14, II.12, III.1, and IV.6–7; *Muṇḍaka* II.1.8 and 10, II.2.1, and III.1.7).
44. For Vaiṣṇava and *Bhāgavata* theology, this indicates that Viṣṇu has no form made of dull matter *prakṛti*. As this narrative establishes, he does, however, possess form (and unlimited forms) made of *Brahman*, pure consciousness, as discussed in part 1.
45. The metaphor of the spider spinning its web goes back to the Upaniṣads (*Bṛhadāraṇyaka* II.1.20; *Śvetāśvatara* VI.10; *Muṇḍaka* I.1.7).
46. Under normal circumstances, all actions performed out of desire generate reactions—the law of *karma* (see *Yoga Sūtras* II.12–14). But actions performed for *Īśvara* are free of *karma* (*Gītā* IX.27–28).
47. As Yoga has its *aṅgas*, limbs (*aṣṭāṅga*), so too does *bhakti*. The notion goes back to the six *aṅgas* of the Vedas that were ancillary to the performance of Vedic ritual.
48. Compare with *Gītā* IX.4–5. The idea in this simile is that the elements preexisted as independent elements prior to becoming ingredients in the forms of created beings. So they both enter creation by being constitutive of all created

objects and also do not, as their own existence predates the things created by them.

49. *Anvaya-vyatireka* is a process of logic that establishes the existence of something through positive and negative concomitance. For example: "Wherever there is consciousness (*ātman*) there is life (positive concomitance), and wherever there is no consciousness there is no life (negative concomitance)."
50. See *Yoga Sūtras* II.30–45 and earlier note.
51. See "Introduction to the Volume," "The *Bhāgavata* as Text."

The *Bhāgavata Purāṇa*: Book III

1. At the end of each cosmic cycle, the universe, and hence the elements of *prakṛti*, dissolve into their finest constituents (which are ultimately the *guṇas*) and lie latent within the manifestation of Viṣṇu, who resides within each universe (as discussed in the introduction, there are multiple forms of Viṣṇu).
2. This refers to the type of *yoga* outlined in the *Yoga Sūtras* that culminates in *nirbīja samādhi*, awareness absorbed in its own pure nature. Hence, in the Yoga tradition, Brahmā is considered the first *yogī* (and reputed author of the original Yoga treatise, the *Hiraṇyagarbha Saṃhitā*).
3. Viśvanātha takes this as one hundred human years but does not comment on the discrepancy with II.9.8 above.
4. Patañjali is considered by tradition to be an incarnation of Śeṣa, also known as Ananta (see commentaries to *Yoga Sūtras* II.47).
5. The sense is that generally ornaments and garments enhance a person's beauty, where here the reverse is true: the beauty of the ornaments is enhanced by the beauty of God.
6. See earlier citation (II.9.15).
7. The imagery of this verse seems to be resonating with that of the banyan tree at the beginning of chapter 15 of the *Gītā*.
8. This mixed metaphor reads awkwardly in English but is not uncommon in stylistic Sanskrit poetics. The wind is the sounds (teachings) of the Vedic texts.
9. The three *dhātus*, dispositions, in Āyurveda are *vāta*, air; *pitta*, fire; and *kapha*, mucus.
10. This is a reference to the *Paramātman*, or *Antaryāmin*, a form of Viṣṇu that pervades the individual *ātman*.
11. This seems to be a reference to *Vedānta Sūtras* (II.1.3), where the author responds to an atheistic opponent (*pūrva-pakṣa*) that a Being who is complete and in possession of everything does not need to create, as people create to obtain something they do not already have. The response is that God creates out of *līlā*, a pure act of joyful spontaneity.
12. The Tale of Ajāmila illustrates such unintentional chanting at the moment of death.
13. *Samādhi* is the final limb of Patañjali's eight limbs of *yoga*. It culminates in consciousness becoming absorbed in its own pure nature, rather than in the permutations of the mind or sensations of the corporeal body (*Yoga Sūtras* I.3).

14. *Tapas* is part of the second limb of *yoga*. Of relevance to this narrative is that extreme forms of austerities can result in the attainment of mystic powers (*Yoga Sūtras* IV.1).
15. The sense is that Viṣṇu, in his form of Time (see *Gītā* XI.32), strips everything from everyone at death. The name used for Viṣṇu here, Urukrama, "the one with a vast stride," is a reference to the Vamana incarnation of Lord Viṣṇu, who covered the entire world with one step and the entire universe with another. In this *līlā*, he stripped King Bali, the regent of the universe, of all his possessions.
16. The *Kāma sūtras* are part of a genre of texts that occupy themselves with "*dharma*, *artha* (resources), and *kāma* (pleasure)," special attention being given to the last (verse 1).
17. This mystic power, *siddhi*, is called *prākāmya*, being unobstructed in fulfilling one's any desire.
18. This mystic power is referred to in *Yoga Sūtras* III.19.
19. The sense here is that although two of the preconditions for *yoga* are nonattachment and celibacy (*Yoga Sūtras* I.15, II.30), which then generate the necessary power to exhibit supernormal powers (*Yoga Sūtras* IV.1), Kardama was not affected by this very sensual situation.
20. The *siddhas* are accomplished *yogis*, who sometimes exhibit mystic powers like flying around the upper realms of the universe.
21. The *Gaṅgā* is held to descend from the celestial realm.
22. Kardama had previously informed Devahūti that he would leave home to take up the life of a wandering ascetic as soon as she conceived a child (III.22.19).
23. Patañjali states that the mind's activities can be either detrimental to the goals of *yoga* or beneficial to it, *kliṣṭa akliṣṭa* (I.5), or, as the *Gītā* puts it, the mind is either the friend of the *ātman* or its enemy (VI.5). The idea is that when the mind becomes attached to Kṛṣṇa or, as in this verse, the *bhāgavatas*, such attachment leads to perfection. Attachment to sensual indulgences, in contrast, leads to bondage and rebirth. See "*Rāga*, *Bhāva*, and *Rasa*" for relevant discussion.
24. This is a reference to III.21.32, where Viṣṇu informs Kardama that a portion of Himself (*aṁśa*) would take birth from Devahūti after she had given birth to nine daughters, in order to teach the truths of Sāṅkhya Yoga.
25. For the five *niyamas*, see *Yoga Sūtras* II.32.
26. The commentor Śrīdhara states that the knot in the heart is the *ahaṅkāra*, ego—considering the inanimate mind to be the self.
27. The *prajāpatis* are the progenitors of the species in the universe. They are born of the creator, Brahmā.
28. This name of Viṣṇu comes from His killing of the Madhu demon (*Mahābhārata Vana Parva* CCVII.16).
29. There are various types of celestial beings: the *gandharvas* are winged warrior celestials renowned for their singing, and *apsaras* are celestial nymphs known for their dancing.
30. Celestials traverse the realms in divine vehicles.

31. Marīci is one of the six sages born from Brahmā's mind.
32. Brahmā is born from a lotus emanating from Viṣṇu's navel.
33. The term *aṁśa* refers to a type of divine manifestation whereby a portion of God's presence or power, rather than the full Godhead, incarnates. There are unlimited divine manifestations in *Bhāgavata* theology, each one manifesting different qualities and potencies.
34. Lotus eyes are a standard motif in Hindu aesthetics to denote beauty. Lotus feet are likewise standard, especially in reference to beings worthy of worship. In addition, incarnations are recognizable by special markings on the soles of their feet and palms, which include the lotus.
35. *Karma*, translated here as "ignorant action," refers to action performed under ignorance of the true self. Ignorance, *avidyā*, is the root cause of *karma* (*Yoga Sūtras* II.4–5), the primary *kleśa* or obstacle to enlightenment indicated in *Yoga Sūtras* II.4–5, namely, action that is performed under the illusion that one is the body and mind by one seeking fulfillment through the body and mind.
36. This is a reference to another demon destroyed by Viṣṇu. The story is narrated in the *Mahābhārata, Śānti Parva*, chapter 348, and the *Devī Bhāgavata*, book 1.
37. Sāṅkhya, perhaps the oldest philosophical system in ancient India, was the speculative metaphysical matrix in matters of analyzing the ingredients of physical reality. (Yoga emerged as one ingredient from this matrix to provide the practical technique of realizing the ultimate reality of *ātman* embedded within this physical reality.) The reference to other teachers here points to the fact that there were numerous Sāṅkhya traditions in circulation (the *Bhāgavata* mentions several).
38. Brahmā is sometimes referred to as the "Swan." His vehicle also happens to be a swan.
39. The universe, in Hindu cosmogony, is schematized as consisting of "three worlds": the celestial, human, and subterranean planes.
40. The four Kumāras are enlightened child *yogīs* whose stories are encountered in book 3, chapter 16.
41. Nārada is one of the greatest devotees of Viṣṇu and travels around the universe chanting the glories of Viṣṇu on his *vīṇā* stringed instrument. He surfaces in many episodes of the *Bhāgavata*, frequently acting as a sort of catalyst to developments in the narrative (see the Tale of Sage Nārada).
42. There are nine sages, *prajāpatis*, born of Brahmā, whose progeny populates this universe.
43. Kardama is demonstrating his humility here, considering himself lowly.
44. See *Gītā* VI.45 for a similar statement pointing to the *yoga* path typically taking many births to reach its full conclusion.
45. The sense here is that Viṣṇu will appear in whatever form is pleasing to His devotee.
46. As noted previously, respect is offered to superiors in Indian culture by honoring or touching or placing one's head on their feet, the idea being that one places the highest part of one's anatomy on the lowest part of the superior's.

This sense of respect is magnified here, by considering even the stool upon which God's feet are placed to be worthy of worship.

47. These are the standard six qualities possessed in absolute fullness by God, Viṣṇu (and in varying lesser degrees by all other beings; see "Definition of *Īśvara*, *Bhagavān*, and *Brahman*").
48. The commentator Śrīdhara takes *tṛi-vṛta* here to refer to the *ahaṅkāra*, the second evolute from *prakṛti*, which, under the influences of the three *guṇas*, manifests respectively the mind, the senses, and the sense objects out of itself.
49. The soul, or pure consciousness, is enveloped in two external and extraneous bodily coverings: gross and subtle. While the gross physical body is changed at each new birth and returns back to *prakṛti* (the gross elements), the subtle mental body is retained life after life until the birth in which enlightenment and liberation is attained, after which it too returns to subtle *prakṛti*.
50. We are reminded here of Kṛṣṇa indicating that the path of Yoga (*buddhi/karma yoga*) that he had formerly imparted to the ancients had become lost, and hence he was rearticulating it to Arjuna (*Gītā* IV.2).
51. *Ātmani ātmanā*. The sense here is that since the self (*ātman*) is pure consciousness, it cannot be perceived by the senses or the mind, which are made of matter (*prakṛti*). It can therefore only know itself in itself by itself (as indicated in the *Gītā* VI.20).
52. Circumambulation (usually of a deity or temple) is an auspicious act of respect and worship.
53. This is a reference to mainstream Vedic religiosity, which, like that of other old-world cultures, involved offering items into the sacred fire for material boons. The ascetic traditions denigrate such materialistic practices (see, for instance, *Muṇḍaka Upaṇisad* 1.7–11; *Gītā* II.42ff.).
54. *Sat-asat* here can mean the real and the nonreal, the true and the false, cause and effect, and other such things. The sense is that God is the ultimate absolute cause of all causes.
55. As pure conscious *Brahman*, Viṣṇu is without material qualities, *guṇas*, yet as a source of matter, *prakṛti*, He is the source of the *guṇas*.
56. This is a major theme in the *Gītā* (see 11.54 and 18.55).
57. The *dvandas* here are Vedānta categories referring to the dualities of the body, such as hot and cold; and of the mind, such as happiness and distress (see, for example, *Gītā* II.14 and 45, IV.22, and VII.28). Since Kardama was absorbed in his true self, the *ātman*, he was transcendent to the dualities of the material body and mind.
58. See the metaphor of the ocean being fed by rivers yet remaining unmoved in *Gītā* II.70. Desires might arise in the mind of the *yogī*, as these are simply *saṁskāras* of past experiences, but the *yogī* does not identify with them, simply witnessing them from a place of detachment without attempting to fulfill them.
59. See *Śvetāśvatara Upaniṣad* (V.2) for an example of this (although later tradition posits two different Kapilas, the one referenced in the *Bhāgavata* and the one in the *Śvetāśvatara*).

60. In fact, the *Yoga Sūtras* of Patañjali cannot really be considered "philosophical" at all; it is aimed primarily at describing meditational states and the methods of attaining them; it is Sāṅkhya, in actual fact, that represents the philosophy and metaphysics of Yoga, sensu stricto. There were various versions of Sāṅkhya in percolation at the time, as exemplified in the highly elaborate theistic strain we find here in the teachings of Kapila in chapter 25 and onward.
61. There are various *prāṇas*, life airs, in Hindu physiology that permeate the body and facilitate the functioning of the senses and organs.
62. In the *Gītā* (XV.15), Kṛṣṇa states that He is both the knower and the compiler of the Vedas.
63. The "I," "me," and "mine" here refers to the false self, namely, the body and its possessions—the *ahaṅkāra* of Sāṅkhya (termed *asmitā* in the *Yoga Sūtras*). Since Viṣṇu is the creator of *prakṛti*, and hence all its evolutes such as ego (*ahaṅkāra*), Kapila, as His incarnation, is indirectly the creator of *ahaṅkāra*.
64. In the *Gītā*, Kṛṣṇa states that He had originally imparted the teachings of *yoga* in primordial time, but over the course of time, they became lost (IV.2).
65. While there are references in, for example, the *Maitrī Upaniṣad* of a six-limbed yoga, the more dominant model became the eight limbs of Patañjali's *Yoga Sūtras*: ethics, morals, posture, breath control, sense withdrawal, concentration, meditation, and *samādhi*, complete meditative absorption.
66. See earlier note to III.23.55 and below.
67. The sense of *udāsīna* here is that *prakṛti* is unconscious and simply acts according to mechanistic principles such as *karma*.
68. See earlier note to III.23.55.
69. The term for virtue here is *sādhu*. Thus a *sādhu* (ascetic) is *sādhu* (virtuous).
70. *Śruta* here refers to the materialistic enticements, both in this world and in the celestial realms, offered in portions of the *Śruti*, the older Vedic sacred texts (more specifically, the ritualistic genre of sacred text known as the *Brāhmanas* and their associated literatures). The Vedic sacrificial rites outlined in these texts were typically performed to fulfill material desires. For similar statements, see *Yoga Sūtras* (I.15) and *Gītā* (II.42ff.).
71. *Nirvāṇa*, in early texts, was a generic term adopted by different schools to refer to liberation (see, for instance, *Gītā* II.72 and IV. 24–26). It was not associated exclusively with Buddhism until later times.
72. See verse 14.
73. We should bear in mind here that most ascetics at the time were male—although we know of women such as Gargī, who outwits the great sage Yajñavalkya in *Bṛhadāraṇyaka Upaniṣad* (III.6), and Maitreyī, who does not allow her husband to fob her off with material inheritances (ibid. II.4). Additionally, as was the case elsewhere in the world in premodern times, the transmission of knowledge systems on technical philosophical matters such as Sāṅkhya would have been a male preserve.
74. *Devānāṁ guṇaliṅgānām* can be translated as senses because the senses are "signs" (*liṅga*)—that is, evolutes of the *guṇas* (for this usage, see *Yoga Sūtras*

II.19); and they are considered controlled by the *devas*, celestial beings. When *sattva* is at its apex, the senses are controlled and one's actions are *dharmic* and free of self-interest (see *Gītā* XVII.17 and XVIII.9).

75. The *Taittirīya Upaniṣad* (II.1–5) speaks of the various *kośas*, subtle sheaths, that cover the soul. Generic liberation ensues once these are removed and the soul can shine forth in its own true autonomous nature.
76. Service to the feet is a standard motif in *bhakti*.
77. As discussed in "The Liberated *Bhakta*: Different Types of *Mokṣa* in the *Bhāgavata*," there are five types of liberation recognized in *bhakti* (see *Bhāgavata* III.29.13, below). From these, the *ekātmatā* of this verse involves merging into God (this is considered to be the lowest level of liberation in Vaiṣṇava traditions). The sense is that devotees desire to serve a personal, separate, and Supreme Divine Being, not merge into Him in oneness, obliterating the personality and individuality both of one's own soul and of God as a distinct Supreme Soul.
78. In Hindu aesthetics, reddish eyes are a sign of beauty.
79. Viṣṇu's abodes, Vaikuṇṭha, are not within the realms of *prakṛti* but are realms within *Brahman*.
80. This refers to another of the five liberations noted above, namely, *sārṣṭī*, having the same opulence as God.
81. There are eight mystic powers referred to in classical texts such as the *Yoga Sūtras* (III.45). They are 1) *aṇimā*, "minuteness": the ability to make one's body atomic in size; this allows one to become so small that one can enter into anything (and hence become invisible to anyone); 2) *laghimā*, "lightness": the ability to make the body as light as one desires in terms of weight; 3) *mahimā*, "largeness": the ability to make the body as heavy in weight as one desires; 4) *prāptiḥ*, "attainment": the ability to attain anything one might desire; 5) *prākāmya*, "freedom of will": the ability to be unobstructed in one's desires; 6) *vaśitva*, "mastery": the ability to control the elements and their qualities and to control other beings; 7) *īśitṛtva*, "lordship": the ability to control the outward appearance, disappearance, and rearrangement of the elements; 8) *yatra-kāmāvasāyitva*: the ability to manipulate the elements at will according to one's fancy.
82. This refers to another of the five liberations noted above, namely, *sārūpya*, having the same form and beauty as God.
83. Viṣṇu's *Brahman* abode, Vaikuṇṭha.
84. The celestial realms, *svarga*, are paradises that pious souls attain in the next life to enjoy the fruits of their good deeds. However, they too are temporary and thus within the cycle of *saṁsāra*. When one's merit is exhausted, one returns again to this world (*Gītā* IX.20–21).
85. Indra is the god of rains, the Indic counterpart of Zeus and Thor in the cognate Indo-European traditions.
86. This common Vedāntic metaphor points to the fact that the sun remains stationary and unmoving in the sky, even as its reflection in a body of water

dances and moves and appears affected by the waves of the water. Likewise, the *ātman* remains unchanged even though it is reflected in the ever-changing mind.

87. The term used here for ego is *ahaṅkriyā*; the more common term is *ahaṅkāra* (*asmitā* in the *Yoga Sūtras*; *abhimāṇa* in the *Sāṅkhya Kārikā*).
88. *Karma-doṣa*: every action generates a reaction, or consequence, good or bad in accordance with the nature of the original action.
89. The previous verse spoke of actions and reactions—cause and effect—that result in the various births in the world of *saṁsāra*. Actually, these are all simply ephemeral—the ever-changing temporary creations of *prakṛti*; the soul is always aloof and transcendental.
90. The *yamas*—nonviolence, truthfulness, celibacy, non-stealing, and nonpossessiveness—are the first of the eight limbs of classical *yoga* (*Yoga Sūtras* II.29–30).
91. This is a reference to the three states of consciousness first outlined in the *Māṇḍūkya Upaniṣad*—waking, dream, and deep sleep. These are followed by pure consciousness, the fourth state (*turīya*), the goal of *yoga*.
92. The idea is that the self, *ātman*, cannot be perceived by the senses or the mind or by any external *prakṛtic* instrument. Therefore it can perceive itself only by means of itself. This phrase, *ātmanātmānam*, occurs elsewhere (see *Gītā* VI.20).
93. *Sad-ābhāsam-asati*. The state alluded to here is called *asmitā samādhi* in the *Yoga Sūtras*. The pure undisturbed mind can become aware of the *ātman* by the reflection of the latter's consciousness upon itself.
94. See earlier note for the mind (here, ego) as mirror.
95. *Sabīja* is when the mind is concentrated on an object in the penultimate stages of *samādhi*, prior to uncoupling from the mind altogether (*Yoga Sūtras* I.46 and preceding verses).
96. For feet as a trope, see earlier note.
97. See earlier citation (II.2n10).
98. We notice that the *Bhāgavata* essentially presents the identical *yamas* and *niyamas* as Patañjali in (II.30ff.), with *yāvad-artha-parigrahaḥ* as a rewording of *aparigrahaḥ*; and *puruṣārcana*, of *Īśvara-praṇidhāna*.
99. The *Haṭha Yoga Pradīpikā* is one source referencing the *cakras*.
100. *Āsana* practices—bodily postures and the like—are solely intended to train the body such that it can sit in a still posture (*āsana*) for prolonged periods of meditation. Thus the term can mean postures or seat.
101. See *Haṭha Yoga Pradīpikā* or commentaries on *Yoga Sūtras* II.49.
102. The term *doṣa* here could refer to imperfections in the balance of the bodily constitution as understood in Āyurveda, but in *yoga* literature, it is more commonly used as a synonym for the *kleśas*, obstacles to *yoga* (*Yoga Sūtras* II.2ff.).
103. See *Gītā* V.27.
104. *Śrīvatsa* is a curl of hair on His chest. These adornments, garments, and other bodily details are all standardized descriptions of the form of Viṣṇu, repeated

frequently to strengthen one's ability to internally visualize the form in meditation practice.

105. The idea here is that the mind is used as a hook to "catch" (contemplate) this vision of *Īśvara*. The supreme *Īśvara*, of course, like the *ātman*, exists beyond the mind.
106. At this point, the *yogī* is not making fresh *karma* and has destroyed all latent *karma*, but the *karma* already activated at birth has to run its course. See *Sāṅkhya Kārikā* (68) for an expression of this.
107. *Mahat* is the first evolute from *prakṛti* (synonymous with *buddhi*).
108. See discussion in "The Rejection of *Brahman*."
109. In Vaiṣṇava theology, a form of *Īśvara*, the *Antaryāmin* or *Paramātman*, pervades and sustains each individual *ātman*.
110. Everything is done by the senses, mind, and intelligence, which are all expressions of *prakṛti* overseen by *Īśvara*.
111. *Kalā*, partial manifestation, in *Bhāgavata* theology refers to the *ātman* as a tiny part of *Bhagavān* (it also refers to other forms of Viṣṇu such as the *Antaryāmī/Parama-ātman*; see discussion in "A Three-Tiered Hierarchy of *Brahman*").
112. *Buddhi* is the first evolute from *prakṛti* and source of all other categories of matter down to the *aṇus*, the smallest elemental particles (see Sāṅkhya chart in appendix 2).
113. I have translated the term *bhinna-dṛś*, literally "one sees differences," variously according to context (for example, in verse 23 as "who does not see others as equal" and so forth).
114. In *Bhāgavata* cosmology, the universe is covered by seven layers—earth, water, fire, air, ether, mind, and ego—each one ten times thicker than the previous layer.
115. Śiva is the deity presiding over *tamas*, Brahmā over *rajas*, and Viṣṇu over *sattva*.
116. A *yojana* is variously estimated to be nine miles or five miles.
117. The various realms of the universe, including the hellish realms, are discussed in the fifth book of the *Bhāgavata*, chapters 16–26.
118. These are the *dhātus* of Āyurveda: chyle, blood, flesh, fat, bone, marrow, and semen.
119. For the three *tāpas*—those pertaining to the body and mind, those ensuing from other living entities, and those inflicted by the environment—see page 564n9 (and the commentaries to *Yoga Sūtras* II.15).
120. See previous citation for *aṁśa* (612n33).
121. The body is described as a city with nine gates in the *Śvetāśvatara Upaniṣad* III.18 and *Gītā* V.13.
122. The gross body changes every birth, but the same subtle body accompanies the *ātman* birth after birth. However, the *saṁskāras* of a *jīva*'s previous birth are covered over by *tamas* in a subsequent birth, even as their effects bear their *karmic* fruits, and they exert subconscious influences.

123. The *ātman* can be perceived only by itself, not by the mind, senses, or any other means. See page 613n51.
124. This verse refers to various evolutes of Sāṅkhya, which envelop the *ātman* with both sense instruments and sense objects. Therefore, the universe is, in this sense, the body of the *ātman*.
125. This refers to a *līlā* where Kṛṣṇa in the form of a baby lies on the waters of the cosmic ocean during the devastation of the universe, sucking His toe.
126. This refers to the Varāha incarnation, who retrieved the Vedas that had been stolen, and thus the knowledge bearing Vedānta teachings of the Upaniṣads, III.13–19.
127. In Vedic orthopraxy, certain rites, such as pressing the sacred *soma* plant to extract the juice for offering to the celestials, could be performed only by the highest *brāhmaṇa* caste, while those outside the Vedic caste system such as dog-eaters were considered so polluted that they were not allowed to even be present in the vicinity of such sacrifices. The idea here is that even those in the lowest rung of the social order, such as dog-eaters, thereby become purified by *bhakti* to *Bhagavān* and surpass the qualifications of those who are assigned the highest social status by birth. In other words, *bhakti* trumps all social and gender stratifications, at least in terms of spiritual possibilities.
128. Viṣṇu's carrier is the great eagle Garuḍa. Kṛṣṇa has Garuḍa as the emblem on His flag (for instance, in the battle of Kurukṣetra).

The *Bhāgavata Purāṇa*: Book IV

1. This tale is dedicated to Michael Ciccone.
2. See, for example, *Yoga Sūtras* II.45; *Gītā* XII.6–7 and XVIII.62.
3. Dhruva controlled his distraught mind by means of intelligence and reasoning. See *Gītā* VI.20 for similar phraseology.
4. Compare with *Yoga Sūtras* I.33.
5. The term for "equilibrium" here is *samaḥ*. *Gītā* II.48 defines *yoga* as *samatvam*, "equanimity."
6. The universe is conceived of as having three realms—higher, middle, and lower. Dhruva's grandfather is Lord Brahmā himself, the engineer of the entire universe, who lives in the highest celestial realm of the universe, so aspiring for an abode higher than his is a seemingly impossible order!
7. Sage Nārada travels around the universe through his mystic powers and is always to be seen playing his *vīṇā* stringed instrument and chanting the glories of Lord Viṣṇu.
8. See verse quoted on page 12–13.
9. The three forms of breath control are *recaka*, suspension after exhalation; *pūraka*, suspension after inhalation; and *kumbhaka*, suspension of both (see *Yoga Sūtras* II.50 and commentaries).
10. We are reminded here of Patañjali referring to *Iśvara* as the Supreme *Guru* in I.26.

11. Kṛṣṇa has certain characteristics, one of which is a curl of hair on His chest called *śrīvatsa*.
12. The heart is the locus of the *ātman* (and the *citta*) in the Upaniṣads and Vedānta traditions (see, for example, *Taittirīya Upaniṣad* I.6). In *Bhāgavata* theology, a form of Viṣṇu, *Antaryāmī* or *Paramātmān*, also resides within the heart with the individual *ātman*.
13. *Japa*, the repetition of *mantra*, is by far the most prominent form of meditation in the Indic traditions (see *Yoga Sūtras* I.27–28).
14. See *Yoga Sūtra*s III.42 for the mystic ability to travel through the air, a *siddhi* that has roots in early Vedic texts (*Āpastamba Sūtras* II.9.23.6–8; *Sāmavidhāna* III.9.1).
15. This verse prescribes the worship of God in the form of a deity. There is great flexibility in terms of time and place in deity worship (see note 17 in this regard).
16. Vaiṣṇavas, devotees of Viṣṇu/Kṛṣṇa, always place leaves from the *tulāsi* plant on their food offerings to the deity.
17. This refers to the eight substances from which deities can be made, discussed in "*Arcana* (Worship)."
18. *Uttama-śloka*, "one whose verses are supreme," can mean that the praises (in the form of *ślokas*, or verses) offered to God are the highest praises, or it can mean that the verses composed by God (such as the *Bhagavad Gītā*) are the highest.
19. For the four goals of human life implied here, see page 602n65.
20. Circumambulation of a person or sacred place is an act of worship and reverence.
21. Nārada is here referring to three of the four goals of life, noted above.
22. Dhruva was meditating on Hari, the Soul of the Universe, and in this sense, he became as if one with this object of concentration—that is, with the universe. In the *Yoga Sūtras*, terms like *samāpatti* and *saṁyama* point to concentrative states where the meditator and object of meditation become as if one by dint of the meditator's intense absorption on the object (see I.41 and III.3), a type of merging of the mind with the subtle substructure of all reality. Therefore Dhruva's state spilled over into the universe: since he had restrained his own breathing, the entire universe became correspondingly choked and deprived of air.
23. Urukrama is a name of Viṣṇu meaning "one whose step is wide." It is taken as a reference to the incarnation of Vāmana in *Bhāgavata* VIII:19.
24. This is most likely a reference to the *Puruṣa-sūkta* hymn of the *Ṛg-Veda*, where the Supreme Being is described as having a thousand heads. *Sahasra-śīrṣā* is also a name of another manifestation of Viṣṇu called Śeṣa, the thousand-headed serpent upon whom Viṣṇu reclines in the ocean of milk. Patañjali, the author of the *Yoga Sūtras*, is considered to be an incarnation of Śeṣa.
25. Most divinities ride a mount, and Viṣṇu's is an enormous eagle, Garuḍa.
26. *Daṇḍa-vat*, like a stick, is full prostration on the ground, with arms extended full length in front.

27. Viṣṇu's form and paraphernalia, such as the conch mentioned here, are made not from *prakṛti*, matter, but from *Brahman*—that is, pure consciousness.
28. The text here is giving a preview of the boon that Viṣṇu will bestow on Dhruva. The name for the polestar in Sanskrit texts is Dhruva, which literally means "that which is fixed."
29. The *mahat-tattva* is primordial *prakṛti*, the material matrix from which all the ingredients of material reality emerge. It consists of the three *guṇas*, *sattva*, *rajas*, and *tamas*. It is Kṛṣṇa's *māyā* (see *Gītā* VII.14).
30. See the Tale and Teachings of Lord Brahmā.
31. The *kalpaka taru* is a tree found in the divine realms, which fulfills any desire.
32. As discussed in part 1, *Brahman* is conscious spiritual energy that emanates from the form of the Lord in *Bhāgavata* theology and contains myriad individual *ātmans*. The individual *ātman* souls are composed of this *Brahman*, and many *yogīs* engage in meditation on their own *ātman* to experience the bliss therein. The sense here is that the bliss of coming in contact with Kṛṣṇa (the Supreme *Ātman*) is far greater than the bliss inherent in the liberated individual *ātman*. See "Hierarchies of Bliss."
33. The celestial realms are temporary realms within the world of *saṁsāra*, which beings with exceptionally good *karma*, meritorious activity, attain until the fruits of their good deeds expire. Residents of those realms are said to move about in celestial air-vehicles.
34. As discussed in part 1, in *Bhāgavata* theology, association of Viṣṇu's devotees is one of the most important ingredients of the spiritual path.
35. Vaikuṇṭha is Viṣṇu's divine eternal abode in Brahman, the kingdom of God.
36. Garuḍa is the eagle carrier of Lord Viṣṇu (and is retained as the name of Indonesian Airlines, reflecting the spread of Indian epic narrative to Southeast Asia during the first millennium C.E.).
37. The four *puruṣārthas*, goals of human life; see earlier note.
38. The four Kumāras—Sanandana, Sanaka, Sanātana, and Sanat—were five-year-old boys who were great devotees of Lord Viṣṇu and eventually attained His abode. Their story is narrated in *Bhāgavata* III:15 and elsewhere.
39. The sense here is that instead of seeing everything as connected to God, Dhruva saw differences (for instance, perceiving his brother as an enemy instead of as a fellow soul).
40. In the *Gītā* (VII.17), Kṛṣṇa states that *daivī-māyā* is His power of illusion (see earlier note), and thus one can overcome it only by surrendering to Him.
41. Dhruva is lamenting his request for the fulfillment of his material desire instead of asking for a spiritual boon.
42. The sense here is that because of poor deeds performed in the past, a person's intelligence is limited or deluded as a consequence.
43. Smelling the head of someone is a sign of intense affection in Hindu aesthetics.
44. We can recall that Brahmā and the progenitors (*prajāpatis*) are empowered to create the forms of the universe. But they are not the primary creators (that is, of matter or the *ātmans*). They are thus more like engineers.

45. Here, as elsewhere, is a reference to the *Antaryāmin* (see "A Three-Tiered Hierarchy of *Brahman*").
46. The idea is that Dhruva is now ready to pursue the fourth goal, *mokṣa*, having fulfilled the preparatory three: *dharma*, duty; *artha*, prosperity; and *kāma*, enjoyment (see earlier reference).
47. While *gandharvas* are celestial beings and themselves not considered illusory, imagining one has seen their city in this world corresponds to the maxim of a castle in the sky (that is, castles exist, but not in the sky).
48. This is known today as Badarīnātha.
49. This form, used in preliminary meditation by conceptualizing a personal form of *Bhagavān* composed of natural phenomena (such as the sun and moon as eyes and so forth), is described in III.6.
50. *Samādhi*, in its highest stage, is contentless awareness in the *Yoga Sūtras*. See "*Smaraṇa* (Remembering)" for comparison with Vaiṣṇava notions of *samādhi*.
51. Circumambulation of shrines, temples, holy objects, and the like is always undertaken in a clockwise direction.
52. The symbolism here should be clear: Dhruva had transcended death.
53. The commentaries take this to be *sapta-ṛṣis*, the seven sages. See V.22.17 for reference to this (and chapters 16–26 of the fifth canto in general for *Bhāgavata* cosmology).
54. According to the *Bhāgavata*, the four Kumāras were born from Brahmā, as was Śiva (III:12).
55. Śrīdhara takes these to be the five *kleśas* of *Yoga Sūtras* II.3ff.—ignorance, ego, desire, aversion, and clinging to life. But there are also five *kośas* first mentioned in the *Taittirīya Upaniṣad* II.2.1 as food, life air, mind, intelligence, and bliss.
56. Compare with *Gītā* II.62–63.
57. Compare with *Bṛhadāraṇyaka Upaniṣad* I.4.8.
58. The commentaries take this to be the *Antaryāmī*, a form of Viṣṇu who permeates and sustains each individual *ātman*. See "The Object of *Bhakti*: *Īśvara*, *Bhagavān*, *Brahman*, and Divine Hierarchies," note 78.
59. Here, the king, in his humility, is indicating that everything belongs to the true *brāhmaṇas*, such as Sanat-kumāra. Needless to say, a true *brāhmaṇa*, by definition, is one who knows *brahman*, as indicated in verse 41, and hence is indifferent to all material possessions.
60. *Karma yoga*, giving up attachments to the fruits (results) of one's actions and acting either from a place of pure selfless duty, *dharma*, or, higher still, by offering all one's activities to Kṛṣṇa, is one of the main teachings of the *Bhagavad Gītā* (for similar language, see II.47–48).
61. The idea here is that realized souls understand that all action is performed by the *prakṛtic* mind and senses; the *ātman* is simply the witness, not the "doer" of deeds.
62. There are four stages of life (*āśramas*), each lasting twenty-five years: *brahmacarya*, celibate studentship; *gṛhastha*, householder; *vānaprastha*, forest dweller; and *sannyāsa*, full ascetic renunciant.

63. In this form of austerity, the *yogī* sits in the middle of four fires placed in each of the cardinal directions, with the fifth, the sun itself, blazing down from above. The idea is to develop detachment from the sensations of the body.
64. Doubt is a function of the intelligence, *buddhi*, associated here with *jñāna*, one of the five *kośas* found in the *Taittirīya Upaniṣad*.
65. The idea here is that even liberating insight is a state of mind and hence it, too, must ultimately be transcended.
66. This type of practice involving the manipulation of the *prāṇa*, life airs, is more typical of the *Śākta* traditions.
67. In Sāṅkhya metaphysics, the subtler elements produce grosser ones sequentially, and the order is reversed when the universe is dissolved, as Pṛthu is here doing on a micro level with the elements of his own body.
68. The *mahat* is the first evolved stage of *prakṛti* after it has been agitated into creativity. In these verses, Pṛthu is progressively involuting, or dissolving every aspect of his material self back into its progressively subtler source, such that only his pure *ātman* remains in its original uncovered nature.
69. The benedictions outlined in the next few verses are not uncommon in the *Bhāgavata*. While they are materialistic in scope, they are clearly a form of "skillful means": enticing those with materialistic ambitions to read the story and thereby become infected with the seed of *bhakti*. The real intended boon is noted in the last verse of the chapter.
70. For the four goals of life, see previous citation.
71. *Karma* here refers to ritualistic activities. The signification of the term covers any form of religiosity that has materialistic (body/mind) benefits as its aim.
72. A subterranean city of celestial serpents, renowned for its beauty (literally "the place of enjoyment").
73. In the aesthetics of Sanskrit poetics, walking like an elephant is a sign of beauty (one needs to consider the graceful sway of an elephant's gait, despite its size, to appreciate this).
74. Śrī, the Goddess of Fortune, holds a lotus in one of her hands.
75. One can recognize celestials, as their feet never touch the ground (they also do not blink, and their garlands never fade!).
76. Kāma, the God of Love, like his Indo-European counterpart, Cupid, shoots arrows of love from his bow. He is "mind-born" because he was born from the mind of Brahmā.
77. It is anathema for a *kṣatriya*, warrior, to beg for anything.
78. *Brāhmaṇas* are exempt from, or receive significantly reduced, punishments (*Manusmṛti* 8.379–81).
79. This refers to the story of Yayāti, whose youngest son accepted his old age from him (*Bhāgavata* IX.18–19).
80. *Mamatā*: from the ultimate perspective, nothing belongs to the real self, the *ātman*, so all notions of ownership (such as "my family") are illusory.
81. As Kṛṣṇa states in the *Gītā*, the state of mind at the moment of death determines the next life (VIII.6).

82. Time is relative in Purāṇic cosmography (see the story of Brahmā in part 3).
83. This is likely a reference to the *Bhagavad Gītā* and/or *Uddhava Gītā* (where Kṛṣṇa imparts a lengthy discourse to Uddhava in the eleventh book of the *Bhāgavata*).
84. We are reminded of I.2.6 in the setting of the *Bhāgavata Purāṇa* chapter, where the highest *dharma* is defined as uninterrupted *bhakti* to Hari that is free of all motives.
85. See note 92 below for the *karmendriyas* of Sāṅkhya.
86. Here (as throughout), I follow the commentators in translating *śakti* as intelligence (*buddhi*).
87. The *ātman* is sometimes metaphorically called "swan."
88. See discussion in "A Three-Tiered Hierarchy of *Brahman*" pertaining to the *ātman* as a part, *aṁśa*, of *Īśvara*.
89. The sense here is that there is only one person, even though he or she may appear to be two—the person looking in the mirror and the face reflected back.
90. Some beings have no legs, such as plants, or one or more, depending on the bodily form.
91. In Sāṅkhya, the five *jñānendriyas* are the organs of hearing, seeing, touching, smelling, and tasting; and the *karmendriyas* are those of speaking, grasping, moving, excreting, and procreation.
92. These are the five *prāṇas*, life airs (*prāṇa, samāna, apāna, vyāna, udāna*).
93. As we find in *Gītā* IX.25, if one worships the gods, one attains the realms of the gods; if one worships the forefathers, one attains that realm. The scriptures teach all manner of things in accordance with the different proclivities and understandings of living beings, so in accordance with what one hears and follows from the scriptures, one attains a corresponding destination.
94. This is an extension of the chariot analogy of the *Kaṭha Upaniṣad* (III.9).
95. These are the standard three types of suffering recognized in many soteriological traditions of ancient India that are inflicted on all beings (see *Yoga Sūtras* II.15 and commentaries).
96. When in ignorance of one's true self, the *ātman*, one thinks one is one's material body and that one actually owns one's possessions.
97. Compare with the black and white *karma* of the *Yoga Sūtras* (IV.7).
98. See *Gīta* (II.42–46) and *Muṇḍaka Upaniṣad* (I.7–11) for similar deprecation of Vedic ritualism.
99. It is only the gross body made of the five elements that is discarded at death. The same subtle body accompanies the *ātman* birth after birth; it is discarded only after the life in which one becomes enlightened. Hence, despite the change of bodies, it is the same entity in the next life who enjoys the fruit of actions performed in a different body by that same agent in a previous life, and not a different person.
100. Dreams, in Yoga psychology, are experiences patched together from imprints (*saṁskāras*) of actions performed when awake. So in dreaming, one may appear

to inhabit a different body, but that dream body is made up of imprints gathered while awake in the physical body. The idea is that just as the experiencer of a dream is the same agent who previously planted the seeds of actions when awake, so the mind of a being in a future body experiences the fruit of action performed by the same mind in a previous birth.

101. As has been noted previously, this phraseology reflecting false notions of the self is common. When one thinks of the self as the body, one thinks in terms of "mine" and "other."
102. Thus, according to this verse, a case (for example) of déjà vu, where one feels a sense of familiarity with, say, a place where one has never been in this life, is explained by dint of the fact that one has been to that place in a previous life and hence there is a subconscious imprint of that place in the mind.
103. The mind might conjure up impossible things in dream or fantasy—the commentators give the examples of a sea on a mountaintop (place), stars in the day (time), or beheading oneself (action), which are in fact experiences that have never taken place—but what the mind is doing is patching together imprints of two things that have been experienced (an imprint of a sea from one place superimposed upon a separate imprint of a mountain from another and so forth). Put differently, they are the confusion of—or, better, fusion of—incompatible times, places, and actions.
104. The commentators take these five parts variously: we have followed Viśvanātha here.
105. This metaphor is probably left truncated because it would have been well-known from its source (*Bṛhadāraṇyaka Upaniṣad* IV.43).
106. Here termed *tat-sāmyatām*. See "The Liberated *Bhakta*: Different Types of *Mokṣa* in the *Bhāgavata*" on the five types of devotional liberation.

The *Bhāgavata Purāṇa*: Book V

1. Consider here the *Gītā*: "The ignorant deride Me when I assume a human-like form. They do not know My higher nature, nor that I am the *Īśvara* of all beings" (IX.11). The Vaiṣṇava traditions hold that when *Īśvara* descends, He does so in a pure *Brahman* body, not in a form made of the *guṇas* (see, for instance, *Bhāgavata* X.14.2).
2. By supporting Bharata as king without envy, his brothers are supporting the well-being of the kingdom and thus of the citizens.
3. The *agni-hotra* is one of the Vedic *yajñas*, fire rituals. Kṛṣṇa, in the *Gītā* (see V.29 and IX.24) and throughout the *Bhāgavata* (see 5.14.30, 45), is the ultimate consumer of sacrifice.
4. The *brāhmaṇas* are consistently eulogized throughout the *Bhāgavata*, as is typical of Vedic literature, so it is pertinent to keep in mind exactly what the text understands to constitute the qualities of this caste; verses 24–25 are particularly noteworthy in this regard.
5. The *āhavanīya* is one of the three fire structures into which oblations were offered (the eastern one) central to certain Vedic sacrificial rites (*yajña*). Be-

ginning with the later Vedic texts such as the *Āraṇyakas* and Upaniṣads, some of the Vedic rites, which were external and materialistic in intention (that is, performed for the purpose of worldly boons), are internalized and reconfigured with esoteric meanings as we find here (for instance, see *Bṛhadāraṇyaka Upaniṣad* I.1 for an example of this).

6. The idea is that Ṛṣabha was so saintly that even his body and its discharges were very *sāttvic* (see *Gītā* XIV.11 for something along these lines).
7. See chapter 3 of the *Yoga Sūtras* for some of these powers.
8. The *Yoga Sūtras* state that "the mystic powers are accomplishments for the mind that is outgoing but obstacles to *samādhi*" (III.37). Typically, they are construed as obstacles to those seeking the *ātman* or *Īśvara* and thus of no interest to real *yogīs*, who are contrasted with other characters depicted in the Purāṇas who performed astonishing austerities simply for the purpose of gaining powers that could be used in malevolent ways (see the Tale of Child Prahlāda).
9. Śiva, the quintessential ascetic, was nonetheless bewildered by Viṣṇu in the latter's female incarnation as Mohiṇī (*Bhāgavata* VIII.12), and the Tale of Saubhari later in this volume recounts his fall-down.
10. As indicated in the *Sāṅkhya Kārikā* (LXVII), the body of the *yogī* who has attained enlightenment continues to function for the remainder of that life, owing to the *saṁskāras* already activated at birth for that life, even as this then becomes the *yogī*'s final life (like the potter's wheel that continues to revolve for a period even after the potter ceases to pump it, because of the kinetic energy already invested in it, even as no further energy is being generated). In Ṛṣabha's case, given his devotional absorption, the functioning of his body continued under the jurisdiction of *yogamāyā* (rather than generic *māyā*; see "*Līlā* and *Yogamāyā*" for discussion). And hence, like an innocent child, says Viśvanātha, he put a stone in his mouth.
11. Mystic powers essentially entail supernormal capabilities and thus are simply enhanced versions of the same temporary, unsatisfying limitations that pertain to mundane sense indulgences.
12. See II.2n10 for the four *puruṣa-arthas*, goals of life. The bliss experienced from the performance of *bhakti* trumps all of these goals, including the fourth, *mokṣa*, the desire for liberation itself (see "The Rejection of *Brahman*" for further discussion).
13. The *brahmacarya āśrama* is the period, up to the age of twenty-five, when students would study Vedic knowledge systems under the tutelage of the teacher, *guru*. For the *brāhmaṇa* caste (see below), this would consist of the sacred Vedic texts. For the warrior caste, as would have been the case with Bharata, the texts and practices pertaining to warfare, *dhanur-śāstras*, and polity, *nīti* and *dharma-śāstras*.
14. The *gṛhastha*, or householder, accepts a wife and raises progeny. In this phase of life, one engages fully in one's caste occupation. These are *brāhmaṇa*, teaching/priestly caste; *kṣatriya*, warrior/administrative cast; *vaiśya*, merchant/landowning caste; *śūdra*, artisan caste, as well as those employed

in service by the other castes (see *Bhāgavata* XI.11 and *Gītā* chapter 18 for discussion).

15. In this third phase of *vānaprastha*, husband and wife practice celibacy, detach themselves from the household, which they entrust to their by now grown-up offspring, and together retire to sacred places to pursue *yogic* practices more fully.
16. Thus, to this day, the name for India in traditional circles is Bhārata.
17. We are reminded here of the *Gītā*: "Whatever is offered to Me with *bhakti*—a leaf, fruit, flower, or water—I accept from one who is devoted, when it is offered with love" (IX.26).
18. These are some of the bodily symptoms of ecstasy ensuing from the advanced stages of devotional meditation.
19. The sense here is that Bharata's mind was focused internally, meditating on Lord Viṣṇu, who is seated in the heart of all beings along with the individual's own *ātman*, rather than on external objects. As early as the Upaniṣads (see *Kaṭha* II.20), the heart is considered to be the seat of both the *ātman* and the mind.
20. The day in ancient India was divided into thirty *muhūrtas*. A *muhūrta* thus corresponds to forty-eight minutes.
21. *Oṁ* is considered the sonic manifestation of *Brahman*, the Absolute Truth, throughout the Upaniṣads, most notably the *Māṇḍūkya*. It is the preferred method of fixing the mind in the *Yoga Sūtras* (I.27–28).
22. The five *yamas* are listed in the *Yoga Sūtras* (II.30) and elsewhere as nonviolence, truthfulness, celibacy, refrainment from stealing, and refrainment from covetousness (the Buddhist *yamas* replace the last one with no intoxication).
23. One of the duties of a king is never to deny protection to a vulnerable and innocent being who approaches for refuge. Although Bharata had renounced the function of kingship, his kingly *saṁskāras* still prompted him to protect a helpless entity.
24. See previous citation (II.12n2).
25. The *kirātas* are a tribe of hunters from a certain area in ancient India who lure animals to trap them. References to them in classical literature tend to be derogatory.
26. The *Ṛg*, *Yajur*, and *Sāma Vedas*.
27. This is a reference to the ancient Vedic fire rites, which even some ascetics in the forest continued to perform (as can also be seen in the Upaniṣads). The fawn nibbled the oblations meant for the offering, thus polluting them. Vedic sacrifices are rigidly bound by regulations pertaining to purity and pollution.
28. The sense here is that owing to some impious or negative actions performed earlier in this or a previous life, Bharata's just fruit or *karmic* reaction manifested in the form of the deer intruding into his life and distracting him from his practices.
29. As noted previously, one attains the same state in which one is absorbed at the moment of death (*Gītā* VIII.6). The idea is that one's strongest attachments

arise in the mind as one is being separated from these objects of attachment during the processs of dying, and these partly determine one's future bodies.

30. The memories of a previous birth normally become dormant in the subsequent birth, and while these memories may exert subconscious influences, they are generally obscured by *tamas*. Because of the devotion Bharata performed before he developed his attachment to the fawn, he was able to retain the memories of his past birth when he became a deer himself.
31. The *śālagrāma* is a sacred stone worshipped by Vaiṣṇavas as a self-manifest form of Viṣṇu Himself. It is found in most Vaiṣṇava temples.
32. Bathing in holy rivers purifies one's *karma*, so the implication is that even as a deer Bharata did everything he could to bring a speedy end to the *karma* that was causing him to be confined in that body, by living in a holy place and taking baths in the sacred river there.
33. The orthodox *brāhmaṇa* caste is considered to comprise eight lineages associated with legendary sages such as Aṅgirā.
34. These are the qualities of the ideal *brāhmaṇa* (see *Gītā* XVIII.42 and throughout).
35. This is a reference to the sacred thread bestowed on *brāhmaṇas* upon completing their Vedic studies. It is worn across the left shoulder, diagonally looping down the right side. The sacred *gāyatrī mantra* is recited with the thumb wrapped in the bottom of this loop thrice daily.
36. After this ceremony, the *āvartana*, *brāhmaṇa* males, are married. The sense here is that the father did not go so far as to marry his son, owing to his apparent retarded state.
37. The *gayatrī* is an invocation to the sun god and begins, *"Oṁ bhūr bhuvaḥ svaḥ,"* the higher, middle, and lower regions of the universe that is illuminated by the sun. This is the *mantra* chanted three times daily by *brāhmaṇas*, as indicated in the note above. The idea is that Bharata could not even learn the twenty-eight syllables of this *mantra* in four months, such was his commitment to appearing retarded so that people would neglect him, thus minimizing his chances of again forming attachments.
38. The sense is that the wife, here referred to as Satī (see the story of Satī in *Bhāgavata* IV.2ff.), entered onto the funeral pyre of the husband. This was a voluntary practice in ancient India, usually undertaken by the wives of certain warrior communities who did not wish to live without their husbands but rather chose to follow them to their next destination.
39. The three Vedas—*Ṛg, Sāma, Atharva*—are chanted during the Vedic fire sacrifices. These sacrifices are usually performed to obtain worldly boons from the celestial beings. The later Vedic texts (see *Muṇḍaka* I.2 and *Gītā* II.42ff.) decry the performance of such sacrifices as foolish, since the boons they provide are temporary and materialistic. A similar critique is intended in this verse.
40. This is a standard and ubiquitous trope in philosophical discourse: the mind is subject to the dualities of such things as honor and dishonor, happiness and

distress; and the body to dualities of hot and cold, pain and pleasure (see *Gītā* II.14 and 38). Thus, one who identifies the self with the body and mind believes that one is happy or distressed, according to the dualities. One who is absorbed in the bliss of the *ātman*, however, which is pure consciousness and a completely different entity from the nonconscious material mind and body that envelops it, transcends these fleeting dualities.

41. The Goddess Kālī, whose worship is today most prominent in East India, is a ferocious form of the Goddess—although she is seen as benevolent (*bhadra*) and motherly to her less *tāmasic* devotees who understand the higher spiritual lessons she imparts through this form. She accepts blood sacrifice in certain contexts. The English word "thug" actually comes from colonial India, where it is derived from a community following ghastly religious practices such as the one referred to in this verse.
42. In other words, their minds were enveloped in greed, ignorance, darkness, violence, and delusion.
43. The companions of the Goddess Kālī, in the *Devī Māhātmya*, are female *śāktis* emanating from the bodies of the primary Gods as well as from the Goddess herself (chapter 8).
44. The term *paramahaṁsa*, supreme swan, used for the enlightened *yogī*, points to the swan's reputed ability to separate milk from water in its beak, an analogy to the realized sage who can distinguish spirit from matter.
45. *Saṁskāras* such as desires prompt action, *karma*, which produces reactions such as the body referenced here.
46. Although *yogīs* burn up all latent seeds of *karma* that have not yet been activated but are lying in storage for future births, *sañcita karma*, and (since they are free of ignorance, ego, and desire) no longer make fresh ongoing *karma*, *sañcīyamāna karma*, they do have to burn up whatever *karma* had already been activated at birth for that particular life, the *prārabdha karma* mentioned here (a clear expression of this principle is found in the *Sāṅkhya Kārikā* LXVII). Hence Bharata was content to again take up the palanquin with this in mind.
47. The term used here, *jñāna-kalā-avatīrṇa*, points to Kapila as an incarnation who descends to teach Sāṅkhya metaphysics, the oldest metaphysical system in the Vedic tradition (see his teachings in this volume). Considered by tradition to be the founder of Sāṅkhya, He therefore especially manifests the knowledge aspect of Viṣṇu's Being. As discussed in "Definition of *Īśvara*, *Bhagavān*, and *Brahman*," the definition of *Bhagavān* is that of the Being who possesses all six qualities in fullness, and some incarnations are specific manifestations of one of these qualities in particular. Kapila is a *jñāna* incarnation.
48. The king is essentially saying that even if one is *ātman*, the body still exists and so does its experience of fatigue on some level; it cannot be fully illusory.
49. The same dismissive language *veda-vāda* is used here as in the *Gītā* (II.42–46), which likewise criticizes those addicted to Vedic rituals. These rituals,

from the earlier Vedic period, are essentially undertaken to secure material gain from higher powers—the Vedic gods. They represent materialistic religiosity—the performance of seemingly religious acts to a higher power, but with a motive of satisfying one's material desires pertaining to one's body and mind. From the perspective of the *ātman*-focused teachings expressed in the later Vedic texts, the Upaniṣads (see *Bṛhadāraṇyaka* 3.8.10; *Muṇḍaka* I.2.6–13), such ritualistic enterprises are therefore acts stemming from ignorance of the true self and of no interest to real seekers of Truth. Hence Bharata criticizes them here and in the next verse.

50. The Vedānta tradition considers the Upaniṣads the *anta*, "conclusion," or higher teachings of the Veda (hence their name, *Veda-anta*).
51. *Vāsanās* are *saṁskāras* from past lives that exert subconscious influence on the mind (see *Yoga Sūtras* IV.8, IV.24).
52. The various categories emanating from primordial *prakṛti* in the Sāṅkhya tradition are enumerated differently in different schools, the most common schema being the twenty-four evolutes. The sixteen noted here, in resonance with *Sāṅkhya Kārikā* (XXIIff.) and *Yoga Sūtras* (II.19), are those from these twenty-four that do not produce any further evolutes from themselves.
53. As the *Gītā* says, the mind is both the friend and the enemy of the living entity (VI.5). Ultimately, both bondage and liberation are states of mind (*Sāṅkhya Kārikā* LXII–LXIII), since the *ātman* is eternally pure and distinct. The *ātman* here is referred to as *kṣetra-jña*, the "field-knower." *Prakṛti* is the field of activities but does not "know"—that is, it is unconscious matter—while the *ātman* as the source of consciousness is "the knower" (chapter 14 of the *Gītā* is about the *kṣetra* and the *kṣetra-jña*).
54. We find here a different schema from the five *vṛttis* of *Yoga Sūtras* (I.5–11). However, as will be seen from the subsequent verses, these are simply schematic differences, not substantial metaphysical ones. There were numerous Sāṅkhya systems in circulation (the *Bhāgavata* mentions several and even notes a variant view in verse 12), given that different sages organized the various evolutes of *prakṛti* differently (reflected here in the two different views noted in verses 9 and 10). But all accepted the same basic categories and shared the ultimate goal of establishing the distinction of the *ātman* from both the mind, senses, and sense objects.
55. Compare *Yoga Sūtras* II.21. One of the arguments used in philosophical discourse to establish the existence of an *ātman*, reflected here, is that the organs of actions and the knowledge-acquiring senses are precisely that—organs and instruments. And instruments exist for the usage of some other entity: they do not exist for themselves.
56. Compare *Yoga Sūtras* I.4 and II.20.
57. In *Bhāgavata* theology (as reflected, for instance, in Vaiṣṇava readings of *Gītā* XV.16–19; *Śvetāśvatara Upaniṣad* IV.4.6), there are two *ātmans* in every embodied being: one is the *ātman* who is the "enjoyer" of experience, who is projected into that body in accordance with the established laws of *karma*;

the other is a form of Viṣṇu (*Antaryāmin*). In other words, Viṣṇu also manifests a personal presence within every embodied *ātman*, which permeates the *ātman* as ether permeates other elements and directs the *ātman* according to the desires it manifests in its mind.

58. We can recall that the king is thinking the *brāhmaṇa* to be Kapila, an incarnation of Viṣṇu, and thus the cause of the universe, disguising his real nature.
59. These are the *mahābhūtas* of Sāṅkhya (and, for that matter, Vaiśeṣiká): the smallest irreducible individualized gross particles (*aṇus*) of earth, water, fire, air, and ether (irreducible in Vaiśeṣiká, although in Sāṅkhya, while these are the smallest individualized entities, they can in fact be further reduced to subtler energies such as the *tanmātras* and, ultimately the finest material essence of everything, the three *guṇas*). The term "atom" for *aṇu* was assigned by early Indologists, since "atom" was the smallest known particle at the time. With the discovery in physics of quarks and other such things, the term is no longer accurate, hence my (still unsatisfactory) rendering of the terms as "subatomic" particles, in an attempt to cover any future such discoveries! (Ironically, the Greek etymology of the term "atom" also in fact refers to the smallest possible entity along similar lines to the term *aṇu*.)
60. This dense verse actually contains standard philosophical concepts. The world of "dualities" is a way of thinking about external reality—things are distinguished from other things along spectrums such as thin and fat and all variants in between. Ultimately, all reality is a manifestation of *prakṛti*, which consists of the three *guṇas*, so things differ from other things only in terms of the proportionality of these *guṇas*. *Prakṛti* manifests in the form of some of the features listed here (which are technical terms of the Indic philosophical traditions): *dravya* are the smallest material substances such as the subatomic particles; *svabhāva*, the essential nature of things (such as liquidity of water); *āśaya*, the reservoir of an individual's *karma*, stored in the subconscious mind, which eventually produces its fruits (*Yoga Sūtras* II.15); *kāla*, the Time factor, which brings the reservoir of *karma* to its fruition in due course; and *karma*, an individual's actual actions themselves, which bear corresponding fruits.
61. Vāsudeva is a name of Kṛṣṇa. As noted in the *Gītā* (VII.19), after many births, a wise person realizes that everything is Vāsudeva.
62. This refers to a practice of extreme asceticism where the *yogī* sits in ice-cold water during the winter and in a circle of several fires in the midday sun of the summer. The idea is to remove consciousness from its attachment and identification with the body and its sensations.
63. In the Vaiṣṇava traditions, love of God is attained only through the medium of the saintly *guru* (see "*Satsaṅga* and the *Guru*").
64. This refers to the enticements of Vedic ritual (see *Yoga Sūtras* I.15 for identical wordage), as expressed more explicitly in *Gītā* II.42–46 and the Upaniṣads (previous citation). The idea is that the successful *yogī* must be free not only from desires for things experienced in this material world, but also from the

enticements of the Vedic scriptures themselves (specifically the *karma khāṇḍa* ritualistic sections, promoting a higher grade of embodied existence in the next life in the subtle celestial realms for those with exceptional *karma*).

65. Śrīdhara states that these are trees whose shade is considered to be inauspicious.
66. *Yakṣas* are a type of superhuman being usually found in forests and other natural settings.
67. The idea here is that, overwhelmed by desire due to firelike *rajas*, a person seeks gold. But since gold is a by-product of the smelting process of fire, it can be analogized as a type of stool excreted by fire and therefore a toxic, noxious, and deadly substance.
68. Since the person is miserly, he does not enjoy the wealth in this world, and since it is not put to proper use for *dharma* as indicated in a prior verse, it is not conducive to a good destination in the next world.
69. Even if one does good deeds, if one does not know the *ātman*, one still needs to return to embodied existence to receive the good fruits. So, ultimately, all embodiment is suffering for the wise (see *Yoga Sūtras* II.15).
70. Devadatta and Viṣṇumitra are the standard names used in Sanskrit commentaries to denote an average person in general.
71. Time is the movement of matter. The *aṇu* is the smallest unit of gross (*mahābhūta*) matter. The time it takes for one atom to move to its immediately adjacent space is the smallest unit of recordable time, the *kṣaṇa*. At the other end of the Time spectrum, the universe is dissolved at the end of Brahmā's life, so this is the largest unit of Time.
72. The *Śruti* is the Vedic corpus, and *Smṛti* is derivative post-Vedic literature (see appendix 1).
73. Almost all *mokṣa* traditions hold ignorance, *avidyā*, as the cause of *saṁsara*, the place where it begins (see, for instance, *Yoga Sūtras* II.4, 12, 24). Therefore, returning to this originating principle and removing it by *vidyā* (knowledge, *viveka*) removes *saṁsāra* (*Yoga Sūtras* II.25–26).
74. This refers to a previous incarnation of Viṣṇu, Hayagrīva, who killed the demons Madhu and Kaiṭabha, after the latter stole the Vedas and hid them in the ocean (referred to in VII.9.37).

The *Bhāgavata Purāṇa*: Book VI

1. In the *Yoga Sūtras,* even as one can fix the mind on an object "according to one's inclination" (I.39), *japa*, the repetition of the name of *Īśvara* (I.27–28), is prioritized. This can be inferred by dint of the fact that *japa* heads the list of objects upon which the mind can be fixed in concentration (*ālambanas*), which according to traditional hermeneutics indicates superiority over other items on the list. Additionally, *Īśvara* as *ālambana* receives eight verses where the five other suggested *ālambanas* receive only one each. Moreover, only *Īśvara* can bestow liberation, where other objects cannot (II.45). Thus Patañjali is tactfully but clearly prioritizing this form of practice.

2. It can be noted, however, that the hells in Hindu and Buddhist cosmographies are temporary places, where torment is inflicted on beings as effects in exact proportionality to the causal acts that generate them (see *Yoga Sūtras* II.14). Once the requisite bad *karma* causing one to spend time there has been accounted for, one moves on to one's next due birth, regaining another chance at a hūman form.
3. The types of negative *karma* performed by humans, and the corresponding hellish realms with their torments that are their appropriate consequences, are outlined in the fifth book of the *Bhāgavata*.
4. The commentators elaborate that one might have seen punishment being meted out by the king and heard about the hellish regions from scriptures.
5. This well-used simile points to the fact that the elephant, immediately after taking his bath, rolls in the sand again, rendering any cleansing useless: thus, suggests the king, with atonement.
6. One might counteract the effects of bad *karma* by atonement, but the roots of sin—desire and the like (the *kleśas*, *Yoga Sūtras* II.3ff.)—remain, so one reengages in bad *karma* all over again. As long as one is ignorant of the true self and thinks one is body/mind, one is inevitably bound by desires to enjoy the body/mind, which all too easily leads to again engaging in bad *karma*. Hence the real solution is knowledge of the true self, which eradicates desire at its roots (*Yoga Sūtras* II.4.24–25).
7. The sense here is that a subtle residue of liquor remains embedded in the liquor pot even after washing, just as the root *saṁskāras* of desire themselves remain latent, even if the mind undertakes atonement for the *karma* created by attempting to fulfill them.
8. From as early as the *Praśna Upaniṣad* (III.6), the *ātman* is said to abide in the region of the heart, as does the mind and subtle body.
9. Of the five types of liberation in Vaiṣṇavism, one is *sārūpya*, having the same form as Viṣṇu, such as His messengers, here (see "The Liberated *Bhakta*: Different Types of *Mokṣa* in the *Bhāgavata*" for discussion).
10. See *Yoga Sūtras* II.14. The "fruit" of action denotes the *karmic* consequences.
11. The present is a consequence of the past and cause of the future and can thus provide a sense of both of these; so with a person's actions (see *Yoga Sūtras* II.12–14).
12. See earlier note for the five *karmendriyas*.
13. We have followed Śrīdhara in taking "the three" to refer to the ingredients outlined in verse 50, but the three could also refer to the three *guṇas* and their products.
14. While the gross body consisting of the five gross atomic elements (earth, water, fire, air, and ether) is discarded at death, the *ātman* soul remains embodied in the subtle body, which consists of the knowledge-acquiring senses and the powers behind the organs of action, noted in verse 50. This subtle body, which transmigrates with the *ātman* birth after birth, is called variously *liṅga* (as in this verse), *sūkṣma śarīra*, or *antaḥ-karaṇa* (or four from the five, *kośas*).

15. The sense here is that, bewildered as to one's real nature, one acts. Bound by the reactions of these acts and, hence, constantly afflicted by inexplicable events unceasingly thrust upon one (in the form of *karmic* fruits), one can see no way out of one's material predicament.
16. This verse is found, verbatim, in *Gītā* III.5.
17. One acts according to one's nature and thus generates corresponding reactions of *karma*, but one's initial nature is itself the product of previous *karma*.
18. This is almost verbatim in *Gītā* III.21.
19. In the *Gītā* (II.45), Kṛṣṇa informs Arjuna that the Vedas deal with goals connected with the three *guṇas*—that is, the normative goal of Vedic culture and of Vedic ritualism is righteous behavior, the fruits of which are the attainment of material prosperity in this life and in the celestial realms of the next (*dharma*, *artha*, *kāma*). Kṛṣṇa exhorts Arjuna to rise above these goals and strive for higher goals (*mokṣa*).
20. For the various types of hell, see V.26.
21. Although the term *svarūpa* here is used by Patañjali in a generic sense to refer to the *ātman* (*Yoga Sūtras* I.3), it takes on an extended sense in the *Bhāgavata* tradition. As discussed in "The Liberated *Bhakta*," the liberated *ātman* in the *Bhāgavata* receives a divine *Brahman* form upon attaining Vaikuṇṭha or Goloka, also called *svarūpa*.
22. This is a reference to activities performed under the three *guṇas*.
23. See *Bṛhadāraṇyaka Upaniṣad* III.6 for the metaphor of the universe being woven.
24. For the term *aṁśa*, see earlier citation (and "Who Is the Supreme *Īśvara*?: The Purāṇic Context").
25. Kṛṣṇa states in the *Gītā* (IV.13) that He created the *varṇāśrama*—the system of four social occupations and four orders of life.
26. These are all different kinds of celestial beings.
27. From the five different types of liberated states or attainments in the *Bhāgavata* tradition, the one noted here, *sārūpya*, involves being bestowed the same form as Viṣṇu (see "The Liberated *Bhakta*").
28. These are the twelve *mahājanas*, the only beings who fully understand *Bhāgavata dharma*.
29. The three sacred fires are the *āhavanīya*, offertorial fire; *dakṣināgni*, southern fire; and *gārhapatya*, householder fire.
30. See *Gītā* II.42 for the flowery words of the Vedas.
31. This and the next verse is a rewording of *Gītā* VII.3.
32. See *Bhāgavata* VI.6–9 for the story of Vṛtra.
33. One version of how Indra's body is covered with eyes is recounted in the *Mahābhārata* I.203.
34. Literally ten million. This is an example of *atiśayokti* or *vakrokti*, exaggeration, in Sanskrit poetics (discussed, for example, in the *Dhvanyāloka* of Ānandavardhana).
35. See the Sāṅkhya chart in appendix 2 for the various coverings that constitute the subtle body of an individual.

36. These are listed in Manu's *Dharma Śāstra* (9.294–95).
37. In the older Vedic traditions, offspring were required to perform offerings (*piṇḍa*) to their departed ancestors at set times, in order to deliver them from hell or other unpleasant afterlife experiences.
38. Tvaṣṭā is a *prajāpati* (progenitor).
39. Subrahmaṇya was the son of Śiva, but the latter's semen was preserved by Agni, god of fire, and he was nursed by the six Kṛttikās (*Rāmāyaṇa*, *Bālakāṇḍa* 37).
40. See earlier note.
41. *Artha* here, among its many meanings, can denote an object of the senses and is glossed by Śrīdhara with earth and the like—that is, the *mahābhūta* atoms perceivable to the senses. Although such atoms in Sāṅkhya (contra Nyāya) are themselves not eternal, since they are products of successively more subtle levels of matter, their ultimate substructure, the *guṇas*, is eternal.
42. The first part of this verse is not entirely clear, given the generic *yoga* position that as a result of discrimination one precisely does realize the distinction between the *ātman* and the body. But it could be suggesting that only the *ātman* is real; the body is ephemeral (or, perhaps, that everything is ultimately the nondual *Brahman*). With regard to the second part, in the school of Nyāya, the logicians, reality is conceived of consisting of seven ultimate and irreducible entities. Two of these are referred to here: an object consists of atoms, which have individuators, a category of reality that preserves their eternal individuality (namely, that prevents them from, for example, merging or dissolving into something else), and a universal "cowness" that allows them to be situated in classes of things (namely, an essence allowing one cow to be grouped with others, and to be perceived as cowness or cowhead). Sāṅkhya traditions like that of the *Bhāgavata* oppose this view and hold that while there may be such things as individuators and universals on a surface level, they are not eternally real entities, as everything can ultimately be reduced to one entity, *prakṛti* (and its three *guṇas*).
43. This is likely a reference to Paraśurāma rather than Lord Rāma.
44. Desires are the results of past actions, *karma*, and although they are mental concoctions, and thus unreal, they nonetheless trigger further action when one strives to fulfill them. Hence the cycle of *saṁsāra* is perpetuated.
45. Saṅkarṣaṇa is a form of Viṣṇu mostly associated with the *pāñcarātrika* Vaiṣṇava traditions.
46. The term *jīva* is used to refer to the soul when it is embodied. In this case, the departed soul of the king's son would be in its subtle body, *sūkṣma-śarīra*, prior to being reembodied in a gross form.
47. In other words, *Īśvara* is beyond description and mental conceptual categories.
48. The *vidyādharas* are a category of celestial beings.
49. Śeṣa is the cosmic serpent upon whom one of the manifestations of Viṣṇu reclines. Patañjali is considered to be an incarnation of Śeṣa (for example, according to certain commentaries on the terms "Ananta," another name for

Śeṣa, in *Yoga Sūtras* II.47 and in the invocation to Patañjali attributed to King Bhoja).

50. The *Sātvatas*, which I have translated here as Vaiṣṇavas, are first noted in literary sources in the *Mokṣadharma* section of the *Mahābhārata* called the *Nārāyaṇīya*, where they are also known as the *Ekāntins*—those who are exclusively devoted to Nārāyaṇa.
51. See earlier citation for *aṁśa*.
52. In the fifth book of the *Bhāgavata*, the structure of the universe is outlined. Although vast, the universe is enveloped in seven sheaths—the seven elements of Sāṅkhya (earth, water, air, fire, ether, ego, and intelligence), each one ten times thicker than the previous one. Thus the sheaths of the universe are vastly more expansive than the universe itself.
53. The sense here is that normally, if one tries to fulfill worldly desires, then one is subject to their corresponding fruits of *karma* and thus is trapped by the world of dualities (like and dislike, and so on; *Gītā* II. 64)—in other words, *saṁsāra*. However, if one worships Viṣṇu, even for selfish sensual reasons to fulfill some worldly desire—the mixed *bhakti* from part 1 ("*Bhakti* Mixed with Attachment to *Dharma* and *Jñāna*")—one is not subject to the fruits normally accruing from the laws of *karma*. Rather, one eventually becomes purified by such worship. This is because Viṣṇu is beyond the *guṇas* (transcendent), and thus anyone absorbed in Viṣṇu (even if originally for mundane motives) eventually also transcends the *guṇas* by dint of the purification ensuing from such meditation.
54. We can recall that in Vaiṣṇava philosophy the *ātman* is a part of the Supreme.

The *Bhāgavata Purāṇa*: Book VII

1. The sense here is that the *ātman* is the hearer behind hearing, and the speaker behind speaking, in the sense of being the consciousness that animates these functions (along the lines of the *Kena Upaniṣad I.2ff.*). So the body and cognitive organs the queens were attached to was still present, but the *ātman* who had animated the body had never been seen by anyone in the first place. So for whom are they lamenting?
2. *Abhiniveśa* is the fifth *kleśa* in the *Yoga Sūtras* (II.9).
3. The sense here is that since his mind was absorbed in Kṛṣṇa and he was not aware of conventional reality, he appeared possessed as if by a ghost or some negative planetary influence.
4. Since the *asuras* are sons of Diti, they are also referred to as *daityas*.
5. The sense here is that the teaching was based on the body, not the universality of the *ātman*, and thus revolved around prioritizing one's self and one's clan, in opposition to others.
6. The household is compared with falling into a "dark well" in the ascetic traditions, as one becomes trapped by duties and responsibilities, with no clear way out.

7. See verse 19.
8. Although there are four goals of life, the *daityas* are interested in these first three (*dharma, artha, kāma*), but not the fourth, *mokṣa*, liberation.
9. This refers to the incarnation of Varāha, who killed Hiraṇyakaśipu's brother Hiraṇyākṣa (*Bhāgavata* III.19).
10. Śunaḥśepa was sold by his father, Ajigarta, for use as a human sacrifice in exchange for one hundred cows (*Aitareya Brāhmaṇa* VII.13–18).
11. Varuṇa is the deity of the waters.
12. The threefold sufferings are *ādhyātmika,* the suffering accruing from one's own mind and body; *ādhibhautika*, from other beings; and *ādhidaivika*, from the environment; (see *Yoga Sūtras* II.15 and commentaries).
13. For the seer and seen, see *Yoga Sūtras* II.17ff.
14. *Siddhis*, mystic powers, can also be attained by *tapas*, austerity (see *Yoga Sūtras* IV.1); hence, with a view of obtaining supernormal powers, many demons also performed *tapas*, such as Rāvaṇa of the Rāmāyaṇa.
15. The eight are *prakṛti*, intelligence, ego, and the five subtle qualities (see *Gītā* VII.4). The sixteen are the eleven senses and the five gross elements (see the Sāṅkhya chart in appendix 2).
16. The Vedānta process of *neti neti*, "it is not this, it is not that," is a method of approaching *ātman/Brahman* by negating everything that it is not—namely, all objects of consciousness (see *Bṛhadāraṇyaka Upaniṣad* II.3.6).
17. *Anvaya-vyatireka* is a form of logical analysis, where something is established based on both the concomitance and the absence of some other thing that is inseparable from it (for example, wherever there is smoke there is fire and wherever there is no fire there is no smoke).
18. See the *Māṇḍūkya Upaniṣad* for the four states of consciousness.
19. The term used here is *svarūpa* (as in *Yoga Sūtras* I.3).
20. The ten directions are N, S, W, E, NE, NW, SE, SW, up, and down.
21. The *cakra*, a disclike weapon, is specific to Viṣṇu. The commentators mention the *vajra*, mostly associated with Indra, as a weapon common to others.
22. See the Tale and Teachings of Lord Brahmā.
23. In Purāṇic cosmography, the ten cardinal points mentioned earlier are guarded by celestial elephants.
24. Where bowing or kneeling denotes respect or submission in the Western epic tradition, the utmost honor afforded to someone in the Indian tradition, which is still exhibited in devotional contexts, is laying the entire body down with arms extended in front, *daṇḍa-vat*, "like a stick."
25. See the Tale of the Elephant *Bhakta*.
26. These are listed in the *Mahābhārata* (V.43.12) as knowledge, truthfulness, control, tranquillity, freedom from malice, modesty, tolerance, freedom from envy, charity, performance of sacrifice, austerity, and sacred learning.
27. The idea here is that the mind is predisposed toward fulfilling desire. In Vedic India, the sanctioned manner of fulfilling certain desires was through Vedic ritualism.

28. According to the *Yoga Sūtras*, the instruments of perception and sense objects of the world are presented so that the *puruṣa* can seek enjoyment (II.18).
29. This is a reference to the ritualistic part of the Vedic corpus (the earlier *Mantra* and *Brāhmaṇa* texts), which pertains to the performance of sacrifices for the good things of life in this world and the attainment of the celestial realms in the next. The *mokṣa* traditions such as the *Bhāgavata* here decry such materialistic religiosity (see, for instance, *Muṇḍaka Upaniṣad* I.2.6ff. and *Gītā* II.42ff.).
30. This is a reference to the *kalpa-vṛkṣa*, a tree said to be found in the celestial realms, which fulfills any wish presented to it by the supplicant.
31. In the cosmology of the *Bhāgavata*, the universe is periodically partially dissolved into its subtlest causal ingredients and eventually completely dissolved, during which it rests within its ultimate cause, Viṣṇu, before a new cycle of creation takes place. See *Bhāgavata* book 2, and *Gītā* VIII.17.
32. These four states, first expressed in the *Māṇḍūkya Upaniṣad*, are waking, dreaming, deep sleep, and enlightenment.
33. This type of discourse sometimes switches from "Him" to "You," as a speaker may be speaking to one form of Viṣṇu, as Prahlāda is doing here, about another form of the same Supreme Being.
34. Ananta is the cosmic serpent Śeṣa. In a verse first found in the eleventh-century commentary on the *Yoga Sūtras* of King Bhoja, Patañjali is considered an incarnation of Śeṣa. It is upon this thousand-hooded snake that Viṣṇu reclines on the waters of dissolution.
35. In Sāṅkhya metaphysics, each of the five gross atomic elements (the *mahābhūtas* of earth, water, fire, air, and ether) has a quality associated with it (the *tanmātras* of smell, taste, sight, touch, and sound, respectively), from which it is generated and therefore by which it is inseparably pervaded. The analogy here indicates that all manifest reality is an inseparable evolute of the finest of all essences, *Īśvara*.
36. In II.1.25ff. and 3.5ff., the various limbs of this particular divine manifestation are each associated with specific realms of the universe.
37. This barely mentioned incarnation is Hayagrīva (noted in passing in II.7.5).
38. Madhu and Kaiṭabha were two demons who stole the Vedas (see previous reference). Although this story is mentioned but not presented in the *Bhāgavata*, it was a well-known narrative (in fact, one of Kṛṣṇa's most common names is Madhusūdana, "killer of Madhu"). It is outlined in the *Mahābhārata* (book 12) and *Devī Bhāgavata* (book 10).
39. See *Gītā* IV.7–8.
40. There are four *yugas*, and each of the first three has an incarnation associated with it. This verse suggests the possibility of a concealed incarnation (*channa*), which the Gauḍīya Vaiṣṇava school takes to be an indirect reference to Caitanya Mahāprabhu, who was born in Bengal in the fifteenth century and spread the chanting of the Hare Kṛṣṇa *mantra* throughout parts of India, especially East India. The distinctive feature of Gauḍīya or Caitanya

Vaiṣṇavism, then, in the greater context of Vaiṣṇavism in general, is this acceptance of Caitanya Mahāprabhu as Kṛṣṇa Himself.

41. The *Vaitaraṇī* river borders the realm of Yama, lord of death.
42. In Sāṅkhya, *prakṛti* is nothing other than the three *guṇas*, from which all reality evolves in sequential fashion. The first evolute is *buddhi* (*mahat*), followed by ego, mind, the powers of the ten organs, the five qualities (sound, touch, sight, taste, and smell), and the five primordial elements (see Sāṅkhya chart in appendix 2).

The *Bhāgavata Purāṇa*: Book VIII

1. All forms of gross matter are ultimately made of the five *mahābhūtas*—the elements of earth, water, fire, air, and ether. At the time of universal dissolution, forms dissolve into their atomic constituents (and then into subtler and subtler energies, until everything dissolves back into the *prakṛtic* matrix). See Sāṅkhya chart in appendix 2.
2. Anything made of *prakṛti* has some sort of identifiable form (*rūpa*) and, therefore, is nameable (*nāma*), albeit both of these are temporal and in this sense ephemeral. *Īśvara*, of course, is transcendent and therefore beyond *nāma-rūpa*.
3. It is standard in eulogies of this sort to slip between "He" and "You" pronominal forms. The sense is: "He who is known as the Supreme Being (etc., etc.) is none other than You."
4. *Kṣetra-jña* (see, for example, *Gītā* XIII.3 and throughout).
5. As the *ātman* can be reflected in the pure mirror of the mind, so can *Īśvara* in His creation.
6. These portions, the *karma kāṇḍa,* deal with satisfying material desires (see "*Bhakti* and *Dharma*").
7. This "inner Seer" is taken by the commentators and *Bhāgavata* philosophy to be one of the manifestations of Viṣṇu who resides in every being as the *Antaryāmī* (*Paramātman*), the inner controller.
8. The Vedic goals of conventional life (see earlier citation).
9. This is a reference to one of the five forms of liberation outlined in the *Bhāgavata* (see "The Liberated *Bhakta*: Different Types of *Mokṣa* in the *Bhāgavata*").
10. For *kalā* (or *aṁśa*), see earlier citation.
11. The sense here is something akin to verses in the *Gītā* (see VII.21 and X.4–5, 10), where Kṛṣṇa states that it is He who provides the appropriate intelligence to all beings that accords with their desires (and appropriate *karma*). For intelligence differentiated by the *guṇas*, see *Gītā* (XVIII.29–32).
12. Gajendra did not address his prayers to a specific *Iśvara* such as Śiva or Viṣṇu.
13. Śrīdhara refers to *itihāsa* (probably the *Mahābhārata*) for the source of this story: Once, the sage Devala was frolicking in a lake with some damsels, when the celestial Hūhū entered the lake, grabbed him by the leg, and pulled him. Devala became enraged and cursed him to become an alligator. Relenting somewhat later, he advised him to grasp the leg of the elephant after he had

taken his alligator birth, so that he would be released by Hari (curses often bear some sort of similarity to the offense that provokes them; they are rarely retracted but can be modified).

14. *Sārūpya* liberation. See "The Liberated *Bhakta*" for the five types of liberated states in *Bhāgavata* theology.
15. We see here a good example of the layerings of stories: present situations are the effects of causes in previous lives, a literary and pedagogical trait so typical of epic and Purāṇic narrative.
16. Compare with the Tale of King Bharata, when the latter was in the body of a deer.
17. This is a reference to Viṣṇu when reclining on the ocean of milk, from whose navel a lotus grows (see the Tale and Teachings of Lord Brahmā).

The *Bhāgavata Purāṇa*: Book IX

1. The *aśvamedha* (horse) sacrifice was performed by the *kṣatriya* warrior caste and was essentially a display of power. It had various functions—for example, for a king with imperatorial aspirations, the horse, followed by the king's army, was let loose to wander through adjacent kingdoms, requiring the neighboring king to either capture it and confront the army or allow it passage and thereby submit to paying tribute. The performance of one hundred *aśvamedhas* generated sufficient *karma* for one to attain the post of the celestial Indra in one's next birth.
2. One of the characteristics of a celestial is that he or she does not blink (additionally, their garlands do not fade, and their feet do not touch the ground).
3. Sacrifices such as the *aśvamedha* are usually motivated by a desire to attain the celestial realms.
4. The *dvādaśī* fast occurs on the twelfth day of the waxing as well as of the waning moon.
5. *Abhiṣeka* involves ritual bathing of a deity—often using various liquids including milk, yogurt, ghee, and honey in addition to water—and, on occasion, of other esteemed personages such as the king at his coronation.
6. The text uses the rhetorical number of six *nyarbuda*, six hundred million.
7. At the end of the universal cycle, a fire consumes the universe (see *Bhāgavata* XII.4).
8. This corresponds to the duration of Brahmā's life.
9. See "The Liberated *Bhakta*: Different Types of *Mokṣa* in the *Bhāgavata*."
10. Eating the remnants of a saint's food (or that of the deity) is called *prasādam* and is considered very purifying.
11. As indicated in the *Yoga Sūtras* (IV.1), mystic powers can accrue in various ways, two of which, referenced here, are through the power of *mantra* and through austerities (*tapas*). Through these means, Saubhari, as was the case with Kardama, was able to create the palaces and such, described here.
12. See the *Gītā* (III.9), where feeding desire is compared with putting fuel on the fire, which simply causes it to rage more intensely.

Śrī Kṛṣṇa's Incarnation: Book X

1. Adapted from Bryant (2003).
2. Vasudeva is the father, Vāsudeva is the son (Kṛṣṇa). See note 17 below.
3. Kṛṣṇa is here exhibiting His form as Viṣṇu.
4. We can recall that in Vaiṣṇavism, *Īśvara*'s body is made not of *prakṛti*, but of pure *Brahman*.
5. Kṛṣṇa incarnates because many *asuras*, demons, had taken birth on earth masquerading as kings.
6. This period corresponds to half of Brahmā's life: ten billion human years.
7. In Sāṅkhya, all the evolutes of *prakṛti*, the manifest, dissolve into their *prakṛtic* matrix, the unmanifest.
8. There is a partial dissolution of the universe at the end of Brahmā's night and also at the end of his day. The complete dissolution occurs at the end of his life of one hundred years (see note 6 above).
9. Each day of Brahmā is divided into fourteen periods, each one governed by a different Manu (progenitor).
10. This refers to the Vāmana incarnation discussed previously with reference to Bali, king of the demons.
11. Yogamāyā is both personality and power. Here, she is the personal Goddess.
12. See previous references to Śeṣa, the snake upon whom Viṣṇu reclines.
13. We encountered Yama in the story of Ajāmila.
14. This is a reference to Rāma crossing the sea to rescue Sītā.
15. There is an astronomical text, the *Garga Saṁhitā*, of which only fragments remain, associated with this sage.
16. These are references to previous incarnations.
17. There are various rules for the creation of patronymics in Sanskrit grammar, one of which is to extend the initial vowel of the parent's name. Thus Vāsudeva is the son of Vasudeva.
18. In other words, Yaśodā saw the various evolutes of *prakṛti* in accordance with Sāṅkhya metaphysics.
19. This is a reference to various demons who tried to kill Kṛṣṇa in previous chapters.
20. This is a reference to Pūtanā, a demon who assumed the form of a beautiful woman and tried to kill Kṛṣṇa by suckling him on her poisoned breast in X.6.
21. This is a reference to the Tṛṇāvarta demon who assumes the form of a whirlwind to kill Kṛṣṇa in X.7.
22. See earlier citation.
23. See discussion in the chapter "Meditating in Enmity," note 36, on this type of liberation attained by Agha.
24. See "The Liberated *Bhakta*: Different Types of *Mokṣa* in the *Bhāgavata*."
25. This refers to the fact that Kṛṣṇa saved Parīkṣit in the womb, when Parīkṣit was about to be incinerated by the *brahmāstra* weapon released against him while still an embryo so as to destroy the last remaining member of the Kuru dynasty.

26. The mothers of the other *gopa* boys in the village, as well as the cows, had all secretly harbored the wish that Kṛṣṇa had been their very own son or calf.
27. The commentator Śrīdhara does not give a reference for this quote.
28. While the parents of the other *gopas* and the cows loved their own children and calves, this love did not compare with their love for Kṛṣṇa, which was unlimited.
29. See "The Practices of *Bhakti*," note 49.
30. Here again we have a reference to the non-*prakṛtic* but rather *Brahman* nature of Viṣṇu's forms.
31. These eleven are the mind, the five knowledge-acquiring senses (eyes, ears, nose, tongue, touch), and the five working senses (arms, legs, genitals, anus, skin).
32. See previous reference for the *neti neti* of the Upaniṣads.
33. Brahmā has four heads. There are various stories as to how he attained these in the Purāṇas.
34. The imagery of the universe being woven like a cloth on threads goes back at least to the *Bṛhadāraṇyaka Upaniṣad* (III.8).
35. *Daṇḍavat*: a full prostration on the ground with arms elongated.
36. The *Aitareya Brāhmaṇa* (VI.9) says that the eating of grains by one who has been consecrated should not occur until the performance of the sacrifice. The *sautrāmaṇī* was a four-day sacrifice to Indra as protector,
37. The *patnīśālā*, women's quarter, was situated in the southwest corner of the *vedī*, or sacrificial arena.
38. Foods are divided as to whether they are licked, swallowed, chewed, or sucked.
39. The participation of the wife was required in certain Vedic rituals.
40. Kṛṣṇa makes numerous statements such as "Abandon all types of *dharma* and simply come exclusively to My shelter; I will free you from all sin, do not worry" (*Gītā* XVIII.66); and "Those who take shelter of Me, even if they be of sinful birth, women, merchants, or laborers, attain the supreme destination" (*Gītā* IX.32).
41. Śrīdhara considers these to be birth from parents, initiation as a *brāhmaṇa* in the sacred-thread ceremony, and initiation for the performance of sacrifice.
42. There are twelve purificatory rites of passage, *saṁskāras* (not to be confused with the word's meaning as memory imprint), incumbent on a male *brāhmaṇa*.
43. Śrīdhara considers these faults to be pride and fickleness: *cañcalā* means the fickle one, since fame and fortune do not stay with anyone for long!
44. Cupid.
45. Both pious and impious deeds are the source of bondage, since both require rebirth in order to fructify.
46. In other words, since their physical bodies were obstructed by their relatives from leaving the house, these *gopīs* simply abandoned their bodies and kept going in their subtle bodies to be with Kṛṣṇa.

47. See discussion in "Meditating in Enmity" on meditation on Kṛṣṇa in enmity and hate.
48. Tulasī is both plant and goddess.
49. Urukrama is Vāmana. See earlier citation.
50. Varāha is the boar incarnation.
51. See note 20 above.
52. This is a reference to Kṛṣṇa's banishing of the Kāliya serpent for poisoning the *Yamunā* river in X.16.
53. This refers to the *līlā* of Kṛṣṇa swallowing the forest fire in X.17.
54. Incarnations typically have such markings on their hands and feet.
55. The word for "worshipped" here is *ārādhitaḥ*, the past passive participle of the verb *ārādh*, "to worship." Gauḍīya Vaiṣṇava commentators see this as a veiled reference to Rādhā, a nominal form of this root, which is the name of Kṛṣṇa's primary consort, who is otherwise not mentioned in the text.
56. This verse is not found in Śrīdhara but is in a number of other versions.
57. Ariṣṭa and Vyomasura were demons killed by Kṛṣṇa in earlier chapters of the tenth book.
58. The idea here is that because one has eyelids, one blinks and, in so doing, is deprived of beholding Kṛṣṇa's beautiful form even if only for a split second.
59. This is a reference to conventional *samādhi.*
60. According to the commentator Śrīdhara, the Vedas, who are both texts and personalities, remain unfulfilled in their ritualistic portions, which pertain to satisfying material desires, but experience bliss in their Upaniṣadic portions, which pertain to the *ātman*.
61. This is not to be confused with *rasa*, discussed in "*Rāga*, *Bhāva*, and *Rasa*."
62. This is a reference to Viṣṇu, whose eternal consort is Lakṣmī, also known as Śrī.
63. See *Gītā* IV.8, where Kṛṣṇa proclaims that He incarnates to reestablish *dharma*.
64. When the gods and the demons churned the ocean of milk, poison was produced as well as valuable things. Śiva drank the poison, as a result of which his throat turned blue (*Bhāgavata* VIII.6–9).
65. The *rāsa līlā* is held to have lasted for the duration of Brahmā's night (for which, see earlier note).

Caitanya's *Śikṣāṣṭakam*: The Eight Verses of Instruction

1. The imagery here is that as the *kairava* is a night-blooming lotus that is nourished by the moon, while other conventional day-blooming lotuses are asleep, so those who chant the names of Kṛṣṇa are awakened to love of God while most entities are asleep under the influence of *avidyā*.
2. See the Tale of Prince Dhruva (IV.12.18) for examples of similar symptoms.

The *Nārada Bhakti Sūtras*

1. For discussion on *yogamāyā* and lack of awareness of God's majesty, see "*Līlā* and *Yogamāyā*."
2. The other practices—Vedic ritualistic specializations, knowledge, and the practice of *yoga*—are to a great extent based on the performer's ego and virtuosity in the techniques of these fields. *Bhakti* involves complete surrender of one's ego and thus involves humility.
3. For *bhakti* under the influence of the *guṇas*, see discussion in "*Bhakti* Mixed with *Karma* and *Jñāna*."
4. See discussion in "*Rāga*, *Bhāva*, and *Rasa*" on *bhāva*.
5. These three could refer, among other possibilities, to the paths of *karma*, *jñāna*, and *bhakti*.

Appendix I

1. The different recensions of the Vedas have been transmitted remarkably intact across the millennia. Indeed, their efficacy as ritualistic texts that can produce tangible effects in the real world (that is, produce the boons associated with sacrificial performance) was held to depend upon the precise preservation and pronunciation of each phoneme.
2. See Śaṅkara on *Vedānta Sūtras* I.2.25.
3. With important differences among the theists, including the *Bhāgavata* tradition, that hold the Vedas to have originally been articulated by *Īśvara*, God (see Gītā XV.15), and the Mīmāṁsakas, who dispense with God as philosophically superfluous and consider the Vedas to be eternally existent but authorless texts (see *Ślokavārtika* 32).
4. The term *kṛṣṇa* does appear occasionally in the hymns in the *Ṛg-Veda*, but simply with its adjectival semantics of "black": there is nothing in these occurrences that allows us to connect these references to the Kṛṣṇa of the Purāṇas. In terms of the *Śruti*, the *Chāndogya Upaniṣad* (III.17.6) of the later Vedic age (circa sixth century B.C.E.) gives us the first plausible, but still questionable, protoreference to the Purāṇic Kṛṣṇa (see Preciado-Solis 1984 for discussion). Even the *Bhāgavata* itself acknowledges that "Kṛṣṇa's activities are not revealed in the Vedas" (I.2.35).
5. If one wishes to embark on an exposition on Truth, then clearly it is essential, from a systematic point of view, to first establish what sources of knowledge one deems relevant to this pursuit right at the beginning of one's treatise (see *Yoga Sūtras* I.7).
6. See *Vedānta Sūtras* I.1.3 and II.1.27; *Mīmāṁsā Sūtras* II and VI–XXIII and commentaries (and in the *Bhāgavata* itself, XI.20.4).
7. It is well-known that the term "Hindu" is not to be found in Sanskrit sources but first occurs, coincidentally, in the hagiography of Caitanya, the founder of Jīva's lineage, mentioned above. While there have been various scholarly discussions as to what exactly the term comprises, there is general agreement

that it refers to traditions that retain some sort of formal allegiance toward the Vedic *Śruti* corpus, even if only nominally, given the innovative directions the later lineages take.

8. Some schools, however, such as Vaiśeṣiká, accepted only scripture and empiricism, Nyāya arguing for four and Mīmāṁsā six distinct methods of knowing something to be true.
9. Although, in point of fact, Navadvīpa, where Caitanya was born, was at the center of new expressions of Nyāya, logic. Caitanya himself was an exceptional teacher in Nyāya prior to becoming an ecstatic (see earlier citation).
10. For *paramparā*, see also *Gītā* IV.4.
11. See II.9.
12. *Ādi parvan* I.267; and *Mokṣa dharma* 340.21.
13. Jīva does not give a reference for this verse, which is not unusual in premodern hermeneutics. However, see *Skanda Purāṇa*, *Prabhāsa-khaṇḍa* V.3.121–24, for a narrative to the same effect.
14. He notes that it is difficult presently to understand the Vedas, and great commentators who have interpreted them have construed contradictory explanations (he has the *Vedānta Sūtras* commentarial tradition in mind here); moreover, there are portions of the Vedas that are unavailable (*anu* 12). The *Bhāgavata* affirms that "the Vedas speak incomprehensibly" (*parokṣa*; XI.3.21). There is a narrative in the *Varāha Purāṇa* (chapter 171) about how the meanings of the Vedas were covered because of the curse of Gautama Muni.
15. See also *Skanda Purāṇa* V.3.17–28 and 5.16.33, 40–44.
16. *Skanda Purāṇa*, reference not given, quoted in *Tattva Sandarbha anu* 16.3.
17. *Śiva Purāṇa* VII.1.1.37–38; *Agni Purāṇa* 60.16–18, 21–22; *Viṣṇu Purāṇa* III.4.2–5.
18. Jīva quotes a verse from the *Garuḍa Purāṇa* here, without verse number (*anu* 21).
19. *Kūrma Purāṇa Pūrva* 52.19–20.
20. A good example of this is the story of Vṛtra (*Bhāgavata* VI.9–12), which takes many varied contours in the chronological progression of the Vedic and post-Vedic texts.
21. See XI.7.24, XV.6.10–12.
22. Much of the endless conjecture and difference of opinion among scholars results from assigning old dates to an entire text on the basis of an archaic reference, which might simply be an ancient, well-preserved fragment in a later compilation. Equally problematic is the reverse tendency of assigning a much later date to an entire text on the basis of a more recent datable reference such as a dynasty of the historical period, which might in fact be a much later interpolation in an older text.
23. The verse deemed most authoritative in this regard is *Bhāgavata* XI.5.32. See Dāsa, *Tattva Sandarbha*, appendix 1, 341, for further references.
24. Most especially in the post-1960s period through ISKCON, popularly known as the Hare Krishna Movement, and its by now various disaffiliated offshoots (see Bryant and Ekstrand 2004 and other scholarship on ISKCON).

Bibliography

Adams, George C. *Bādarāyaṇa's Brahma Sūtras*. Delhi: Motilal Banarsidass, 1993.

Alter, Joseph S. *Yoga in Modern India*. Princeton, NJ: Princeton University Press, 2004.

Balagangadhara, S. N. *Reconceptualizing India Studies*. New York: Oxford University Press, 2012.

Beck, Guy. *Sonic Theology: Hinduism and Sacred Sound*. Columbia: University of South Carolina Press, 1993.

———. *Alternative Krishnas: Regional and Vernacular Variations on a Hindu Deity*. Albany: State University of New York Press, 2005.

Bhattacharya, Ramkrishna. *Studies on the Cārvāka/Lokāyata*. London: Anthem, 2011.

Bhattacharya, Siddhesvara. *The Philosophy of Śrīmad Bhāgavata*. Vols. 1 and 2. Calcutta: Visva Bharati, 1960–62.

Bronkhurst, Johannes. *The Two Traditions of Meditation in Ancient India*. Delhi: Motilal Banarsidass, 1993.

Brooks, Douglas Renfrew. *The Secret of the Three Cities*. Chicago: Chicago University Press, 1990.

———. *Auspicious Wisdom*. Albany: State University of New York Press, 1992.

Brown, C. M. "The Origin and Transmission of the Two *Bhāgavata Purāṇas*: A Canonical and Theological Dilemma." *Journal of the American Academy of Religion* 51 (1983): 551–67.

———. *Hindu Perspectives on Evolution: Darwin, Dharma and Design*. New York: Routledge, 2012.

Bryant, Edwin. *The Quest for the Origins of Vedic Culture: The Indo-Aryan Migration Debate*. New York: Oxford University Press, 2001.

———. "The Date and Provenance of the *Bhāgavata Purāṇa* and the Vaikuṇṭha Perumāl Temple." *Journal of Vaishnava Studies* 11, no. 1 (2002): 51–80.

———. *Krishna: The Beautiful Legend of God (Śrīmad Bhāgavata Purāṇa Book X)*. New York: Penguin Books, 2003.

———, ed. *Krishna: A Source Book*. New York: Oxford University Press, 2007.

———. *The Yoga Sūtras of Patañjali (with Insights from the Traditional Commentators)*. New York: North Point Press, 2009.

———, and Maria Ekstrand, eds. *The Hare Krishna Movement: The Post-Charismatic Fate of a Religious Transplant*. New York: Columbia University Press, 2004.

———, and Laurie L. Patton, eds. *The Indo-Aryan Controversy: Evidence and Inference in Indian History*. Richmond, UK: Routledge, 2005.

Buchta, David. "Dependent Agency and Hierarchical Determinism in the Theology of Madhva." In *Free Will, Agency, and Selfhood in Indian Philosophy*, edited by Matthew Dasti and Edwin Bryant, 255–78. New York: Oxford University Press, 2013.

Case, Margaret. *Seeing Krishna*. Oxford: Oxford University Press, 2000.

Chari, Srinivasa. *The Philosophy of the Vedāntasūtra*. Delhi: Munshiram Manoharlal, 1998.

Coleman, Tracy. "Viraha-Bhakti and Strīdharma: Re-reading the Story of Kṛṣṇa and the Gopīs in the *Harivaṁśa* and the *Bhāgavata Purāṇa*." *Journal of the Oriental Society* 130, no. 3 (2010): 385–412.

Cornell, Judith. *Amma*. London: Piatkus Books, 2001.

Cowell, E. B., and A. E. Gough, trans. *Sarva Darṣana Saṅgraha of Mādhava Ācārya*. London: Kegan Paul, Trench, Trübner & Co., 1908.

Cremo, Michael. *Human Devolution*. Los Angeles: Bhaktivedanta Book Trust, 2003.

Das, Shukavak. *Hindu Encounter with Modernity*. Calcutta: Sri, 1999.

Dāsa, Gopīparānadhana. *Śrī Bṛhad Bhāgavatāmṛta*. Los Angeles: Bhaktivedanta Book Trust, 2002.

Dāsa, Sarvabhāvana. *Śrī Caitanya-bhāgavata*. Vrindavan: Rasbiharilal, n.d.

Dāsa, Satyanārāyana. *Śrī Tattva Sandarbha*. Vrindavan: Jiva, 1995.

———. *Śrī Bhakti Sandarbha*. Vrindavan: Jiva, 2005.

———. "The Six Sandarbhas of Jiva Gosvami." In *Krishna: A Source Book*, edited by Edwin Bryant, 373–408. New York: Oxford University Press, 2007.

Dasgupta, Surendranath. *A History of Indian Philosophy*. Delhi: Motilal, 1922.

Dasti, Matthew. "Indian Rational Theology: Proof, Justification, and Epistemic Liberality in Nyāya's Argument for God." *Asian Philosophy* 21, no. 1 (2011): 1–21.

———, and Edwin Bryant, eds. *Free Will, Agency, and Selfhood in Indian Philosophy*. New York: Oxford University Press, 2013.

Davis, Richard. *The Bhagavad Gītā: A Bibliography*. Princeton, NJ: Princeton University Press, 2014.

De, S. K. *Early History of the Vaishnava Faith and Movement in Bengal*. Calcutta: KLM Ltd., 1986.

De Michelis, Elizabeth. *A History of Modern Yoga*. London: Continuum, 2004.

Deutsch, Eliot. *Advaita Vedānta: A Philosophical Reconstruction*. Honolulu: East-West Center Press, 1969.

———, and J. A. B. van Buitenen. *A Source Book of Advaita Vedānta*. Honolulu: University Press of Hawaii, 1971.

Dimock, Edward C., Jr., and Tony Stewart, trans. *Caitanya Caritāmṛta of Kṛṣṇadāsa Kavirāja*. Harvard Oriental Series 56. Cambridge: Harvard University Press, 2000.

Doniger, Wendy, and Brian Smith. *The Laws of Manu*. London: Penguin Books, 1991.

Dyczkowski, Mark. *The Doctrine of Vibration*. Albany: State University of New York Press, 1987.

Edelmann, J. "Hindu Theology as Churning the Latent." *Journal of the American Academy of Religion* 81, no. 2 (2013): 427–66.

———. *Hindu Theology and Biology: The Bhāgavata Purāṇa and Contemporary Theory*. New York: Oxford University Press, 2014.

Edgerton, Franklin. "The Meaning of Sāṅkhya and Yoga." *American Journal of Philosophy* 45, no. 1 (1924): 1–46.

Entwhistle, A. W. *Braj: Center of Krishna Pilgrimage*. Groningen, Netherlands: Egbert Forsten, 1987.

Fort, Andrew. *Living Liberation*. Albany: State University of New York Press, 1996.

Ganeri, Jonardon. *The Lost Age of Reason: Philosophy in Early Modern India, 1450–1700*. New York: Oxford University Press, 2011.

Gopal, Sarvepalli. *Anatomy of a Confrontation*. Chicago: University of Chicago Press, 1992.

Goswami, C. L., trans. *Śrīmad Bhāgavata Mahāpurāṇa*. Gorakhpur: Gita Press, n.d.

Goswami, Tamal Krishna. *A Living Theology of Krishna Bhakti*. Oxford: Oxford University Press, 2012.

Gupta, Ravi, and Kenneth Valpey, eds. *The Bhāgavata Purāṇa: Sacred Text and Living Tradition*. New York: Columbia University Press, 2013.

Haberman, David. *Acting as a Way to Salvation: A Study of Rāgānugā Bhakti Sādhana*. New York: Oxford University Press, 1988.

———. "Divine Betrayal: Krishna-Gopal of Braj in the Eyes of Outsiders." *Journal of Vaishnava Studies* 3, no. 1 (1994): 83–112.

———. *Journey Through the Twelve Forests: An Encounter with Krishna*. New York: Oxford University Press, 1994.

———. *The Bhaktirasāmṛtasindhu of Rūpa Gosvāmin*. Delhi: Indira Gandhi Center for the Arts, 2003.

Halbfass, Wilhelm. *India and Europe*. Albany: State University of New York Press, 1988.

Hastie, W. *Hindu Idolatry and English Enlightenment*. Calcutta: Thacker, Spink & Co., 1882.

Hawley, John Stratton. *The Memory of Love: Sūrdās Sings to Krishna*. New York: Oxford University Press, 2009.

Holdredge, Barbara. *Bhakti and Embodiment: Fashioning Divine Bodies and Devotional Bodies in Kṛṣṇa Bhakti*. New York: Routledge, 2012.

Hopkins, Thomas. "The Social Teachings in the *Bhāgavata Purāṇa*." In *Krishna: Myths, Rites, and Attitudes*, edited by Milton Singer. Honolulu: East-West Center Press, 1966.

Jain, Andrea. *Selling Yoga: From Counterculture to Pop Culture*. New York: Oxford University Press, 2015.

Jamison, Stephanie. *Sacrificed Wife/Sacrificer's Wife*. New York: Oxford University Press, 1996.

King, Richard. *Early Advaita Vedānta and Buddhism*. Albany: State University of New York Press, 1995.

———. *Orientalism and Religion*. New York: Routledge, 1999.

Larson, Gerald James. *Classical Sāṅkhya*. Encyclopedia of Indian Philosophies. Delhi: Motilal Banarsidass, 1979.

Lawrence, David. *Rediscovering God with Transcendental Argument*. New York: State University of New York Press, 1999.

Lipner, Julius. *The Face of Truth: A Study of Meaning and Metaphysics in the Vedāntic Theology of Rāmāṇuja*. New York: State University of New York Press, 1986.

M [*sic*]. *The Gospel of Sri Ramakrishna*. New York: Ramakrishna-Vivekananda Center, 1942.

Maas, Philipp. *Samādhipāda: Das erste Kapitel des* Pātañjalayogaśāstra *zum ersten Mal kritisch ediert (The First Chapter of the* Pātañjalayogaśāstra, *for the First Time Critically Edited*). Aachen, Germany: Shaker, 2006.

———. "On the Written Transmission of the *Patañjalayogaśāstra*." In *From Vasubandhu to Caitanya: Studies in Indian Philosophy and Its Textual History*, edited by Johannes Bronkhorst and Karin Preisendanz, 157–72. Delhi: Motilal Banarsidass, 2010.

Masuzawa, Tomoko. *The Invention of World Religions*. Chicago: University of Chicago Press, 2005.

Muktānanda, Swami. *Play of Consciousness: A Spiritual Biography*. South Fallsburg, NY: Siddha Yoga Publications, 1978.

Muller-Ortega, Paul. *The Triadic Heart of Śiva*. Albany: State University of New York Press, 1989.

Nelson, Lance. "Krishna in Advaita Vedanta: The Divine in Human Form." In *Krishna: A Source Book*, edited by Edwin Bryant. New York: Oxford University Press, 2007.

Nicholson, Andrew. *Unifying Hinduism*. New York: Columbia University Press, 2010.

———. *Lord Śiva's Song: The Iśvara Gītā*. New York: State University of New York Press, 2014.

Oddie, Geoffrey. *Imagined Hinduism*. New Delhi: Sage, 2006.

Olivelle, Patrick. *Upaniṣads*. Oxford: Oxford University Press, 1996.

———. *Dharmasūtras*. Oxford: Oxford University Press, 1999.

Patil, Parimal. *Against a Hindu God: Buddhist Philosophy of Religion in India.* New York: Columbia University Press, 2009.

Pennington, Brian. *Was Hinduism Invented?* New York: Oxford University Press, 2005.

Preciado-Solis, Benjamin. *The Kṛṣṇa Cycle in the Purāṇas.* Delhi: Motilal Banarsidass, 1984.

Raghavachar, S. S. *Vedārtha Saṅgraha of Sri Rāmāṇujācarya.* Mysore: Ramakrishna Ashram, 1978.

Rocher, Ludo. *The Purāṇas.* Wiesbaden, Germany: Otto Harrassoqitz, 1986.

Roy, Raja Rammohun. "A Letter on the Prospects of Christianity." In *The English Works of Raja Rammohun Roy.* Part IV. Calcutta: Sadharan Brahmo Samaj, 1947.

———. "Second Appeal to the Christian Public." In *The English Works of Raja Rammohun Roy.* Part VI. Calcutta: Sadharan Brahmo Samaj, 1951.

Rukmani, T. S. *A Critical Study of the Bhāgavata Purāṇa.* Varanasi, India: Chowkhamba, 1975.

Sardella, Ferdinando. *Modern Hindu Personalism: The History, Life, and Thought of Bhaktisiddhānta Sarasvatī.* New York: Oxford University Press, 2013.

———, and Abhishek Ghosh. "Modern Reception and Text Migration of the *Bhāgavata Purāṇa.*" In *The Bhāgavata Purāṇa: Sacred Text and Living Tradition*, edited by Ravi M. Gupta and Kenneth Russell Valpey. New York: Columbia University Press, 2013.

Sarma, Deepak. *An Introduction to Mādhva Vedānta.* Aldershot, UK: Ashgate Publishers, 2003.

———. *Epistemologies and the Limitations of Philosophical Inquiry: Doctrine in Mādhva Vedānta.* New York: RoutledgeCurzon Press, 2004.

Sastri, Suryanarayana. *The Śivādvaita Nirṇaya of Appayya Dikṣita.* Madras: University Press, 1974.

Schomerus, H. W. *Śaiva Siddhānta.* Edited by Humphrey Palmer. Translated by Mary Law. Delhi: Motilal Banarsidass, 1979.

Schweig, Graham. *Dance of Divine Love: The Rāsa Līlā of Krishna from the Bhāgavata Purāṇa.* Princeton, NJ: Princeton University Press, 2005.

Sharma, B.N.K. *The Brahmasūtras and Their Principal Commentaries.* 3 vols. Delhi: Munshiram Manoharlal, 1971, 1974, and 1978.

———. *History of the Dvaita School of Vedānta and Its Literature.* Delhi: Motilal Banarsidass, 1981.

Sharpe, Eric. *The Universal Gītā.* La Salle, IL: Open Court Publishing, 1985.

Shastri, M. D. "History of the Word Ishvara and Its Idea." *Proceedings and Transactions of the All-India Oriental Conference* 7 (1935): 487–503.

Sheth, Noel. "Kṛṣṇa as a Portion of the Supreme." *Purāṇa* 24, no. 1 (1982): 79–90.

Singleton, Mark. *Yoga Body: The History of Modern Posture Practice.* New York: Oxford University Press, 2010.

———, and Jean Byren, eds. *Yoga in the Modern World.* London: Routledge, 2008.

Sivananda, Swami. *Autobiography of Swami Sivananda*. Rishikesh, India: Yoga-Vedanta Forest Academy, 1958.

Sjoman, N. E. *The Yoga Tradition of the Mysore Palace*. New Delhi: Abhinav, 1996.

Strauss, Sarah. *Positioning Yoga*. Oxford: Berg, 2005.

Strensi, Ivan. *Thinking About Religion: An Introduction to Theories of Religion*. Oxford: Blackwell Publishing, 2006.

Swami, H. H. Bhanu, trans. *Śrīmad Bhāgavatam: Śārārtha Darṣinī*. Vols. 1–9. Chennai, India: Sri Vaikuntha Enterprises, 2008–11.

Syman, Stefanie. *The Subtle Body: The Story of Yoga in America*. New York: Farrar, Straus and Giroux, 2010.

Tagare, Ganesh Vasudeo, trans. *The Bhāgavata Purāṇa*. Vols. 7–11. Ancient Indian Tradition and Mythology Series. Delhi: Motilal Banarsidass, 1976–78.

Thibaut, George. *The Vedānta Sūtras with the Commentary of Rāmānuja*. Vol. 48. Sacred Books of the East. Oxford: Oxford University Press, 1904.

Thompson, Richard L. *Mechanistic and Nonmechanistic Science: An Investigation into the Nature of Consciousness and Form*. Lynbrook, NY: Bala Books, 1981.

———. *Computer Simulations of Self-Organizations in Biological Systems*. London: Croom Helm, 1988.

———. *Vedic Cosmography and Astronomy*. Los Angeles: Bhaktivedanta Book Trust, 1989.

———. *Māyā: The World as Virtual Reality*. Alachua, FL: Govardhan Hill Publishing, 2003.

———. *The Cosmology of the Bhāgavata Purāṇa: Mysteries of the Sacred Universe*. Delhi: Motilal Banarsidass, 2006.

———. *God and Science: Divine Causation and the Laws of Nature*. Delhi: Motilal Banarsidass, 2007.

Vyasa, Ramnarayan. *The Synthetic Philosophy of the Bhāgavata*. Delhi: Meharchand, 1974.

Yogananda, Paramahansa. *Autobiography of a Yogi*. Los Angeles: Self-Realization Fellowship, 1946.